T0198302

HEALTH BEHAVIOR
THEORY, RESEARCH, AND PRACTICE

Fifth Edition

Karen Glanz
Barbara K. Rimer
K. Viswanath
EDITORS

JB **JOSSEY-BASS**™
A Wiley Brand

Published by Jossey-Bass
A Wiley Brand
One Montgomery Street, Suite 1000, San Francisco, CA 94104-4594   www.josseybass.com

Jossey-Bass books and products are available through most bookstores. To contact Jossey-Bass directly call our Customer Care Department within the U.S. at 800-956-7739, outside the U.S. at 317-572-3986, or fax 317-572-4002.

Wiley publishes in a variety of print and electronic formats and by print-on-demand. Some material included with standard print versions of this book may not be included in e-books or in print-on-demand. If this book refers to media such as a CD or DVD that is not included in the version you purchased, you may download this material at http://booksupport.wiley.com. For more information about Wiley products, visit www.wiley.com.

Library of Congress Cataloging-in-Publication Data
Health behavior and health education
    Health behavior : theory, research, and practice / Karen Glanz, Barbara K. Rimer, K. Viswanath, editors.—Fifth edition.
        pages cm.—(Jossey-Bass public health)
    Revision of: Health behavior and health education. 2008. 4th ed.
    Includes index.
    ISBN 978-1-118-62898-0 (hardback)—ISBN 978-1-118-62905-5 (pdf)—ISBN 978-1-118-62900-0 (epub)
    1. Health behavior. 2. Health education. 3. Health promotion. I. Glanz, Karen. II. Rimer, Barbara K. III. Viswanath, K. (Kasisomayajula). IV. Title.
    RA776.9.H434 2015
    613—dc23

                                                                                            2015007625

Printed in the United States of America
FIFTH EDITION

CONTENTS

TABLES AND FIGURES

Tables

Figures

In memory of my father, Michael Glanz, who lived so well and so long, and whose unconditional love and support helped me to succeed in work and in life.

K. G.

In memory of Irving Rimer, my father, who did so much to reduce smoking rates in the U.S. He inspired me and others through his love, courage, conscience, and creativity. And with thanks to my husband, Bernard Glassman, whose support enables me to accomplish more than I could achieve alone.

B.K.R.

To my parents and their parents who modeled a life of honesty, industry, and kindness to their children and grandchildren.

K. V.

Health is inseparable from behavior. According to one CDC study, individuals who engaged in one or more of three healthy behaviors—not smoking, eating a healthy diet, and getting adequate physical activity—substantially reduced their risk of death within the next six years. The greatest benefit was seen among those who engaged in all three healthy behaviors. But if the benefits of a healthy lifestyle are so clear, why aren't these behaviors more common, and why are they so difficult to change.

This fifth edition of *Health Behavior: Theory, Research, and Practice* provides a compelling and practical response to these difficult questions. This volume is compelling because it provides vivid illustrations of the multiple determinants and complex mechanisms underlying health behavior. It is practical in that it provides a feasible roadmap for conceptualizing, measuring, and changing health behaviors within everyday contexts.

The challenges faced by any individual or organization that seeks to influence health behaviors are many. Where should we focus? What strategies should we use? What outcomes should we measure? Whether we are working in a local or national context, the temptation often is to rely on intuition or the least controversial strategy. But as this book demonstrates, such an approach is not only inappropriate but inexcusable. Given the scarcity of resources to support health behavior programs and the scale of the problems to be addressed, it is essential that we rely on sound research evidence and a rigorous and explicit conceptualization of both the target behaviors and the strategies required to modify them. A complete understanding of behavior is not a prerequisite to action, but action uninformed by the best available theory and evidence concerning the determinants of that behavior is foolish.

The unique role that this and previous editions of this classic text are playing in the evolution of health behavior theory, research, and application cannot be underestimated. For many years, an unfortunate schism between research and practice existed, and to some extent, it still exists. Much of the literature in the field has been either too esoteric and theoretical or too limited in its rigor and generalizability. Current and future leaders in the field need to learn how best to balance the conceptual with the practical. This book is designed precisely to fill that gap. The chapters throughout this book recognize and appreciate this fundamental challenge but then go on to demonstrate the practical utility of theory in a variety of public health contexts. The solutions are imperfect and evolving, but as in all fields of science, progress has been facilitated through the development of new methods, the testing and refinement of theories, and the diversification of our workforce. The growth of transdisciplinary team science has continued to challenge traditional ways of thinking within the research community while the substantive engagement of community stakeholders has informed the application of theories to implementation strategies.

Within the context of other books in the field, this one does not focus on one problem domain, nor does it focus on one theoretical approach. The goal instead is to provide students and practitioners with a diverse set of theories and applications in order to illustrate how to rigorously conceptualize problems and how best to address them in ways that test these conceptualizations. Rather than advocating one "best theory," this book illustrates the reciprocal nature of understanding and action, encouraging the reader to consider the context of the problem, the relevant levels of analysis, and the importance of measuring key constructs. Generalizable knowledge depends on the careful assessment of mechanisms underlying behavior change, and the work described here indicates that there is an ongoing need for basic behavioral science. That work is described elsewhere, as is purely applied work that focuses entirely on a particular health behavior or problem context. The achievement of this book is that it provides the reader with foundational knowledge concerning the theory-intervention interface in a manner that is relevant to both researchers and practitioners.

As in previous editions, the editors have enlisted an impressive group of experienced scholars who have conducted some of the best theoretically based intervention research. The scope of the volume has expanded, in terms of both the theories covered and the increased emphasis on disparities and theory utilization. Given rapid changes in information technology and the information environment, the current edition also reflects changes in how health communication strategies are conceptualized. As new sources of *big data*, such as social media, become available to health behavior scientists, the tension between atheoretical exploratory analysis methods and more focused, theoretically driven research is likely to grow. Although exploratory analytic methods will continue to uncover unanticipated relationships and generate hypotheses, the work described in this book demonstrates the unique value of theory in establishing priorities for measurement and targeted intervention.

Perhaps no other policy context in recent years has generated as much discussion and debate as health insurance and health care reform. Much of the debate surrounding how best to improve the quality and efficiency of health care focuses on strategies for changing the behavior of patients, providers, administrators, and health care systems. It is worth noting that many of the discussions suffer from a lack of appreciation for many of the key themes and challenges addressed in this book. What are the theories of change underlying the predictions and interventions offered by proponents and critics of reform? Are assumptions clearly and explicitly stated so that they can be tested against the data? If so, to what degree does the evidence support predictions derived from the theory? Do theories adequately address behavior change at multiple levels of the organization? How do changes in the context of patient care influence behaviors at the individual patient and provider level? In order to test theories of health reform, we need valid measures of theoretical constructs such as coordinated care, patient-centered care, and the value of care. Do these measures exist, and if so, are they being used appropriately?

The example of health care reform illustrates how vital the knowledge and skills afforded by this volume are in a complex and contentious policy environment. Our progress against obesity, tobacco use, diabetes, asthma, alcohol abuse, and many other health problems will depend on our ability to thoughtfully utilize and evaluate theories of health behavior in order to maximize the impact of health behavior interventions. Policies can serve as constraints or facilitators at any level and we urgently need more evidence concerning the impact of policies on individual behaviors. We also need more theory-based policy, tested in many cases through natural experiments such as state-to-state variation. By reviewing the research evidence and theories described here, the reader will be in a much stronger position to contribute thoughtfully and substantially to some of the most important health policy debates facing nations around the world. Just as global health has served as a catalyst for the growth of implementation science, debates concerning the most effective strategies for preventing disease will only strengthen the demand for individuals who are knowledgeable about health behavior theory, research, and practice. This book provides a timely and essential foundation for students, researchers, or practitioners who want to make meaningful and long-lasting contributions to the health and vitality of their fellow citizens.

Robert T. Croyle
Bethesda, Maryland
July 2015

Programs to influence health behavior, including health promotion and education programs and interventions, are more likely to benefit participants and communities when guided by a theory or theories of health behavior. Theories of health behavior can help program planners to consider in a systematic way the sources of influence on particular health behaviors, and to identify the targets for behavior change and methods for accomplishing these changes. Theories also can inform the evaluation of change efforts by helping planners, evaluators, and others to specify the outcomes to be measured, as well as the timing and methods of study to be used. Although the evidence is not unequivocal, when they are developed and implemented thoughtfully and systematically, theory-driven health promotion and education efforts stand in contrast to programs based primarily on precedent, tradition, intuition, or general principles.

Theory-driven health behavior change interventions and programs require an understanding of the components of health behavior theories, as well as the operational or practical forms of the theories. The first edition of *Health Behavior and Health Education: Theory, Research, and Practice*, published in 1990, was the first text to provide an in-depth analysis of a variety of theories of health behavior relevant to health education in a single volume. It brought together dominant health behavior theories, research based on those theories, and examples of health education practice derived from theory that had been tested through evaluation and research. The second (1996), third (2002), and fourth (2008) editions of *Health Behavior and Health Education* updated and improved upon the earlier volumes. People around the world are using this book. It has been translated into multiple languages, including, most recently, Japanese, Korean, and Chinese editions.

It has been over six years since the release of the fourth edition of this book. We are confident that the fifth edition of *Health Behavior: Theory, Research, and Practice* improves upon the preceding edition, as each earlier edition has done. We have shortened the title to reflect the broad influence of health behavior theory and research, which is not limited to health education and health promotion. The main purpose of the book is the same: to advance the science of understanding health behavior and the practice of health behavior change through the informed application of theories of health behavior. Likewise, this book serves as the definitive text for students, practitioners, and scientists in these areas and in education in three ways: by analyzing the key components of theories of health behavior, describing current applications of these theories in selected public health and health promotion programs and interventions, and identifying important future directions for research and practice in health behavior change.

The fifth edition responds to new developments in health behavior theories and the application of theories in new settings, to new populations, and in new ways. We have moved the chapter on ecological models to the first section of the book to set the stage for the subsequent chapters grouped into individual-, interpersonal-, and community-level theories and models. The previous edition's chapter on social networks and social support is now two separate chapters, reflecting the increasing activity and maturation of theory-driven research on social networks. We have added a chapter on behavioral economics and its application to understanding and improving health behavior. Three chapters in the fourth edition do not appear in this edition: "The Precaution Adoption Process Model," "Mobilizing Organizations for Health Promotion: Theories of Organizational Change," and "Evaluation of Theory-Based Interventions." However, key elements from these earlier chapters are integrated into other chapters in this volume.

This edition includes an enhanced focus on the application of theories for diverse populations and settings; an expanded section on using theory, including its translation for program planning; and chapters on additional theories of health behavior. More global applications from both developing and developed countries are included. As new information and communication technologies have opened up an unprecedented range of strategies for health behavior change, this edition integrates coverage of e-health into health intervention examples throughout the book. Issues of culture and health disparities are also integrated into many chapters. These issues are of broad and growing importance across many theories and models. We believe that these additions strengthen the book and increase its appropriateness for use in settings around the world.

Audiences

Health Behavior: Theory, Research, and Practice is written for graduate students, practitioners, and scientists who spend part or all of their time in the broad arenas of health behavior change, public health, health promotion, and health education; this text will assist them both to understand the theories and to apply them in practical settings. Practitioners, as well as students, should find this text a major reference for the development and evaluation of theory-driven health behavior change programs and interventions. Researchers should emerge with a recognition of areas where empirical support is deficient and theory testing is required, helping to set the research agenda for health behavior going forward.

This book is intended to assist all professionals who value the need to influence health behavior positively. Their fields include health promotion and education, health communication, medicine, nursing, public health, health psychology, behavioral medicine, health communications, nutrition and dietetics, dentistry, pharmacy, social work, exercise science, clinical psychology, and occupational and physical therapy.

Overview of the Book

This volume presents an up-to-date understanding of both theory and its application in a variety of settings that characterize the diverse practice of health behavior change, public health, and health promotion: for example, worksites, hospitals, ambulatory care settings, community-based organizations, schools, and communities. The chapters, written expressly for this fifth edition, address theories and models of health behavior at the individual, interpersonal, group, organization, and community levels and present approaches that are integrated across multiple levels.

This book is organized into five parts. Part One defines key terms and concepts and introduces ecological models. The next three parts reflect important units of health behavior and education practice: the individual, the interpersonal or group level, and the community or aggregate level. Each of these parts has several chapters and begins with an introductory chapter to orient readers to the subsequent chapters and their interrelationships. Part Two focuses on theories of individual health behavior, and its chapters focus on variables within individuals that influence their health behavior and response to health promotion and education interventions. Three bodies of theory are reviewed in separate chapters that address the Health Belief Model; the Theory of Reasoned Action, Theory of Planned Behavior, and the Integrated Behavioral Model; and The Transtheoretical Model. Part Three examines interpersonal theories, which emphasize elements in the interpersonal environment that affect individuals' health behavior. Five chapters examine social cognitive theory, social support, social networks, stress and coping, and interpersonal communication. Part Four covers models for the community or aggregate level of change, and includes chapters on community engagement; implementation, dissemination, and diffusion of innovations; and media communications. Part Five explores using theory and presents the key components and applications of overarching planning and process models, and integrated models and approaches to health behavior change. It includes chapters on theory-based planning models, behavioral economics (new with this edition), and social marketing.

The major emphasis of *Health Behavior: Theory, Research, and Practice* is on the analysis and application of health behavior theories to public health and health promotion practice. The introductory chapters for Parts Two, Three, and Four introduce the theories discussed in each section; summarize their potential application to the development of health behavior change interventions; and highlight strengths, weaknesses, gaps, and areas for future development and research, and promising strategies. Each core chapter in Parts Two, Three, and Four begins with a discussion of the background of the theory or model and a presentation of the theory or model; reviews empirical support for it; and concludes with one or two applications.

Chapter authors are established researchers and practitioners who draw on their experience in state-of-the-art research to critically analyze and apply the theories to understanding health behavior and the practice of health behavior change. This text makes otherwise lofty theories accessible and practical, and advances understanding and practice in the process.

No single book can be truly comprehensive and still be concise and readable. Decisions about which theories to include were made with both an appreciation of the evolution of the study of health behavior and a vision of its future (see Chapter Two). We purposely chose to emphasize theories and conceptual frameworks that encompass a range from the individual to the societal level. We acknowledge that there is substantial variability in the extent to which various theories and models have been codified, tested, and supported by empirical evidence. Of necessity, some promising emerging theories were not included.

The first four editions of *Health Behavior and Health Education* grew out of the editors' own experiences, frustrations, and needs, as well as their desire to synthesize many literatures and to draw clearly the linkages between theory, research, and practice in health behavior and education. We have sought to show how theory, research, and practice interrelate and to make each accessible and practical. In this edition, we have attempted to respond to changes in the science and practice of public health and health promotion, and to update the coverage of these areas in a rapidly evolving field. Substantial efforts have been taken to present findings from health behavior change interventions based on the theories that are described and to illustrate the adaptations needed to successfully reach diverse and unique populations.

Through the preceding four editions, *Health Behavior and Health Education* has become established as a widely used text and reference book. It is our sincere hope that the fifth edition will continue to be relevant and useful and to stimulate readers' interest in theory-based health behavior and health education. We aspire to provide readers with the information and skills to ask critical questions, think conceptually, and stretch their thinking beyond using formulaic strategies to improve health. Ultimately, we aim to encourage users to use, test, refine, and even develop theories with the goal of improving health for people around the world and to benefit especially those populations that have suffered disproportionately from the conditions that predispose to poor health.

Acknowledgments

We owe deep gratitude to all the authors whose work is represented in this book. They worked diligently with us to produce an integrated volume, and we greatly appreciate their willingness to tailor their contributions to realize the vision of the book. Their collective depth of knowledge and experience across the broad range of theories and topics far exceeds the expertise that the editors can claim.

We pay special tribute to Drs. Martin Fishbein and Noreen Clark, luminaries in our broad field, whose work in applied health behavior theory taught and inspired us, and whose bodies of work cut across several chapters in this book. Along with many colleagues, we were saddened by Marty's death in 2009 and Noreen's passing in 2013. Their work will continue to be influential in using theory to improve research, practice, and health.

We also wish to acknowledge authors who contributed to the first four editions of this text; although some of them did not write chapters for this edition, their intellectual contributions form an important foundation for the present volume.

The staff at Jossey-Bass have provided valuable support to us for development, production, and marketing from the time that the first edition was released through completion of this edition. Our editors at Jossey-Bass, Andy Pasternack and Seth Schwartz, have provided encouragement and assistance throughout. We were deeply saddened by Andy's death in 2013, as he had steered us through two previous editions and the development of this edition. We also are grateful to Alice Petersen for her exceptional technical editing support for this edition.

The editors are also indebted to their colleagues and students who, over the years, have taught them the importance of both health behavior theories and the cogent and precise representation of those theories. They have challenged us to stretch, adapt, and continue to learn through our years of work at the University of Michigan, University of North Carolina (UNC) at Chapel Hill, University of Pennsylvania (UPenn), Emory University, Harvard, the University of Minnesota, Ohio State University, The Johns Hopkins University, Temple University, Fox Chase Cancer Center, Duke University, the University of Hawai'i, and the National Cancer Institute (NCI). Laura Bach at UNC and Beth Stelson at UPenn helped with an updated review of theory use for this edition.

Hana Hayashi and Rachel McLoud at Harvard/Dana-Farber provided invaluable editorial contributions to Vish Viswanath. Further, completion of this manuscript would not have been possible without the dedicated assistance of Angelica Figueroa and Pamela Lee at UNC, Nancy Klockson at Harvard/Dana-Farber, and Alyssa Yackle and David Buff at UPenn.

We would like to thank proposal reviewers Christopher Coutts, Brandon M. Eggleston, Mary J. Findorff, Mir M. Ali, Lynn Carol Miller, Janine M. Jurkowski, Jean Peteet, Michelle S. Harcrow, John Korkow, Laura Carlin Cochran, and Dan Gerber.

We also wish to express our thanks to our colleagues, staffs, friends, and families, whose patience, good humor, and encouragement sustained us through our work on this book.

Instructor resources and supplementary materials are available at www.wiley.com/go/glanz5e. Additional materials such as videos, podcasts, and readings can be found at www.josseybasspublichealth.com. Comments about this book are invited and can be sent to publichealth@wiley.com.

Karen Glanz
Philadelphia, Pennsylvania

Barbara K. Rimer
Chapel Hill, North Carolina

K. Viswanath
Boston, Massachusetts

July 2015

ABOUT THE EDITORS

Karen Glanz is George A. Weiss University Professor, professor of epidemiology in the Perelman School of Medicine, professor of nursing in the School of Nursing, and director of the Prevention Research Center and the Center for Health Behavior Research at the University of Pennsylvania. She is a Senior Fellow of the Leonard Davis Institute of Health Economics and of the Center for Public Health Initiatives, a Distinguished Fellow of the Annenberg Public Policy Center, and a Fellow of the Penn Institute for Urban Research. She was previously at Emory University (2004–2009), the University of Hawai'i (1993–2004), and Temple University (1979–1993). She received her MPH degree (1977) and PhD degree (1977) in health behavior and health education from the University of Michigan School of Public Health and Rackham Graduate School, respectively.

A globally influential public health scholar whose work spans psychology, epidemiology, nutrition, and other disciplines, her research in community and health care settings focuses on obesity, nutrition, and the built environment; cancer prevention and control; chronic disease management and control; the reduction of health disparities; and health communication technologies. Her research and publications, ranging from the 1980 to the present, about understanding, measuring, and improving healthy food environments have been widely recognized and replicated. She is a member of the U.S. Community Preventive Services Task Force. Her scholarly contributions consist of more than 400 journal articles and book chapters.

Karen Glanz has a long history of leading community-based health research and programs, and currently serves in several related roles at the University of Pennsylvania. She is director of the Community Engagement and Research (CEAR) Core of the UPenn Clinical and Scientific Translational Award (CTSA); director of the Pro-CEED Community Engagement and Dissemination Core of the NIMHD-funded P60 Center to Reduce Health Disparities in Prostate Cancer; scientific director of the Recruitment, Outcomes and Assessment Resource (ROAR) Core of the Abramson Cancer Center; and director of research for the Center for Public Health Initiatives (CPHI).

Dr. Glanz has been recognized with local and national awards for her work, including being elected to membership in the Institute of Medicine of the National Academy of Sciences in 2013. She was named a Fellow of the Society for Behavioral Medicine and received the Elizabeth Fries Health Education Award. She was designated a Highly Cited Author by ISIHighlyCited.com, in the top 0.5% of authors in her field over a twenty-year period.

Barbara K. Rimer is dean and Alumni Distinguished Professor of Health Behavior and Health Education at the School of Public Health at the University of North Carolina at Chapel Hill. Dr. Rimer received an MPH degree (1973) from the University of Michigan, with joint majors in health education and medical care organization, and a DrPH degree (1981) in health education from the Johns Hopkins School of Hygiene and Public Health. Previously, she served as deputy director for population sciences at the Lineberger Comprehensive Cancer Center at UNC-Chapel Hill (2003–2005), director of the Division of Cancer Control and Population Sciences at the National Cancer Institute (part of the National Institutes of Health) (1997–2002), professor of community and family medicine at Duke University (1991–1997), and director of behavioral research and a full member at the Fox Chase Cancer Center in Philadelphia (1987–1991).

Dr. Rimer has conducted research in a number of areas, including informed decision making, long-term maintenance of behavior changes (in such areas as diet, cancer screening, and tobacco use), interventions to increase adherence to cancer prevention and early detection, dissemination of evidence-based interventions, and use of new technologies for information, support, and behavior change.

Dr. Rimer is the author of over 265 peer-reviewed articles, fifty-five book chapters, and six books and serves on several journal editorial boards. She is the recipient of numerous awards and honors; in 2013, she was awarded the American Cancer Society's Medal of Honor for her cancer research, which has guided national research, practice, and policy for more than twenty years.

Dr. Rimer was the first woman and behavioral scientist to lead the National Cancer Institute's National Cancer Advisory Board, a presidential appointment. Dr. Rimer was elected to the Institute of Medicine in 2008 and appointed by President Obama to chair the President's Cancer Panel in 2011, a position she still holds.

K. "Vish" Viswanath is professor of health communication in the Department of Social and Behavioral Sciences at the Harvard School of Public Health (HSPH) and in the McGraw/Patterson Center for Population Sciences at the Dana-Farber Cancer Institute.

Dr. Viswanath's work, drawing from literatures in communication science, social epidemiology, and social and health behavior sciences, focuses on translational communication science to influence public health policy and practice. His primary research is in documenting the relationships among communication inequalities, poverty and health disparities, and knowledge translation to address health disparities. He has written more than 170 journal articles and book chapters concerning communication inequalities and health disparities, knowledge translation, public health communication campaigns, e-health and the digital divide, public health preparedness, and the delivery of health communication interventions to underserved populations. He is the coeditor of three books: *Mass Media, Social Control, and Social Change* (Iowa State University Press, 1999), *The Role of Media in Promoting and Reducing Tobacco Use* (National Cancer Institute, 2008), and the present volume. He was also the editor of the Social and Behavioral Research section of the twelve-volume *International Encyclopedia of Communication* (Blackwell Publishing, 2008).

Dr. Viswanath has been recognized with several awards, including the Joseph W. Cullen Memorial Award for Excellence in Tobacco Research from the American Society of Preventive Oncology (2014), the Dale E. Brashers Distinguished Mentorship Award from the National Communication Association (2013), the Outstanding Health Communication Scholar Award from the International Communication Association and the National Communication Association (2010), and the Mayhew Derryberry Award from the American Public Health Association for his contribution to health education research and theory (2009). He has been elected Fellow of the International Communication Association (2011), the Society for Behavioral Medicine (2008), and the Midwest Association for Public Opinion Research (2006). He chaired the Board of Scientific Counselors for the National Center for Health Marketing at the Centers for Disease Control and Prevention (CDC), Atlanta, from 2007 to 2010 and has served on three Institute of Medicine committees. Currently, he is a member of the National Vaccine Advisory Committee (NVAC) of the U.S. Department of Health and Human Services and chairs NVAC's Working Group on Vaccine Acceptance, and a member of the Board of Scientific Counselors, Office of Public Health Preparedness and Response, CDC.

Alice Ammerman is professor in the Gillings School of Global Public Health and director of the Center for Health Promotion and Disease Prevention at the University of North Carolina at Chapel Hill.

David Asch is professor in the Perelman School of Medicine and the Wharton School and the executive director of the Penn Medicine Center for Health Care Innovation at the University of Pennsylvania.

Magdalena Avila is assistant professor in the Department of Health, Exercise, and Sports Sciences at the University of New Mexico.

L. Kay Bartholomew is professor and associate dean for academic affairs at the University of Texas School of Public Health.

Noel T. Brewer is associate professor in the Department of Health Behavior at the Gillings School of Global Public Health at the University of North Carolina at Chapel Hill.

Ross C. Brownson is Bernard Becker Professor of Public Health and holds joint appointments at the Brown School of Social Work and the School of Medicine at Washington University in St. Louis.

Lori Carter-Edwards is deputy director for research and operations for the University of North Carolina Center for Health Promotion and Disease Prevention.

Victoria L. Champion is distinguished professor at the Indiana University School of Nursing and associate director of population science research at the IU Simon Cancer Center.

Ashley Duggan is associate professor in the Communication Department at Boston College.

Kerry E. Evers is senior vice president of research and product development at Pro-Change Behavior Systems, Inc., in Rhode Island.

María E. Fernández is associate professor in the Division of Health Promotion and Behavioral Sciences at the University of Texas School of Public Health.

John R. Finnegan Jr. is professor and dean of the School of Public Health at the University of Minnesota.

Sarah Gollust is assistant professor in the Division of Health Policy and Management at the University of Minnesota School of Public Health.

Catherine A. Heaney is associate professor (teaching) in the Stanford Prevention Research Center, the Department of Psychology, and the Program in Human Biology at Stanford University.

Ronald Hess is with the Johns Hopkins Center for Communication Programs and served as chief of party of the Communication for Healthy Living (CHL) project in Egypt, from 2003 to 2010.

Deanna Hoelscher is John P. McGovern Professor in Health Promotion and director of the Michael and Susan Dell Center for Healthy Living at the University of Texas School of Public Health.

Julianne Holt-Lunstad is associate professor of psychology at Brigham Young University.

Danuta Kasprzyk is associate professor in the Department of Family and Child Nursing at the University of Washington School of Nursing.

Steven H. Kelder is Beth Toby Grossman Professor in Spirituality and Healing and co-director of the Michael and Susan Dell Center for Healthy Living at the University of Texas School of Public Health.

George Loewenstein is professor of economics and psychology in the Department of Social and Decision Sciences at Carnegie Mellon University.

Christine Markham is associate professor in the Division of Health Promotion and Behavioral Sciences at the University of Texas School of Public Health.

Meredith Minkler is professor of health and social behavior in the School of Public Health at the University of California, Berkeley.

Daniel E. Montaño is associate professor in the Department of Family and Child Nursing at the University of Washington School of Nursing.

Pat Mullen is professor in the Division of Health Promotion and Behavioral Sciences at the University of Texas School of Public Health.

Neville Owen is professor in and head of the Behavioural and Generational Change Program at the Baker IDI Heart and Diabetes Institute in Melbourne, Australia.

Cheryl L. Perry is professor and regional dean at the University of Texas School of Public Health, Austin Regional Campus.

James O. Prochaska is professor and director of the Cancer Prevention Research Center at the University of Rhode Island.

Colleen A. Redding is research professor in the Cancer Prevention Research Center at the University of Rhode Island.

Gary Saffitz is with Gary Saffitz Consulting.

James F. Sallis is Distinguished Professor of Family Medicine and Public Health at the University of California, San Diego.

Victoria Sánchez is associate professor of public health at the University of New Mexico.

Marc D. Schwartz is professor of oncology and co-leader of the Cancer Prevention and Control program at the Georgetown University Lombardi Comprehensive Cancer Center in Washington, DC.

Celette Sugg Skinner is professor of clinical sciences, division chief of behavioral and communication sciences, and associate director for population sciences at the Harold C. Simmons Cancer Center at the University of Texas Southwestern Medical Center.

Katherine A. Stamatakis is associate professor in the Departments of Epidemiology and Behavioral Science and Health Education at Saint Louis University, College for Public Health and Social Justice.

J. Douglas Storey is director for communication science and research at the Center for Communication Programs in the Johns Hopkins University Bloomberg School of Public Health.

Richard L. Street Jr. is professor in the Department of Communication at Texas A&M University, professor of medicine at the Baylor College of Medicine, and chief of the Health Decision-Making and Communication Program at the Michael E. DeBakey VA Medical Center in Houston.

Rachel G. Tabak is research assistant professor at the Prevention Research Center and the George Warren Brown School of Social Work at Washington University in St. Louis.

Jasmin Tiro is assistant professor in the Department of Clinical Sciences at the University of Texas Southwestern Medical Center.

Bert N. Uchino is professor of psychology at the University of Utah.

Thomas W. Valente is professor in the Department of Preventive Medicine and director of the Master of Public Health Program at the University of Southern California's Keck School of Medicine.

Kevin Volpp is professor of medicine in the Perelman School of Medicine and professor of health care management in the Wharton School at the University of Pennsylvania. He is also director of the Center for Health Incentives and Behavioral Economics and vice chairman for health policy in the Department of Medical Ethics and Health Policy at the University of Pennsylvania.

Nina Wallerstein is professor in the Public Health Program and director of the Center for Participatory Research at the University of New Mexico in Albuquerque.

Elaine Wethington is professor in the Departments of Human Development and Sociology and an associate director of the Brofenbrenner Center for Translational Research at Cornell University.

PART ONE

HEALTH BEHAVIOR: THE FOUNDATIONS

CHAPTER 1

THE SCOPE OF HEALTH BEHAVIOR

The Editors

In the past few years, wearable tracking devices have become commonplace in the United States. These devices enable users to count steps, track calories burned and miles covered, be reminded when they have been sitting too long, share data with others, and examine trends over time. More and more, consumers have accessible tools to assess their own health behaviors and health risks in ways that once were available only through health providers. For example, researchers at the Massachusetts Institute of Technology have produced sensor-infused bands that send alerts when a person may be about to suffer an epileptic seizure (Poh et al., 2012). This is an example of how the frontiers of communication and behavior have expanded far beyond what we imagined twenty-five years ago, when we wrote the first edition of this book.

It is an exciting time to contemplate behavior change. Perhaps never before have there been so many demands on those who aim to facilitate positive changes in health behaviors and so many potential strategies from which to choose. Whether it is the need to reduce the rate of hospital readmissions in order to avoid costly penalties from Medicare or communities faced with increased rates of childhood obesity, there is growing recognition that health behavior changes are needed across the world if population health is to improve. Where professionals once might have seen their roles as working at a particular level of intervention (such as changing organizational or individual health behaviors) or employing a specific type of behavior change strategy (such as group interventions or individual counseling), we now realize that multiple kinds of interventions at different levels often are needed to initiate and sustain behavior change effectively. Once, health behavior experts might have relied on intuition, experience, and their knowledge of the literature. Increasingly, however, professionals are expected to act on the basis of evidence. In the time since the first edition of this book in 1990, the evidence base for health behavior change has grown dramatically. Along with the evidence base on behavior change interventions is growing interest in using and assessing the impact of theories of behavior change.

Many systematic reviews have examined whether using theory in crafting interventions can lead to more powerful effects than interventions developed without theory (Glanz & Bishop, 2010; Michie, West, Campbell, Brown, & Gainforth, 2014). Reviews have varied in how they code theory use and specific theories, and how they interpret findings related to the theory use–impact question. Some reviews found that using theoretical foundations for interventions was associated with better outcomes (Albada, Ausems, Bensing, & van Dulmen, 2009; Ammerman, Lindquist, Lohr, & Hersey, 2002; Legler et al., 2002; Noar, Benac, & Harris, 2007; Noar, Black, & Pierce, 2009; Taylor, Conner, & Lawton, 2011). Some reviews found no association or mixed results (Gardner, Wardle, Poston, & Croker, 2011; Prestwich et al., 2013).

As the body of literature of systematic reviews and meta-analyses of interventions that examine theory use grows, the picture becomes more complex. Our interpretation from a "review of reviews" to date suggests that outcomes are better when theory is applied or more thoroughly applied. But this is not a simple, strong, or unequivocal conclusion. Nonetheless, there are many reasons for both researchers and practitioners to be well versed in the theoretical foundations of health behavior and facile with applying them in their work. It is even more important to become skilled at using and testing theories, because some equivocal results may be due to failures in theory specification and testing.

Today we have many tools and strategies for improving our understanding of the role that health behavior theories can play in producing effective, sustained behavior changes. These tools and strategies are more and more accessible from web-based repositories. Furthermore, the stage for health behavior change research and practice has changed from one that was primarily local and country-specific to one that is *both* global and local, in a world that is increasingly interconnected.

These exciting opportunities are occurring at a propitious time. The positive and rapid changes in medical innovations, a strong evidence base, and increasingly accessible tools for health promotion are buffeted by countercurrents of increasing globalization, urbanization, industrialization, and inequalities that may deter us from fulfilling the promise of advances in medicine and health promotion. Major challenges include the billions of dollars spent yearly across the world on the promotion of unhealthy lifestyles, such as tobacco use and sugary beverage consumption, and also the challenges of physical inactivity, increasing pollution, and health problems associated with poverty, including overcrowding, lack of safe drinking water, unsafe neighborhoods, and limited access to health care.

Unhealthy behaviors continue to account for a disproportionate share of deaths in countries around the world. And the rise of noncommunicable diseases globally is a major threat to world health, pushing many below the poverty line (Choi, 2012; Lueddeke, 2015). National and global health policies must encourage and enable people to practice healthy habits (Lueddeke, 2015). Improved health is not dependent on medicine or health care alone; it is the sum of multiple factors at multiple levels of societies.

The topics on which health professionals and health behavior specialists focus have grown and evolved as health problems have changed around the world (Fisher et al., 2011). Professionals may counsel people at risk for AIDS about safe sex; help children avoid tobacco, alcohol, and drugs; assist adults to stop smoking; teach patients to manage and cope with their chronic illnesses; and organize communities and advocate policy changes aimed at fostering health improvement. Health professionals also may address environmental concerns, such as safe, accessible water and healthy air. Over the next decade, more behavior change interventions around the world will be directed at changing individual and community behaviors related to basic hygiene and clean water consumption (Briscoe & Aboud, 2012) while also trying to reduce noncommunicable diseases around the world. The former problems are often a result of poverty and poor living conditions while the latter stem, in part, from growing influence of the developed world on developing nations.

Public health professionals work all over the world and in a variety of settings, including schools, worksites, nongovernmental organizations (including voluntary health organizations), medical settings, and communities. And professional fields other than health may also influence health behavior.

Since the time of the first edition of this book, there has been increased recognition that what happens in one part of the world affects us all, wherever we may be. Rapid changes in communication technologies have made the world a much smaller place and have accelerated the pace of sharing information and ideas. To the extent that public health is global health, and global health is local, we are committed in this volume to explore the use of health behavior theories around the world and to discuss the potential relevance of what is learned in one setting to other areas. While many of our examples are from research conducted in the United States, our perspective is decidedly global.

Since the fourth edition of this book was published seven years ago, the growth of new information and communication technologies has opened up an unprecedented range of strategies for health behavior change programs. Through the Internet, mobile devices, and wearables, health behavior change interventions are accessible to people all over the world, regardless of location. The result could be positive changes in health behaviors and health on a scale never before imagined, potentially reaching millions of people rather than hundreds or thousands.

There also is increased recognition that the fruits of research take too long to reach people who could benefit from them (Glasgow & Emmons, 2007; Viswanath, 2006). This has led to an increased emphasis on the dissemination of evidence-based interventions and attention to how interventions are implemented and scaled and to the growing field of implementation science. Part of the rationale for this book is to speed the dissemination of knowledge about how to use theory, so that theory can inform those who develop and use health behavior interventions around the world.

Health experts are challenged to disseminate the best of what is known in new situations. They may also forge and test fundamental theories that drive research and practice in public health, health education, and health care. A premise of *Health Behavior: Theory, Research, and Practice* is that a dynamic exchange among theory, research, and practice is most likely to produce positive health behaviors. The editors believe, fundamentally, that theory and practice should coexist in a healthy dialectic; they are not dichotomies. The best theory is likely to be grounded in real lessons from practice. Similarly, best practices should be grounded in theory.

Kanfer and Schefft (1988) observed that "as science and technology advance, the greatest mystery of the universe and the least conquered force of nature remains the human being and his actions and human experiences." The body of research in health behavior has grown rapidly over the past two and a half decades, and health behavior change is increasingly recognized as critical to meeting public health objectives of the United States and improving the success of public health and medical interventions around the world. While this expanding body of literature improves the science base of health behavior, knowledge management is becoming both a growing challenge and an imperative.

The science and art of health behavior and health behavior change are eclectic, are rapidly evolving, and reflect an amalgamation of approaches, methods, and strategies from the social and health sciences. They draw on the theoretical perspectives, research, and practice tools of such diverse disciplines as psychology, sociology, anthropology, communications, nursing, economics, and marketing. Health behavior research and practice are also dependent on epidemiology, statistics, and medicine. Big data are now a tool of health behavior and other fields. There is greater emphasis on developing and testing evidence-based interventions and disseminating them widely (Rimer, Glanz, & Rasband, 2001). Evidence-based groups like the Cochrane Collaboration (http://www.cochrane.org) and the CDC's Guide to Community Preventive Services (http://www.thecommunityguide.org) offer regular syntheses of behavioral interventions, some of which include theoretical constructs as variables in analyses of effectiveness.

Many kinds of professionals contribute to and conduct health behavior research and intervention programs. Ultimately, their practice is strengthened by the close collaboration among professionals of different disciplines, each concerned with the behavioral and social intervention process, and each contributing a unique perspective. New emphases on interprofessional education may provide the educational foundation to achieve better collaboration across disciplines. While health behavior professionals often have worked this way, there is an increasing emphasis on an interdisciplinary or even a transdisciplinary focus (Turkkan, Kaufman, & Rimer, 2000). Psychology brings to health education a rich legacy of over one hundred years of research and practice on individual differences, motivation, learning, persuasion, and attitude and behavior change (Matarazzo, Weiss, Herd, Miller, & Weiss, 1984), as well as the perspectives of organizational and community psychology. Physicians are important collaborators and are in key roles for effecting change in health behaviors (Grol, Bosch, Hulscher, Eccles, & Wensing, 2007). Likewise nurses and social workers contribute their particular expertise in working with individual patients and patients' families to facilitate learning, adjustment, and behavior change and to improve quality of life. Other health, education, and human service professionals contribute their special expertise as well, along with those in the information sciences and related fields. Increasingly, there are partnerships with genetic counselors, neuroscientists, and other specialists in this rapidly developing field.

Health, Disease, and Health Behavior: The Changing Context

The greatest causes of death in the United States and globally are chronic diseases, including heart disease, cancer, lung diseases, and diabetes (Lozano et al., 2012). Behavioral factors, particularly tobacco use, diet and activity patterns, alcohol consumption, sexual behavior, and avoidable injuries, are among the most prominent contributors to mortality (Fisher et al., 2011). Projections of the global burden of disease for the next two decades include increases in noncommunicable diseases, high rates of tobacco-related deaths, and a dramatic rise in deaths from HIV/AIDS (Abegunde, Mathers, Adam, Ortegon, & Strong, 2007; Mathers & Loncar, 2006). Worldwide, the major causes of death by 2030 are expected to be HIV/AIDS, depressive disorders, and heart disease (Mathers & Loncar, 2006).

At the same time, in many parts of the world, infectious diseases pose grim threats, especially for the very young, the old, and those with compromised immune systems. Malaria, diarrheal diseases, and other infectious diseases, such as Ebola, SARS (severe acute respiratory syndrome), MERS (Middle East respiratory syndrome), and tuberculosis, in addition to AIDS, are increasing health threats to the poorest people around the world (The *PLoS Medicine* Editors, 2007). And as with chronic diseases, their trajectory may be influenced by the application of effective health behavior interventions as well as by social determinants that influence health and illness. Substantial suffering, premature mortality, and medical costs can be avoided by positive changes in behavior at multiple levels.

During the past twenty years, there has been a dramatic increase in public, private, and professional interest in preventing disability and death through changes in lifestyle and participation in screening programs. Country and global population health goals are an essential part of the strategy (e.g., U.S. Healthy People goals and WHO goals). Much of this interest in disease prevention and early detection has been stimulated by the epidemiologic transition from infectious to chronic diseases as leading causes of death, the aging of the global population, rapidly escalating health care costs, and data linking individual behaviors to increased risk of morbidity and mortality. The evidence that early detection can save lives from highly prevalent conditions such as breast and colorectal cancer has also been influential. The AIDS epidemic has also contributed. Moreover, around the world, communicable diseases and malnutrition exist alongside increasing problems such as obesity among the middle class (Abegunde et al., 2007).

Landmark reports in Canada and the United States during the 1970s and 1980s heralded the commitment of governments to health education and promotion (Epp, 1986; Lalonde, 1974; U.S. Department of Health, Education, and Welfare, 1979). In the United States, federal initiatives for public health education and monitoring population-wide behavior patterns were spurred by the development of the *Health Objectives for the Nation* (U.S. Department of Health and Human Services [DHHS], 1980) and their successors, *Healthy People 2000: National Health Promotion and Disease Prevention Objectives* (DHHS, 1991), *Healthy People*

2010 (DHHS, 2000), and *Healthy People 2020* (DHHS, 2014b). Similarly, international agencies are drawing attention to the global burden of diseases and health inequalities (World Health Organization [WHO], 2014b). Increased interest in behavioral and social determinants of health behavior change has spawned numerous training programs and public and commercial service programs.

Data systems and surveillance initiatives now make it feasible to track trends in risk factors, health behaviors, and healthy environments and policies in the United States and developed countries and, in some cases, to tie these changes to disease incidence and mortality (WHO, 2014a). Indeed, positive change has occurred in several areas. Deaths from coronary heart disease and cancer have declined in the United States, though disparities between racial and economic groups persist. Blood pressure control has improved and mean population blood cholesterol levels have declined. Alcohol-related motor vehicle deaths and overall deaths due to automobile crashes and also deaths from drowning have continued to decrease. Following major litigation against the tobacco industry and a multistate settlement, there are increased restrictions on tobacco advertising and enforcement of laws against selling tobacco to minors (Glanz, Jarrette, Wilson, O'Riordan, & Jacob Arriola, 2007). In the United States, fewer adults are using tobacco products—the reduction in adult smoking from 42.4 percent to 18.1 percent between 1965 and 2012 (Centers for Disease Control and Prevention, 2014) is hailed as one of the top public health achievements of the past century. Rates of HIV/AIDS in the United States have leveled off and transfusion-related HIV infections have decreased markedly. The proportion of women aged forty and older who have had mammograms within the previous two years reached 67.1 percent in 2010 (DHHS, 2013). The collective efforts of those in health care, health education, and public health have made a difference.

While this progress is encouraging, much work remains to be done in the United States and other countries. More adults and children are overweight. Diabetes is increasing to near-epidemic proportions. More adolescents are sexually active. Ten percent of children under three years old have not received a basic series of vaccinations for polio, measles, diphtheria, and other diseases. The proportion of adults under sixty-five years of age with no health insurance coverage has declined recently but still exceeds 15 percent. Ethnic minorities and those in poverty still experience a disproportionate burden of preventable disease and disability, and the gap persists between disadvantaged and affluent groups in the use of preventive services (National Commission on Prevention Priorities, 2007).

Reducing the global disease burden is critical to the future of the planet. Data from Popkin (2007) and others show that, like the tobacco epidemic, the obesity epidemic has taken on global proportions. One study of the burden of chronic diseases in twenty-three low- and middle-income countries posits that chronic disease is responsible for 50 percent of the disease burden in 2005, and estimates an economic loss of almost US$84 billion between 2006 and 2015 if nothing is done to address this burden (Mathers & Loncar, 2006).

Changes in health care systems are providing new supports and opportunities for health behavior change. Respect for patients' rights and more participatory, patient-centered communications can lead to improved health outcomes (Arora, 2003; Epstein & Street, 2007). The U.S. Patient Protection and Affordable Care Act included expectations for health care systems to increase patients' engagement and to measure their success in achieving this outcome. Increasingly, patients are driving their own searches for health information by using the Internet (see, e.g., Hesse et al., 2005; Rimer et al., 2005), though disparities remain in information seeking between those of higher and lower socioeconomic status (Ramanadhan & Viswanath, 2006). Clinical prevention and behavioral interventions are often considered cost effective but are neither universally available nor equally accessible across racial and socioeconomic groups (Gostin & Powers, 2006; Schroeder, 2007).

The rapid emergence of new communication technologies and new models of use for older technologies, such as the telephone, also provide new opportunities and dilemmas. Just a few years ago, "new" electronic media for interactive health communications consisted mainly of the Internet, CD-ROMs, and personal digital assistants. Today, social media, tablets, wireless communications, and personal monitoring devices are widespread. They can serve as sources of individualized health information, reminders, and social support for health behavior change (see Chapter Seventeen). These new technologies also may connect individuals with similar health concerns around the world (Bukachi & Pakenham-Walsh, 2007). This may be especially important for people with rare or stigmatized health conditions. However, the new products of the communication revolution have not reached affluent and disadvantaged populations equally (Viswanath, 2006).

E-health and m-health strategies are becoming important behavior change strategies. Internet and computer-based applications—along with wireless technologies—support many of the strategies based on theories presented in this book. Use of new technologies should be based on theories of health behavior and evaluated (Webb, Joseph, Yardley, & Michie, 2010). In the end, emphasis should be on desired health outcomes. Technology can enable behavior change and measurement of change but should not be an end in itself.

At the same time, new technologies have the potential to cause harm through misleading or deceptive information, promotion of inappropriate self-care, and interference in the patient-provider relationship, although the empirical evidence on harms remains to be documented. Interactive health communications provide new options for behavioral medicine and preventive medicine, and are altering the context of health behavior and health education as they unfold and as their effects are studied (Hesse et al., 2005). Viswanath, Finnegan, and Gollust (Chapter Seventeen in this book) also have cautioned about the potential for new technologies to exacerbate health disparities.

Health Behavior and Health Behavior Change

Health Behaviors

Positive, informed changes in health behaviors are typically the ultimate aims of health behavior change programs. If behaviors change but health is not subsequently improved, the result is a paradox that must be resolved by examining other issues, such as the link between behavior and health status, or the ways in which behavior and/or health are measured. Informed decision making is a desirable endpoint for problems involving medical uncertainty, and studies suggest that shared decision making may lead to improved patient satisfaction and health outcomes (Rimer, Briss, Zeller, Chan, & Woolf, 2004). Likewise, environmental or structural interventions to change presumed social environmental determinants of health behaviors are intended to improve health by changing behavior (Smedley & Syme, 2000; Story, Kaphingst, Robinson-O'Brien, & Glanz, 2008). Thus efforts to improve environments, policies, and other outcomes should ultimately be evaluated for their effects on health behaviors and health. If a policy changes but does not lead to measurable changes in behavior, the change may be either too weak, too short-lived, ineffectively implemented, or only a limited determinant of behavior.

In its broadest sense, *health behavior* refers to the actions of individuals, groups, and organizations as well as those actions' determinants, correlates, and consequences, including social change, policy development and implementation, improved coping skills, and enhanced quality of life (Parkerson et al., 1993). This is similar to the working definition of *health behavior* that Gochman proposed (although his definition emphasized individuals): it includes not only observable, overt actions but also the mental events and feeling states that can be reported and measured. Gochman defined health behavior as "those personal attributes such as beliefs, expectations, motives, values, perceptions, and other cognitive elements; personality characteristics, including affective and emotional states and traits; and overt behavior patterns, actions, and habits that relate to health maintenance, to health restoration, and to health improvement" (Gochman, 1982, 1997).

Gochman's definition is consistent with and embraces the definitions of specific categories of overt health behavior proposed by Kasl and Cobb in their seminal articles (1966a, 1966b). Kasl and Cobb defined three categories of health behavior:

Preventive health behavior: any activity undertaken by an individual who believes himself (or herself) to be healthy, for the purpose of preventing or detecting illness in an asymptomatic state.

Illness behavior: any activity undertaken by an individual who perceives himself to be ill, to define the state of health, and to discover a suitable remedy (Kasl & Cobb, 1966a).

Sick-role behavior: any activity undertaken by an individual who considers himself to be ill, for the purpose of getting well. It includes receiving treatment from medical providers, generally involves a whole range of dependent behaviors, and leads to some degree of exemption from one's usual responsibilities (Kasl & Cobb, 1966b).

Disciplinary Influences on Health Behavior Change over Time

Health behavior change has been the focus of multiple fields and professions, including health education, public health, psychology, social work, and various health and medical specialties. Clinical psychologists have traditionally focused on changing individuals, and social work tends to address individuals within their social and family contexts. In the field of health education, the emphasis during the 1970s and 1980s on individuals' behaviors as determinants of health status eclipsed attention to the broader social determinants of health. Advocates of system-level changes to improve health called for renewal of a broad vision of health education and promotion (Minkler, 1989; also see Chapter Three). These calls for moving health education toward social action heralded a tighter connection to the broad field of public health. They are consistent with the longstanding concern of public health with the impact of social, economic, and political forces on health. Thus the idea that focusing on downstream (individual) causes of poor health to the exclusion of the upstream causes risks missing important opportunities to improve health (McKinlay & Marceau, 2000) is not new in public health and health education and promotion, but continues to receive increasing attention.

The view of health behavior change strategies as instruments of social change has been renewed and invigorated during the past decade. Policy, advocacy, and organizational change have been adopted as central activities of public health and health education. Most recently, experts have explicitly recommended that interventions on social and behavioral factors related to health should link multiple levels of influence, including the individual, interpersonal, institutional, community, and policy levels (Smedley & Syme, 2000). This volume purposefully includes chapters on community and societal influences on health behavior and strategies to effect community and social policy changes in addition to the individual-level theories (McLeroy, Bibeau, Steckler, & Glanz, 1988; also see Chapter Three).

Settings and Audiences for Health Behavior Change

During the past century, and more specifically during the past few decades, the scope and methods of health behavior change strategies have broadened and diversified dramatically. This section briefly reviews the range of settings and audiences for health behavior change today.

Settings: Where Are Health Behavior Change Strategies Provided?

Seven major settings are particularly relevant to contemporary health behavior: schools, communities, worksites, health care settings, homes, the consumer marketplace, and the communication environment.

Schools

Health behavior change programs in schools include classroom teaching, teacher training, and changes in school environments that support healthy behaviors (A. Franks et al., 2007; Luepker et al., 1996). To support long-term health enhancement initiatives, theories of dissemination and implementation can be used to encourage adoption of comprehensive smoking control programs in schools. Diffusion of Innovations theory and the Theory of Reasoned Action have been used to analyze factors associated with adoption of AIDS prevention curricula in Dutch schools (Paulussen, Kok, Schaalma, & Parcel, 1995).

Communities

Community-based health promotion draws on social relationships and organizations to reach large populations with media and interpersonal strategies. Models of community engagement and community mobilization enable program planners both to gain support for and to design suitable health messages and delivery mechanisms (see Chapter Fifteen). Community interventions in churches, clubs, recreation centers, and neighborhoods have been used to encourage healthful nutrition, reduce risk of cardiovascular disease, and use peer influences to promote breast cancer detection among minority women.

Worksites

Since its emergence in the mid-1970s, worksite health promotion has grown and has spawned new tools for health behavior change. Because people spend so much time at work, the workplace is a source of both stress and social support (Israel & Schurman, 1990). Effective worksite programs can harness social support as a buffer to stress, with the goal of improving worker health and health practices. Today many businesses, particularly large corporations, provide health promotion programs for their employees. The U.S. Affordable Care Act provides incentives for employees to alter health behaviors, further advancing worksite health behavior change initiatives (see Chapter Twenty). Both high-risk and population-wide strategies have been used in worksite health behavior change programs to reduce chronic disease risk factors. Systematic reviews of worksite programs to prevent or reduce obesity have shown success using a variety of strategies (Anderson et al., 2009).

Health Care Settings

Health behavior change programs for high-risk individuals, patients, their families, and the surrounding community and in-service training for health care providers are all part of health care today. The changing nature of health service delivery has stimulated greater emphasis on implementing health behavior change and provider-focused quality improvement strategies in physicians' offices and medical homes, health maintenance organizations, public health clinics, and hospitals (Grol et al., 2007; Powell et al., 2012). Primary care settings, in particular, provide an opportunity to reach a substantial number of people (Campbell et al., 1994) and to achieve goals of improved population health. The use of community health workers for patients discharged from hospitals is increasingly considered a strategy for reducing readmission rates (Kangovi et al., 2014).

Homes

Health behavior change interventions can be delivered to people in their homes, both through traditional public health means—home visits—and through a variety of communication channels and media, such as the Internet, telephone calls, and mail (McBride & Rimer, 1999). Strategies, such as mailed tailored messages (Glanz, Schoenfeld, & Steffen, 2010) and motivational interviewing by telephone (Emmons & Rollnick, 2001), make it possible to reach larger groups and high-risk groups in a convenient way that reduces barriers to their receiving motivational messages. In-home coaching that helps people improve their home health environments to support health behavior change has also shown promise (Kegler et al., 2012).

The Consumer Marketplace

The advent of home health and self-care products, as well as the use of "health" appeals to sell consumer goods, has created new opportunities for health education but also means of misleading consumers about the potential health effects of items they can purchase (Glanz et al., 1995). Social marketing, with its roots in consumer behavior theory, is used increasingly by health educators to enhance the salience of health messages and to improve their persuasive impact (see Chapter Twenty-One). Health information policies intended to support informed consumer decision making, such as policies that encourage adding calorie information to menus (Swartz, Braxton, & Viera, 2011) and require graphic warning labels on cigarette packs (Huang, Chaloupka, & Fong, 2014), have emerged prominently in the past few years.

The Communication Environment

There have been striking and rapid changes in the availability and use of new information and communication technologies (ICTs), ranging from mass media changes (e.g., online versions of newspapers and podcasts of radio programs) to personalized, mobile, and interactive media and a host of wireless tools in homes, businesses, and communities (see Chapter Seventeen). These channels can be used in any of the settings described above. Yet they are unique, increasingly prominent and specialized, and provide opportunities for intervention as well as requiring evaluation of their reach and impact on health behaviors (Ahern, Phalen, Le, & Goldman, 2007).

Audiences: Who Are the Recipients of Health Behavior Change Interventions?

For health behavior change interventions to be effective, strategies should be designed with an understanding of the recipients, or target audiences; their health, cultural context, and social characteristics; and their beliefs, attitudes, values, skills, and past behaviors. These audiences consist of people who may be reached as individuals, in groups, through organizations, as communities or sociopolitical entities, or through some combination of these approaches. They may be health professionals, clients, people at risk for disease, or patients. This section discusses four dimensions along which potential audiences can be characterized: sociodemographic characteristics, ethnic or racial background, life cycle stage, and disease or at-risk status.

Sociodemographic Characteristics and Ethnic/Racial Background

Socioeconomic status has been linked with both health status and health behavior, with less affluent persons consistently experiencing higher morbidity and mortality (Berkman & Kawachi, 2000). Recognition of differences in disease and mortality rates across socioeconomic and ethnic or racial groups has led to increased efforts to reduce or eliminate health disparities (Smedley, Stith, & Nelson, 2003; World Health Organization, Commission on Social Determinants of Health, 2007). For example, it has long been known that African Americans die at earlier ages than whites. Life expectancy for African American males is almost seven years less than for white males. The difference of five years for African American versus white women is smaller but still alarmingly discrepant. The gaps have grown over the past three decades and are even greater for those with lower levels of education and income (P. Franks, Muennig, Lubetkin, & Jia, 2006).

A variety of sociodemographic characteristics, such as gender, age, race, marital status, place of residence, and employment, characterize audiences for changes in health behaviors. The United States has experienced a rapid influx of new immigrant populations, especially from Africa and Europe, and the proportion of nonwhite minority residents continues to climb. These factors, while generally not *modifiable* within the bounds of health education programs, are important to understand in order to guide the targeting of strategies and educational materials, and to identify channels and media through which to reach consumers. Health behavior interventions should be appropriate to the educational and reading levels of particular target audiences and be compatible with their ethnic and cultural backgrounds (Resnicow, Braithwaite, DiIorio, & Glanz, 2002), and their access to and facility with technology.

Life Cycle Stage

Health education is provided for people at every stage of the life cycle, from childbirth education whose beneficiaries are not yet born to self-care education and rehabilitation for the very old. Developmental perspectives help to guide the choice of intervention and research methods. Children may have misperceptions about health and illness, such as thinking that illnesses are a punishment for bad behavior (Armsden & Lewis, 1993). Knowledge of children's cognitive development helps provide a framework for understanding these beliefs and ways to respond to them. Adolescents may feel invulnerable to accidents and chronic diseases. The Health Belief Model (see Chapter Five) is a useful framework for understanding the factors that may predispose youth to engage in unsafe sexual practices. Healthy People 2020 goals stress reaching people in every stage of life, with a special focus on vulnerabilities that may affect people at various life cycle stages (DHHS, 2014b).

Disease and At-Risk Status

People who are diagnosed with life-threatening diseases often experience not only symptoms but also the distress associated with their prognosis and having to make decisions about medical care (see Chapter Twelve). Illness may compromise their ability to attend to new information or develop new skills at critical points. Because of this, timing, channels, and audiences for patient education should be carefully considered. Successful patient education depends on a sound understanding of the patient's view of the world (Glanz & Oldenburg, 2001). For individuals at high risk due to family history or identified risk factors, health behavior change interventions may have heightened salience when linked to strategies for reducing individual risk (Weinstein, Sandman, & Blalock, 2008). Even so, strategies used to enable initial changes in behavior, such as quitting smoking, may be insufficient to maintain behavior change over the long term, even in these people. Models and theories of health behavior can suggest strategies to prevent relapse and enhance maintenance of recommended practices for high-risk individuals (Glanz & Oldenburg, 2001).

Progress in Health Behavior Research and Practice

Over the past three decades, many studies, large and small, have been conducted to identify and test the most effective methods to achieve health behavior change (e.g., Carleton, Lasater, Assaf, Feldman, & McKinlay, 1995; Farquhar et al., 1990; Glasgow, Terborg, Hollis, Severson, & Boles, 1995; Luepker et al., 1994; Sorensen et al., 1996; Winkleby, 1994). More precise quantification of personal health behaviors and improved health outcomes have grown from partnerships among behavioral scientists, biomedical experts, and people from other fields, including education and the information sciences.

Although many large studies were disappointing in the lack of significant results or smaller results than expected, several behavior change campaigns produced behavior changes conducive to health (Hornik, 2002). These experiences suggest that health education interventions must be carefully planned, developed from strong formative research, and theory-based (Randolph & Viswanath, 2004; also see Chapter Nineteen). While randomized controlled trials provide the most rigorous test of health behavior interventions, the past two decades have been marked by an increase in carefully designed evaluation research in health education, which combines quantitative and qualitative methods. Evaluations of community-based AIDS prevention projects (Janz et al., 1996) and coalitions for prevention of alcohol, tobacco, and other drug abuse (Butterfoss, Goodman, & Wandersman, 1996) exemplify applications of community research methodologies that offer in-depth process information across multiple programs in diverse settings. Similarly, new statistical methods and adaptive trials may ultimately permit faster answers and the capacity to answer more questions through more efficient trial design.

Overall, there has been a growing recognition of the importance of building an evidence base in the domain of health-related behavior change interventions (Rimer, Glanz, & Rasband, 2001). Today, systematic reviews and meta-analyses of health behavior change studies are both common and expected to guide future work. It has been nearly twenty years since the uptick in quantitative synthesis began to grow. A review of health education research between 1994 and 2003 found a significant increase in use of quantitative statistics, while also finding that the most common types of articles were those that addressed cross-sectional studies and review articles (Merrill, Lindsay, Shields, & Stoddard, 2007). That review was limited to three health education journals. Other reviews of research design and statistics also found a preponderance of correlational and descriptive studies (Noar & Zimmerman, 2005; Painter, Borba, Hynes, Mays, & Glanz, 2008; Weinstein, 2007). As the research literature grows, it is critical that the evidence base and the methods behind the evidence are accessible to both researchers and practitioners around the world (Von Elm et al., 2007). Evidence reviews are defined as those using formalized methods to collect, prioritize, and weigh the findings of intervention research. Important progress has been made over the past ten to fifteen years in improving the process of and guidance for conducting systematic reviews and meta-analyses (Hoffman et al., 2014; Moher, Liberati, Tetzlaff, Altman, & the PRISMA Group, 2009). The U.S. Task Force on

Community Preventive Services is defining, categorizing, summarizing, and rating the quality of evidence on the effectiveness of population-based interventions for disease prevention and control; providing recommendations on these interventions and methods for their delivery based on the evidence; and identifying and summarizing research gaps (Briss et al., 2000; DHHS, 2014a). Parallel efforts are underway in other countries as well, such as the work in England being conducted by the National Institute for Health and Clinical Excellence (NICE) (2014).

Observations by McGinnis (1994) are still relevant today: the challenge of understanding and improving health behavior is "one of the most complex tasks yet confronted by science. To competently address that challenge, the . . . research community must simply do more and do it better" in certain key areas of behavioral research. A coordinated and focused effort is essential to resolve many of the most vexing health issues facing our society (Smedley & Syme, 2000). Integration of the best available knowledge from theory, research, and behavior change practice can advance that agenda in the years ahead.

Health Behavior Foundations for Theory, Research, and Practice

This chapter has discussed the dynamic nature of health behavior today in the context of changing patterns of disease and trends in social interaction and communication, health care, health education, and disease prevention in the United States and globally. It has provided definitions of health behavior and described the broad and diverse parameters of this maturing field. Although thousands more studies of health behavior change have been conducted and reported since the last edition of this book, their variable and sometimes disappointing results raise new questions and pose methodological, theoretical, and substantive challenges. The importance of theory, research, and practice and the interrelationships among them are set against the backdrop of the urgent, growing, and complex imperative to improve the health of populations around the world and to do so in a context that recognizes that health services are only some of the forces that influence health status. Today's students, researchers, and practitioners can make a difference in the burden of illness and in the potential to develop effective, scalable interventions to improve health.

References

Abegunde, D. O., Mathers, C. D., Adam, T., Ortegon, M., & Strong, K. (2007). The burden and costs of chronic diseases in low-income and middle-income countries. *Lancet, 370*(9603), 1929–1938.

Ahern, D. K., Phalen, J. M., Le, L. X., & Goldman, R. (Eds.). (2007). *Childhood obesity prevention and reduction: Role of eHealth.* Boston: Health e-Technologies Initiative.

Albada, A., Ausems, M. G., Bensing, J. M., & van Dulmen, S. (2009). Tailored information about cancer risk and screening: A systematic review. *Patient Education and Counseling, 77*(2), 155–171.

Ammerman, A. S., Lindquist, C. H., Lohr, K. N., & Hersey, J. (2002). The efficacy of behavioral interventions to modify dietary fat and fruit and vegetable intake: A review of the evidence. *Preventive Medicine, 35*(1), 25–41.

Anderson, L. A., Quinn, T., Glanz, K., Ramirez, G., Kahwati, L. C., Johnson, D. B., . . . Task Force on Community Preventive Services. (2009). The effectiveness of worksite nutrition and physical activity interventions for controlling employee overweight and obesity: A systematic review. *American Journal of Preventive Medicine, 37*(4), 340–357.

Armsden, G., & Lewis, F. (1993). The child's adaptation to parental medical illness: Theory and clinical implications. *Patient Education and Counseling, 22*, 153–165.

Arora, N. K. (2003). Interacting with cancer patients: The significance of physicians' communication behavior. *Social Science & Medicine, 57*(5), 791–806.

Berkman, L. F., & Kawachi, I. (2000). *Social epidemiology.* New York: Oxford University Press.

Briscoe, C., & Aboud, F. (2012). Behaviour change communication targeting four health behaviours in developing countries: A review of change techniques. *Social Science & Medicine, 75*(4), 612–621.

Briss, P., Zaza, S., Pappaioanou, M., Fielding, J., Wright-De Agüero, L., Truman, B. I., . . . Harris, J. R. (2000). Developing an evidence based Guide to Community Preventive Services—methods. *American Journal of Preventive Medicine, 18*(Suppl. 1), 35–43.

Bukachi, F., & Pakenham-Walsh, N. (2007). Information technology for health in developing countries. *Chest, 132*(5), 1624–1630.

Butterfoss, F. D., Goodman, R., & Wandersman, A. (1996). Community coalitions for prevention and health promotion: Factors predicting satisfaction, participation, and planning. *Health Education Quarterly, 23*(1), 65–79.

Campbell, M., DeVellis, B. M., Strecher, V. J., Ammerman, A. S., DeVellis, R. F., & Sandler, R. F. (1994). Improving dietary behavior: The effectiveness of tailored messages in primary care settings. *American Journal of Public Health, 84*(5), 783–787.

Carleton, R., Lasater, T. M., Assaf, A. R., Feldman, H. A., & McKinlay, S. (1995). The Pawtucket Heart Health Program: Community changes in cardiovascular risk factors and projected disease risk. *American Journal of Public Health, 85*(6), 777–785.

Centers for Disease Control and Prevention. (2014). Current cigarette smoking among adults—United States, 2005–2012. *Morbidity and Mortality Weekly Report, 63*(2), 29–34.

Choi, B. C. (2012). The past, present, and future of public health surveillance. *Scientifica.* doi: 10.6064/2012/875253

Emmons, K. M., & Rollnick, S. (2001). Motivational interviewing in health care settings: Opportunities and limitations. *American Journal of Preventive Medicine, 20*(1), 68–74.

Epp, L. (1986). *Achieving health for all: A framework for health promotion in Canada.* Toronto: Health and Welfare Canada.

Epstein, R. M., & Street, R. L., Jr. (2007). *Patient-centered communication in cancer care: Promoting healing and reducing suffering* (NIH Publication No. 07-6225). Bethesda, MD: National Cancer Institute.

Farquhar, J. W., Fortmann, S. P., Flora, J. A., Taylor, C. B., Haskell, W. L., Williams, P. T., . . . Wood, P. D. (1990). Effect of communitywide education on cardiovascular disease risk factors: The Stanford Five-City Project. *JAMA, 264*(3), 359–365.

Fisher, E. B., Fitzgibbon, M. L., Glasgow, R. E., Haire-Joshu, D., Hayman, L. L., Kaplan, R. M., . . . Ockene, J. K. (2011). Behavior matters. *American Journal of Preventive Medicine, 40*(5), e15–e30.

Franks, A., Kelder, S. H., Dino, G. A., Horna, K. A., Gortmaker, S. L., Wiecha, J. L., & Simoes, E. J. (2007). School-based programs: Lessons learned from CATCH, Planet Health, and Not-On-Tobacco. *Preventing Chronic Disease, 4*(2), A33.

Franks, P., Muennig, P., Lubetkin, E., & Jia, H. (2006). The burden of disease associated with being African-American in the United States and the contribution of socio-economic status. *Social Science & Medicine, 62*(10), 2469–2478.

Gardner, B., Wardle, J., Poston, L., & Croker, H. (2011). Changing diet and physical activity to reduce gestational weight gain: A meta-analysis. *Obesity Reviews, 12*(7), e602–e620.

Glanz, K., & Bishop, D. (2010). The role of behavioral science theory in development and implementation of public health interventions. *Annual Review of Public Health, 31*, 399–418.

Glanz, K., Jarrette, A. D., Wilson, E. A., O'Riordan, D. L., & Jacob Arriola, K. R. (2007). Reducing minors' access to tobacco: Eight years' experience in Hawaii. *Preventive Medicine, 44*(1), 55–58.

Glanz, K., Lankenau, B., Foerster, S., Temple, S., Mullis. R., & Schmid, T. (1995). Environmental and policy approaches to cardiovascular disease prevention through nutrition: Opportunities for state and local action. *Health Education Quarterly, 22*(4), 512–527.

Glanz, K., & Oldenburg, B. (2001). Utilizing theories and constructs across models of behavior change. In R. Patterson (Ed.), *Changing patient behavior: Improving outcomes in health and disease management*. San Francisco: Jossey-Bass.

Glanz, K., Schoenfeld, E. R., & Steffen, A. (2010). Randomized trial of tailored skin cancer prevention messages for adults: Project SCAPE. *American Journal of Public Health, 100*(4), 735–741.

Glasgow, R. E., & Emmons, K. M. (2007). How can we increase translation of research into practice? Types of evidence needed. *Annual Review of Public Health, 28*, 413–433.

Glasgow, R. E., Terborg, J. R., Hollis, J. F., Severson, H. H., & Boles, S. M. (1995). Take Heart: Results from the initial phase of a work-site wellness program. *American Journal of Public Health, 85*(2), 209–216.

Gochman, D. S. (1982). Labels, systems, and motives: Some perspectives on future research. *Health Education Quarterly, 9*, 167–174.

Gochman, D. S. (1997). Health behavior research: Definitions and diversity. In D. S. Gochman (Ed.), *Handbook of health behavior research: Vol. I. Personal and social determinants*. New York: Plenum Press.

Gostin, L. O., & Powers, M. (2006). What does social justice require for the public's health? Public health ethics and policy imperatives. *Health Affairs, 25*(4), 1053–1060.

Grol, R., Bosch, M. C., Hulscher, M. E., Eccles, M. P., & Wensing, M. (2007). Planning and studying improvement in patient care: The use of theoretical perspectives. *Milbank Quarterly, 85*(1), 93–138.

Hesse, B. W., Nelson, D. E., Kreps, G. L., Croyle, R. T., Arora, N. K., Rimer, B. K., & Viswanath, K. (2005). Trust and sources of health information: The impact of the Internet and its implications for health care providers: Findings from the first Health Information National Trends Survey. *Archives of Internal Medicine, 165*(22), 2618–2624.

Hoffman, T. C., Glasziou, P. P., Milne, R., Moher, D., Altman, D. G., Barbour, V., . . . Michie, S. (2014). Better reporting of interventions: Template for Intervention Description and Replication (TIDieR) checklist and guide. *BMJ, 348*, g1687.

Hornik, R. (2002). Public health communication: Making sense of contradictory evidence. In R. Hornik (Ed.), *Public health communication: Evidence for behavior change*. Mahwah, NJ: Erlbaum.

Huang, J., Chaloupka, F. J., & Fong, G. T. (2014). Cigarette graphic warning labels and smoking prevalence in Canada: A critical examination and reformulation of the FDA regulatory impact analysis. *Tobacco Control, 23*(Suppl. 1), i7–i12.

Israel, B., & Schurman, S. (1990). Social support, control, and the stress process. In K. Glanz, F. M. Lewis, & B. K. Rimer (Eds.), *Health behavior and health education: Theory, research, and practice*. San Francisco: Jossey-Bass.

Janz, N. K., Zimmerman, M. A., Wren, P. A., Israel, B. A, Freudenberg, N., & Carter, R. J. (1996). Evaluation of 37 AIDS prevention projects: Successful approaches and barriers to program effectiveness. *Health Education Quarterly, 23*(1), 80–97.

Kanfer, F. H., & Schefft, B. (1988). *Guiding the process of therapeutic change.* Champaign, IL: Research Press.

Kangovi, S., Mitra, N., Grande, D., White, M. L., McCollum, S., Sellman, J., . . . Long, J. A. (2014). Patient-centered community health worker intervention to improve posthospital outcomes: A randomized clinical trial. *JAMA Internal Medicine, 174*(4), 535–543.

Kasl, S. V., & Cobb, S. (1966a). Health behavior, illness behavior, and sick-role behavior: I. Health and illness behavior. *Archives of Environmental Health, 12*(2), 246–266.

Kasl, S. V., & Cobb, S. (1966b). Health behavior, illness behavior, and sick-role behavior: II. Sick-role behavior. *Archives of Environmental Health, 12*(4), 531–541.

Kegler, M. C., Alcantara, I., Veluswamy, J. K., Haardorfer, R., Hotz, J. A., & Glanz, K. (2012). Results from an intervention to improve rural home food and physical activity environments. *Progress in Community Health Partnerships: Research, Education, and Action, 6*(3), 265–277.

Lalonde, M. (1974). *A new perspective on the health of Canadians: A working document.* Toronto: Health and Welfare Canada.

Legler, J., Meissner, H. I., Coyne, C., Breen, N., Chollette, V., & Rimer, B. K. (2002). The effectiveness of interventions to promote mammography among women with historically lower rates of screening. *Cancer Epidemiology, Biomarkers and Prevention, 11*(1), 59–71.

Lozano, R., Naghavi, M., Foreman, K., Lim, S., Shibuya, K., Aboyans, V., . . . Memish, Z. A. (2012). Global and regional mortality from 235 causes of death for 20 age groups in 1990 and 2010: A systematic analysis for the Global Burden of Disease Study in 2010. *Lancet, 380*(9859), 2095–2128.

Lueddeke, G. (2015). *Global population health and well-being in the 21st century.* New York: Springer.

Luepker, R. V., Murray, D. M., Jacobs, D. R., Mittelmark, M. B., Bracht, N., Carlaw, R., . . . Blackburn, H. (1994). Education for cardiovascular disease prevention: Risk factor changes in the Minnesota Heart Health Program. *American Journal of Public Health, 84*(9), 1383–1393.

Luepker, R. V., Perry, C. L., McKinlay, S. M., Nader, P. R., Parcel, G. S., Stone, E. J., . . . Verter, J. (1996). Outcomes of a trial to improve children's dietary patterns and physical activity: The Child and Adolescent Trial for Cardiovascular Health (CATCH). *JAMA, 275*(10), 768–776.

Matarazzo, J. D., Weiss, S. M., Herd, J. A., Miller, N. E., & Weiss, S. M. (Eds.). (1984). *Behavioral health: A handbook of health enhancement and disease prevention.* New York: Wiley.

Mathers, C. D., & Loncar, D. (2006). Projections of global mortality and burden of disease from 2002 to 2030. *PLoS Medicine, 3*(11), 2011–2030.

McBride, C. M., & Rimer, B. K. (1999). Using the telephone to improve health behavior and health service delivery. *Patient Education and Counseling, 37*(1), 3–18.

McGinnis, J. M. (1994). The role of behavioral research in national health policy. In S. Blumenthal, K. Matthews, & S. Weiss (Eds.), *New research frontiers in behavioral medicine: Proceedings of the national conference.* Bethesda, MD: NIH Health and Behavior Coordinating Committee.

McKinlay, J. B., & Marceau, L. D. (2000). Upstream healthy public policy: Lessons from the battle of tobacco. *International Journal of Health Services, 30*(1), 49–69.

McLeroy, K. R., Bibeau, D., Steckler, A., & Glanz, K. (1988). An ecological perspective on health promotion programs. *Health Education Quarterly, 15*(4), 351–377.

Merrill, R. M., Lindsay, C. A., Shields, E. D., & Stoddard, J. (2007). Have the focus and sophistication of research in health education changed? *Health Education & Behavior, 34*(1), 10–25.

Michie, S., West, R., Campbell, R., Brown, J., & Gainforth, H. (2014). *ABC of theories of behaviour change.* London: Silverback.

Minkler, M. (1989). Health education, health promotion, and the open society: A historical perspective. *Health Education Quarterly, 16*(1), 17–30.

Moher, D., Liberati, A., Tetzlaff, J., Altman, D. G., & the PRISMA Group. (2009). Preferred reporting items for systematic reviews and meta-analyses: The PRISMA statement. *Annals of Internal Medicine, 151*(4), 264–269.

National Commission on Prevention Priorities. (2007). *Preventive care: A national profile on use, disparities, and health benefits.* Washington, DC: Partnership for Prevention.

National Institute for Health and Clinical Excellence. (2014). [Home page.] Retrieved from http://www.nice.org.uk

Noar, S. M., Benac, C. N., & Harris, M. S. (2007). Does tailoring matter? Meta-analytic review of tailored print health behavior change interventions. *Psychological Bulletin, 133*(4), 673–693.

Noar, S. M., Black, H. G., & Pierce, L. B. (2009). Efficacy of computer technology-based HIV prevention interventions: A meta-analysis. *AIDS (London, England), 23*(1), 107–115.

Noar, S. M., & Zimmerman, R. S. (2005). Health behavior theory and cumulative knowledge regarding health behaviors: Are we moving in the right direction? *Health Education Research, 20*(3), 275–290.

Painter, J. E., Borba, C. P., Hynes, M., Mays, D., & Glanz, K. (2008). The use of theory in health behavior research from 2000 to 2005: A systematic review. *Annals of Behavioral Medicine, 35*(3), 358–362.

Parkerson, G., Connis, R. T., Broadhead, W. E., Patrick, D. L., Taylor, T. R., & Tse, C. K. (1993). Disease-specific versus generic measurement of health-related quality of life in insulin dependent diabetic patients. *Medical Care, 31*(7), 629–637.

Paulussen, T. G., Kok, G., Schaalma, H. P., & Parcel, G. S. (1995). Diffusion of AIDS curricula among Dutch secondary school teachers. *Health Education Quarterly, 22*(2), 227–243.

The *PLoS Medicine* Editors. (2007). Thirty ways to improve the health of the world's poorest people. *PLoS Medicine, 4*(10), e310.

Poh, M. Z., Loddenkemper, T., Reinsberger, C., Swenson, N. C., Goyal, S., & Picard, R. W. (2012). Convulsive seizure detection using a wrist-worn accelerometer biosensor. *Epilepsia, 53*(5), e93–e97.

Popkin, B. M. (2007). The world is fat. *Scientific American, 297*(3), 88–95.

Powell, B. J., McMillen, J. C., Proctor, E. K., Carpenter, C. R., Griffey, R. T., Bunger, A. C., . . . York, J. L. (2012). A compilation of strategies for implementing clinical innovations in health and mental health. *Medical Care Research and Review, 69*(2), 123–157.

Prestwich, A., Sniehotta, F. F., Whittington, C., Dombrowski, S. U., Rogers, L., & Michie, S. (2013). Does theory influence the effectiveness of health behavior interventions? Meta-analysis. *Health Psychology, 33*(5), 465–474.

Ramanadhan, S., & Viswanath, K. (2006). Health and the information non-seekers: A profile. *Health Communication, 20*(2), 131–139.

Randolph, W., & Viswanath, K. (2004). Lessons from mass media public health campaigns: Marketing health in a crowded media world. *Annual Review of Public Health, 25*, 419–437.

Resnicow, K. K., Braithwaite, R. L., DiIorio, C., & Glanz, K. (2002). Applying theory to culturally diverse and unique populations. In K. Glanz, B. K. Rimer, & F. M. Lewis (Eds.), *Health behavior and health education: Theory, research, and practice* (3rd ed.). San Francisco: Jossey-Bass.

Rimer, B. K., Briss, P. A., Zeller, P. K., Chan, E. C., & Woolf, S. H. (2004). Informed decision making: What is its role in cancer screening? *Cancer, 101*(Suppl. 5), 1214–1228.

Rimer, B. K., Glanz, K., & Rasband, G. (2001). Searching for evidence about health education and health behavior interventions. *Health Education & Behavior, 28*(2), 231–248.

Rimer, B. K., Lyons, E. J., Ribisl, K. M., Bowling. J. M., Golin, C. E., Forlenza, M. J., & Meier, A. (2005). How new subscribers use cancer-related online mailing lists. *Journal of Medical Internet Research, 7*(3), e32.

Schroeder, S. A. (2007). We can do better—improving the health of the American people. *New England Journal of Medicine, 357*, 1221–1228.

Smedley, B. D., Stith, A. Y., & Nelson, A. R. (Eds.). (2003). *Unequal treatment: Confronting racial and ethnic disparities in health care.* Committee on Understanding and Eliminating Racial and Ethnic Disparities in Health Care. Washington, DC: National Academies Press.

Smedley, B. D., & Syme, S. L. (Eds.). (2000). *Promoting health: Intervention strategies from social and behavioral research.* Washington, DC: National Academies Press.

Sorensen, G., Thompson, B., Glanz, K., Feng, Z., Kinne, S., DiClemente, C., . . . Lichtenstein, E. (1996). Working Well: Results from a worksite-based cancer prevention trial. *American Journal of Public Health, 86*, 939–947.

Story, M., Kaphingst, K., Robinson-O'Brien, R., & Glanz, K. (2008). Creating healthy food and eating environments: Policy and environmental approaches. *Annual Review of Public Health, 29*, 253–272.

Swartz, J. J., Braxton, D., & Viera, A. J. (2011). Calorie menu labeling on quick-service restaurant menus: An updated systematic review of the literature. *International Journal of Behavioral Nutrition and Physical Activity, 8*, 135.

Taylor, N., Conner, M., & Lawton, R. (2011). The impact of theory on the effectiveness of worksite physical activity interventions: A meta-analysis and meta-regression. *Health Psychology Review, 6*(1), 33–73.

Turkkan, J. S., Kaufman, N. J., & Rimer, B. K. (2000). Transdisciplinary tobacco use research centers: A model collaboration between public and private sectors. *Nicotine and Tobacco Research, 2*(1), 9–13.

U.S. Department of Health, Education, and Welfare. (1979). *Healthy people: The surgeon general's report on health promotion and disease prevention* (Public Health Service Publication No. 79-55071). Washington, DC: U.S. Government Printing Office.

U.S. Department of Health and Human Services. (1980). *Promoting health and preventing disease: Health objectives for the nation.* Washington, DC: U.S. Government Printing Office.

U.S. Department of Health and Human Services. (1991). *Healthy People 2000: National health promotion and disease prevention objectives* (DHHS Publication No. PHS 91-50213). Washington, DC: U.S. Government Printing Office.

U.S. Department of Health and Human Services. (2000). *Healthy People 2010: Understanding and improving health.* Washington, DC: U.S. Government Printing Office.

U.S. Department of Health and Human Services. (2013). *Health United States, 2013.* Table 83. Washington, DC: U.S. Government Printing Office.

U.S. Department of Health and Human Services. (2014a). *The community guide.* Retrieved from http://www.thecommunityguide.org

U.S. Department of Health and Human Services. (2014b). *Healthy People* 2020. Retrieved from http://www.healthypeople.gov

Viswanath, K. (2006). Public communications and its role in reducing and eliminating health disparities. In G. E. Thomson, F. Mitchell, & M. B. Williams (Eds.), *Examining the health disparities research plan of the National Institutes of Health: Unfinished business* (pp. 215–253). Washington, DC: Institute of Medicine.

Von Elm, E., Altman, D. G., Egger, M., Pocock, S. J., Gøtzsche, P. C., & Vandenbroucke, J. P., for the STROBE Initiative. (2007). The Strengthening of Reporting of Observational Studies in Epidemiology (STROBE) statement: Guidelines for reporting observational studies. *Annals of Internal Medicine, 147*(8), 573–577.

Webb, T. L., Joseph, J., Yardley, L., & Michie, S. (2010). Using the Internet to promote health behavior change: A systematic review and meta-analysis of the impact of theoretical basis, use of behavior change techniques, and mode of delivery on efficacy. *Journal of Medical Internet Research, 12*(1), e4.

Weinstein, N. D. (2007). Misleading tests of health behavior theories. *Annals of Behavioral Medicine, 33*(1), 1–10.

Weinstein, N. D., Sandman, P. M., & Blalock, S. J. (2008). The precaution adoption process model. In K. Glanz, B. K. Rimer, & K. Viswanath (Eds.), *Health behavior and health education: Theory, research, and practice* (4th ed., pp. 123–147). San Francisco: Jossey-Bass.

Winkleby, M. A. (1994). The future of community-based cardiovascular disease intervention studies. *American Journal of Public Health, 84*(9), 1369–1372.

World Health Organization. (2014a). *Data and statistics.* Retrieved from http://www.who.int/research/en

World Health Organization. (2014b). *Global burden of disease.* Retrieved from http://www.who.int/healthinfo/global_burden_disease/gbd/en

World Health Organization, Commission on Social Determinants of Health. (2007). *Achieving health equity: From root causes to fair outcomes* (Interim report). Retrieved from http://whqlibdoc.who.int/publications/2007/interim_statement_eng.pdf

CHAPTER 2

THEORY, RESEARCH, AND PRACTICE IN HEALTH BEHAVIOR

The Editors

Theory, Research, and Practice: Interrelationships

Aristotle distinguished between *theoria* and *praxis*. *Theoria* signifies those sciences and activities concerned with knowing for its own sake, whereas *praxis* corresponds to action or doing. This contrast between theory and practice (Bernstein, 1971) permeates Western philosophical and scientific thought from Aristotle to Marx and on to Dewey and other contemporary twentieth-century philosophers. Theory and practice have long been regarded as opposites with irreconcilable differences. Within academic departments, there is often a hierarchical split between those who conduct theoretical work and those who pursue practice. Dewey attempted to resolve the dichotomy by focusing on similarities and continuities between theoretical and practical judgments and inquiries. He described *experimental knowing* as essentially an art that involves a conscious, directed manipulation of objects and situations. "The craftsman perfects his art, not by comparing his product to some 'ideal' model, but by the cumulative results of experience—experience which benefits from tried and tested procedures but always involves risk and novelty" (Bernstein, 1971). Dewey thus described empirical investigation, that is, research, as the ground between theory and practice and the testing of theory in action.

Although the perception of theory and practice as a dichotomy has a long tradition in intellectual thought, we follow in Dewey's tradition and focus on the similarities and continuities rather than on the differences. Theory, research, and practice are a continuum along which the skilled professional should move with ease. Not only are they related but they are each essential to understanding health behavior and health behavior change. There is a tension between theory and practice that one must navigate continually, but they are not in opposition. Theory and practice enrich one another by their dynamic interaction. The best theory is informed by practice; the best practice should be grounded in theory. There is too little of both in health behavior. And as Green (2006) has written compellingly, there is also a need for more practice-based evidence. Researchers and practitioners may differ in their priorities, but the relationship between research and its application can and should move in both directions. There is a critical need for more "reflective practitioners," professionals who can ensure that theories and practice build on each other (Schön, 1983).

Among the most important challenges facing us is to understand health behavior and to transform knowledge about behavior into effective strategies for health enhancement. Research in health behavior ultimately will be judged by its contributions to improving the health of populations. Although basic behavioral research is important in developing theories, we must ultimately test our theories iteratively in real-world contexts (Green, 2006). When we do so, theory, research, and practice begin to converge. The authors of this book examine theories in light of their applicability. By including an explanation of theories and their application in each chapter, we aim to break down the dichotomy between theory and practice.

Relationships among theory, research, and practice are not simple or linear. The larger picture of health improvement and disease reduction is better described as a cycle of interacting types of endeavors, including fundamental research (research into determinants as well as development of methodologies), intervention research (research aimed toward change), surveillance research (research that tracks population-wide trends, including maintenance of change), and application and program delivery (Hiatt & Rimer, 1999). At the heart of this cycle is knowledge synthesis. Regularly updated critical appraisals of the available literature are central to identifying interventions that should be disseminated in order to reduce the burden of disease (Rimer, Glanz, & Rasband, 2001). There is increasing recognition that, as Green has stated, "if we want more evidence-based practice, we need more practice-based evidence" (Green & Glasgow, 2006).

This fifth edition of *Health Behavior: Theory, Research, and Practice* aims to help health care providers, public health professionals, behavior change experts, and educators—whatever their backgrounds or disciplines—to understand some of the most important theoretical underpinnings of health behavior and to use theory to inform research and practice. The authors of this volume believe that "there is nothing so useful as a good theory" (Lewin, 1935). Each chapter demonstrates the practical value of theory; each summarizes what was learned through conceptually sound research and practice; and each draws the linkages between theory, research, and practice.

Professionals charged with responsibility for improving health behavior are, by and large, interventionists. They are action oriented. They use their knowledge to design and implement programs to improve health. This is true whether they are working to encourage health-enhancing changes in individual or community behavior or conditions. It is equally true of most health behavior research. Often, in the process of attempting to change behavior, environments, or policies, researchers must do precisely what practitioners do—develop and deliver interventions. At some level, both practitioners and researchers are accountable for results, whether these are measured in terms of participants' satisfaction with programs or changes in awareness, knowledge, attitudes, beliefs, or health behaviors; improved decision making; institutional norms; community integration; or more distal results, including morbidity, mortality, and quality of life. They may assess these results anecdotally, complete in-depth qualitative assessments, or conduct rigorous empirical evaluations.

The design of interventions that yield desirable changes can be improved when it is done with an understanding of theories of behavior change and an ability to use them skillfully in research and practice (Grol, Bosch, Hulscher, Eccles, & Wensing, 2007). Most public health educators and managers, and behavior change clinicians, work in situations in which resources are limited. This makes it essential that they reach evidence-informed judgments about the choice of interventions, both in the interest of efficiency and to improve the odds of success. There may be no second chance to reach a critical target audience.

A synthesis of theory, research, and practice will advance what is known about health behavior. A health behavior change agent without a theory is like a mechanic or a technician, whereas the professional who understands theory and research comprehends the "why" and can design and craft well-tailored interventions. In health behavior, the circumstances include the nature of the target audience and the setting, resources, goals, and constraints (Bartholomew, Parcel, Kok, & Gottlieb, 2006). There are a number of good planning models available to help professionals and communities decide which problems and variables to focus on and also help them understand key elements of the background situation (see Chapter Nineteen for examples).

An understanding of theory may guide users to measure more carefully and astutely in order to assess the impact of interventions (Glasgow & Linnan, 2008; Grol et al., 2007). Learning from successive interventions and from published evidence strengthens the knowledge base of individual health professionals. Over time, such cumulative learning also contributes to the knowledge base of all.

The health professional in a health maintenance organization who understands how to use the Transtheoretical Model or Social Cognitive Theory (SCT) may be able to design better interventions to help patients lose weight or stop smoking. The community health educator who understands principles of social marketing and media communication can make better use of the mass media than one who does not. The nurse who recognizes that observational learning is important to how people learn, as postulated in SCT, may do a better job of teaching diabetics how to administer their injections. A working knowledge of community organization can help the educator identify and mobilize key individuals and groups to develop or maintain a health promotion program. The physician who understands interpersonal influence can communicate more effectively with patients. The health psychologist who understands the Transtheoretical Model of change will know how to design better smoking cessation and exercise interventions and how to tailor them to the needs of his or her patients.

What Is Theory?

A *theory* is a set of interrelated concepts, definitions, and propositions that present a *systematic* view of events or situations by specifying relations among variables, in order to *explain* and *predict* events or situations. The notion of *generality*, or broad application, is important, as is *testability* (van Ryn & Heaney, 1992). Theories are by their nature *abstract*: that is, they do not have a specified content or topic area. Like an empty coffee cup, they have a shape and boundaries but nothing concrete inside. They only come alive in public health and health behavior when they are filled with practical topics, goals, and problems.

A formal theory—more an ideal than a reality—is a completely closed deductive system of propositions that identifies the interrelationships among the concepts and is a systematic view of the phenomena (Blalock, 1969; Kerlinger, 1986). In reality, there is no such system in the social sciences or health promotion and education; it can only be approximated (Blalock, 1969). Theory has been defined in a variety of ways, each consistent with Kerlinger's definition. Table 2.1 summarizes several definitions of theory. These definitions, put forth in the 1970s and 1980s, have stood the test of time. They have been articulated in more recent works without substantive changes (Isaac & Michael, 1995; Sussman, 2001).

Theories are useful during the various stages of planning, implementing, and evaluating interventions. Program planners can use theories to shape the pursuit of answers to *why? what?* and *how?* That is, theories can be used to guide the search for *why* people are not following public health and medical advice or not caring for themselves in healthy ways. They can help pinpoint *what* one needs to know before developing and organizing an intervention program. They can provide insight into *how* to shape program strategies to reach people and organizations and make an impact on them. They can also help to identify *what* should be monitored, measured, and/or compared in a program evaluation (Glanz, Lewis, & Rimer, 1996; Glanz, Rimer, & Lewis, 2002; Glasgow & Linnan, 2008).

Thus theories and models *explain* behaviors and suggest ways to achieve behavior *change*. Explanatory theories, often called a *theory of the problem*, help to describe and identify why

Table 2.1   Definitions of Theory

Definition	Source
A set of interrelated constructs (concepts), definitions, and propositions that presents a systematic view of phenomena by specifying relations among variables, with the purpose of explaining and predicting phenomena	Kerlinger, 1986, p. 9
A systematic explanation for the observed facts and laws that relate to a particular aspect of life	Babbie, 1989, p. 46
Knowledge writ large in the form of generalized abstractions applicable to a wide range of experiences	McGuire, 1983, p. 2
A set of relatively abstract and general statements which collectively purport to explain some aspect of the empirical world	Chafetz, 1978, p. 2
An abstract, symbolic representation of what is conceived to be reality—a set of abstract statements designed to "fit" some portion of the real world	Zimbardo, Ebbesen, & Maslach, 1977, p. 53

a problem exists. These theories also predict behaviors under defined conditions. They guide the search for modifiable factors like knowledge, attitudes, self-efficacy, social support, lack of resources, and so on. Change theories, or *theories of action*, guide the development of interventions. They also form the basis for evaluation, pushing the evaluator to make explicit her or his assumptions about how a program should work. Implementation theories are change theories that link theory specifically to a given problem, audience, and context (Institute of Medicine, 2002; also see Chapter Sixteen). These two types of theories often have different foci but are complementary.

Even though various theoretical models of health behavior may reflect the same general ideas, each theory employs a unique vocabulary to articulate the specific factors considered important. The *why* tells us about the processes through which changes occur in particular target variables. Theories vary in the extent to which they have been conceptually developed and empirically tested. Bandura (1986) stressed that "theories are interpreted in different ways depending on the stage of development of the field of study; in some younger fields, theories specify the determinants governing the phenomena of interest." The term *theory* is used in the latter sense in *Health Behavior: Theory, Research, and Practice*, because this field is still relatively young.

As we discuss later in this chapter, many new theories and models have been and continue to be proposed in health behavior (Michie, West, Campbell, Brown, & Gainforth, 2014). The proliferation of theories in health behavior poses a challenge: When do we accept a theory as truly advancing our understanding of a phenomenon? Lakatos and Musgrave (1970), though referring to theories in physics, offer some rules of thumb. A new theory can be considered acceptable if it explains everything that the prior theories explain, provides explanations for phenomena that could *not* be explained by prior theories, and identifies conditions under which the theory could be falsified. Another expectation of an established theory is that there should be a body of research testing it, and supporting it, by multiple scientists beyond the original developer(s).

Concepts, Constructs, and Variables

Concepts are the major components of a theory; they are its building blocks or primary elements. Concepts can vary in the extent to which they have meaning, or can be understood outside the context of a specific theory. When concepts are developed or adopted for use in a particular theory, they are called *constructs* (Kerlinger, 1986). The term *subjective normative belief* is an example of a construct within Ajzen and Fishbein's (1980) Theory of Reasoned Action (see Chapter Six); this specific construct has a precise definition in the context of that theory. Another example of a construct is *perceived susceptibility* in the Health Belief Model (see Chapter Five).

Variables are the empirical counterparts, or operational forms, of constructs. They specify how a construct is to be measured in a specific situation. *Variables* should be matched to *constructs* when identifying what should be assessed in the evaluation of a theory-driven program.

Principles

Theories go beyond principles. Principles are general guidelines for action. They are broad and nonspecific and may actually distort realities or results based on research. Principles may be based on precedent or history *or* on research. At their best, principles are based on accumulated research. In this best form, principles are the basis for hypotheses, "leading ideas" in the words of Dewey, and serve as our most informed hunches about how or what we should do to obtain a desired outcome in a target population. Principles should not be so broad that they invite multiple interpretations and are therefore unreliable. Nor should they be ambiguous so that they can be all things to all people.

Models

Health behavior and the guiding concepts for influencing it are far too complex to be explained by a single, unified theory. *Models* draw on a number of theories to help understand a specific problem in a particular setting or context. They are often informed by more than one theory, as well as by empirical findings (Earp & Ennett, 1991). Several models that support program planning processes are widely used in health promotion and education: Green and Kreuter's PRECEDE-PROCEED Model (2005; also see Chapter Nineteen) and social marketing (see Chapter Nineteen) and ecological models (McLeroy, Bibeau, Steckler, & Glanz, 1988; also see Chapter Three).

Paradigms for Theory and Research in Health Behavior

A *paradigm* is a basic schema that organizes our broadly based view of something (Babbie, 1989). Paradigms are widely recognized scientific achievements that, for a time, provide model problem-solving approaches to a community of practitioners and scientists. They include theory, application, and instrumentation and constitute models that represent coherent traditions of scientific research (Kuhn, 1962). Paradigms gain status because they are more successful than their competitors at solving pressing problems (Kuhn, 1962), but they can also impede scientific progress by protecting inconsistent findings until a crisis point is reached; these crisis points lead to scientific revolutions.

Paradigms create boundaries within which the search for answers occurs. They do not answer particular questions, but they do direct the search for answers (Babbie, 1989). Paradigms circumscribe or delimit what is important to examine in a given field of inquiry. The collective judgments of scientists define the dominant paradigm that constitutes the body of science (Wilson, 1952).

In the science of health behavior (and in this text), the dominant paradigm that supports the largest body of theory and research is *logical positivism*, or *logical empiricism*. This basic view, developed in the Vienna Circle from 1924 to 1936, has two central features: (1) an emphasis on the use of induction, or sensory experience, feelings, and personal judgments as the source of knowledge; and (2) the view that deduction is the standard for verification or confirmation of theory so that theory must be tested through empirical methods and systematic observation of phenomena (Runes, 1984). Logical empiricism reconciles the deductive and inductive extremes; it prescribes that the researcher begin with a hypothesis deduced from a theory and then test it, subjecting it to the jeopardy of disconfirmation through empirical testing (McGuire, 1983).

An alternative worldview that is also important in health behavior relies more heavily on induction and is often identified as a predominantly *constructivist* paradigm. This perspective argues that the organization and explanation of events should be revealed through a process of discovery rather than organized into prescribed conceptual categories before a study begins. In this paradigm, data collection methods such as standardized questionnaires and predetermined response categories have a limited place. Ethnography, phenomenology, and grounded theory are examples of approaches using a constructivist paradigm (Kendler, 2005; Strauss, 1987). It has become increasingly common in the health behavior field for work to originate in a constructivist paradigm and shift toward a focus on answering specific research questions using methodologies from the logical positivist paradigm. The use of mixed methods that include both qualitative and quantitative measures has gained traction in health behavior, psychological research, and other social sciences (Cacioppo, Semin, & Berntson, 2004; Creswell, 2013). However, without quantitative data, a theory is unlikely to be accepted.

Lewin's meta-theory stipulates the rules to be followed for building good theory. The rules are consistent with logical positivism but focus on his view that the function of social psychology is to further understanding of the interrelationships between the individual and the social environment (Gold, 1992). This meta-theory is an orientation, or approach, distinct from Lewin's specific field theory (Gold, 1992), and it has been influential in health behavior theory since the earliest attempts to use social science to solve public health problems (Rosenstock, 1990). Key rules of Lewin's "meta-theory" include analysis that starts with the situation as a whole, contemporaneity, a dynamic approach, a constructive method, a mathematical representation of constructs and variables, and a psychological approach that explains both inner experiences and overt actions from the actor's perspective (Lewin, 1951). The last of these rules implies a single level of analysis requiring "closed theory" and poses a serious limitation to solving the problems of contemporary health behavior. It raises the issue—one that those concerned with health behavior often grapple with—that we must often trade off theoretical elegance in favor of relevance (Gold, 1992).

Ultimately, those who study and practice in fields that involve health behavior are generally concerned with approaches to solving social problems, and in many cases, solving some of the most significant threats and problems facing the world today. In other words, they are grappling with fundamental challenges of behavior change in the health domain. Considerable scholarly and practitioner effort has been devoted to developing techniques that change behavior. Although these efforts grew out of a desire to produce a better world, techniques that "push" people to change were experienced by many as manipulative, reducing freedom of choice, and sustaining a balance of power in favor of the "change agent" (Kipnis, 1994). A paradigm shift occurred, and many techniques for promoting individual behavior change (e.g., social support, empowerment, and personal growth) shifted focus to become based on *reducing obstacles to change* and promoting informed decision making, rather than on pushing people to change.

New paradigms for understanding, studying, and applying knowledge about human behavior continue to arise and may be influential in the future of applied social sciences in health behavior and education. The Institute of Medicine's Committee on Capitalizing on Social Science and Behavioral Research to Improve the Public's Health recommended strongly that "interventions on social and behavioral factors should link multiple levels of influence" rather than focusing on a single or limited number of health determinants (Smedley & Syme, 2000, p. 7). Today, this recommendation is echoed as health educators and social scientists struggle with some of the most challenging health behavior issues, such as tobacco control and obesity prevention, at a time when ecological models are beginning to be more clearly articulated and studied (see Chapter Three).

Trends in Use of Health Behavior Theories and Models

Theories that gain recognition in a discipline shape the field, help to define the scope of practice, and influence the training and socialization of its professionals. Today, no single theory or conceptual framework dominates research or practice for understanding and changing health behavior. Instead, one can choose from a multitude of theories.

Previous Reviews of the Most Often Used Theories

For the first four editions of this book, we reviewed a sample of publications to identify the most often used theories. In a review of 116 theory-based articles published between 1986 and 1988 in two major health education journals, conducted during planning for the first edition of this book, we found fifty-one distinct theoretical formulations. At that time, the three most frequently mentioned theories were Social Learning Theory, the Theory of Reasoned Action, and the Health Belief Model (Glanz, Lewis, & Rimer, 1990).

To plan for the second edition of this book, we reviewed 526 articles from twenty-four journals in health education, medicine, and behavioral sciences, published from mid-1992 to mid-1994. Sixty-six theories and models were identified, and twenty-one of these were mentioned eight times or more. Two-thirds of the total instances of theory use in the 497 articles involving one or more of the twenty-one most common theories/models were accounted for by the first eight: the Health Belief Model, Social Cognitive Theory, self-efficacy (Bandura, 1997), the Theory of Reasoned Action/Theory of Planned Behavior, community organization, the Transtheoretical Model/Stages of Change, social marketing, and social support/social networks (Glanz et al., 1996).

In our review of all issues of twelve journals in health education, health behavior, and preventive medicine published in 1999 and 2000, conducted for the third edition of this book (Glanz et al., 2002), ten theories or models clearly emerged as the most often used. The first two, and by far the most dominant, were Social Cognitive Theory and the Transtheoretical Model/Stages of Change. The remainder of the top ten theories and models were the Health Belief Model, social support and social networks, patient-provider communication, the Theory of Reasoned Action and Theory of Planned Behavior, stress and coping, community organization, ecological models/social ecology, and Diffusion of Innovations.

In a review of theory use in published research between 2000 and 2005, we found that the most often used theories were the Transtheoretical Model, Social Cognitive Theory, and the Health Belief Model (Painter, Borba, Hynes, Mays, & Glanz, 2008). Overall, the same theories found to be dominant in 1999 and 2000 were still dominant. Like previous reviews, this review revealed that dozens of theories and models were used, though only a few of them were used in multiple publications and by several authors. Some were minor variations of another theory. Several key constructs cut across the most often cited models for understanding behavior and behavior change: the importance of the individual's view of the world, multiple levels of influence, behavior change as a process, motivation versus intention, intention versus action, and changing behavior versus maintaining behavior change (Glanz & Oldenburg, 2001).

Updated Review of the Most Often Used Theories

There has been a continuing proliferation of theories and models up to the present. Rather than conducting a new literature review for the fifth edition of this book, we looked to published reviews. We identified several reviews that examined the use of theory for behavior change in specific behavioral categories, such as dietary change, cancer screening, and reducing sexual risk (Albada, Ausems, Bensing, & van Dulmen, 2009; Ammerman, Lindquist, Lohr, & Hersey, 2002; Gardner, Wardle, Poston, & Croker, 2011; Glanz & Bishop, 2010; Legler et al., 2002; Noar, Benac, & Harris, 2007; Noar, Black, & Pierce, 2009; Prestwich et al., 2013; Taylor, Conner, & Lawton, 2011; Webb, Joseph, Yardley, & Michie, 2010). A recently published compendium of behavior change theories, using clearly defined inclusion criteria, provides summaries of eighty-three theories and models (Michie et al., 2014). As these reviews assessed primarily individual outcomes of behavior change interventions, we also examined reviews of strategies for implementation and dissemination in health and mental health services (Powell et al., 2012; Tabak, Khoong, Chambers, & Brownson, 2012) and a review of social ecological contextual levels of health promotion interventions across a twenty-year period (Golden & Earp, 2012).

These reviews point to several key conclusions about the use of theories and models for health behavior change research. The first is the inescapable observation that there are *many* available theories and models. For example, the (acknowledged) selective review of eighty-three theories in Michie and others' book (2014); the sixty-eight distinct strategies identified by Powell and others (2012); and the sixty-one models included in Tabak and others' dissemination and implementation research review (2012). These theories and models are not mutually exclusive. As Tabak and colleagues have stated, "there is substantial overlap between models, as the included constructs are often similar" (2012). Review authors have used different coding schemes to classify the theories in their reviews. A novel approach taken by Michie and others (2014) to examine the interconnectedness of the eighty-three theories summarized in their book was to use network analysis methods to examine contributions, links, and patterns among the theories they describe.

Our synthesis of the various reviews, and the Michie et al. network analysis (2014), leads to the conclusion that, indeed, only a small number of theories and models have been widely used and/or have informed numerous other theories. In fact, those theories are the same ones identified in the last three editions of this book: the Health Belief Model, Social Cognitive Theory (and Social Learning Theory, its predecessor), Theory of Planned Behavior (and Theory of Reasoned Action, its predecessor), social support, Diffusion of Innovations, and the Social Ecological Model.

A third issue in examining the use of theories and models for health behavior change is the level at which they seek to understand and/or influence behavior and its determinants (see Chapter Three). Golden and Earp reviewed 157 intervention articles published in the journal *Health Education & Behavior* (and its predecessor through 1997, *Health Education Quarterly*) between 1989 and 2008. They coded intervention levels of focus according to the Social Ecological Model and found that, across all settings, theories, topics, and time periods, the intervention strategies and targets for change were most likely to be at the individual and interpersonal levels, and were less often at the institutional, community, and policy levels (Golden & Earp, 2012). In contrast, Tabak and colleagues (2012) found that most of the models for dissemination and implementation research that they identified were distributed across all levels of the Social Ecological Model. The focus and scope of the two reviews was very different—with Golden and Earp looking at a single journal over time, and the Tabak review examining inherently multilevel issues (dissemination and implementation) across a wide range of sources. Viewing these contrasting findings through the interdisciplinary lens of health behavior research and practice, an important conclusion is that broader exposure across topics and published sources appears to be associated with greater application across multiple levels of study and intervention.

How Are Theories Being Used in Health Behavior Research and Practice?

Along with the published observations about *which* theories are being used, concerns have been raised about *how* theories are used (or not used) in research and practice. A common refrain is that researchers may not understand how to measure and analyze constructs of health behavior theories (Marsh, Johnson, & Carey, 2001; Rejeski, Brawley, McAuley, & Rapp, 2000) or that they may pick and choose variables from different theories in a way that makes it difficult to ascertain the role of theory in intervention development and evaluation (Michie et al., 2014). Considerable conceptual confusion—among both researchers and practitioners—about interrelationships among related theories and variables has also been observed (Rosenstock, Strecher, & Becker, 1988; Weinstein, 1993). Others have cautioned about the limitations of theory testing because of overreliance on correlational designs (Weinstein, 2007), and the paucity of studies that empirically compare more than one theory (Noar & Zimmerman, 2005; Weinstein & Rothman, 2005). The difficulty of reliably translating theory into interventions to improve clinical effectiveness has led to calls for more pragmatic trials, and increasing attention to the generalizability and translation of interventions into real-world clinical practice (Rothwell, 2005) and community settings (Rohrbach, Grana, Sussman, & Valente, 2006). These are reasonable questions that should encourage us all to question *how* we use theory, how we test theory, how we turn theories into interventions, and what conclusions we draw from research.

Building on our distinctions among the type and degree of theory use (Glanz, 2002, p. 546), our review of theory used from 2000 to 2005 classified articles that employed health behavior theory along a continuum consisting of these four categories: (1) *informed by theory:* a theoretical framework was identified, but no or limited application of the theory was used in specific study components and measures; (2) *applied theory:* a theoretical framework was specified and several of the constructs were applied in components of the study; (3) *tested theory:* a theoretical framework was specified and more than half the theoretical constructs were measured and explicitly tested, or two or more theories were compared to one another in a study; or (4) *building/creating theory:* new or revised/expanded theory was developed using constructs specified, measured, and analyzed in a study.

Of all the theories used in the sample of articles ($n = 69$ articles using 139 theories), 69.1 percent used theory to inform a study, 17.9 percent of theories were "applied," 3.6 percent were tested, and 9.4 percent involved building/creating theory (Painter et al., 2008). These findings lead us to reaffirm calls by Noar and Zimmerman (2005) and Weinstein and Rothman (2005) for thorough application and testing of health behavior theories to advance science and move the field forward. Similar observations have been made by Michie and others (2014) as well.

Selection of Theories for This Book

Our selection of theories and models for inclusion in the fifth edition of *Health Behavior: Theory, Research, and Practice* was based on the published information summarized above, including an updated synthesis of reviews of theory use in the health behavior literature. Each of the most often cited theories and models is the focus of a chapter in this volume. They have been selected to provide readers with a range of theories representing different units of intervention (e.g., individuals, groups, and communities). They were also chosen because they represent, as in the case of Social Cognitive Theory, the Transtheoretical Model, and the Health Belief Model, dominant theories of health behavior and health behavior change. Others, like social marketing, Intervention Mapping and the PRECEDE/PROCEED Model, and community organization, were chosen for their practical value in applying theoretical formulations in a way that has demonstrated usefulness to professionals concerned with health behavior change.

Our selection of theories also reflects some difficult editorial decisions. Three criteria helped us to define our selection. First, we determined that, to be included, a theory must meet basic standards of adequacy for research and practice, thus having the potential for effective use by health education practitioners. Second, there must be evidence that the theory is being used in *current* health behavior research. (That is why, e.g., we include the Health Belief Model rather than Lewin's Field Theory.) The third criterion is that there must be at least promising, if not substantial, empirical evidence supporting the theory's validity in predicting or changing health behaviors. This does not preclude the possibility of mixed findings and critiques of the evidence, which we believe are important to bring to light.

In the later sections of the book, a purpose, theme, or focus rather than a theory is the identifying title for a chapter—as in the case of Chapter Thirteen, on interpersonal communication, which describes theories of interpersonal communication and social influence and illustrates their utility for health behavior. Chapter Fifteen on community engagement and community organization is named for this approach to intervention strategies rather than for the convergent theoretical bases that form the foundation for community organization work. Chapters in Part Five present the Intervention Mapping and the PRECEDE-PROCEED Model for program planning, social marketing, and behavioral economics, each of which draws on multiple theories to understand health behavior and assist in development of effective intervention programs and strategies.

We recognize the lack of consensus regarding the definition and classification of theories. We have taken a liberal, ecumenical stance toward theory. We concede that the lowest common denominator of the theoretical models herein might be that they are all *conceptual or theoretical frameworks, models,* or broadly conceived perspectives used to organize ideas. Nevertheless, we have not abandoned the term *theory*, because it accurately describes the spirit of this book and describes the goal to be attained for developing frameworks and tools for refining health education research and practice.

Fitting Theory to Research and Practice: Building Bridges and Forging Links

Effective health behavior change depends on marshaling the most appropriate theory and practice strategies for a given situation. Different theories are best suited to different units of practice, such as individuals, groups, and organizations. For example, when one is attempting to overcome women's personal barriers to obtaining mammograms, the Health Belief Model may be useful. The Transtheoretical Model may be especially useful in developing smoking cessation interventions. When trying to change physicians' mammography practices by instituting reminder systems, dissemination and implementation science approaches are more suitable. At the same time, physicians might use the Transtheoretical Model to inform their discussions with individual patients about getting a first mammogram or annual screening. The choice of a suitable theory or theories should begin with identifying the problem, goal, and units of practice (Sussman & Sussman, 2001; van Ryn & Heaney, 1992), *not* with selecting a theoretical framework because it is intriguing, familiar, or in vogue. As Green and Kreuter (2005) have argued, one should start with a logic model of the problem and work backward to identify potential solutions.

The adequacy of a theory is most often assessed in terms of three criteria: (1) its *logic,* or *internal consistency,* in not yielding mutually contradictory derivations; (2) the extent to which it is *parsimonious,* or broadly relevant, while using a manageable number of concepts, and (3) its *plausibility* in fitting with prevailing theories in the field (McGuire, 1983).

Theories are also judged in the context of practitioners' and researchers' activities. Practitioners may apply the pragmatic criterion of *usefulness* to a theory and thus be concerned with its consistency with everyday observations. Researchers make scientific judgments of a theory's *ecological validity,* or the extent to which it conforms to observable reality when empirically tested (McGuire, 1983). We should test our theories iteratively in the field

(Rosenstock, 1990) as well as in more controlled settings. When we do so, theory, research, and practice begin to converge.

Researchers and practitioners of health behavior change benefit from and are challenged by the multitude of theoretical frameworks and models from the social sciences available for their use, because the best choices and direct translations may not be immediately evident. The inherent danger in a book like this is that one can begin to think that the links between theory, research, and health outcomes are easily forged. They are not. For the unprepared, the choices can be overwhelming, but for those who understand the commonalities and differences among theories of health behavior and health education, the growing knowledge base can provide a firm foundation upon which to build. We find that one of the most frequent questions students around the world ask is, "What theory should I use?" It is an important question, whose answer, we believe, will be found not just in the readings contained in this book but also in the experience and judgment that equip readers to apply what is learned here: *theory into practice and research*. We hope that *Health Behavior: Theory, Research, and Practice* will provide and strengthen that foundation for readers.

Science is, by definition, cumulative, with periods of paradigm shifts that come more rarely as a result of crises when current theories fail to explain some phenomena (Kuhn, 1962). This applies as well to the science base that supports long-standing as well as innovative health behavior interventions. More research is needed at all points along the research continuum—more basic research to develop and test theories, more intervention research to develop and test evidence-based interventions, more implementation science research and more practice to understand and apply the processes of implementation, and more concerted attention to dissemination of evidence-based interventions (Institute of Medicine, 2002; Rimer et al., 2001; Rohrbach et al., 2006; Weinstein, 2007).

Moreover, the health behavior research and practice communities are sorely in need of more rigor and precision in theory development and testing—in measures, in assessment of mediating variables, and in specification of theoretical elements (Rejeski et al., 2000). We encourage more care and attention to how theories are tested, and especially to the way variables are measured and analyzed. Building a solid, cumulative base of theory development is very difficult when one researcher's findings cannot be compared to another's. However, we also caution that while rigor is critically important in the verification of the component parts of theories and in testing hypotheses, we eschew a one-size-fits-all approach to rigor. As Potter and Green (2012) have cautioned: the social and behavioral sciences continue to fall short in the theories and methods they bring to the systems needs identified by public health today; many of their methods and theories have been dominated by psychology and have not dealt adequately with the broader ecological understanding of causal webs and systems interventions that we seek today.

The gift of theory is that it provides the conceptual underpinnings for well-crafted research and informed practice. "The scientist values research by the size of its contribution to that huge, logically articulated structure of ideas which is already, though not half built, the most glorious accomplishment of mankind" (Medawar, 1967).

In this book, we aim to demystify theory and to communicate theory and theoretically inspired research alongside their implications for practice. We encourage informed criticism of theories. Only through rigorous scrutiny will theories improve. The ultimate test of these ideas and this information rests on its use over time, critical assessment, refinement, and application. The process is circular in that it doesn't end with publication of a particular study. The goal of a theory, for a small number of people, may be proof of that theory. But for most readers of this book, it will be improved health. Theory, then, is a tool for improving health outcomes. Thus we should think about theory *and* practice, not theory *or* practice. Green (2006) said it well: the translational gap between research and practice has long been discussed, often as a one-way street—get practitioners to recognize and utilize the research that is being conducted. While that is important, equally important is the reverse—integrating practice-based evidence and context into the research conducted. We need a bridge between the two, not a pipeline. Achieving this vision, as would be the case for sustaining any health behavior, will require social support, supportive environments, and periodic reinforcement. The beneficiaries will be practitioners, researchers, and participants in health education programs.

As this chapter and the preceding one demonstrate, health behavior is a concern of ever-increasing importance to the well-being of humankind worldwide. As scholars, researchers, and practitioners, we grapple with the complexities of human beings in populations and societies. We press forward within the limits of current methodologies while striving to build a cumulative body of knowledge in a fast-changing world. Our efforts do not always achieve successful results, but this should motivate, not deter, us in pursuing high-quality work. Continual dialogue between theory, research, and practice involves compromise, creativity, healthy criticism, appreciation of others' skills, and a willingness to cooperate to learn and to set high standards. "We must learn to honor excellence in every socially accepted human activity, however humble the activity, and to scorn shoddiness, however exalted the activity. An excellent plumber is infinitely more admirable than an incompetent philosopher. The society that scorns excellence in plumbing because plumbing is a humble activity and tolerates shoddiness in philosophy because it is an exalted activity will have neither good plumbing nor good philosophy. Neither its pipes nor its theories will hold water" (Gardner, 1984).

Limitations of This Book

No text can be all inclusive nor can it meet the needs of all potential audiences, and that is true for this book as well. Some theories and frameworks presented in previous editions of this book do not appear in this edition: consumer information processing (Rudd & Glanz, 1990), Multiattribute Utility Theory (Carter, 1990), Attribution Theory (Lewis & Daltroy, 1990), media advocacy (Wallack, 1990), organizational change (Butterfoss, Kegler, & Francisco, 2008), and the Precaution Adoption Process Model (Weinstein, Sandman, & Blalock, 2008). These theories and frameworks remain important, but they are less widely used than those included in this edition. We did not update the chapters in the third edition on communication technology and health behavior change (Owen, Fotheringham, & Marcus, 2002) and applying theory to culturally diverse and unique populations (Resnicow, Braithwaite, DiIorio, & Glanz, 2002). Rather, these issues are woven throughout various chapters in this edition. Interested readers should refer to the first, third, and fourth editions of this book for coverage of these frameworks.

Other important theories and conceptual frameworks could not be included because of space limitations. These include Self-Regulation Theory (Leventhal, Zimmerman, & Gutmann, 1984), Protection Motivation Theory (Rogers, 1975), and more familiar classical theories such as Field Theory (Lewin, 1935) and cognitive consistency (Festinger, 1957). Some of these are described as part of the historical origins of the various theories discussed in this book. Others are discussed in the introductory chapters. Some are summarized in Michie and others' recent book (2014).

This book is not a how-to guide or manual for program planning and development in health education and health behavior. Other books in health education, nursing, medicine, psychology, and nutrition serve that purpose, and readers should seek out key sources in each discipline for more on the nuts and bolts of practice. This volume will be most useful when it is included as part of a problem-oriented learning program, whether in a formal professional education setting or continuing education venues. Besides using search engines, there are a number of useful sources of evidence reviews that include assessments of the use of theory on various health outcomes. These include the *Guide to Community Preventive Services* (www.thecommunityguide.org) and the Cochrane Collaborative (www.cochrane.org). For specific programs and tools, see, for example, Cancer Control P.L.A.N.E.T. (cancer controlplanet.cancer.gov) and the National Cancer Institute's Research-Tested Intervention Programs (rtips.cancer.gov/rtips/index.do), which provide information relevant to cancer prevention and control. The National Registry of Evidence-Based Programs and Practices (nrepp.samhsa.gov) is a searchable, online registry of mental health and substance abuse interventions that have been scientifically tested and can be readily disseminated.

The editors intend that readers emerge with a critical appreciation of theory and with the curiosity to pursue not only the theories presented in this book but other promising theories as well. Thus *Health Behavior: Theory, Research, and Practice* should be regarded as a starting point, not the end.

Theories—or conceptual frameworks—can be and *are* useful because they enrich, inform, and complement the practical technologies of health promotion and education. Thus the readers of this book should "pass with relief from the tossing sea of Cause and Theory to the firm ground of Result and Fact" (Churchill, 1898). As the ocean meets the shore, so we hope you will find that theory, research, and practice can converge in a single landscape of improved health for all.

References

Albada, A., Ausems, M. G., Bensing, J. M., & van Dulmen, S. (2009). Tailored information about cancer risk and screening: A systematic review. *Patient Education and Counseling, 77*(2), 155–171.

Ajzen, I., & Fishbein, M. (1980). *Understanding attitudes and predicting social behavior*. Englewood Cliffs, NJ: Prentice Hall.

Ammerman, A. S., Lindquist, C. H., Lohr, K. N., & Hersey, J. (2002). The efficacy of behavioral interventions to modify dietary fat and fruit and vegetable intake: A review of the evidence. *Preventive Medicine, 35*(1), 25–41.

Babbie, E. (1989). *The practice of social research* (5th ed.). Belmont, CA: Wadsworth.

Bandura, A. (1986). *Social foundations of thought and action: A social cognitive theory.* Englewood Cliffs, NJ: Prentice Hall.

Bandura, A. (1997). *Self-efficacy: The exercise of control.* New York: Freeman.

Bartholomew, L. K., Parcel, G. S., Kok, G., & Gottlieb, N. H. (2006). *Planning health promotion programs: An intervention mapping approach.* San Francisco: Jossey-Bass.

Bernstein, R. (1971). *Praxis and action.* Philadelphia: University of Pennsylvania Press.

Blalock, H. M., Jr. (1969). *Theory construction, from verbal to mathematical constructions.* Englewood Cliffs, NJ: Prentice Hall.

Butterfoss, F. D., Kegler, M. C., & Francisco, V. T. (2008). Mobilizing organizations for health promotion: Theories of organizational change. In K. Glanz, B. K. Rimer, & K. Viswanath (Eds.), *Health behavior and health education: Theory, research, and practice* (4th ed., pp. 335–361). San Francisco: Jossey-Bass.

Cacioppo, J. T., Semin, G. R., & Berntson, G. G. (2004). Realism, instrumentalism, and scientific symbiosis: Psychological theory as a search for truth and the discovery of solutions. *American Psychologist, 59*(4), 214–223.

Carter, W. (1990). Health behavior as a rational process: Theory of Reasoned Action and Multiattribute Utility Theory. In K. Glanz, F. M. Lewis, & B. K. Rimer (Eds.), *Health behavior and health education: Theory, research, and practice* (pp. 63–91). San Francisco: Jossey-Bass.

Chafetz, J. (1978). *A primer on the construction of theories in sociology.* Itasca, IL: Peacock.

Churchill, W. (1898). *The Malakand Field Force.* London: Longmans Green.

Creswell, J. W. (2013). *Research design: Qualitative, quantitative, and mixed methods approaches.* Thousand Oaks, CA: Sage.

Earp, J. A., & Ennett, S. T. (1991). Conceptual models for health education research and practice. *Health Education Research, 6*(2), 163–171.

Festinger, L. (1957). *A theory of cognitive dissonance.* Stanford, CA: Stanford University Press.

Gardner, B., Wardle, J., Poston, L., & Croker, H. (2011). Changing diet and physical activity to reduce gestational weight gain: A meta-analysis. *Obesity Reviews, 12*(7), e602–e620.

Gardner, J. W. (1984). *Excellence: Can we be equal and excellent too?* (Rev. ed.). New York: Norton.

Glanz, K. (2002). Perspectives on using theory. In K. Glanz, F. M. Lewis, & B. K. Rimer (Eds.), *Health behavior and health education: Theory, research, and practice* (3rd ed.). San Francisco: Jossey-Bass.

Glanz, K., & Bishop, D. (2010). The role of behavioral science theory in development and implementation of public health interventions. *Annual Review of Public Health, 31*, 399–418.

Glanz, K., Lewis, F. M., & Rimer, B. K. (Eds.). (1990). *Health behavior and health education: Theory, research, and practice.* San Francisco: Jossey-Bass.

Glanz, K., Lewis, F. M., & Rimer, B. K. (Eds.). (1996). *Health behavior and health education: Theory, research, and practice* (2nd ed.) San Francisco: Jossey-Bass.

Glanz, K., & Oldenburg, B. (2001). Utilizing theories and constructs across models of behavior change. In R. Patterson (Ed.), *Changing patient behavior: Improving outcomes in health and disease management.* San Francisco: Jossey-Bass.

Glanz, K., Rimer, B. K., & Lewis, F. M. (Eds.). (2002). *Health behavior and health education: Theory, research, and practice* (3rd ed.). San Francisco: Jossey-Bass.

Glasgow, R. E., & Linnan, L. A. (2008). Evaluation of theory-based interventions. In K. Glanz, B. K. Rimer, & K. Viswanath (Eds.), *Health behavior and health education: Theory, research, and practice* (4th ed., pp. 487–508). San Francisco: Jossey-Bass.

Gold, M. (1992). Metatheory and field theory in social psychology: Relevance or elegance? *Journal of Social Issues, 48*(2), 67–78.

Golden, S., & Earp, J. A. (2012). Social ecological approaches to individuals and their contexts: Twenty years of health education and behavior interventions. *Health Education & Behavior, 39*(3), 364–372.

Green, L. W. (2006). Public health asks of systems science: To advance our evidence-based practice, can you help us get more practice-based evidence? *American Journal of Public Health, 96*(3), 406–409.

Green, L. W., & Glasgow, R. E. (2006). Evaluating the relevance, generalization, and applicability of research: Issues in external validation and translation methodology. *Evaluation and the Health Professions, 29*(1), 126–153.

Green, L. W., & Kreuter, M. W. (2005). *Health promotion planning: An educational and ecological approach* (4th ed.). New York: McGraw-Hill.

Grol, R., Bosch, M. C., Hulscher, M. E., Eccles, M. P., & Wensing, M. (2007). Planning and studying improvement in patient care: The use of theoretical perspectives. *Milbank Quarterly, 85*(1), 93–138.

Hiatt, R. A., & Rimer, B. K. (1999). A new strategy for cancer control research. *Cancer Epidemiology, Biomarkers and Prevention, 8*(11), 957–964.

Institute of Medicine, Committee on Communication for Behavior Change in the 21st Century: Improving the Health of Diverse Populations. (2002). *Speaking of health: Assessing health communication strategies for diverse populations.* Washington, DC: National Academies Press.

Isaac, S., & Michael, W. B. (1995). *Handbook of research and evaluation* (3rd ed.). San Diego, CA: Educational and Industrial Testing Services.

Kendler, H. H. (2005). Psychology and phenomenology: A clarification. *American Psychologist, 60,* 318–324.

Kerlinger, F. N. (1986). *Foundations of behavioral research* (3rd ed.). New York: Holt, Rinehart & Winston.

Kipnis, D. (1994). Accounting for the use of behavior technologies in social psychology. *American Psychologist, 49*(3), 165–172.

Kuhn, T. S. (1962). *The structure of scientific revolutions.* Chicago: University of Chicago Press.

Lakatos, I., & Musgrave, A. (Eds.). (1970). *Criticism and the growth of knowledge.* Cambridge, UK: Cambridge University Press.

Legler, J., Meissner, H. I., Coyne, C., Breen, N., Chollette, V., & Rimer, B. K. (2002). The effectiveness of interventions to promote mammography among women with historically lower rates of screening. *Cancer Epidemiology, Biomarkers and Prevention, 11*(1), 59–71.

Leventhal, H., Zimmerman, R., & Gutmann, M. (1984). Compliance: A self-regulation perspective. In D. Gentry (Ed.), *Handbook of behavioral medicine.* New York: Guilford Press.

Lewin, K. (1935). *A dynamic theory of personality.* New York: McGraw-Hill.

Lewin, K. (1951). Field theory and learning. In *Field theory in social science: Selected theoretical papers* (D. Cartwright, ed.). New York: Harper.

Lewis, F. M., & Daltroy, L. (1990). How causal explanations influence health behavior: Attribution theory. In K. Glanz, F. M. Lewis, & B. K. Rimer (Eds.), *Health behavior and health education: Theory, research, and practice.* San Francisco: Jossey-Bass.

Marsh, K. L., Johnson, B. T., & Carey, M. P. (2001). Conducting meta-analyses of HIV prevention literatures from a theory-testing perspective. *Evaluation and the Health Professions, 24,* 255–276.

McGuire, W. J. (1983). A contextualist theory of knowledge: Its implications for innovation and reform in psychological research. *Advances in Experimental Social Psychology, 16,* 1–47.

McLeroy, K. R., Bibeau, D., Steckler, A., & Glanz, K. (1988). An ecological perspective on health promotion programs. *Health Education Quarterly, 15*, 351–377.

Medawar, P. B. (1967). *The art of the soluble.* New York: Methuen.

Michie, S., West, R., Campbell, R., Brown, J., & Gainforth, H. (2014). *ABC of theories of behaviour change.* London: Silverback.

Noar, S. M., Benac, C. N., & Harris, M. S. (2007). Does tailoring matter? Meta-analytic review of tailored print health behavior change interventions. *Psychological Bulletin, 133*(4), 673–693.

Noar, S. M., Black, H. G., & Pierce, L. B. (2009). Efficacy of computer technology-based HIV prevention interventions: A meta-analysis. *AIDS (London, England), 23*(1), 107–115.

Noar, S. M., & Zimmerman, R. S. (2005). Health behavior theory and cumulative knowledge regarding health behaviors: Are we moving in the right direction? *Health Education Research, 20*, 275–290.

Owen, N., Fotheringham, M. J., & Marcus, B. H. (2002). Communication technology and health behavior change. In K. Glanz, B. K. Rimer, & F. M. Lewis (Eds.), *Health behavior and health education: Theory, research, and practice* (3rd ed., pp. 510–529). San Francisco: Jossey-Bass.

Painter, J. E., Borba, C. P., Hynes, M., Mays, D., & Glanz, K. (2008). The use of theory in health behavior research from 2000 to 2005: A systematic review. *Annals of Behavioral Medicine, 35*(3), 358–362.

Potter, M., & Green, L. W. (2012). *Bridging research and reality: Practice-based evidence and evidence-based practice, a cyber seminar.* National Cancer Institute. Retrieved from https://researchtoreality.cancer.gov/cyber-seminars/bridging-research-and-reality-practice-based-evidence-evidence-based-practice

Powell, B. J., McMillen, J. C., Proctor, E. K., Carpenter, C. R., Griffey, R. T., Bunger, A. C., . . . York, J. L. (2012). A compilation of strategies for implementing clinical innovations in health and mental health. *Medical Care Research and Review, 69*(2), 123–157.

Prestwich, A., Sniehotta, F. F., Whittington, C., Dombrowski, S. U., Rogers, L., & Michie, S. (2013). Does theory influence the effectiveness of health behavior interventions? Meta-analysis. *Health Psychology, 33*(5), 465–474.

Rejeski, W. J., Brawley, L. R., McAuley, E., & Rapp, S. (2000). An examination of theory and behavior change in randomized clinical trials. *Controlled Clinical Trials, 21*(Suppl. 5), 164S–170S.

Resnicow, K., Braithwaite, R. L., DiIorio, C., & Glanz, K. (2002). Applying theory to culturally diverse and unique populations. In K. Glanz, B. K. Rimer, & F. M. Lewis (Eds.), *Health behavior and health education: Theory, research, and practice* (3rd ed.). San Francisco: Jossey-Bass.

Rimer, B. K., Glanz, K., & Rasband, G. (2001). Searching for evidence about health education and health behavior interventions. *Health Education & Behavior, 28*(2), 231–248.

Rogers, R. (1975). A protection motivation theory of fear appeals and attitude change. *Journal of Psychology, 91*, 93–114.

Rohrbach, L. A., Grana, R., Sussman, S., & Valente, T. W. (2006). Type II translation: Transporting prevention interventions from research to real-world settings. *Evaluation and the Health Professions, 29*(3), 302–333.

Rosenstock, I. M. (1990). The past, present, and future of health education. In K. Glanz, F. M. Lewis, & B. K. Rimer (Eds.), *Health behavior and health education: Theory, research, and practice* (pp. 405–420). San Francisco: Jossey-Bass.

Rosenstock, I. M., Strecher, V. J., & Becker, M. H. (1988). Social learning theory and the health belief model. *Health Education Quarterly, 15*(2), 175–183.

Rothwell, P. M. (2005). External validity of randomized controlled trials: "To whom do the results of this trial apply?" *Lancet, 365*, 82–93.

Rudd, J., & Glanz, K. (1990). How individuals use information for health action: Consumer information processing. In K. Glanz, F. M. Lewis, & B. K. Rimer (Eds.), *Health behavior and health education: Theory, research, and practice.* San Francisco: Jossey-Bass.

Runes, D. (1984). *Dictionary of philosophy.* Totowa, NJ: Rowman and Allanheld.

Schön, D. (1983). *The reflective practitioner: How professionals think in action.* London: Temple Smith.

Smedley, B. D., & Syme, S. L. (Eds.). (2000). *Promoting health: Intervention strategies from social and behavioral research.* Washington, DC: National Academies Press.

Strauss, A. L. (1987). *Qualitative analysis for social scientists.* Cambridge, UK: Cambridge University Press.

Sussman, S. (Ed.). (2001). *Handbook of program development for health behavior research and practice.* Thousand Oaks, CA: Sage.

Sussman, S., & Sussman, A. N. (2001). Praxis in health behavior program development. In S. Sussman (Ed.), *Handbook of program development for health behavior research and practice.* Thousand Oaks, CA: Sage.

Tabak, R. G., Khoong, E. C., Chambers, D. A., & Brownson, R. C. (2012). Bridging research and practice: Models for dissemination and implementation research. *American Journal of Preventive Medicine, 43*(3), 337–350.

Taylor, N., Conner, M., & Lawton, R. (2011). The impact of theory on the effectiveness of worksite physical activity interventions: A meta-analysis and meta-regression. *Health Psychology Review, 6*(1), 33–73.

van Ryn, M., & Heaney, C. A. (1992). What's the use of theory? *Health Education Quarterly, 19*(3), 315–330.

Wallack, L. (1990). Media advocacy: Promoting health through mass communication. In K. Glanz, F. M. Lewis, & B. K. Rimer (Eds.), *Health behavior and health education: Theory, research, and practice.* San Francisco: Jossey-Bass.

Webb, T. L., Joseph, J., Yardley, L., & Michie, S. (2010). Using the Internet to promote health behavior change: A systematic review and meta-analysis of the impact of theoretical basis, use of behavior change techniques, and mode of delivery on efficacy. *Journal of Medical Internet Research, 12*(1), e4.

Weinstein, N. D. (1993). Testing four competing theories of health-protective behavior. *Health Psychology, 12*(4), 324–333.

Weinstein, N. D. (2007). Misleading tests of health behavior theories. *Annals of Behavioral Medicine, 33*(1), 1–10.

Weinstein, N. D., & Rothman, A. J. (2005). Commentary: Revitalizing research on health behavior theories. *Health Education Research, 20*(3), 294–297.

Weinstein, N. D., Sandman, P., & Blalock, S. (2008). The precaution adoption process model. In K. Glanz, B. K. Rimer, & K. Viswanath (Eds.), *Health behavior and health education: Theory, research, and practice* (4th ed., pp. 123–147). San Francisco: Jossey-Bass.

Wilson, E. B. (1952). *An introduction to scientific research.* New York: McGraw-Hill.

Zimbardo, P. G., Ebbesen, E. B., & Maslach, C. (1977). *Influencing attitudes and changing behavior* (2nd ed.). Reading, MA: Addison-Wesley.

CHAPTER 3

ECOLOGICAL MODELS OF HEALTH BEHAVIOR

James F. Sallis
Neville Owen

In this chapter we provide a brief history of ecological models as applied to health behavior and describe ecological models as contemporary frameworks for integrating the theories and models outlined in the following four parts of this book. We propose principles of ecological models that can be used to guide research and applications. We present selected applications of ecological models for health behavior research, reflecting on lessons from the comprehensive, multilevel approaches that have characterized tobacco control interventions. Examples from physical activity and sedentary behavior illustrate applications of ecological models and how the principles are being evaluated. Finally, we review the strengths and limitations of ecological models, along with the challenges of applying them.

History and Background of Ecological Models

The term *ecology* is derived from biological science and refers to the interrelationships between organisms and their environments. Ecological models, as they have evolved in the behavioral sciences and public health, focus on the nature of people's transactions with their physical and sociocultural environments (Stokols, 1992). The environmental and policy levels of influence distinguish ecological models from widely used behavioral models and theories that emphasize individual characteristics, skills, and proximal social influences, such as family and friends, but do not explicitly consider the broader

KEY POINTS

This chapter will:

- Define the core concept of ecological models.

- Explain how ecological models of health behavior can integrate multiple theories and be applied to improving the understanding of health behaviors and intervention effectiveness.

- Propose five core principles of ecological models of health behavior:

  1. There are multiple levels of influence on health behaviors.

  2. Environmental contexts are significant determinants of health behaviors.

  3. Influences on behaviors interact across levels.

  4. Ecological models should be behavior-specific.

  5. Multilevel interventions should be most effective in changing behaviors to improve health.

- Discuss the challenges of evaluating multilevel interventions based on ecological models.

community, organizational, and policy influences on health behaviors. Ecological models can be used to incorporate constructs from theories and models that focus on psychological, social, and organizational levels of influence (as described in the chapters in the subsequent parts of this book). Ecological models can provide a framework for integrating multiple theories and serve as a meta-model to ensure that environmental and policy factors are considered in developing comprehensive approaches to studying and intervening on health behaviors.

Healthy behaviors are thought to be maximized when environments and policies support healthful choices, and individuals are motivated and educated to make those choices (Canadian Public Health Association, 1986). Education about healthful choices when environments are not supportive is believed to produce weak and short-term effects on behavior. Yet, providing plentiful vegetables, sidewalks, or accessible condoms is no guarantee that people will make use of those resources (Sallis et al., 2006). Thus a central proposition of ecological models is that it usually takes the combination of *both* individual-level and environmental- and policy-level interventions to achieve substantial positive changes in health behaviors that are then maintained.

A general acceptance of and enthusiasm for a broad, multilevel, ecological perspective on health behaviors is reflected in authoritative documents that guide public health programs nationally and internationally. These documents include the Healthy People 2020 goals and objectives (U.S. Department of Health and Human Services, 2010), Institute of Medicine reports on health behaviors (Institute of Medicine, 2001), and childhood obesity prevention findings and recommendations (Koplan, Liverman, & Kraak, 2005), the Australian National Preventative Health Strategy (National Preventative Health Taskforce, 2009), the World Health Organization's *WHO Framework Convention on Tobacco Control* (WHO, 2003), and the WHO strategy for diet, physical activity, and health (WHO, 2004). These calls for application of ecological models on a widespread scale create an urgency to (1) ensure that researchers and practitioners are well informed about the nature, strengths, and weaknesses of ecological models, and (2) provide evidence about multilevel correlates and interventions to guide the applications.

Ecological Models Can Integrate Multiple Theories

Most theories and models presented in this book *describe* how variables within one level can influence behavior or *guide* intervention approaches that target one level of influence. These theories and models provide useful guidance in developing interventions, and there is evidence of effectiveness for all of them. However, adoption of a single theory or model as the basis for a study or intervention is not likely to be optimal. The central tenet of ecological models is that all levels of influence are important. Thus multilevel studies of correlates or determinants should explain behaviors better than studies of one level, and multilevel interventions generally should be more effective than single-level interventions. The weaknesses of ecological models are that they do not necessarily specify the variables or processes at each level expected to be most influential on behavior, they do not specify how such influences may vary for different behaviors, and it may not be feasible to intervene on all levels. Ecological models present research design and measurement challenges, and implementing multilevel studies and interventions may be difficult or even impossible, in part because investigators are unlikely to have control of all relevant interventions.

An important strength of ecological models is that they can provide a framework for integrating other theories and models to create a comprehensive approach to study design and interventions. Instead of choosing one model to guide a study or intervention, a multilevel ecological framework can lead investigators to select individual, social, and organizational models that can guide the development of comprehensive studies and interventions.

Ecological models do not displace other health behavior theories but place them in a broader context that recognizes the value of each theory. Thus an ecological model can be considered a meta-model that can organize other models into a coherent whole. They can help us develop a more comprehensive understanding of the factors that influence particular behaviors and what might be necessary to alter those behaviors. Ecological models can help us use all of the tools available, whether the tools are concepts, measures, or intervention strategies. A challenge in using ecological models of health behavior is to identify, from the available theories and models, which are most appropriate and influential for the purpose, behavior, and population of interest. While reading the subsequent parts of this book, consider how several theories or models might be combined in a comprehensive ecological framework to suit your needs.

History of Ecological Models

The proliferation of contemporary ecological models in public health is based on a rich conceptual tradition in the behavioral and social sciences, as described in a previous version of the present chapter (Sallis & Owen, 2002) and summarized in Table 3.1. There has been a progression from the early concept that only *perceptions* of environments were important (Lewin, 1951) to an emphasis on *direct effects* of environments on behaviors (Barker, 1968). Earlier models were developed to apply broadly across behaviors, but more recent models were created to inform the development of health promotion programs and strategies, such as those proposed by Cohen, Scribner, and Farley (2000); Fisher, Brownson, Heath, Luke, and Sumner (2004); Flay and Petraitis (1994); Glanz, Sallis, Saelens, and Frank (2005); Glass and McAtee (2006); McLeroy, Bibeau, Steckler, and Glanz (1988); Stokols (1992); Stokols, Grzywacz, McMahan, and Phillips (2003); and Story, Kaphingst, Robinson-O'Brien, and Glanz (2008). Categories and hierarchies of behavioral influences have been described in numerous ways, including Bronfenbrenner's (1979) micro-, meso-, and exo-system approach and McLeroy and colleagues' five levels of influence: intrapersonal, interpersonal, institutional, community, and policy (McLeroy et al., 1988). The first part of Table 3.1 describes models mainly designed to explain behavior, and the second part contains models primarily intended to guide interventions. Some models are designed to be applicable to many health behaviors (Cohen et al., 2000; Glass & McAtee, 2006; Lohrmann, 2010; Stokols, 1992; Stokols et al., 2003), whereas others are designed for specific behaviors (Fisher et al., 2004; Flay & Petraitis, 1994; Glanz et al., 2005; Story et al., 2008).

Table 3.1   Historical and Contemporary Ecological Models

Author, Citation, Model	Key Concepts
Models designed mainly to explain behavior	
Kurt Lewin (1951): ecological psychology	*Ecological psychology* is the study of the influence of the outside environment on the person.
Roger Barker (1968): environmental psychology	*Behavior settings* are the social and physical situations in which behaviors take place. Concludes that behaviors could be predicted more accurately from the situations people are in than from people's individual characteristics.
Rudolph Moos (1980): social ecology	Defines four categories of environmental factors. (1) Physical settings: features of the natural (weather, etc.) and built (buildings, etc.) environment. (2) Organizational settings: size and function of worksites and schools. (3) The *human aggregate*: sociocultural characteristics of the people in an environment. (4) The *social climate*: supportiveness of a social setting for a particular behavior.
Urie Bronfenbrenner (1979): systems theory	Identifies three levels of environmental influences. (1) The *microsystem* consists of interactions among family members and work groups. (2) The *mesosystem* consists of physical family, school, and work settings. (3) The *exosystem* consists of the larger social system of economics, culture, and politics.
Thomas Glass and Matthew McAtee (2006): ecosocial model	Conceptualizes hierarchies of influences on behavior within biology and society, which have social and physical environment dimensions. Structural contingencies provide opportunities and constraints, and biological processes regulate expression of behavior.
Models designed mainly to guide behavioral interventions	
B. F. Skinner (1953): operant learning theory	Primary model is environment → behavior. Reinforcers and cues in the environment directly control behavior. Recently, Hovell, Wahlgren, and Gehrman (2002) proposed a behavioral ecological model that draws heavily on Skinner.
Albert Bandura (1986): social learning and social cognitive theories	Proposes environmental and personal influences on behavior. Bandura referred mainly to social environments and rarely addressed the role of physical, community, or organizational environments. (See Chapter 9.)
Kenneth McLeroy et al. (1988): ecological model of health behavior	Identifies five sources of influence on health behaviors: intrapersonal factors, interpersonal processes and primary groups, institutional factors, community factors, and public policy.
Daniel Stokols (1992, 2003): social ecology model for health promotion	Based on four assumptions. (1) Health behavior is influenced by physical environments, social environments, and personal attributes. (2) Environments are multidimensional, with such dimensions as social or physical, actual or perceived, discrete attributes (spatial arrangements) or constructs (social climate). (3) Human-environment interactions occur at varying levels of aggregation: individual, family, cultural group, or the whole population. (4) People influence their settings, and the changed settings then influence health behaviors.
Deborah Cohen et al. (2000): structural-ecological model	Defines four categories of structural influences. (1) Availability of protective or harmful consumer products. (2) Physical structures (or physical characteristics of products). (3) Social structures and policies. (4) Media and cultural messages.
Brian Flay and John Petraitis (1994): theory of triadic influence	Genes and environment are assumed to affect all behaviors. The three streams of influence on behavior are intrapersonal, social, and sociocultural.
Karen Glanz et al. (2005): model of community food environments	Proposes key constructs that affect eating behaviors: availability, price, placement, and promotion of foods, as well as nutrition information. Applies to restaurants and food stores.

Table 3.1   *(Continued)*

Author, Citation, Model	Key Concepts
Edwin Fisher et al. (2005): self-management model	Based on integration of individuals' skills and choices with support they receive from the social environment, as well as the physical and policy environments of communities.
David Lohrmann (2010)	Describes an ecological model for a coordinated school health program, emphasizing the complex interrelationships between intrapersonal factors, interpersonal processes and primary groups, institutional factors, community factors, and public policy.
David Ogilvie et al. (2011)	In relation to improving infrastructure for walking and cycling, developed an applied ecological framework with which current theories about the behavioral effects of environmental change may be tested in heterogeneous and complex intervention settings.
Takemi Sugiyama et al. (2012)	Extends the principle of specificity of environmental influence, classifying the built environment determinants of utilitarian and recreational walking in terms of destinations (presence, proximity, quality) and route attributes (sidewalks, connectivity, aesthetics, traffic, safety).
Neville Owen et al. (2011)	Extends the principle of behavior-specific ecological models, through adapting the ecological model of four domains of active living (see Figure 3.1) to address a newly identified health risk: sedentary behavior (put simply, too much sitting, as distinct from too little exercise)

A recent trend has been the development of ecological models tailored not only to particular health behaviors but also to subsets of behaviors and classes of environmental attributes. For example, the ecological model of Ogilvie et al. (2011) specifies the infrastructure requirements for walking and cycling. Sugiyama, Neuhaus, Cole, Giles-Corti, and Owen (2012) take an even more specific perspective on the route and environmental attributes associated with walking. A multilevel model of sedentary behavior is based on the idea that sitting is a class of behavior that is distinct from physical inactivity and with its own antecedents and consequences (Owen et al., 2011). This growing diversity and move toward specialized models illustrates the practical appeal, adaptability, and robustness of ecological models.

There is a consensus that ecological models are a useful framework for conceptualizing multiple levels of determinants of health behaviors, and they are used widely as guides for the design of comprehensive multilevel interventions. Health promotion program coordinators—at least in the United States and the Netherlands—endorse the utility of ecological models (Kok, Gottlieb, Commers, & Smerecnik, 2008). However, an examination of the ecological levels that health promotion programs targeted, based on 157 intervention articles from the past twenty years of the journal *Health Education & Behavior*, found that articles were much more likely to describe interventions focused on individual and interpersonal characteristics rather than institutional, community, or policy factors (Golden & Earp, 2012). Though there might be broad agreement about the importance of ecological perspectives for addressing major public health issues, such as tobacco control, HIV/AIDS, and obesity, in a comprehensive manner, the operationalization and implementation of ecological models in research and practice is not yet consistent with the rhetoric.

There is a reason we refer to ecological *frameworks*, *perspectives*, and *models* instead of *theories*. Theories specify variables and the relations among them. Ecological models have a heuristic value in prompting investigators to consider multiple levels of influence and intervention, but ecological models do not specify constructs or variables that generalize across behaviors. The lack of specificity of the broader ecological framework can be considered a weakness, but it is also a strength that leads to development of behavior-specific models. To improve the utility of ecological models, we have identified generalizable principles that can be applied across behaviors.

Ecological Perspectives on Health Behavior: Five Principles

Principle 1: There Are Multiple Levels of Influence on Health Behaviors

Ecological models specify that factors at multiple levels, often including intrapersonal, interpersonal, organizational, community, and public policy levels, can influence health behaviors, although the relative influence may vary by target behavior and context. Sociocultural factors and physical environments may apply to more than one level, such as organizational and community levels. Inclusion of all these levels of influence distinguishes ecological models from theories that primarily focus on one or two levels.

Principle 2: Environmental Contexts Are Significant Determinants of Health Behaviors

Behaviors may be predicted more accurately from the situations people are in than from their individual characteristics, according to environmental psychologists (Wicker, 1979). Inclusion of social and physical environment variables is a defining feature of ecological models. *Behavior settings* (Barker, 1968) are the social and physical situations in which behaviors take place, and ecological models open the possibility of intervening on these environments. "The importance of behavior settings is they restrict the range of behavior by promoting and sometimes demanding certain actions and by discouraging or prohibiting others" (Wicker, 1979, p. 4). Environmental contexts can shape or constrain individual and interpersonal determinants of health behaviors.

Principle 3: Influences on Behaviors Interact Across Levels

The interaction of influences means that variables work together. *Interaction* does not refer directly to statistical interactions; however, cross-level influences or interplay can be studied through statistical interactions or moderator effects. For example, individuals with high motivation to avoid weight gain may react differently from those with lower motivation do to driving past fast food restaurants. Education to be physically active may work better when policies support active living through physician counseling, insurance discounts for engaging in regular activity, and sidewalks on all streets. Because ecological models specify multiple levels of influence, and there are likely to be multiple variables at each level, it may be difficult to discern which of the possible interactions are most important. Thus a challenge for research is to advance our understanding of these interactions across levels.

Principle 4: Ecological Models Should Be Behavior-Specific

Ecological models appear most useful for guiding research and intervention when they are tailored to specific health behaviors. Often, environmental and policy variables are behavior-specific. The availability of condoms in nightclubs has little relevance to dietary behaviors, the presence of cycling trails in suburban neighborhoods is unlikely to affect alcohol intake, and policies related to food subsidies have little relevance to sun protection behaviors. By contrast, the key constructs in individual theories (see Part Two of this book), such as self-efficacy and outcome expectations, apply across many behaviors. The need to identify environmental and policy variables that are specific to each behavior is a challenge in the development and use of ecological models, because lessons learned with one behavior (e.g., promoting jogging) may not translate to an apparently similar behavior (e.g., walking to work).

Principle 5: Multilevel Interventions Should Be Most Effective in Changing Behaviors

The superiority of multilevel interventions over single-level interventions follows from the principle that there are important influences at all levels of influence. There are many examples of interventions that targeted only individuals and showed small and short-term effects. Educational interventions designed to change beliefs and behavioral skills are likely to work better when policies and environments support the targeted behavior changes. Similarly, environmental changes by themselves may be insufficient to change behaviors. Putting more fruits and vegetables in all convenience stores may have little impact unless that environmental change is supported by pricing policies and educational and motivational campaigns. Individually oriented interventions can be intensive and have large effects on a few people who choose to participate in the programs, though changes tend to be temporary unless those people are already in supportive environments and/or are affected by health-promoting policies. Organizational, environmental, and policy changes can be sustained over the long term and affect many more people, even though individual changes may be modest.

Applications of Ecological Models to Health Behaviors

This section describes applications of ecological models in health behavior research and interventions, reflecting, first, on lessons from comprehensive, multilevel interventions for tobacco control and, second, on the ways that ecologically based studies of physical activity and sedentary behavior are improving understanding about these behaviors and evaluating the principles of ecological models.

Ecological Models Applied to Tobacco Control

Several decades of tobacco control have produced remarkable success, with decreases in smoking prevalence to below 20 percent in some industrialized countries. Systematic studies of the outcomes of tobacco control efforts have identified the effective components of tobacco control as wide availability of clinical smoking cessation programs, mass media campaigns, regulatory efforts to restrict opportunities for smoking, economic approaches that make cigarettes more expensive, and comprehensive multilevel programs combining these approaches (Borland, Young, Coghill, & Zhang, 2010; Mercer et al., 2003). Tobacco control provides strong support for Principle 5 (*multilevel interventions should be most effective in changing behavior*).

Tobacco control, while by no means providing a precise template for intervening on other health behaviors, provides a powerful example of the effectiveness of changing the health promotion agenda from an individual responsibility and personal change focus to broader environmental and policy initiatives (Fisher et al., 2004). Population-wide activities in tobacco control began with programs designed to influence the individual smoker through public education and counter-advertising in the mass media. A broader public awareness developed about the addictive properties of tobacco. With widespread dissemination of information about industry efforts to manipulate those addictive properties and the effects of secondhand smoke, public support for widespread change developed, including workplace smoking bans. Evidence that the tobacco industry was specifically targeting uptake of smoking among youth through its advertising led to support for mandated advertising restraints on the tobacco industry (Green et al., 2006). Thus mass media interventions to educate individuals supported policy changes, illustrating Principle 3 (*influences on behaviors interact across levels*).

As social acceptance of tobacco control initiatives gained momentum, policy and environmental interventions were enacted that affected millions of people, such as tobacco taxes, limited vending machine access, and smoke-free workplaces and restaurants (Principle 2—*environmental contexts are significant determinants of health behaviors*). Complementary educational campaigns were designed to build on this momentum, so as to denormalize smoking and highlight tobacco industry deceptions to generate support for policy changes (Principle 5—*multilevel interventions should be most effective in changing behavior*).

Consistent with these principles of ecological models of health behavior, Borland et al. (2010) describe a framework for examining the social ecology of tobacco use. As is appropriate for addressing strategies to control the delivery of a legal but highly addictive substance, they focus on regulatory actions, such as pricing, smoking bans, and limiting access, that have widespread impact and have been shown to be effective.

Tobacco control, while it exemplifies so much of the guidance that can be derived from ecological models as comprehensive approaches that emphasize environmental and policy interventions, may not provide direct guidance regarding what will be effective for other health behaviors. For example, the food, electronic entertainment, and automobile industries that appear to be contributing to the obesity epidemic cannot realistically be portrayed as complete villains, as has been the case for the tobacco industry (Sallis & Green, 2012). Nevertheless, in tobacco control we have a model for highly effective comprehensive approaches to population-wide and long-term health behavior change, showing the key role for multilevel interventions.

The remarkable success of tobacco control, replicated over many countries, illustrates three important lessons that can be applied to other health behaviors (Green et al., 2006):

- Focusing change efforts solely on educating and motivating individuals is unlikely to create population change, as was the case for group-based smoking cessation programs.
- For some behaviors and some groups, there may be levels of influence that are particularly powerful. In the case of tobacco control, this has been observed for pricing policies.
- Even when health risks are well understood and severe, widespread changes in social norms and support for environmental and policy initiatives can take decades to develop.

Ecological Models Applied to Physical Activity and Sedentary Behavior

The physical activity field has advanced from broad recognition of the importance of environmental influences to development and testing of behavior-specific, multilevel ecological models and implementation of multilevel interventions. In light of the intensive use of ecological models in physical activity research, we describe an ecological model of physical activity and highlight several areas of advancement in evaluating the model and developing interventions.

Multilevel Intervention and Multisectoral Approaches

In the *Lancet Physical Activity Series*, Lee et al. (2012) identified physical inactivity as a major contributor to noncommunicable diseases in countries of all income levels, contributing to the deaths of more than five million people each year. Bauman et al. (2012) explained how a comprehensive understanding of why people are physically active or inactive can contribute to evidence-based planning of multilevel interventions for whole populations, with the most effective programs likely targeting multiple risk factors for inactivity (Principle 1—*there are multiple levels of influence on health behaviors*). They argued that ecological models appropriately focus attention on the environments where people can perform physical activity, which emphasizes the need to partner with groups traditionally outside the health sector with responsibility for those environments, including the urban planning, transportation, parks and trails, architecture, and education sectors (Principle 2—*environmental contexts are significant determinants of health behaviors*).

Ecological Models of Physical Activity

Several ecological models specific to physical activity have been published, including one developed to guide community interventions in a Latin American context (Matsudo et al., 2004). The example shown in Figure 3.1 synthesizes findings and concepts from the fields of public health, behavioral science, transportation and city planning, policy studies and economics, and the leisure sciences (Sallis et al., 2006). The model has a commonly used layered, or "onion," structure to represent the multiple levels of influence, but with three distinguishing features. First, the model is organized around four domains of physical activity: active transport,

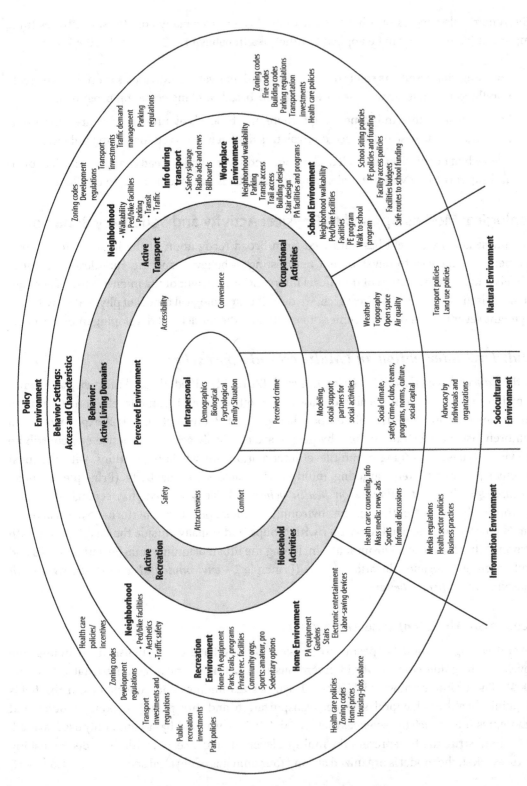

Figure 3.1 Ecological Model of Four Domains of Active Living

Source: J. F. Sallis, R. B. Cervero, W. Ascher, K. A. Henderson, M. K. Kraft, and J. Kerr (2006), "An Ecological Approach to Creating Active Living Communities." *Annual Review of Public Health, 27,* 297–322. Reprinted with permission from the *Annual Review of Public Health.*

Note: PA = physical activity.

occupational activities, household activities, and active recreation. This reflects Principle 4 (*ecological models should be behavior-specific*). Second, some types of relevant influences are not tied to settings where behavior takes place. For example, information environments are ubiquitous, and counseling in health care settings may influence physical activity done elsewhere. A third feature is that social and cultural environments operate at multiple levels. Other ecological models can be developed for specific physical activity behaviors (e.g., walking to school, use of parks) and population subgroups (e.g., low-income groups, rural residents).

An Ecological Model of Sedentary Behavior

The model portrayed in Figure 3.1 has been adapted to understanding multiple levels of influences on sedentary behaviors (Owen et al., 2011). Recent research has documented increased risk of type 2 diabetes, cardiovascular disease, and breast and colon cancer associated with high volumes of sedentary behavior—put simply, too much sitting, as distinct from too little physical activity (Owen, 2012). There are few studies of correlates of sedentary behavior, but there were lower levels of television viewing time among Australian women living in high-walkable neighborhoods (Sugiyama, Salmon, Dunstan, Bauman, & Owen, 2007), and those in low-walkable neighborhoods increased their TV viewing time over four years (Ding, Sugiyama, et al., 2012).

The Need for Empirical Evidence Supporting Ecological Models

While ecological models have been widely used in physical activity research and intervention, it is important to test the principles of ecological models empirically. Bauman et al. (2012) systematically reviewed the literature and found evidence for consistent correlates of physical activity at all ecological levels, supporting Principle 1 (*there are multiple levels of influence [at least correlates] on health behaviors*). Below, we provide examples of studies that evaluate principles of ecological models and illustrate how multilevel models are guiding major interventions.

Understanding Multiple Levels of Influence

Few studies have examined the relative importance of individual, social, and environmental correlates of physical activity. Early studies found that built environment variables, such as the presence of sidewalks and nearby destinations, accounted for the least variance (De Bourdeaudhuij, Sallis, & Saelens, 2003; Giles-Corti & Donovan, 2002). An Australian study showed that built environment factors remained significant correlates of walking for transport after controlling for personal attributes, such as individuals' reasons for choosing to live in their neighborhoods (Owen et al., 2007). A U.S. study documented significant correlates of total physical activity at the demographic/biological (age and gender), psychological (self-efficacy), and environmental levels, but not the social level (Saelens et al., 2012). The latter study found that an objectively measured built environment variable, retail floor area ratio (retail FAR), was as strong a correlate as gender. The seldom studied retail FAR reflects both proximity to retail destinations and whether they are designed for pedestrians. Retail FAR is the ratio of store floor space to land area of the parcel, so if the ratio is high it probably means pedestrians enter the store directly from the sidewalk. If the ratio is low, it likely means the store is surrounded by parking. Thus the observed strength of environmental variables in relation to psychosocial variables is likely to depend on the variables studied.

Research addressing Principle 2 (*environmental contexts are significant determinants of health behaviors*) has benefited from advances in objective measures of environmental attributes using geographic information systems (GIS) (also see the Supplementary Web Materials). *Environmental measures are central to progress in applying ecological models to physical activity.* The urban planning concept of *walkability* refers to neighborhood designs that allow residents to easily walk from their homes to everyday destinations such as shops and schools. Research on walkability has been advanced by a multicomponent walkability measure in GIS that combines residential density, mix of land uses (e.g., homes, shops, and government services near each other), street connectivity (connected streets provide direct paths for pedestrians), and retail FAR (floor area ratio—if the ratio of building area to land area is high, it usually means the building opens onto the sidewalk, instead of being surrounded by parking lots) (Frank et al., 2010). This technology allows for the assessment and mapping of walkability across entire regions, which can support planning to target improvements to specific neighborhoods.

Exploring Interactions Across Ecological Levels

The principle of interactions across levels is important because understanding such interactions could help in the design of efficient packages of interventions. Studies of cross-level interactions are now emerging, but different interactions may occur, depending on participant characteristics. Ding, Sallis, et al. (2012) studied adults aged twenty to sixty-five and found few significant interactions of psychosocial and environmental variables for total physical activity or walking for transport. However, several interactions in analyses of walking for leisure all had the same pattern. Favorable environmental conditions, such as having a park nearby or good aesthetics, seemed to be most helpful for people with unfavorable psychosocial conditions, such as many perceived barriers or low enjoyment of activity. Thus improving built environments might be most helpful for those less inclined to be active.

A study of adults sixty-six years old and older found psychosocial by environmental variable interactions for total physical activity, walking for transport, and walking for leisure, but the pattern was different for older adults (Carlson et al., 2012). For older adults, supportive environments, such as walkability and sidewalks, seemed to be more important for those with *favorable* psychosocial variables, such as social support and self-efficacy. The implication was that the combination of improving environments and individual interventions may be most effective for older adults. Additional studies are needed to determine whether these findings are replicated.

Improving Study Designs: Prospective and Quasi-Experimental Studies

A primary criticism of built environment and physical activity research based on ecological models is the reliance on evidence from studies examining cross-sectional associations. There is the likelihood of self-selection bias because people who like to walk may choose to live in a walkable neighborhood. The literature indicates that self-selection does not account for the whole association between neighborhood environments and physical activity (Cao, Mokhtarian, & Handy, 2009), but stronger study designs provide better evidence of causality. Recent studies are reporting prospective relationships of environmental attributes with physical activity and sedentary behaviors. For example, in high-walkable neighborhoods, Shimura, Sugiyama, Winkler, and Owen (2012) showed less decline over four years in those middle- to older-aged adults walking for transport. Ding, Sugiyama, et al. (2012) demonstrated interactions between neighborhood walking and individual-level attributes in explaining changes in television viewing time over four years in Australian adults.

Project RESIDE in Perth, Australia

The most ambitious prospective study in this area, Project RESIDE in Perth, Australia, was conducted to evaluate a livable neighborhood policy that was consistent with walkable community designs (Giles-Corti et al., 2013). About 1,400 adults were measured before and twelve months after they moved to new neighborhoods that were built under either the livable neighborhoods policy or the previous policy favoring less-walkable, more car-oriented designs. Changes in neighborhood characteristics were assessed by self-report and objectively, and environmental differences across "before" and "after" neighborhoods were significantly related to changes in walking for transportation and leisure in each neighborhood. For each type of additional destination in their new neighborhoods, such as food store, clothing store, or library, adults increased walking for transport by about six minutes per week. For each type of additional recreational facility in their new neighborhoods, such as a park or health club, residents increased walking for leisure by about seventeen minutes per week. The RESIDE results enhance confidence in the findings of many observational and cross-sectional studies that neighborhood environments can shape physical activity (Bauman et al., 2012; Mumford, Contant, Weissman, Wolf, & Glanz, 2011). However, the authors noted a challenge in that it takes several years for all the amenities in livable neighborhoods to be built, so a full evaluation will require measuring people for years.

Lessons from International Studies

A central problem for ecologically based studies of environmental attributes is that there may be too little variation in social, environmental, and policy variables in studies conducted in single countries (Giles-Corti & Donovan, 2002; Kerr et al., 2013). For example, a random sample of residents of a U.S. city might yield few adults who value active transport (walking and bicycling), limited social support for walking for transportation, and few high-walkable neighborhoods. A random sample in many European cities would likely produce few participants with negative attitudes, widespread social support for active transportation, and few low-walkable neighborhoods. Within one study region, there may be no variation at all in policies related to park resources or zoning laws. Lack of variation can lead to underestimation of effect sizes and an inability to test important hypotheses. Thus studies that include assessments of environmental and policy variables must be designed to ensure variation in those factors. One method of increasing environmental variability is to conduct international studies.

One study combined data from eleven environmentally diverse countries to examine perceived environmental correlates of overall physical activity, using common methods. The results showed five of seven environmental variables to be significantly related to meeting physical activity guidelines, supporting the international relevance of built environment variables such as mixed land use, sidewalks, and park access (Sallis et al., 2009). Associations were stronger than those reported in single-country studies, probably because data from multiple countries provide a wider range of environmental variability.

A series of analyses using data from the United States, Australia, and Belgium examined associations of perceived neighborhood environmental attributes with adults' recreational physical activity (Van Dyck et al., 2013), transport-related walking and cycling (Van Dyck et al., 2012b), sitting time (Van Dyck et al., 2012a), and the interacting psychosocial and environmental correlates of leisure-time activity (Van Dyck et al., 2014). Across these studies, associations of environments and activity-related outcomes were generally similar for the United States and Australia but different for Belgium. For example, Van Dyck and colleagues (2013) found that a "recreational walking-friendliness" index and a "leisure-time activity friendliness" index had positive linear associations respectively with recreational walking and with leisure-time physical activity. The associations were significant in all study sites except Belgium. Even this sample of three countries identified important differences that may reflect varying environmental and cultural contexts, which illustrates the value of ecological models that support the examination of context.

Ecological Models Applied to Physical Activity Interventions

Ecological models are used explicitly or implicitly to guide the design of many physical activity interventions, as shown by a summary of national physical activity plans from six countries (Bornstein, Pate, & Pratt, 2009). All plans reflected use of ecological models in recommending interventions at multiple levels, emphasis on environmental and policy strategies, and targeting multiple sectors of society (e.g., education, health care, transportation, and parks). Application of ecological models has become standard for community-based, physical activity interventions. One example is Active Living by Design, which supported interventions in twenty-five communities throughout the United States, most of them with low-income or mostly minority populations (Bors et al., 2009). Communities developed coalitions to implement interventions based on the program's 5P model. The 5P's encompass a multilevel approach: preparation (developing partnerships), promotions (to change perceptions and knowledge), programs (targeting individuals or organizations), policy (usually at organizational or local government levels), and physical projects (built environments).

The difficulties of evaluating multilevel interventions are illustrated by the bicycling literature. Bicycling interventions evaluated by transportation researchers include mainly bike lanes, bike paths, parking, integration with public transit, bike rentals, signage, education and promotion, incentives, and policies to increase penalties for automobile collisions with cyclists.

Two reviews of the scientific literature concluded that few if any of these specific interventions had strong evidence for increasing cycling (Pucher, Dill, & Handy, 2010; Yang, Sahlqvist, McMinn, Griffin, & Ogilvie, 2010). However, Pucher et al. (2010) collected unpublished data on cycling for transportation in about twenty cities around the world before and after multicomponent, long-term cycling interventions. Virtually all of these case studies demonstrated notable increases in cycling, whether the baseline was 1 percent or 20 percent of trips by cycling. The case studies were not randomized and comparison cities were not presented, so conclusions must be drawn cautiously. However, one interpretation of these findings is that single-level interventions were usually not effective, but multilevel interventions had some evidence of effects, consistent with Principle 5 (*multilevel interventions should be most effective in changing behavior*). The intervention literature is intriguing but far from definitive. In absence of controlled studies of single- versus multilevel interventions, we are left with inadequate tests of Principle 5 of ecological models.

Critique of Ecological Models

Strengths and Limitations

Ecological models have been central to health promotion practice for several decades. Health groups and government agencies rely increasingly on multilevel interventions to solve the most pressing health problems. Based in part on success in reversing the epidemic of tobacco use, there are high expectations that interventions consistent with the principles of ecological models can reverse the obesity epidemic by improving environments and policies that drive physical activity and nutrition behaviors. The Institute of Medicine (2001); Koplan et al. (2005), and the World Health Organization (2004) propose solutions to obesity that require policy and environmental change. The increasing emphasis on applications of ecological models creates a need for a critical examination of their strengths and weaknesses. Enthusiasm for the potential of ecological models does not reduce the need to understand the benefits and limitations of multilevel interventions, test hypotheses derived from ecological models, and continue to refine the concepts and methods used in research and practice informed by ecological models.

A key strength of ecological models is their focus on multiple levels of influence, which broadens options for interventions. Policy and environmental changes are expected to affect virtually entire populations, in contrast to programs that reach only individuals who choose to participate. Policy and environmental interventions establish settings and incentives that can persist in sustaining behavior changes, helping to solve the problem of poor maintenance of many individually directed interventions. Expanding the range of behavioral determinants studied and directing development of multilevel interactions are likely to be strengths, though the value of multilevel interventions has not been definitively demonstrated by direct comparisons to single-level approaches.

A weakness of many ecological models of health behavior is their lack of specificity about the most important hypothesized influences. This puts a greater burden on health promotion professionals to identify critical factors for each behavioral application. However, some ecological models provide more guidance about behavioral influences, such as Figure 3.1. A related weakness—even for behavior-specific ecological models—is the lack of information about how the broader levels of influence operate or how constructs interact across levels. Thus the models broaden *perspectives* without identifying specific constructs or providing guidance about how to use ecological models to improve research or interventions. By contrast, individual-level psychosocial theories of health behavior are more likely to specify the constructs and the mechanisms by which those constructs are expected to influence behavior (see Part Two in this book). A major challenge for those working with ecological models is to develop more sophisticated models that lead to testable hypotheses and useful guidance for interventions. Intervening on multiple levels simultaneously may be constrained by budgetary and practical limitations, such as policies and environments not being under the control of investigators. However, even if one must choose a particular level on which to intervene, ecological models can be helpful in placing specific behaviors and interventions in the larger context of a comprehensive understanding of the multiple determinants of particular behaviors.

Tests of Principles Have Been Progressing

In the past few years, empirical support for most of the principles of ecological models has accumulated for some behaviors, as illustrated by the earlier section on physical activity. Regarding Principle 1, research in many topic areas indicates there are multiple levels of influence on (or at least correlation with) health behaviors. Many ecologically based studies include environmental variables and support Principle 2, that environmental contexts are significant determinants of health behaviors. This support for Principles 1 and 2 demonstrates the need for multilevel models and emphasizes the value of ensuring that organizational, built environment, and policy levels of influence are considered in designing studies and interventions. Integrating other theories and models into ecological frameworks is justified by the evidence.

Principle 3 (*influences on behaviors interact across levels*) has received only preliminary support in the physical activity field (Carlson et al., 2012; Ding, Sallis, et al., 2012). It is not yet possible to make informed hypotheses about how variables might interact across levels, and additional research is warranted because understanding cross-level interactions can inform the design of efficient multilevel interventions. At least in the physical activity field, Principle 4, about behavior-specific models, is well supported. There is good evidence that psychosocial variables are related mainly to leisure-time physical activity and that there are different environmental correlates of physical activity for leisure and transport purposes (Bauman et al., 2012; Saelens & Handy, 2008; Sugiyama et al., 2012). Principle 5, regarding the expected superiority of multilevel interventions, is both the most important and least supported principle. It is most important because it has the potential to improve health interventions. But the relevant evidence is all circumstantial, as illustrated by the bicycling interventions described above (Pucher et al., 2010). Just demonstrating that multilevel interventions are effective does not adequately test the principle. The complexity of comparing single- and multilevel interventions in controlled studies is a major challenge.

Challenges of Applying and Evaluating Ecological Models

Ecological principles point to complex interactions of personal, social, and community characteristics that are difficult to manipulate experimentally. The typical goal of experimental designs—to isolate a single intervention from the effects of its context—is conceptually at odds with the ecological emphasis on studying how intervention components interact with their context. Although controlled experiments with multilevel interventions are challenging to design and conduct, rigorous analytic strategies can be applied productively (Bull, Eakin, Reeves, & Kimberly, 2006). For example, a community program to promote childhood asthma management intervened on personal, social, and community factors (Fisher et al., 2004). The program was evaluated with a nonrandomized design using structural equation modeling. Individual-level factors like parents' attitudes toward asthma predicted children's medical utilization. Social support from lay asthma workers and asthma management classes predicted reduced emergency room and hospital care. Thus interventions targeted at multiple levels predicted relevant outcomes.

Research based on ecological models is, by definition, more demanding than behavioral research at a single level. Developing and collecting measures of influences at multiple levels, expanding the number of disciplines represented in investigative teams, conceptualizing and implementing interventions at multiple levels, and using more sophisticated statistical strategies, all place substantial demands on investigators and program evaluators. However, multilevel studies are the only way to generate knowledge that will lead to effective multilevel interventions.

The practical difficulty of implementing multilevel interventions should not be underestimated. The length of time required to change policies and environments is a deterrent to program directors called on to make changes to meet legislators' schedules or grant timelines. Few environmental variables and policies of interest are controlled by health professionals, and change requires a political process that is unpredictable in timing and outcome. To implement multilevel interventions, public health professionals must become more skilled in advocacy and political change, or partner with those who have such skills. Nevertheless, the consensus that multilevel interventions are required to solve the critical health problems of the twenty-first century is leading governmental and nongovernmental health agencies to design and implement multilevel interventions to combat tobacco use, obesity, diabetes, inactivity, poor diet, alcohol and drug abuse, violence, HIV/AIDS, and other public health scourges. The imperative for public health action creates an urgent demand for researchers to conduct the difficult studies required to build the evidence base for continued improvement of multilevel interventions.

Complex Systems Models for Conceptualizing Multiple Influences on Health Behaviors and Interventions

Ecological models have helped to broaden perspectives on both the causes and solutions of health behaviors, and they are being used to guide the development of multilevel interventions worldwide. It could be argued that in the past decade or so, ecological models have stimulated a paradigm shift, at least with some health behaviors and problems such as obesity. Though ecological models tell us that variables interact across levels, the models say nothing about *how* those variables interact or *which* variables interact. This is an important limitation that points to the need for the next step in improving our conceptual models.

Complex systems models can be useful in trying to understand systems of heterogeneous components that are nonlinearly interrelated, have feedback loops, and are adaptive to changes in context (Finegood, 2011; Hammond, 2009). This is a good description of the many and diverse influences on most health behaviors and chronic diseases. Complex models have been used to predict weather patterns and climate change for years, and they have also been used to study infectious disease outbreaks. The most relevant and well-known application of complex systems models to chronic disease is a diagram of over 100 biological, psychological, behavioral, environmental, economic, and policy influences on obesity, with 300 arrows of influence and 100 feedback loops, developed in the United Kingdom (UK Government Office for Science, 2007). The process of developing a complex systems model forces investigators to specify all the relevant variables and make explicit hypotheses about how the variables interact. Computational methods can be used to estimate the effects of changing one or more components on other components and outcomes (Hammond, 2009). Thus the effects of different intervention strategies can be modeled as an aid to decision making. Such models could help us identify synergies among intervention components, likely unintended consequences, and how the systems could evolve over time. Thus complex systems models may be able to take the multilevel frameworks of ecological models and make them more explicit and quantitative, leading, we can hope, to better recommendations for multilevel interventions.

Application of complex systems models to obesity is mostly conceptual to date. This means the models use simulated data, with investigators specifying the variables and types of interactions. To the authors' knowledge, the models have not been validated in their ability to predict real-world outcomes. A next step is to systematically build models with multilevel data, then test different types of interactions in their ability to predict empirical outcomes. There is a great deal of enthusiasm for complex systems models, but they have not yet demonstrated their concrete value for studying and improving health behaviors and outcomes.

Summary

Ecological models are particularly helpful in our efforts to understand how people interact with their environments. Ecological models are likely to be especially important in understanding behaviors with complex etiology that must be maintained over time, such as physical activity, nutrition, sun protection, and substance use. Ecological models direct us to examine multiple levels of influence on health behaviors, including community, environmental, and policy levels that are absent from most other models of health behavior. Better understanding can be used to develop effective multilevel approaches to improve health behaviors. Other theories and models oriented to individual, social, and organizational influences and interventions can be integrated within a multilevel ecological framework to guide development of comprehensive intervention approaches. Multilevel interventions hold promise for producing greater and longer-lasting changes in health behaviors than single-level approaches, and ecological models are guiding major public health interventions for a variety of behaviors. There are logistical challenges in implementing multilevel studies and interventions, and it will be difficult to definitively demonstrate that multilevel interventions are better than single-level approaches.

The basic premise of the ecological perspective is simple. Providing individuals with the motivation and skills to change behavior cannot be effective if environments and policies make it difficult or impossible to choose healthful behaviors. Rather, we should create environments and policies that make it convenient, attractive, and economical to make healthful choices, and then motivate and educate people to make those healthy choices.

References

Bandura, A. (1986). *Social foundations of thought and action: A social cognitive theory*. Englewood Cliffs, NJ: Prentice Hall.

Barker, R. G. (1968). *Ecological psychology*. Stanford, CA: Stanford University Press.

Bauman, A. E., Reis, R. S., Sallis, J. F., Wells, J. C., Loos, R. J., & Martin, B. W., for the Lancet Physical Activity Series Working Group. (2012). Correlates of physical activity: Why are some people physically active and others not? *Lancet, 380*(9838), 258–271.

Borland, R., Young, D., Coghill, K., & Zhang, J. Y. (2010). The tobacco use management system: Analyzing tobacco control from a systems perspective. *American Journal of Public Health, 100*(7), 1229–1236.

Bornstein, D. B., Pate, R. R., & Pratt, M. (2009). A review of the national physical activity plans of six countries. *Journal of Physical Activity and Health, 6*(Suppl. 2), S245–S264.

Bors, P., Dessauer, M., Bell, R., Wilkerson, R., Lee, J., & Strunk, S. (2009). The Active Living by Design national program: Community initiatives and lessons learned. *American Journal of Preventive Medicine, 37*(6, Suppl. 2), S313–S321.

Bronfenbrenner, U. (1979). *The ecology of human development*. Cambridge, MA: Harvard University Press.

Bull, S., Eakin, E., Reeves, M., & Kimberly, R. (2006). Multi-level support for physical activity and healthy eating. *Journal of Advanced Nursing, 54*, 585–593.

Canadian Public Health Association. (1986). *Ottawa Charter for Health Promotion*. Ottawa: Author.

Cao, X. Y., Mokhtarian, P. L., & Handy, S. L. (2009). Examining the impacts of residential self-selection on travel behaviour: A focus on empirical findings. *Transport Reviews, 29*, 359–395.

Carlson, J. A., Sallis, J. F., Conway, T. L., Saelens, B. E., Frank, L. D., Kerr, J., ... King, A. C. (2012). Interactions between psychosocial and built environment factors in explaining older adults' physical activity. *Preventive Medicine, 54*(1), 68–73.

Cohen, D. A., Scribner, R. A., & Farley, T. A. (2000). A structural model of health behavior: A pragmatic approach to explain and influence health behaviors at the population level. *Preventive Medicine, 30*, 146–154.

De Bourdeaudhuij, I., Sallis, J. F., & Saelens, B. E. (2003). Environmental correlates of physical activity in a sample of Belgian adults. *American Journal of Health Promotion, 18*, 83–92.

Ding, D., Sallis, J. F., Conway, T. L., Saelens, B. E., Frank, L. D., Cain, K. L., & Slymen, D. J. (2012). Interactive effects of built environment and psychosocial attributes on physical activity: A test of ecological models. *Annals of Behavioral Medicine, 44*(3), 365–74.

Ding, D., Sugiyama, T., Winkler, E., Cerin, E., Wijndaele, K., & Owen, N. (2012). Correlates of change in adults' television viewing time: A four-year follow-up study. *Medicine & Science in Sports & Exercise, 44*, 1287–1292.

Finegood, D. T. (2011). The complex systems science of obesity. In J. Cawley (Ed.), *The Oxford handbook of the social science of obesity* (pp. 208–236). New York: Oxford University Press.

Fisher, E. B., Brownson, C. A., O'Toole, M. L., Shetty, G., Anwuri, V. V., & Glasgow, R. E. (2005). Ecologic approaches to self management: The case of diabetes. *American Journal of Public Health, 95*(9), 1523–1535.

Fisher, E. B., Brownson, R. C., Heath, A. C., Luke, D. A., & Sumner, W., II. (2004). Cigarette smoking. In J. Raczynski, L. Bradley, & L. Leviton (Eds.), *Health behavior handbook* (Vol. 2, pp. 75–120). Washington, DC: American Psychological Association.

Flay, B. R., & Petraitis, J. (1994). The theory of triadic influence: A new theory of health behavior with implications for preventive interventions. In G. S. Albrecht (Ed.), *Advances in medical sociology: A reconsideration of models of health behavior change* (Vol. 4, pp. 19–44). Greenwich, CT: JAI Press.

Frank, L. D., Sallis, J. F., Saelens, B. E., Leary, L., Cain, K., Conway, T. L., & Hess, P. M. (2010). The development of a walkability index: Application to the Neighborhood Quality of Life Study. *British Journal of Sports Medicine, 44*, 924–933.

Giles-Corti, B., Bull, F., Knuiman, M., McCormack, G., Van Niel, K., Timperio, A., ... Boruff, B. (2013). The influence of urban design on neighborhood walking following residential relocation: Longitudinal results from the RESIDE study. *Social Science & Medicine, 77*, 20–30.

Giles-Corti, B., & Donovan, R. J. (2002). The relative influence of individual, social, and physical environment determinants of physical activity. *Social Science & Medicine, 54*, 1793–1812.

Glanz, K., Sallis, J. F., Saelens, B. E., & Frank, L. D. (2005). Healthy nutrition environments: Concepts and measures. *American Journal of Health Promotion, 19*, 330–333.

Glass, T. A., & McAtee, M. J. (2006). Behavioral science at the crossroads in public health: Extending horizons, envisioning the future. *Social Science & Medicine, 62*(7), 1650–1671.

Golden, S. D., & Earp, J. A. (2012). Social ecological approaches to individuals and their contexts: Twenty years of health education & behavior health promotion interventions. *Health Education & Behavior, 39*(3), 364–372.

Green, L. W., Orleans, C. T., Ottoson, J. M., Cameron, R., Pierce, J. P., & Bettinghaus, E. P. (2006). Inferring strategies for disseminating physical activity policies, programs, and practices from the successes of tobacco control. *American Journal of Preventive Medicine, 31*(Suppl. 4), S66–S81.

Hammond, R. A. (2009). Complex systems modeling for obesity research. *Preventing Chronic Disease, 6*(3), A97.

Hovell, M. F., Wahlgren, D. R., & Gehrman, C. A. (2002). The behavioral ecological model: Integrating public health and behavioral science. In R. J. DeClemente, R. A. Crosby, & M. Kegler (Eds.), *Emerging theories in health promotion practice and research: Strategies for improving public health* (pp. 347–384). San Francisco: Jossey-Bass.

Institute of Medicine. (2001). *Health and behavior: The interplay of biological, behavioral, and societal influences.* Washington, DC: National Academies Press.

Kerr, J., Sallis, J. F., Owen, N., De Bourdeaudhuij, I., Cerin, E., Reis, R., ... Bracy, N. (2013). Advancing science and policy through a coordinated international study of physical activity and built environments: IPEN methods. *Journal of Physical Activity and Health, 10*(4), 581–601.

Kok, G., Gottlieb, N. H., Commers, M., & Smerecnik, C. (2008). The ecological approach in health promotion programs: A decade later. *American Journal of Health Promotion, 6*, 437–442.

Koplan, J. P., Liverman, C. T., & Kraak, V. I. (Eds.). (2005). *Preventing childhood obesity: Health in the balance.* Washington, DC: National Academies Press.

Lee, I.-M., Shiroma, E. J., Lobelo, F., Puska, P., Blair, S. N., Katzmarzyk, P. T., for the Lancet Physical Activity Series Working Group. (2012). Effect of physical activity on major non-communicable diseases worldwide: An analysis of burden of disease and life expectancy. *Lancet, 380*(9838), 219–229.

Lewin, K. (1951). *Field theory in social science: Selected theoretical papers* (D. Cartwright, ed.). New York: Harper.

Lohrmann, D. K. (2010). A complementary ecological model of the coordinated school health program. *Journal of School Health, 80*(1), 1–9.

Matsudo, S. M., Matsudo, V. R., Andrade, D. R., Araújo, T. L., Andrade, E., de Oliveira, L., & Braggion, G. (2004). Physical activity promotion: Experiences and evaluation of the Agita São Paulo program using the ecological mobile model. *Journal of Physical Activity and Health, 1*, 81–97.

McLeroy, K. R., Bibeau, D., Steckler, A., & Glanz, K. (1988). An ecological perspective on health promotion programs. *Health Education Quarterly, 15*(4), 351–377.

Mercer, S. L., Green, L. W., Rosenthal, A. C., Husten, C. G., Khan, L. K., & Dietz, W. H. (2003). Possible lessons from the tobacco experience for obesity control. *American Journal of Clinical Nutrition, 77*(Suppl. 4), 1073S–1082S.

Moos, R. H. (1980). Social-ecological perspectives on health. In G. C. Stone, F. Cohen, & N. E. Adler (Eds.), *Health psychology: A handbook* (pp. 523–547). San Francisco: Jossey-Bass.

Mumford, K. G., Contant, C. K., Weissman, J., Wolf, J., & Glanz, K. (2011). Changes in physical activity and travel behaviors in residents of a mixed-use development. *American Journal of Preventive Medicine, 41*(5), 504–507.

National Preventative Health Taskforce. (2009). *Australia: The healthiest country by 2020: National Preventative Health Strategy—the roadmap for action.* Canberra: Australian Government, Preventative Health Taskforce.

Ogilvie, D., Bull, F., Powell, J., Cooper, A. R., Brand, C., Mutrie, N., . . . iConnect Consortium. (2011). An applied ecological framework for evaluating infrastructure to promote walking and cycling: The iConnect study. *American Journal of Public Health, 101*(3), 473–481.

Owen, N. (2012). Sedentary behavior: Understanding and influencing adults' prolonged sitting time. *Preventive Medicine, 55*(6), 535–539.

Owen, N., Cerin, E., Leslie, E., duToit, L., Coffee, N., Frank, L. D., . . . Sallis, J. F. (2007). Neighborhood walkability and the walking behavior of Australian adults. *American Journal of Preventive Medicine, 33*(5), 387–395.

Owen, N., Sugiyama, T., Eakin, E. E., Gardiner, P. A., Tremblay, M. S., & Sallis J. F. (2011). Adults' sedentary behavior: Determinants and interventions. *American Journal of Preventive Medicine, 41*(2), 189–196.

Pucher, J., Dill, J., & Handy, S. (2010). Infrastructure, programs, and policies to increase bicycling: An international review. *Preventive Medicine, 50*(Suppl. 1), S106–S125.

Saelens, B. E., & Handy, S. L. (2008). Built environment correlates of walking: A review. *Medicine & Science in Sports & Exercise, 40*(Suppl. 7), S550–S566.

Saelens, B. E., Sallis, J. F., Frank, L. D., Cain, K. L., Conway, T. L., Chapman, J. E., . . . Kerr, J. (2012). Neighborhood environmental and psychosocial correlates of adults' physical activity. *Medicine & Science in Sports & Exercise, 44*(4), 637–646.

Sallis, J. F., Bowles, H. R., Bauman, A. E., Ainsworth, B. E., Bull, F. C., Craig, C. L., . . . Bergman, P. (2009). Neighborhood environments and physical activity among adults in 11 countries. *American Journal of Preventive Medicine, 36*, 484–490.

Sallis, J. F., Cervero, R. B., Ascher, W., Henderson, K. A., Kraft, M. K., & Kerr, J. (2006). An ecological approach to creating active living communities. *Annual Review of Public Health, 27,* 297–322.

Sallis, J. F., & Green, L. W. (2012). Active Living by Design and its evaluation: Contributions to science. *American Journal of Preventive Medicine, 43*(5, Suppl. 4), S410–S412.

Sallis, J. F., & Owen, N. (2002). Ecological models of health behavior. In K. Glanz, B. K. Rimer, & F. M. Lewis (Eds.), *Health behavior and health education: Theory, research, and practice* (3rd ed., pp. 462–484). San Francisco: Jossey-Bass.

Shimura, H., Sugiyama, T., Winkler, E.A.H., & Owen, N. (2012). High neighborhood walkability mitigates declines in middle-to-older aged adults' walking for transport. *Journal of Physical Activity and Health, 9*(7), 1004–1008.

Skinner, B. F. (1953). *Science and human behavior.* New York: Macmillan.

Stokols, D. (1992). Establishing and maintaining healthy environments: Toward a social ecology of health promotion. *American Psychologist, 47*(1), 6–22.

Stokols, D., Grzywacz, J. G., McMahan, S., & Phillips, K. (2003). Increasing the health promotive capacity of human environments. *American Journal of Health Promotion, 18*(1), 4–13.

Story, M., Kaphingst, K., Robinson-O'Brien, R., & Glanz, K. (2008). Creating healthy food and eating environments: Policy and environmental approaches. *Annual Review of Public Health, 29,* 253–272.

Sugiyama, T., Neuhaus, M., Cole, R., Giles-Corti, B., & Owen, N. (2012). Destination and route attributes associated with adults' walking: A review. *Medicine & Science in Sports & Exercise, 44,* 1275–1286.

Sugiyama, T., Salmon, J., Dunstan, D. W., Bauman, A. E., & Owen, N. (2007). Neighborhood walkability and TV viewing time among Australian adults. *American Journal of Preventive Medicine, 33,* 444–449.

UK Government Office for Science. (2007). *Tackling obesities: Future choices–project report* (2nd ed.). Retrieved from https://www.gov.uk/government/publications/reducing-obesity-future-choices

U.S. Department of Health and Human Services. (2010). *Healthy People 2020.* Retrieved from https://www.healthypeople.gov

Van Dyck, D., Cerin, E., Conway, T. L., De Bourdeaudhuij, I., Owen, N., Kerr, J., ... Sallis, J. F. (2012a). Associations between perceived neighborhood environmental attributes and adults' sedentary behavior: Findings from the USA, Australia and Belgium. *Social Science & Medicine, 74*(9), 1375–1384.

Van Dyck, D., Cerin, E., Conway, T. L., De Bourdeaudhuij, I., Owen, N., Kerr, J., ... Sallis, J. F. (2012b). Perceived neighborhood environmental attributes associated with adults' transport-related walking and cycling: Findings from the USA, Australia and Belgium. *International Journal of Behavioral Nutrition and Physical Activity, 9,* 70.

Van Dyck, D., Cerin, E., Conway, T. L., De Bourdeaudhuij, I., Owen, N., Kerr, J., ... Sallis, J. F. (2013). Perceived neighborhood environmental attributes associated with adults' leisure-time physical activity: Findings from Belgium, Australia and the USA. *Health & Place, 19,* 59–68.

Van Dyck, D., Cerin, E., Conway, T. L., De Bourdeaudhuij, I., Owen, N., Kerr, J., ... Sallis, J. F. (2014). Interacting psychosocial and environmental correlates of leisure-time physical activity: A three-country study. *Health Psychology, 33*(7), 699–709.

Wicker, A. W. (1979). *An introduction to ecological psychology.* Monterey, CA: Brooks/Cole.

World Health Organization. (2003). *WHO Framework Convention on Tobacco Control.* Geneva: Author.

World Health Organization. (2004). *Global strategy on diet, physical activity and health.* Geneva: Author.

Yang, L., Sahlqvist, S., McMinn, A., Griffin, S. J., & Ogilvie, D. (2010). Interventions to promote cycling: Systematic review. *BMJ, 341,* c5293.

MODELS OF INDIVIDUAL HEALTH BEHAVIOR

CHAPTER 4

INTRODUCTION TO HEALTH BEHAVIOR THEORIES THAT FOCUS ON INDIVIDUALS

Barbara K. Rimer
Noel T. Brewer

The chapters in Part Two address the Health Belief Model (HBM), the Theory of Planned Behavior (TPB)/Theory of Reasoned Action (TRA) and the companion Integrated Behavioral Model (IBM), and the Transtheoretical Model (TTM). These theories can help researchers and practitioners to identify antecedents to health behaviors and to design and evaluate effective health behavior change interventions. Theories covered in this section have some common constructs and somewhat different strengths and limitations. All have weathered the test of time. The TRA/TPB/IBM and the HBM share the assumption that health behaviors reflect expected value. Behavioral motivation and barriers to change are inherent in all the models, although not always explicitly stated. While the theories reviewed here are robust, many interesting questions remain to be answered for each of these theories.

A Closer Look at Individual-Level Theories

Health Belief Model (HBM)

The HBM (see Chapter Five) has an intuitive logic and clearly stated central tenets. It was developed to answer the very practical question, why did people not seek

We thank Drs. Seth Noar and Neil Weinstein for their ideas and feedback on an earlier draft of this chapter and Dr. Pascal Sheeran for sharing unpublished manuscripts.

tuberculosis screening when it was available to them? The model assumes that people will engage in a health behavior or take a recommended action when they believe that doing so can reduce a threat that is both likely and would have severe consequences. Expectancy and value apply to the health threat (perceived likelihood and severity of harm) and the health behavior (perceived benefit of and barriers to taking action). Cues to action—a construct not based on expectancy or value—may be as diverse as medical symptoms, a doctor's recommendation, mailed reminders from a health plan, or a media campaign. Self-efficacy, a construct proposed well after the model was formulated, is also not derived directly from an expectancy-value approach. Although substantial research has shown that self-efficacy is a strong predictor of many health behaviors (see Chapter Nine), as Skinner and colleagues note in Chapter Five, no studies have examined the predictive utility achieved by adding self-efficacy to the HBM.

As Skinner, Tiro, and Champion discuss, constructs in the HBM have received substantial empirical support for their strength in predicting health behaviors in cross-sectional and, to some extent, experimental intervention studies (Albarracín et al., 2005). The construct of cues to action is perhaps unique among health behavior models, other than the Common Sense Model (Leventhal, Brissette, & Leventhal, 2003), in providing a specific place for the potent effect of health symptoms in motivating behavior.

The HBM is a parsimonious model, requiring as few as six questions to assess its key constructs. The model is a proven way to identify correlates of health behavior that may be important in behavior changes and is useful for informing intervention design and evaluation.

Theory of Planned Behavior (TPB), Theory of Reasoned Action (TRA), and Integrated Behavioral Model (IBM)

The TRA/TPB/IBM (Chapter Six) assume that attitudes, subjective norms, and perceived behavioral control all affect behavioral intentions, which in turn are linked to behavior. Because many important attitudes *are* changeable, they are ideal targets for intervention. The TRA first aimed to explain health and nonhealth behaviors, such as condom use, organ donation, and voting. Later models (TPB and IBM) retained this general focus.

The TRA/TPB/IBM provide a systematic method for identifying issues most important to decisions about performing specific behaviors. Appropriate measurement methods require precision and detailed preliminary work to assess the populations in which interventions are to be conducted. Behavioral intention measures should closely match the target behaviors. While potentially time consuming, this groundwork is especially important when intervening in new topic areas and with populations from different cultures, both in the United States and globally.

Longitudinal correlational studies have found strong intention-behavior relationships (Sheeran, 2002), while more rigorous experiments indicate small to moderate effects that still have substantive significance (Webb & Sheeran, 2006). Intentions are often an important step along the pathway to behavior change. However, because intentions do not always translate into behavior changes, they usually are not an adequate proxy for behavior change, especially in large behavior change trials. The TPB/TRA are well supported by data from laboratory experiments and health behavior intervention studies. When confronting the goal of large-scale behavior changes needed to reduce risks for AIDS, Fishbein (2000) extended the TRA/TPB to create the Integrated Behavioral Model (IBM). The IBM refines the conceptualization of perceived behavioral control by dividing it into two component parts, leaving self-efficacy early in the model to predict intentions, and specifying environmental constraints and skills as moderators of the intention-behavior pathway. More research is needed to determine the viability of this expanded model, but it appears promising.

The Transtheoretical Model (TTM)

The Transtheoretical Model (Chapter Seven) evolved from theories of psychoanalysis as a way to consolidate these varied approaches and to understand how people change health behaviors, such as smoking. The TTM quickly became one of the most widely used behavior change models.

The TTM posits that people are in different stages of readiness to make health behavior changes. The stages are qualitatively different with respect to the constructs and processes that move people closer to behavior. Thus, according to the TTM, people should receive interventions appropriate for their stage in the behavior change process. A persistent and still unresolved question is whether stage-matched interventions are more effective than those not matched on stage (e.g., Dijkstra, Conijn, & De Vries, 2006). The answer today still is very much, "it depends." Some studies have found support for the effectiveness of stage-matched over non-stage-matched interventions (Robinson & Vail, 2012), whereas other studies do not confirm such a conclusion (e.g., Aveyard, Massey, Parsons, Manaseki, & Griffin, 2009).

Among people who have yet to engage in a given health behavior, stage of change and behavioral intentions are often correlated highly, suggesting substantial overlap in the two constructs (de Vet, de Nooijer, De Vries, & Brug, 2007). In correlational studies, intention measures do as well as stages of change in predicting subsequent behavior (Abrams, Herzog, Emmons, & Linnan, 2000). For more detailed discussions of stage models, including the TTM, see work by others (Sutton, 2001; Weinstein, 2007; Weinstein & Rothman, 2005; West, 2005). As with measurement of behavioral intentions, stage change toward contemplation or preparation in the Transtheoretical Model (TTM) may be a reasonable proxy for actual behavior change in early studies. For most areas of study today, behavior should be the outcome of interest.

The inclusion of *processes* of change, a diverse set of activities that people naturally engage in, is a special strength of the TTM. While not interventions per se, data about processes of change used by individuals and populations can provide useful insights for intervention development. However, processes of change are often not assessed in TTM-based studies or practice applications, and it is not clear whether a subset of processes could be used rather than the full set (Marshall & Biddle, 2001). More methodological research is needed.

Commonalities and Differences Across the Theories

The theories in this section of the book have much in common. Perceived barriers inhibit behavior change in the HBM and TRA/TPB/IBM. Perceived risk is important in the HBM and, depending on the results of pilot work for a given study, may be important in the TPB.

In the TTM, analyses of processes of change can help in identifying strategies to overcome particular types of barriers. Self-efficacy is embodied in the TTM and IBM and included in updated versions of the HBM and TPB. Although not identical, the TTM's decisional balance construct, which reflects the tension between the pros and cons of behavior change, has some similarity to the concepts of barriers and benefits in the HBM. Both theories recognize that if the negatives, or barriers, associated with behavior change are greater than perceived benefits, the likelihood of change decreases. Intentions are explicit in the TRA/TBM and the IBM, but similar motivational constructs appear in the conceptualization of HBM (orientation toward health as a goal) and the stages of TTM, increasing readiness to make and maintain behavior changes. Greater attention should be paid to the ways that motivation is more or less likely to yield behavior in different settings and populations (Webb & Sheeran, 2006).

Measurement of key variables in each of the theories requires careful attention. Theory users should use standard questions and question formats, when available, and make their questions openly available through web-based repositories, an increasingly common practice. Doing so can benefit others engaged in theory testing and refinement. It is difficult to compare the results of one study to another when different measures are used.

Which Theory to Use?

We encourage health behavior students, researchers, and practitioners to use theories, to be explicit about the constructs they use, and to be critical consumers of health behavior theories. We suggest some strategies for choosing among health behavior theories that focus on individuals.

A starting point is to think about the specific behavior being studied or intervened on. Vaccination behavior, screening, and symptom-prompted health care seeking may fit especially well with the Health Belief Model, given its origins and inclusion of cues to action. HPV vaccination and colon cancer screening are timely applications provided in Chapter Five. Smoking cessation and habitual behaviors may be particularly well suited to the TTM, consistent with its development in studying the behavior of smokers who quit successfully. The TRA/TPB/IBM may be useful for deliberative behaviors that have a strong intention-behavior link (Webb & Sheeran, 2006). Chapter Six uses the example of using condoms to prevent HIV transmission in global settings. That said, the models in this section all could be adapted to study and intervene on the behaviors mentioned above and others.

Some theories have a finite set of well-defined constructs and thus are easier to use and apply. The HBM is one of these. For other health behavior theories, including the TRA/TPB/IBM, there are well-developed measurement tools for many different behaviors, but using them requires real commitment to data collection. Still, the knowledge gained through this process may be more than worth the added effort. Finally, some theories, like TTM, facilitate the transition from concepts and constructs to intervention strategies (Noar & Zimmerman, 2005).

The choice of theoretical constructs may be as important as selection of a particular theory. Certain constructs, drawn from theories in this section, may be more predictive of behavior change than others. For example, Sheeran, Harris, and Epton (2014) examined the roles of various constructs in behavior change. Interventions that successfully changed perceived severity led to small changes in health behavior. A bigger effect was achieved when the interventions also increased perceived likelihood. Interventions that changed self-efficacy led to even larger changes in health behaviors.

When choosing among individual-level theories, it is also important to consider the array of higher-level influences that affect health behaviors, including social determinants. Selective use of different interventions from multiple domains may create the strongest force for change. It is common for researchers and practitioners to combine or blend theories, an approach that can be fruitful when done systematically and thoughtfully. An important aid in doing so is the creation of a logic model, as described by Bartholomew and colleagues in Chapter Nineteen of this book. Thoughtful combinations of constructs may improve the effectiveness of interventions over those built upon the foundation of single theories.

Another useful strategy is to map measures directly onto intervention components (Michie, Johnston, Francis, Hardeman, & Eccles, 2008). A trial to increase repeat mammograms used several theories (including the HPM, TRA, TTM, and Goal-Directed Behavior) to guide intervention development (DeFrank et al., 2009; Gierisch et al., 2010). To check that the intervention and measures included all relevant constructs from these theories, the researchers created a table of key constructs and examined them in relation to each intervention's key components.

Challenges

The dominant health behavior theories that focus on individuals have remained remarkably similar for the past fifty years. Few studies have compared theories (Brewer & Gilkey, 2012). That is understandable, since doing so requires the inclusion of more measures than would be needed for a study based on one theory. However, comparative research is important for understanding the relative strength of different theories and their constructs.

Emotions can play an important role in health behavior, but they are not included in the theories in Part Two. Some researchers have called for a separate and more central role for affect (Fredrickson, 2000). Research suggests at least four ways that emotions affect decisions related to health: focusing people's attention on a threat, helping people choose among several courses of action, facilitating decisions about dissimilar outcomes such as money and health, and prompting people to spring into action (Peters, Lipkus, & Diefenbach, 2006; Sandberg & Connor, 2008). Emotions like anticipated regret from not taking a recommended health action may also influence health behaviors and are covered in the chapter on behavioral economics in this volume (Chapter Twenty).

The execution or implementation of behavior change and maintenance of change merits greater attention to interventions, though this is a special strength of the TTM. A growing body of work shows that implementation intentions may amplify the impact of behavior change interventions (Bargh, Gollwitzer, & Oettingen, 2010; Gollwitzer & Sheeran, 2006; Webb & Sheeran, 2005, 2006). *Implementation intention* interventions encourage people to specify exactly when and under what conditions they will engage in a particular behavior (e.g., using if-then statements to identify what one will do if a particular situation occurs). Implementation intentions are a potent point of intervention, stronger than having people form more general intentions to act (Webb & Sheeran, 2006). Implementation intentions may also enable inclusion of other factors that may influence behavior, such as community context. This concept may be especially important in improving the predictive utility of behavioral theories, because implementation intentions appear to be one step closer to behavior.

The TTM explicitly includes maintenance of behavior changes, and the HBM and TRA/TPB/IBM do not exclude it. However, conceptualization and prediction of maintenance may require refinement of constructs and measures or other theories altogether (Rothman, 2000). One study found that the TPB was useful in predicting attendance at health screenings but did not reliably differentiate people who delayed attending or initially attended and then relapsed (Sheeran, Conner, & Norman, 2001). These apparent nuances are important, not only in classifying and describing health behaviors but also in developing effective interventions. Because maintenance of many health behaviors is required for optimal health benefit, and repeated, infrequent behaviors, such as mammography, are likely controlled by deliberative reasoning processes and past experiences, understanding the basis for behavioral enaction is important (Gierisch et al., 2010). The HBM and TRA/TPB/IBM identify factors that motivate behavior change, such as perceptions of disease susceptibility and severity, assessments of barriers and benefits to engaging in a behavior, self-efficacy, and intentions. The IBM also includes skills, an important precondition for enacting many behaviors. In a meta-analysis of internet-delivered interventions, Webb, Joseph, Yardley, and Michie (2010) found not only that studies indicating use of theory had larger effect sizes but also that TRA/TPB studies tended to have larger effect sizes than interventions based on TTM, which were in turn larger than SCT-based interventions.

The HBM, TTM, and TRA/TPB/IBM might be augmented by the Model of Goal-Directed Behavior (Bargh et al., 2010), which focuses on strategies for translating motivation to action and differentiating habitual behaviors, like getting regular exercise, from those performed infrequently, such as mammography. Model of Goal-Directed Behavior strategies include elaboration on the positive consequences of engaging in and negative consequences of not engaging in a behavior. As Webb and Sheeran (2010) remind us, theoretical constructs must be turned into intervention techniques and interventions. How well this is done may affect intervention outcomes.

Summary

Theories that emphasize individual health behaviors are important in understanding how to improve human health, but they are not the answer to all health problems. Even though many health problems are complex and warrant interventions at multiple levels (as Chapter Three, on ecological models, has discussed), understanding individuals' behaviors remains important.

Imagine a situation, unfortunately common, in which people in a village who lack access to clean water and sanitation are advised to use a new household water purification system.

It will prevent diarrheal diseases that are endemic and life threatening. The system is cheap, simple, and effective. But people in the village don't use it or use it initially and then stop. Then they're given household systems for free, but use is not sustained. When community workers visit households, they see the systems abandoned outside. Finally, the workers realize that they not only need to change individuals' beliefs and motivations but also must alter community norms through peer interventions and a social marketing campaign. Individual behavior is part of the equation for change, but it is not all there is. One must nearly always consider the relevant social and community contexts to understand where beliefs come from and find ways to change both beliefs and external constraints. Still, individuals exert volitional control over many of the health behaviors we seek to change, and understanding how to influence them is a strength of the theories in this section. Students, researchers, and health professionals should consider the nature of the health problem or condition on which they wish to intervene. That will then lead to selecting the most appropriate theory or theories and the corresponding constructs to implement interventions at one or multiple levels.

References

Abrams, D. B., Herzog, T. A., Emmons, K. M., & Linnan, L. (2000). Stages of change versus addiction: A replication and extension. *Nicotine Addiction Research, 2*(3), 223–229.

Albarracín, D., Gillette, J. C., Earl, A. N., Glasman, L. R., Durantini, M. R., & Ho, M. H. (2005). A test of major assumptions about behavior change: A comprehensive look at the effects of passive and active HIV prevention interventions since the beginning of the epidemic. *Psychological Bulletin, 131*(6), 856–897.

Aveyard, P., Massey, L., Parsons, A., Manaseki, S., & Griffin, C. (2009). The effect of transtheoretical model based interventions on smoking cessation. *Social Science & Medicine, 68*(3), 397–403.

Bargh, J. A., Gollwitzer, P. M., & Oettingen, G. (2010). Motivation. In S. T. Fiske & G. Lindzay (Eds.), *Handbook on Social Psychology* (5th ed.). Hoboken, NJ: Wiley.

Brewer, N. T., & Gilkey, M. B. (2012). Comparing theories of health behavior using data from longitudinal studies: A comment on Gerend and Shepherd. *Annals of Behavioral Medicine, 44*(2), 147–148.

DeFrank, J. T., Rimer, B. K., Gierisch, J. M., Bowling, J. M., Farrell, D., & Skinner, C. S. (2009). Impact of mailed and automated telephone reminders on receipt of repeat mammograms: A randomized controlled trial. *American Journal of Preventive Medicine, 36*(6), 459–467.

de Vet, E., de Nooijer, J., De Vries, N. K., & Brug, J. (2007). Comparing stage of change and behavioral intention to understand fruit intake. *Health Education Research, 22*(4), 599–608.

Dijkstra, A., Conijn, B., & De Vries, H. (2006). A match-mismatch test of a stage model of behaviour change in tobacco smoking. *Addiction, 101*(7), 1035–1043.

Fishbein, M. (2000). The role of theory in HIV prevention. *AIDS Care, 12*(3), 273–278.

Fredrickson, B. L. (2000). Cultivating positive emotions to optimize health and well-being. *Prevention and Treatment, 3*(1).

Gierisch, J. M., DeFrank, J. T., Bowling, J. M., Rimer, B. K., Matuszewski, J. M., Farrell, D., & Skinner, C. S. (2010). Finding the minimal intervention needed for sustained mammography adherence. *American Journal of Preventive Medicine, 39* (4), 334–344.

Gollwitzer, P. M., & Sheeran, P. (2006). Implementation intentions and goal achievement: A meta-analysis of effects and processes. *Advances in Experimental Social Psychology, 38*, 69–119.

Leventhal, H., Brissette, I., & Leventhal, E. A. (2003). The common-sense model of self-regulation of health and illness. In L. D. Cameron & H. Leventhal (Eds.), *The self-regulation of health and illness behaviour* (pp. 42–65). New York: Routledge.

Marshall, S. J., & Biddle, S. J. (2001). The transtheoretical model of behavior change: A meta-analysis of applications to physical activity and exercise. *Annals of Behavioral Medicine, 23*(4), 229–246.

Michie, S., Johnston, M., Francis, J., Hardeman, W., & Eccles, M. (2008). From theory to intervention: Mapping theoretically derived behavioural determinants to behaviour change techniques. *Applied Psychology, 57*(4), 660–680.

Noar, S. M., & Zimmerman, R. S. (2005). Health behavior theory and cumulative knowledge regarding health behaviors: Are we moving in the right direction? *Health Education Research, 20*(3), 275–290.

Peters, E., Lipkus, I., & Diefenbach, M. A. (2006). The functions of affect in health communications and in the construction of health preferences. *Journal of Communication, 56*(Suppl. 1), S140–S162.

Robinson, L. M., & Vail, S. R. (2012). An integrative review of adolescent smoking cessation using the transtheoretical model of change. *Journal of Pediatric Health Care, 26*(5), 336–345.

Rothman, A. J. (2000). Toward a theory-based analysis of behavioral maintenance. *Health Psychology, 19,* 64–69.

Sandberg, T., & Conner, M. (2008). Anticipated regret as an additional predictor in the theory of planned behaviour: A meta-analysis. *British Journal of Social Psychology, 47*(4), 589–606.

Sheeran, P. (2002). Intention-behavior relations: A conceptual and empirical review. *European Review of Social Psychology, 12*(1), 1–36.

Sheeran, P., Conner, M., & Norman, P. (2001). Can the theory of planned behavior explain patterns of health behavior change? *Health Psychology, 20*(1), 12–19.

Sheeran, P., Harris, P., & Epton, T. (2014). Does heightening risk appraisals change people's intentions and behavior? A meta-analytic review of the experimental evidence. *Psychological Bulletin, 140*(2), 511–543.

Sutton, S. (2001). Back to the drawing board? A review of applications of the transtheoretical model to substance use. *Addiction, 96*(1), 175–186.

Webb, T. L., Joseph, J., Yardley, L., & Michie, S. (2010). Using the Internet to promote health behavior change: A systematic review and meta-analysis of the impact of theoretical basis, use of behavior change techniques, and mode of delivery on efficacy. *Journal of Medical Internet Research, 12*(1), e4.

Webb, T. L., & Sheeran, P. (2005). Integrating goal theories to understand the achievement of personal goals. *European Journal of Social Psychology, 35,* 69–96.

Webb, T. L., & Sheeran, P. (2006). Does changing behavioral intentions engender behavior change? A meta-analysis of the experimental evidence. *Psychological Bulletin, 132*(2), 249–268.

Webb, T. L., & Sheeran, P. (2010). A viable, integrative framework for contemporary research in health psychology: Commentary on Hall and Fong's temporal self-regulation theory. *Health Psychology Review, 4,* 79–82.

Weinstein, N. D. (2007). Misleading tests of health behavior theories. *Annals of Behavioral Medicine, 33,* 1–10.

Weinstein, N. D., & Rothman, A. J. (2005). Revitalizing research on health behavior theories. *Health Education Research, 20*(3), 294–297.

West, R. (2005). Time for a change: Putting the transtheoretical (stages of change) model to rest. *Addiction, 100,* 1036–1039.

CHAPTER 5

THE HEALTH BELIEF MODEL

Celette Sugg Skinner
Jasmin Tiro
Victoria L. Champion

Since the 1950s, the Health Belief Model (HBM) has been one of the most widely used conceptual frameworks in health behavior research, both to explain change of health-related behaviors and as a guiding framework for interventions. Over the decades, the HBM has been expanded, compared, and contrasted to other frameworks and used to inform interventions to change health behavior.

In this chapter, we review the HBM's historical development, core constructs, hypotheses, relationships of constructs to each other and to specific health behaviors, and empirical evidence. The HBM has been used with many different behaviors. We provide in-depth examples from interventions to increase colon cancer screening and descriptive/correlational studies using HBM constructs to understand HPV vaccine uptake. Finally, we discuss how researchers can advance understanding and use of the HBM to predict behavior and the theory's utility in designing health behavior interventions. We also discuss limitations of the theory.

KEY POINTS

This chapter will:

- Discuss origins of the Health Belief Model (HBM) and its relationship to psychosocial theories.

- Describe key components and critical assumptions of the HBM.

- Present empirical evidence about the HBM.

- Give examples of applications of the HBM to colorectal cancer screening and human papillomavirus (HPV) vaccination.

Background on the Health Belief Model

Origins of the Health Belief Model

The Health Belief Model was developed in the 1950s by social psychologists in the U.S. Public Health Service to explain the widespread failure of people to participate in programs to prevent and detect disease (Hochbaum, 1958; Rosenstock, 1960). At that time, researchers and health professionals were concerned because few people were getting screened for tuberculosis (TB), even though mobile X-ray vans came to their neighborhoods. Later, the model was extended to study people's behavioral responses to opportunities to detect diseases when people are treatable and potentially curable and when diagnosed with illnesses. Research on response to illnesses has focused particularly on adherence to medical regimens that would alleviate symptoms (Becker, 1974; Kirscht, 1974). The HBM's constructs were built on tenets of Cognitive Theory, briefly reviewed below.

During the first half of the twentieth century, social psychologists developed two major approaches for explaining behavior: Stimulus-Response Theory (Watson, 1925) and Cognitive Theory (Lewin, 1951; Tolman, 1932). Stimulus-response theorists believed that events (termed *reinforcements*) affect physiological drives that activate behavior. B. F. Skinner formulated the widely accepted hypothesis that frequency of a behavior is determined by its consequences or reinforcements (Skinner, 1938). For Skinner, the mere temporal association between a behavior and an immediately following reward was thought to be sufficient to increase the probability that the behavior would be repeated. According to Stimulus-Response Theory, behavior is automatic and does not require mental processes, such as *reasoning* or *thinking*.

Conversely, cognitive theorists believed that reinforcements operated by influencing expectations rather than by influencing behavior directly. Mental processes such as thinking, reasoning, hypothesizing, or expecting are critical components of cognitive theories, which are often termed *value-expectancy* models, because they propose that behavior is a function of the degree to which individuals *value* an outcome and their assessment of the probability, or *expectation*, that a particular action will achieve that outcome (Kohler, 1925; Lewin, Dembo, Festinger, & Sears, 1944). For health-related behaviors, the *value* is avoiding illnesses and staying or getting well. The *expectation* is that a specific health action may prevent (or ameliorate) an illness or condition for which people believe they might be at risk.

Key Components of the HBM

The Health Belief Model contains several primary components (or constructs) that predict whether and why people will take action to prevent, detect, or control illness conditions. These constructs include perceived *susceptibility*, perceived *severity*, perceived *benefits* and *barriers* to engaging in a behavior, *cues to action*, and *self-efficacy*. Self-efficacy is rooted in Bandura's Social Cognitive Theory which, unlike other concurrent theories, emphasizes the role of learning and human agency in behavior. That is, according to Social Learning Theory, behavior is guided by cognitive and affective factors as well as biological and external events (Bandura, 2005). (See Chapter Nine for an extended discussion of self-efficacy.) Findings from Hochbaum's (1958) initial study of participation in TB screening were striking. Among individuals who believed that they were more susceptible to tuberculosis and that there were benefits from early detection, 82 percent had at least one voluntary chest X-ray. In contrast, only 21 percent of those who perceived lower personal susceptibility and benefits obtained X-rays.

The overall premise of the HBM is that people are likely to engage in a health behavior if they believe that:

1. They are susceptible to a condition (at risk for a disease).

2. The condition could have potentially serious consequences.

3. A course of action (behavior) available to them could be of benefit in reducing either their susceptibility to or the severity of the condition.

4. There are benefits to taking action.

5. Their perceived barriers (or costs) are outweighed by the benefits and are not strong enough to prevent action.

The model applies to behaviors with the potential to reduce risk of developing a disease as well as the effects of an existing disease (e.g., medication adherence). Definitions of HBM constructs are summarized in Table 5.1. Figure 5.1 illustrates relationships among constructs.

Perceived susceptibility is defined as belief about the likelihood of getting a disease or condition. For instance, a woman must believe that she is at risk of getting colon cancer before she is willing to take action by getting screened.

Perceived severity is a belief about the seriousness of contracting an illness or condition or of leaving it untreated, including physical consequences (e.g., death, disability, and pain) and social consequences (e.g., having the ability to work, maintaining relationships with others, or feeling stigmatized).

Perceived threat is the construct formed by the combination of susceptibility and severity. Perceived susceptibility should be multiplied by perceived severity to calculate perceived threat; thus if either of these components is zero, the perceived threat would be zero.

Perceived benefits are beliefs about positive features or advantages of a recommended action to reduce threat. These benefits might reduce threat of a disease or its consequences. Other non-health-related benefits might be tangible (such as the financial savings related to quitting smoking) or social (such as the satisfaction that may come from doing what a physician recommends or pleasing a family member who has expressed concern about one's lung cancer risk).

Perceived barriers are defined as possible obstacles to taking action, which can include negative consequences resulting from an action. These perceived obstacles and negative consequences impede action or subsequent engagement in the behavior. Obstacles may include inconvenience, cost, or fear of a screening procedure. Consequences may be tangible ("if I quit, I will be ridiculed by my still-smoking friends") or psychological ("trying to quit smoking might cause me to become anxious").

Cues to action. Early formulations of the HBM included the concept of cues that can trigger actions. For example, Hochbaum (1958) proposed that perceived susceptibility and perceived benefits were relevant only when activated by other factors he termed *cues* to instigate action. Cues could be internal (e.g., feeling a symptom that increased perceived threat) or external (e.g., media publicity, a recommendation from a physician during an office visit, receipt of a free sample, or even a friend's diagnosis). Cues have not been well defined (Hochbaum, 1958) nor systematically studied. This is a deficit in our understanding of the HBM.

Strecher and Rosenstock (1997) suggested that cues operate mainly through perceived threat. A painful sunburn might prompt one to feel at increased risk of skin cancer and to

Table 5.1   Key HBM Components, Conceptual Definitions, and Intervention Strategies

Concepts	Concept Definition	Intervention Strategy to Influence Concept
Perceived susceptibility	Beliefs about the likelihood of getting a disease or condition	• Define population(s) at risk and risk, and levels. • Personalize risk based on person's individual characteristics or behaviors. • Make an individual's perceptions more consistent with his or her actual risk.
Perceived severity	Beliefs about the seriousness of contracting a disease or condition, including consequences	• Specify consequences of risks and conditions. • Trigger emotions like distress and regret with images.
Perceived benefits	Beliefs about the positive aspects of adopting a health behavior (e.g., efficacy of the behavior for reducing risk or serious consequences)	• Shift individual's perspective by highlighting others' beliefs about the behavior and its effects. • Provide knowledge and arguments in favor of the behavior.
Perceived barriers	Beliefs about obstacles to performing a behavior, and the negative aspects (both tangible and psychological costs) of adopting a health behavior	• Identify and reduce perceived barriers through reassurance, correction of misinformation, incentives, and assistance.
Cues to action	Internal or external factors that could trigger the health behavior	• Promote awareness. • Use appropriate reminder and recall systems.
Self-efficacy	Beliefs that one can perform the recommended health behavior (confidence)	• Provide training and guidance in performing the recommended action. • Use progressive goal setting. • Give verbal reinforcement. • Demonstrate or model desired behaviors. • Reduce anxiety about taking action.

add sunscreen to the shopping list. Hochbaum also suggested scenarios through which a cue directly prompted behaviors, without operating through beliefs. His often-used classroom example was a point-of-purchase display at the drugstore counter that prompts a person to throw a tube of sunscreen in his basket, without changing his perceptions. That is, the person believed in the benefits of sunscreen but would have left the store without it were it not for the prompt and easy access at the cash register.

Other variables. An assumption of HBM is that demographic, structural, and psychosocial factors may affect beliefs and indirectly influence health behaviors. For example, sociodemographic factors, such as educational attainment, can indirectly influence behaviors by altering perceptions of susceptibility, severity, benefits, and barriers (Rosenstock, 1974; Salloway, Pletcher, & Collins, 1978). However, the model does not specify *how* such factors operate or interact with other constructs. This is a major gap in the HBM.

Efficacy expectations. Years after the Health Belief Model was developed, Bandura articulated the constructs of self-efficacy and outcome efficacy expectations. (See Chapter Nine for a more thorough discussion of self-efficacy.) *Outcome efficacy*—beliefs about the extent to which a particular behavior will lead to a certain outcome (Bandura, 1997, 1999)—is similar to the HBM construct of perceived benefits. But the construct of *self-efficacy*—the conviction that one can successfully execute a behavior—was not clearly represented by an HBM construct (although lack of self-efficacy was sometimes added as a barrier to taking action) (Mahoney, Thombs, & Ford, 1995). In 1988, Rosenstock, Strecher, and Becker suggested that self-efficacy be added to the HBM as a separate construct.

Operationalization of the HBM (Critical Assumptions and Hypotheses)

Health Belief Model components are depicted in Figure 5.1. Arrows indicate pathways through which constructs are linked to each other and to health behaviors. As shown, sociodemographic variables, such as age, sex, race, education, or socioeconomic issues, such as insurance status, may moderate relationships between health beliefs and health behaviors. For example, because cancer is more prevalent among older people, a person's age may moderate the relationship between perceived threat and cancer screening behavior, with the result that older individuals may believe themselves to be at greater risk for cancer and rate cancer as a more severe disease than younger adults do. Gender may moderate the effects of perceived susceptibility

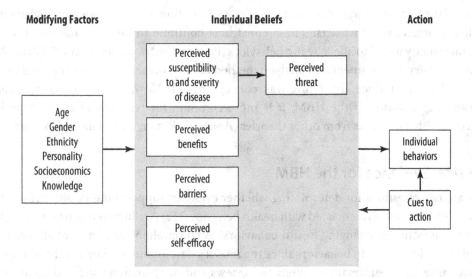

Figure 5.1 Components of the Health Belief Model

and benefits on HPV vaccination because females are more aware of the link between HPV infection and cervical cancer, whereas males may not know that HPV infection can lead to cancers that affect males, such as anal, penile, and oropharyngeal cancers. Cues to action may affect health behaviors either directly or indirectly through their influence on health beliefs.

The HBM clearly specifies that health beliefs collectively affect behaviors, but precise combinations, weights, and relationships among variables are not delineated (Abraham & Sheeran, 2005). This ambiguity has led to variation in how the HBM is applied in research. For example, while many studies have evaluated the direct path of beliefs to a given health behavior, others have tested mathematical combinations of constructs that were not part of the model's original specifications.

Some researchers have evaluated whether barriers should be subtracted from benefits (Becker & Maiman, 1975). They have argued that, conceptually, a kind of unconscious, cost-benefit analysis occurs wherein individuals weigh the behavior's expected benefits against perceived barriers: "It could help me, but it may be expensive, painful, unpopular, unpleasant, or inconvenient," and so forth. This combination of benefits and barriers is similar to the Transtheoretical Model's proposition that pros and cons are weighed against each other to form a single decisional balance score. (See Chapter Seven for a more thorough discussion of decisional balance defined as weighing the pros/benefits against the cons/barriers of a health behavior.) In contrast, Weinstein (1988) argued that benefits and barriers are qualitatively different and should be treated as distinct constructs with the potential to have different pathways linking them to other HBM constructs and behavior. Weinstein's position has been borne out in the HBM context through psychometric testing of barrier and benefit scales, showing that they act as separate factors (Champion, 1984, 1993, 1999; Champion & Scott, 1997; Tiro et al., 2005). Recent studies using structural equation modeling to test multiple pathways also show that benefits and barriers have independent effects on behavior (Gerend & Shepherd, 2012; Murphy, Vernon, Diamond, & Tiro, 2014).

The HBM initially was designed to explain adoption of health-related behaviors by identifying predictive constructs. These constructs continue to be used, because they have been consistently found to affect health behaviors (Painter, Borba, Hynes, Mays, & Glanz, 2008). However, theory development and analytic methods to test theories have become significantly more sophisticated since the HBM was conceptualized. Now, instead of comprehensive application and testing of the HBM, it is more common for researchers to combine HBM constructs with constructs from other theories (Brewer & Rimer, 2008; Glanz & Bishop, 2010).

Empirical Evidence for the HBM

There are two questions for determining whether evidence supports the Health Belief Model: (1) Are HBM constructs associated with health behaviors? (2) Are interventions targeting HBM constructs effective in changing health behaviors? A comprehensive review of all work using the HBM to address health behaviors since the model's development is beyond the scope of this chapter. Instead, we summarize systematic reviews and meta-analyses focused on answering these two key questions. We also describe limitations in the model's application.

Do HBM Constructs Influence Health Behaviors?

Critical reviews of the HBM's predictive validity were published at four different times and covered different studies. In addition, each review used slightly different methods (Table 5.2) and, because they were published at different times (Carpenter, 2010; Harrison, Mullen, & Green, 1992; Janz & Becker, 1984; Zimmerman & Vernberg, 1994), included different sets of studies. Janz and Becker (1984) and Zimmerman and Vernberg (1994) calculated a significance ratio for each construct, defined as the number of studies that found a significant association divided by the total number of studies measuring the construct. Zimmerman and Vernberg (1994) examined the model as a whole (e.g., all the constructs added together) for predicting behavior. Carpenter covered the literature from 1982 to 2007 and focused on moderators. Three of the four reviews (Carpenter, 2010; Harrison et al., 1992; Zimmerman & Vernberg, 1994) calculated a weighted mean effect size, which is a summary measure of the magnitude of each construct's relationship with behaviors, taking into account differences in studies' sample size and design. All of these reviewers were interested in quantifying each construct's direct effects on behaviors and did not examine whether HBM constructs also have indirect effects on behavior through other variables. Collectively, these quantitative reviews have combined the results of more than eighty-nine studies for an overall assessment of the model's performance.

Results of these critical reviews have provided substantial empirical support for HBM constructs, from both prospective and retrospective research. However, the magnitude of each of the constructs' effects is small (Table 5.2 summarizes the range of effects). *Perceived barriers* are the most powerful single construct predictor across all studies and behaviors (Carpenter, 2010; Harrison et al., 1992). *Perceived benefits* are the second most important construct, with the magnitude of effect higher for prevention and risk reduction behaviors (influenza vaccination, child safety restraints) versus treatment behaviors (adherence to a drug or medical regimen). *Perceived susceptibility* follows the same pattern as benefits, being a stronger predictor of preventive health behaviors (Janz & Becker, 1984), most of which are one-time or periodic actions, like having a screening test, rather than behaviors like smoking cessation or physical activity that must be maintained over time. Janz and Becker (1984) and Harrison et al. (1992) concluded that perceived severity is the weakest predictor, whereas Carpenter (2010) identified susceptibility as weakest.

It is unclear why susceptibility and benefits differ in magnitude across the various analyses. An explanation may lie, in part, in the debate whether perceived susceptibility and severity should be combined additively or multiplicatively to create the overarching construct of perceived threat. Lewis (1994) proposed a multiplicative combination (or interaction) where severity has to achieve a certain threshold to influence health behavior. Once that severity threshold has been reached, perhaps only susceptibility predicts behavior (threat = susceptibility + [susceptibility × severity]). This hypothesis might explain why studies that have tested only direct pathways between HBM constructs and behaviors found that severity had weak or nonexistent predictive power (Carpenter, 2010; Janz & Becker, 1984). Others have suggested that low variance in perceived severity (e.g., most individuals consider diseases like cancer to be very severe) empirically leads to small effect sizes (Harrison et al., 1992).

Table 5.2 Summary Measures from Four Critical Reviews of HBM Constructs

Review (Publication Year)	Study Selection Process	Study N/ Participant N	Summary Measure[2]	Perceived Susceptibility	Perceived Severity	Perceived Benefits	Perceived Barriers
Janz & Becker (1984)	Cross-sectional and longitudinal studies published between 1974 and 1984 that measured *at least 1* of the HBM constructs	46 studies[1]/Not reported	Significance ratio[2]	30/37 (81%)	24/37 (65%)	29/37 (78%)	25/28 (89%)
Zimmerman & Vernberg (1994)	Cross-sectional and longitudinal studies published between 1980 and 1991 that measured *at least 1* of the HBM constructs	30 studies[1]/Not reported	Significance ratio[2]	9/25 (36%)	6/22 (27%)	10/18 (56%)	10/17 (59%)
			Weighted mean effect size[2] measured as β (beta) or Pearson's r	0.37^3	0.18^3	0.13^3	0.52^3
Harrison et al. (1992)	Cross-sectional and longitudinal studies published between 1966 and 1987 that measured *all 4* HBM constructs	16 studies/ 3,515 adults	Weighted mean effect size[2] measured as Pearson's r	0.15	0.08	0.13	−0.21
Carpenter et al. (2010)	Longitudinal non-intervention studies published between 1982 and 2007 that measured *at least 2* of the HBM constructs	18 studies/ 2,702 adults	Weighted mean effect size[2] measured as Pearson's r	0.15^3	0.05^3	0.27^3	0.30^3

Note: The four critical reviews covered overlapping time periods; some studies were included in two or more reviews.

[1] Some studies included in the review did not measure all of the HBM constructs.

[2] The critical reviews used two different summary measures (significance ratio and mean effect size) to evaluate whether HBM constructs were good predictors of behavior. *Significance ratio* is the number of significant findings for each construct divided by the total number of studies measuring the construct. *Mean effect size* is the average magnitude of a relationship between HBM construct and behavioral outcome across all studies, weighted by the number of individuals in each study.

[3] Of the 18 studies in the meta-analysis, the number included in the summary measure for perceived susceptibility was 18; for severity, 17; for benefits, 15; and for barriers, 17.

No reviews have evaluated the contribution of cues to action, due in part to the fact that few studies have explained whether or how cues were measured or used for intervention (Abraham & Sheeran, 2005). Finally, no reviews have evaluated whether the addition of self-efficacy has increased the HBM's predictive validity. This is an important gap.

Are Interventions That Use HBM Effective at Changing Health Behaviors?

The fact that HBM constructs are fairly intuitive has made the use of this model popular in community-based interventions conducted among underserved groups with lower levels of formal education, and with interventions delivered by lay health advisors who assess their peers' HBM-related perceptions—often with questions such as, "What is the main reason you would/would not [engage in the health behavior]?"—and who then address those factors and facilitate behavior change (Campbell et al., 2004; Earp et al., 2002). The constructs are perhaps more intuitive than those of other models because they are relatively easily defined and related to real-life experiences. HBM constructs have been used as tailoring variables not only in face-to-face communications but also in computer-tailored interventions that are "intended to reach one specific person, based on characteristics . . . unique to that person, related to an outcome of interest, and derived from an individual assessment" (Kreuter & Farrell, 2000, p. 277). Noar, Benac, and Harris's 2007 review of tailored print communications found the HBM was second only to the Transtheoretical Model (Chapter Seven) in its use for tailoring.

Assessing an individual's perceived barriers to action is a fairly straightforward process. Intervention components to reduce specific barriers can then be designed and delivered to individuals for whom they are important. The HBM was developed such that interventions would be effective only if they addressed a person's *specific* perceptions about susceptibility, benefits, barriers, and efficacy. For example, people who already believe they are at risk for developing cancer do not need messages to convince them about their susceptibility. Those who want to get free HIV testing and know where to go but can't find a way to get there need interventions tailored to address transportation, not cost. Just as it is important to validly *measure* HBM constructs, tailoring technology has allowed interventions to *address* the HBM constructs most relevant for individuals. Noar et al. (2007) found that interventions tailored on self-efficacy were among those with largest effect sizes for behavior change, but that tailoring on susceptibility was associated with significantly decreased effects. The authors speculated, "It may be that in a number of health domains, messages that focus on increasing positive views and feelings toward a health behavior (e.g., attitudes), and those that increase one's confidence in performing the behavior (i.e., self-efficacy) are more motivating to health behavior change than messages that raise the threat of a disease," or that, "if most individuals in a given study believe that they have high perceived susceptibility but continue the behavior despite this, then perceived susceptibility may not be the most effective concept for tailoring because of a lack of variability" (Noar et al., p. 15). Unfortunately, this study did not assess effects associated with tailoring to particular perceived benefits or barriers.

In summary, reviews of empirical evidence of the HBM highlight several important issues. First, because cross-sectional and retrospective studies have found markedly larger effect sizes for all of the HBM constructs when compared to prospective studies, researchers should interpret cross-sectional studies with caution. For a discussion of how cross-sectional studies may overestimate strengths of relationships between HBM constructs and behavior, see Weinstein (2007). Also, there has been little testing of researchers' proposals to use mathematical combinations of HBM constructs, or explore more complex pathways linking HBM constructs to each other (Becker & Maiman, 1975; Lewis, 1994; Strecher, Champion, & Rosenstock, 1997). Although many studies demonstrate relationships of HBM constructs to various health behaviors, we still do not understand *how* the constructs operate to influence health behaviors.

Measurement of HBM Constructs

One of the most important limitations in both descriptive and intervention research using the Health Belief Model has been variability in measurement of its central constructs (Carpenter, 2010; Harrison et al., 1992; Janz & Becker, 1984). Several important principles have guided HBM measurement development. Construct definitions should be consistent with HBM theory as originally conceptualized. Measures also should be specific to the behavior being addressed (e.g., barriers to mammography may be quite different from barriers to colonoscopy) and relevant to the population among whom they will be used (e.g., groups with lower versus higher health literacy). To ensure content validity, it is important to measure the full range of factors that may influence behaviors. Formative research is often required to identify factors perceived as particular benefits, barriers, and susceptibility beliefs for particular health behaviors, among particular populations, and in particular settings. Once identified, these beliefs may be incorporated into scales that include multiple items for each construct. Using a scale rather than a single item reduces measurement error and increases the probability of including all relative components for each construct. However, scales should not be applied to different groups without being tested for reliability and validity. Cultural and population differences make applying scales without such examination prone to error. Despite notable exceptions (Champion, 1984, 1993; Champion & Scott, 1997; King et al., 2012; Rawl et al., 2001; Rawl, Menon, Champion, Foster, & Skinner, 2000; Russell, Champion, & Perkins, 2003; Vernon, Myers, & Tilley, 1997), it appears that most studies using the HBM have not conducted adequate reliability and validity of measures testing prior to research. This lack of scientific rigor in measurement stems in part from the model's lack of specificity regarding relationships among its constructs. A major component of construct validity in most models is the determination of relationships between constructs and the relationship of constructs to the behavior they are predicting.

Applications of the Health Belief Model

In this section, we discuss how the HBM has been applied to research on two health behaviors—for interventions to increase use of colorectal cancer (CRC) screening and, descriptively, for uptake of human papillomavirus (HPV) vaccination.

HBM and Colon Cancer Screening

Several reviews of colon cancer screening interventions were published between 2010 and 2012. Morrow, Dallo, and Julka (2010) reviewed community-based trials, while Naylor, Ward, and Polite (2012) focused on interventions for minority populations; Rawl, Menon, Burness, and Breslau (2012) evaluated all available randomized controlled trials, and Holden et al. (2010) looked at factors associated with appropriate use and quality of available screening tests. Only Rawl, Menon, et al. (2012) reported the interventions' theoretical frameworks, showing that, from 1997 to 2007, HBM was the most widely used theoretical model for interventions that were effective in increasing use of fecal occult blood testing (FOBT) and colonoscopy.

The positive finding from reviews of HBM constructs and screening tests led Rawl, Skinner, et al. (2012) to develop and test an HBM-based, tablet-based, interactive, computer-tailored intervention promoting colorectal cancer screening (CRC) to be used by African American patients while waiting for their primary care appointments. In a randomized trial, study participants waiting to see their providers were assigned to use the tailored, interactive program or to receive nontailored, usual care CRC screening information developed by the American Cancer Society.

The intervention program, titled *Colon Testing: Celebrate Life for Years to Come*, uses narrative vignettes that show friends interacting in the context of a fiftieth birthday party. The man celebrating his fiftieth birthday has recently been to see his doctor, who recommended CRC screening. The program's introductory scene shows friends around a table discussing birthdays and health as one ages. As the man's wife sets a birthday cake with lighted candles in front of her husband, a narrator says:

> Mr. Robert Gibson celebrates his fiftieth birthday today with his family and friends. Robert's in good health—he watches what he eats, stays active, and takes his blood pressure medicine. But there's something else he'll need to start doing to STAY healthy in the years ahead. Colon testing is something EVERYONE needs to think about when they get to be Robert's age. Some of his friends and family members have had their colon tested but others, like Robert, haven't even thought about it. Let's see what YOU think . . .

The interactive program then asks a number of questions based on HBM constructs. Based on users' responses, the program selects narration, graphics, and video from a library of all potential versions. The measures of HBM perceptions in the program were developed and tested for reliability and validity in Rawl and colleagues' previous research (Rawl et al., 2000, 2001). Program messages and graphics were developed through extensive formative research, input from a community advisory board, and pretesting with African American primary care patients to determine whether messages addressed the constructs as intended by intervention developers and were both understandable and culturally relevant. *Colon Testing: Celebrate Life for Years to Come* is described in detail elsewhere (Rawl, Skinner, et al., 2012). A few examples from the tailored message library follow.

Program users whose *perceived susceptibility* is so low they think they do not need screening receive messages emphasizing their personal risk factors. One of the messages, created for those with a close relative diagnosed with CRC, shows a graph with the number of affected relatives on the x axis and the percentage chance of getting CRC on the y axis. There is a stationary bar on the x axis at 6 percent—the risk of someone with no family history. Then, a second bar appears at 0 percent and grows to 18 percent—the risk for someone with a close relative diagnosed before the age of sixty. As users watch the second bar grow, the narrator says, "This picture shows how your chances of getting colon cancer go up when someone in your family has it." Messages for those without family history mention other risk factors, such as age and race. Therefore, in addition to tailored text, the messages were tailored in numeric percentages and in visual representations of magnitude.

There are also messages addressing potential *barriers*, *benefits*, and *self-efficacy*. In one example, those who say they would put off screening because they don't want to know if something is wrong see this dialogue between two of the programs' characters:

James   Why would I want to take a test to find something wrong? I don't go looking for trouble. If it ain't broke, don't fix it.

Emmett   I used to think the same way. But then, I had the test. All I know is if I hadn't had the test they wouldn't have found those two polyps that may have turned into cancer.

Program users who say a colonoscopy would be painful or embarrassing watch this dialogue:

Mary   It sounds to me like a colonoscopy would just hurt, and I would just be too embarrassed.

Patricia Well, you know Mary, I thought the same thing. I went, they gave me some medicine, I dozed off, when I woke up it was over. I didn't have time to be embarrassed. I didn't even know what had happened.

As hypothesized, participants in the randomized trial who received the interactive program tailored on HBM constructs had greater increases in perceived susceptibility and benefits and reductions in perceived barriers (Rawl, Skinner, et al., 2012) than those who received the nontailored material. They were also more likely to report discussions with their health care providers about CRC screening, perhaps consequentially, and to have provider recommendations for CRC screening documented in their electronic medical records (Christy et al., 2013). The intervention group also completed significantly more FOBTs compared to the group receiving usual care.

HBM and HPV Vaccine Adoption

Human papillomavirus (HPV) infections cause the overwhelming majority of cervical cancers—about 400,000 cases per year out of a total of 600,000 cases per year worldwide—and account for a large proportion of several other cancers, including oropharyngeal cancers, which are increasing among both males and females. Even before the first HPV vaccine was approved by the U.S. Food and Drug Administration in 2006, several investigators had examined HBM constructs' association with vaccine acceptability among mothers and their intentions to vaccinate their daughters (Brewer & Fazekas, 2007). Since the HPV vaccine was recommended for routine administration to adolescent and young adult females in 2006 (Markowitz et al., 2007) and extended to similar age males in 2011 (Dunne et al., 2011), fifteen studies have assessed one or more HBM constructs and actual vaccine uptake (Allen et al., 2009, 2010; Bastani et al., 2011; Brewer et al., 2011; Bynum, Brandt, Sharpe, Williams, & Kerr, 2011; Conroy et al., 2009; Gerend & Shepherd, 2012; Gerend, Weibley, & Bland, 2009; Juraskova, Bari, O'Brien, & McCaffery, 2011; Krawczyk et al., 2012; Licht et al., 2010; Manhart et al., 2011; Naleway et al., 2012; Reiter, Brewer, Gottlieb, McRee, & Smith, 2009; Roberts, Gerrard, Reimer, & Gibbons, 2010). Seven of the fifteen studies were explicitly designed to measure all five HBM constructs (Brewer et al., 2011; Bynum et al., 2011; Gerend & Shepherd, 2012; Juraskova et al., 2011; Krawczyk et al., 2012; Manhart et al., 2011; Reiter et al., 2009), whereas five measured selected HBM constructs along with constructs from other theories, such as the Theory of Planned Behavior, Social Cognitive Theory, and the Transtheoretical Model (Allen et al., 2009, 2010; Bastani et al., 2011; Gerend et al., 2009; Roberts et al., 2010). Most studies were descriptive, looking at constructs' direct association with initiation, defined as getting the first of the three-dose vaccination series, although Manhart et al. (2011) also examined three-dose series completion. Four studies used longitudinal designs (Brewer et al., 2011; Conroy et al., 2009; Gerend & Shepherd, 2012; Juraskova et al., 2011), with a range of two (Juraskova et al., 2011) to sixteen months (Brewer et al., 2011) between measurement of HBM constructs and vaccine behavior. Only Gerend and Shepherd (2012) and Juraskova et al. (2011) measured the HBM in the context of a vaccine-promotion intervention. Gerend and Shepherd (2012) used structural equation modeling to examine whether cues to action indirectly influenced behavior through susceptibility, benefits, and the perceived barrier of vaccine cost; the others assessed direct relationships between each HBM construct and vaccination behavior. Table 5.3 reports the significance ratios for perceived susceptibility, severity, benefits, barriers, and cues to action. Variations in the studies' comprehensiveness and quality of construct measurement may have affected findings.

Perceived susceptibility was measured most frequently, but inconsistent measurement may have contributed to discrepancies in findings. Half the studies used a multi-item scale with reported validity or reliability (Allen et al., 2009; Brewer et al., 2011; Bynum et al., 2011; Conroy et al., 2009; Gerend & Shepherd, 2012; Juraskova et al., 2011; Krawczyk et al., 2012). Several investigators used single items that measured perceptions of risks for different health outcomes—acquiring an HPV infection (Manhart et al., 2011), transmitting HPV (Licht et al., 2010), or developing cervical cancer (Naleway et al., 2012)—and under different conditions, such as risk given past sexual behavior (Bynum et al., 2011), risk relative to others (Bastani et al., 2011), or risk with versus without vaccination (Gerend et al., 2009; Roberts et al., 2010). Several cross-sectional studies measured perceived susceptibility postvaccination,

Table 5.3 Summary of Fifteen Studies Measuring HBM Constructs and HPV Vaccine Initiation

Summary Measure	Perceived Susceptibility	Perceived Severity	Perceived Benefits	Perceived Barriers	Cues to Action
Significance ratio[1]	7/10 (70%)	2/9 (22%)	4/10 (40%)	4/7 (57%)	5/7 (71%)

Note: The fifteen studies did not measure all of the HBM constructs. Three studies were not included in the significance ratio calculations because of their methods. Allen et al. (2009, 2010) used stage of adoption as the outcome variable. Naleway et al. (2012) surveyed only those who had initiated the vaccine series.
[1] *Significance ratio* is the number of significant findings for each construct divided by the total number of studies measuring the construct.

when susceptibility should have decreased (Weinstein, 2007). Thus it is not surprising that patterns of association between perceived susceptibility and vaccination were inconsistent. The significance ratio was 70 percent (Table 5.3), with five studies finding a positive association (Gerend & Shepherd, 2012; Gerend et al., 2009; Juraskova et al., 2011; Licht et al., 2010; Roberts et al., 2010), two finding negative associations (Krawczyk et al., 2012; Reiter et al., 2009), and three finding no associations (Bastani et al., 2011; Brewer et al., 2011; Bynum et al., 2011).

Perceived severity was assessed in eleven studies. Multi-item scales focused on seriousness of both HPV infection and cervical cancer. Among the nine studies that measured HPV vaccine initiation, most found no association between severity and HPV vaccine initiation (significance ratio = 22%).

Perceived benefits and barriers were measured in ten studies. Operational definitions of benefits mainly focused on the vaccine's effectiveness (significance ratio = 40%). However, investigators assessed a variety of potential barriers, including cost, difficulty finding a health care provider, concern about side effects, pain, and worry that the vaccine might cause fertility problems or encourage sexual activity at an earlier age. Most researchers looked at independent associations between each of these barriers and vaccination behavior. Two studies reported factor analyses to determine whether the barriers' responses could be combined into a summary score, but results showed that they did not load onto one latent factor and thus could not be used as a scale (Brewer et al., 2011; Gerend & Shepherd, 2012). As with susceptibility and benefits, findings for barriers were mixed (significance ratio = 57%).

Cues to action were explicitly measured in six studies, with four using a single-item measure—physician recommendation. While this is an incomplete assessment of cues in terms of the HBM developers' conceptualization described above, it mirrors measurement of cues for other behaviors (e.g., cancer screening). Physician recommendation was directly or indirectly associated with vaccine uptake in four of the six studies (Bynum et al., 2011; Gerend & Shepherd, 2012; Krawczyk et al., 2012; Reiter et al., 2009).

Summary of HBM Application Examples

These two examples of Health Belief Model application to colon cancer screening and HPV vaccination highlight the process of applying the model to new behaviors. Colon cancer screening has been available since the 1980s, although guidelines and recommended methods for screening have shifted over this time period (Levin et al., 2008; Lieberman, 2009; McFarland et al., 2008; U.S. Preventive Services Task Force, 2008; Whitlock, Lin, Liles, Beil, & Fu, 2008). In ensuing years, research has described HBM constructs associated with screening uptake, including specific perceived benefits and barriers associated with the different kinds of colon cancer testing options and among different populations. Measures of HBM constructs have been developed and tested, and interventions based on the HBM have been tested in randomized screening-promotion trials. However, HPV vaccines have been available and recommended only since 2006 for females and later for males (Markowitz et al., 2007). Most published research to date has been descriptive, to determine what constructs are associated with vaccination uptake. In these studies, measures and operational definitions of HBM constructs have varied widely, as has timing of measurement (e.g., some studies measured perceived susceptibility before vaccination with others measuring it after). Although results from a wave of intervention trials now under way will be published in the next few years, we currently lack examples of how HBM constructs are being operationalized for HPV vaccine promotion interventions and whether they are successful.

Challenges for Future HBM Research

The HBM has been used for more than half a century to predict health-related behaviors and inform the development of interventions to change behaviors. As indicated by the research reviewed here, the HBM has been useful in predicting and explaining cancer screening and HPV vaccination. Its intuitive conceptualizations have made its modifiable beliefs popular for use in interventions. HBM constructs are also often used in tailored interventions to modify individuals' beliefs. For instance, when individuals do not perceive benefits to an action, the interventions seek to strengthen their perception of benefits. Many studies have found that interventions tailored to address specific barriers predict adherence to recommended health behaviors.

However, even after all this model's use, we still know relatively little about relationships among HBM constructs, such as whether they all directly predict behavior or whether some beliefs mediate the relationships to behavior. (Notable recent exceptions are studies by Gerend et al., 2009, and Murphy et al., 2014). In addition, few have investigated factors that moderate HBM constructs' effect on behavior (e.g., Li et al., 2003). Key questions about the HBM remain. For example, does self-efficacy add unique variance for predicting behavior? Does self-efficacy influence behavior both directly and indirectly through barriers? Advances in statistical analysis, such as structural equation modeling, provide theorists and researchers who use and/or test theory with new opportunities to extend understanding about HBM relative to other commonly used health behavior theories featured in this edition of this book. New empirical studies evaluating unique contributions of HBM constructs and building consensus across theories (Noar & Zimmerman, 2005; Weinstein & Rothman, 2005) may further enhance our understanding of how HBM constructs affect behavior. This has the potential to advance even more effective use of the model in the future. For instance, although many studies have examined individual relationships between constructs and outcome behaviors, fewer have identified relationships between constructs or identified moderator or mediator effects. (See Brewer & Gilkey, 2012, and Weinstein, 2007, for further discussion about study designs and methods to test health behavior theories.)

Summary

In this chapter, we described origins of the Health Belief Model, reviewed and defined its key components and hypothesized relationships, summarized critical reviews of the HBM, and provided examples of how the HBM has been applied to colorectal cancer screening and HPV vaccination. The HBM is a model focused on cognitions that does not consider the emotional component of behavior. This latter component, along with cues to action and self-efficacy, should be more systematically incorporated into HBM research.

References

Abraham, C., & Sheeran, P. (2005). The health belief model. In M. Conner & P. Norman (Eds.), *Predicting health behavior* (2nd ed., pp. 28–80). Philadelphia: Open University Press.

Allen, J. D., Mohllajee, A. P., Shelton, R. C., Othus, M. K., Fontenot, H. B., & Hanna, R. (2009). Stage of adoption of the human papillomavirus vaccine among college women. *Preventive Medicine, 48,* 420–425.

Allen, J. D., Othus, M. K., Shelton, R. C., Li, Y., Norman, N., Tom, L., & del Carmen, M. G. (2010). Parental decision making about the HPV vaccine. *Cancer Epidemiology, Biomarkers and Prevention, 19*(9), 2187–2198.

Bandura, A. (1997). *Self-efficacy: The exercise of control.* New York: Freeman.

Bandura, A. (1999). *Social learning theory.* Englewood Cliffs, NJ: Prentice Hall.

Bandura, A. (2005). The primacy of self-regulation in health promotion. *Applied Psychology, 54*(2), 245–254.

Bastani, R., Glenn, B. A., Tsui, J., Chang, L. C., Marchand, E. J., Taylor, V. M., & Singhal, R. (2011). Understanding suboptimal human papillomavirus vaccine uptake among ethnic minority girls. *Cancer Epidemiology, Biomarkers and Prevention, 20*(7), 1463–1472.

Becker, M. H. (1974). The health belief model and personal health behavior. *Health Education Monographs, 2,* 409–419.

Becker, M. H., & Maiman, L. A. (1975). Sociobehavioral determinants of compliance with health and medical care recommendations. *Medical Care, 13*(1), 10–24.

Brewer, N. T., & Fazekas, K. I. (2007). Predictors of HPV vaccine acceptability: A theory-informed, systematic review. *Preventive Medicine, 45*(2–3), 107–114.

Brewer, N. T., & Gilkey, M. B. (2012). Comparing theories of health behavior using data from longitudinal studies: A comment on Gerend and Shepherd. *Annals of Behavioral Medicine, 44*(2), 147–148.

Brewer, N. T., Gottlieb, S. L., Reiter, P. L., McRee, A. L., Liddon, N., Markowitz, L., & Smith, J. S. (2011). Longitudinal predictors of human papillomavirus vaccine initiation among adolescent girls in a high-risk geographic area. *Sexually Transmitted Diseases, 38*(3), 197–204.

Brewer, N. T., & Rimer, B. K. (2008). Perspectives on theories of health behavior that focus on individuals. In K. Glanz, B. K. Rimer, & V. Viswanath (Eds.), *Health behavior and health education: Theory, research, and practice* (4th ed., pp. 149–165). San Francisco: Jossey Bass.

Bynum, S. A., Brandt, H. M., Sharpe, P. A., Williams, M. S., & Kerr, J. C. (2011). Working to close the gap: Identifying predictors of HPV vaccine uptake among young African American women. *Journal of Health Care for the Poor and Underserved, 22*(2), 549–561.

Campbell, M. K., James, A., Hudson, M. A., Carr, C., Jackson, E., Oakes, V., . . . Tessaro, I. (2004). Improving multiple behaviors for colorectal cancer prevention among African American church members. *Health Psychology, 23*(5), 492–502.

Carpenter, C. J. (2010). A meta-analysis of the effectiveness of health belief model variables in predicting behavior. *Health Communication, 25*(8), 661–669.

Champion, V. L. (1984). Instrument development for health belief model constructs. *Advances in Nursing Science, 6*(3), 73–85.

Champion, V. L. (1993). Instrument refinement for breast cancer screening behaviors. *Nursing Research, 42*(3), 139–143.

Champion, V. L. (1999). Revised susceptibility, benefits, and barriers scale for mammography screening. *Research in Nursing & Health, 22*(4), 341–348.

Champion, V. L., & Scott, C. R. (1997). Reliability and validity of breast cancer screening belief scales in African American women. *Nursing Research*, *46*(6), 331–337.

Christy, S. M., Perkins, S. M., Tong, Y., Krier, C., Champion, V. L., Skinner, C. S., . . . Rawl, S. M. (2013). Promoting colorectal cancer screening discussion: A randomized controlled trial. *American Journal of Preventive Medicine*, *44*(4), 325–329.

Conroy, K., Rosenthal, S. L., Zimet, G. D., Jin, Y., Bernstein, D. I., Glynn, S., & Kahn, J. A. (2009). Human papillomavirus vaccine uptake, predictors of vaccination, and self-reported barriers to vaccination. *Journal of Women's Health*, *18*(10), 1679–1686.

Dunne, E. F., Markowitz, L. E., Chesson, H., Curtis, C. R., Saraiya, M., Gee, J., & Unger, E. (2011). Recommendations on the use of quadrivalent human papillomavirus vaccine in males—Advisory Committee on Immunization Practices (ACIP), 2011. *Morbidity and Mortality Weekly Report*, *60*(50), 1705–1708.

Earp, J. A., Eng, E., O'Malley, M. S., Altpeter, M., Rauscher, G., Mayne, L., . . . Qaqish, B. (2002). Increasing use of mammography among older, rural African American women: Results from a community trial. *American Journal of Public Health*, *92*(4), 646–654.

Gerend, M. A., & Shepherd, J. E. (2012). Predicting human papillomavirus vaccine uptake in young adult women: Comparing the health belief model and theory of planned behavior. *Annals of Behavioral Medicine*, *44*(2), 171–180.

Gerend, M. A., Weibley, E., & Bland, H. (2009). Parental response to human papillomavirus vaccine availability: Uptake and intentions. *Journal of Adolescent Health*, *45*(5), 528–531.

Glanz, K., & Bishop, D. B. (2010). The role of behavioral science theory in development and implementation of public health interventions. *Annual Review of Public Health*, *31*, 399–418.

Harrison, J. A., Mullen, P. D., & Green, L. W. (1992). A meta-analysis of studies of the health belief model with adults. *Health Education Research*, *7*(1), 107–116.

Hochbaum, G. M. (1958). *Public participation in medical screening programs: A socio-psychological study*. Washington, DC: U.S. Department of Health, Education and Welfare.

Holden, D. J., Harris, R., Porterfield, D. S., Jonas, D. E., Morgan, L. C., Reuland, D., . . . Lyda-McDonald, B. (2010). Enhancing the use and quality of colorectal cancer screening. *Evidence Report/Technology Assessment*, *190*, 1–195.

Janz, N. K., & Becker, M. H. (1984). The health belief model: A decade later. *Health Education Quarterly*, *11*(1), 1–47.

Juraskova, I., Bari, R. A., O'Brien, M. T., & McCaffery, K. J. (2011). HPV vaccine promotion: Does referring to both cervical cancer and genital warts affect intended and actual vaccination behavior? *Women's Health Issues*, *21*(1), 71–79.

King, R. B., Champion, V. L., Chen, D., Gittler, M. S., Heinemann, A. W., Bode, R. K., & Semik, P. (2012). Development of a measure of skin care belief scales for persons with spinal cord injury. *Archives of Physical Medicine and Rehabilitation*, *93*(10), 1814–1821.

Kirscht, J. P. (1974). The health belief model and illness behavior. *Health Education & Behavior*, *2*(4), 387–408.

Kohler, W. (1925). *The mentality of apes*. New York: Harcourt Brace.

Krawczyk, A. L., Perez, S., Lau, E., Holcroft, C. A., Amsel, R., Knauper, B., & Rosberger, Z. (2012). Human papillomavirus vaccination intentions and uptake in college women. *Health Psychology*, *31*(5), 685–693.

Kreuter, M. W., & Farrell, D. (2000). *Tailoring health messages: Customizing communication with computer technology*. Mahwah, NJ: Erlbaum.

Levin, B., Lieberman, D. A., McFarland, B., Andrews, K. S., Brooks, D., Bond, J., . . . American College of Radiology Colon Cancer Committee. (2008). Screening and surveillance for the early detection of colorectal cancer and adenomatous polyps, 2008: A joint guideline from the American Cancer Society, the U.S. Multi-Society Task Force on Colorectal Cancer, and the American College of Radiology. *Gastroenterology, 134*(5), 1570–1595.

Lewin, K. (1951). The nature of field theory. In M. H. Marx (Ed.), *Psychological theory: Contemporary readings*. New York: Macmillan.

Lewin, K., Dembo, T., Festinger, L., & Sears, P. S. (1944). Level of aspiration. In J. Hunt (Ed.), *Personality and the behavior disorders* (pp. 333–378). Somerset, NJ: Ronald Press.

Lewis, K. S. (1994). *An examination of the health belief model when applied to diabetes mellitus* (Unpublished doctoral dissertation), University of Sheffield.

Li, C., Unger, J. B., Schuster, D., Rohrbach, L. A., Howard-Pitney, B., & Norman, G. (2003). Youths' exposure to environmental tobacco smoke (ETS): Associations with health beliefs and social pressure. *Addictive Behaviors, 28*(1), 39–53.

Licht, A. S., Murphy, J. M., Hyland, A. J., Fix, B. V., Hawk, L. W., & Mahoney, M. C. (2010). Is use of the human papillomavirus vaccine among female college students related to human papillomavirus knowledge and risk perception? *Sexually Transmitted Infections, 86*(1), 74–78.

Lieberman, D. (2009). Colon cancer screening and surveillance controversies. *Current Opinion in Gastroenterology, 25*(5), 422–427.

Mahoney, C. A., Thombs, D. L., & Ford, O. J. (1995). Health belief and self-efficacy models: Their utility in explaining college student condom use. *AIDS Education and Prevention, 7*(1), 32–49.

Manhart, L. E., Burgess-Hull, A. J., Fleming, C. B., Bailey, J. A., Haggerty, K. P., & Catalano, R. F. (2011). HPV vaccination among a community sample of young adult women. *Vaccine, 29*(32), 5238–5244.

Markowitz, L. E., Dunne, E. F., Saraiya, M., Lawson, H. W., Chesson, H., Unger, E. R., . . . Advisory Committee on Immunization Practices. (2007). Quadrivalent human papillomavirus vaccine: Recommendations of the Advisory Committee on Immunization Practices (ACIP). *Morbidity and Mortality Weekly Report: Recommendations and Reports, 56*(RR-2), 1–24.

McFarland, E. G., Levin, B., Lieberman, D. A., Pickhardt, P. J., Johnson, C. D., Glick, S. N., . . . American College of Radiology. (2008). Revised colorectal screening guidelines: Joint effort of the American Cancer Society, U.S. Multi-Society Task Force on Colorectal Cancer, and American College of Radiology. *Radiology, 248*(3), 717–720.

Morrow, J. B., Dallo, F. J., & Julka, M. (2010). Community-based colorectal cancer screening trials with multi-ethnic groups: A systematic review. *Journal of Community Health, 35*(6), 592–601.

Murphy, C. C., Vernon, S. W., Diamond, P. M., & Tiro, J. A. (2014). Competitive testing of health behavior theories: How do benefits, barriers, subjective norm, and intention influence mammography behavior? *Annals of Behavioral Medicine, 47*(1), 120–129.

Naleway, A. L., Gold, R., Drew, L., Riedlinger, K., Henninger, M. L., & Gee, J. (2012). Reported adverse events in young women following quadrivalent human papillomavirus vaccination. *Journal of Women's Health, 21*(4), 425–432.

Naylor, K., Ward, J., & Polite, B. N. (2012). Interventions to improve care related to colorectal cancer among racial and ethnic minorities: A systematic review. *Journal of General Internal Medicine, 27*(8), 1033–1046.

Noar, S. M., Benac, C. N., & Harris, M. S. (2007). Does tailoring matter? Meta-analytic review of tailored print health behavior change interventions. *Psychological Bulletin, 133*(4), 673–693.

Noar, S. M., & Zimmerman, R. S. (2005). Health behavior theory and cumulative knowledge regarding health behaviors: Are we moving in the right direction? *Health Education Research, 20*(3), 275–290.

Painter, J. E., Borba, C. P., Hynes, M., Mays, D., & Glanz, K. (2008). The use of theory in health behavior research from 2000 to 2005: A systematic review. *Annals of Behavioral Medicine*, *35*(3), 358–362.

Rawl, S., Champion, V., Menon, U., Loehrer, P. J., Vance, G. H., & Skinner, C. S. (2001). Validation of scales to measure benefits of and barriers to colorectal cancer screening. *Journal of Psychosocial Oncology*, *19*(3–4), 47–63.

Rawl, S. M., Menon, U., Burness, A., & Breslau, E. S. (2012). Interventions to promote colorectal cancer screening: An integrative review. *Nursing Outlook*, *60*(4), 172–181.

Rawl, S. M., Menon, U., Champion, V. L., Foster, J. L., & Skinner, C. S. (2000). Colorectal cancer screening beliefs: Focus groups with first-degree relatives. *Cancer Practice*, *8*(1), 32–37.

Rawl, S. M., Skinner, C. S., Perkins, S. M., Springston, J., Wang, H. L., Russell, K. M., . . . Champion, V. L. (2012). Computer-delivered tailored intervention improves colon cancer screening knowledge and health beliefs of African-Americans. *Health Education Research*, *27*(5), 868–885.

Reiter, P. L., Brewer, N. T., Gottlieb, S. L., McRee, A. L., & Smith, J. S. (2009). Parents' health beliefs and HPV vaccination of their adolescent daughters. *Social Science & Medicine*, *69*(3), 475–480.

Roberts, M. E., Gerrard, M., Reimer, R., & Gibbons, F. X. (2010). Mother-daughter communication and human papillomavirus vaccine uptake by college students. *Pediatrics*, *125*(5), 982–989.

Rosenstock, I. M. (1960). What research in motivation suggests for public health. *American Journal of Public Health and the Nation's Health*, *50*, 295–302.

Rosenstock, I. M. (1974). Historical origins of the health belief model. *Health Education Monographs*, *2*, 1–8.

Rosenstock, I. M., Strecher, V. J., & Becker, M. H. (1988). Social learning theory and the health belief model. *Health Education & Behavior*, *15*(2), 175–183.

Russell, K. M., Champion, V. L., & Perkins, S. M. (2003). Development of cultural belief scales for mammography screening. *Oncology Nursing Forum*, *30*(4), 633–640.

Salloway, J. C., Pletcher, W. R., & Collins, J. J. (1978). Sociological and social psychological models of compliance with prescribed regimen: In search of a synthesis. *Sociological Symposium*, *23*, 100–121.

Skinner, B. F. (1938). *The behavior of organisms*. Englewood Cliffs, NJ: Appleton-Century-Crofts.

Strecher, V. J., Champion, V. L., & Rosenstock, I. M. (1997). The health belief model and health behavior. In D. S. Goschman (Ed.), *Handbook of health behavior research* (Vol. 1, pp. 71–91). New York: Plenum Press.

Strecher, V. J., & Rosenstock, I. M. (1997). The health belief model. In K. Glanz, F. M. Lewis, & B. K. Rimer (Eds.), *Health behavior and health education: Theory, research, and practice* (2nd ed., pp. 41–59). San Francisco: Jossey-Bass.

Tiro, J. A., Diamond, P. M., Perz, C. A., Fernandez, M., Rakowski, W., DiClemente, C. C., & Vernon, S.W. (2005). Validation of scales measuring attitudes and norms related to mammography screening in women veterans. *Health Psychology*, *24*(6), 555–566.

Tolman, E. C. (1932). *Purposive behavior in animals and men*. New York: Appleton-Century-Crofts.

U.S. Preventive Services Task Force. (2008). Screening for colorectal cancer: U.S. Preventive Services Task Force recommendation statement. *Annals of Internal Medicine*, *149*(9), 627–638.

Vernon, S. W., Myers, R. E., & Tilley, B. C. (1997). Development and validation of an instrument to measure factors related to colorectal cancer screening adherence. *Cancer Epidemiology, Biomarkers & Prevention*, *6*(10), 825–832.

Watson, J. B. (1925). *Behaviorism*. New York: Norton.

Weinstein, N. D. (1988). The precaution adoption process. *Health Psychology*, *7*(4), 355–386.

Weinstein, N. D. (2007). Misleading tests of health behavior theories. *Annals of Behavioral Medicine*, *33*(1), 1–10.

Weinstein, N. D., & Rothman, A. J. (2005). Commentary: Revitalizing research on health behavior theories. *Health Education Research*, *20*(3), 294–297.

Whitlock, E. P., Lin, J. S., Liles, E., Beil, T. L., & Fu, R. (2008). Screening for colorectal cancer: A targeted, updated systematic review for the U.S. Preventive Services Task Force. *Annals of Internal Medicine*, *149*(9), 638–658.

Zimmerman, R. S., & Vernberg, D. (1994). Models of preventive health behavior: Comparison, critique, and meta-analysis. In G. Albrecht (Ed.), *Advances in medical sociology, health behavior models: A reformulation* (pp. 45–67). Greenwich, CT: JAI Press.

CHAPTER 6

THEORY OF REASONED ACTION, THEORY OF PLANNED BEHAVIOR, AND THE INTEGRATED BEHAVIORAL MODEL

Daniel E. Montaño
Danuta Kasprzyk

The Theory of Reasoned Action (TRA) and the Theory of Planned Behavior (TPB) focus on theoretical constructs concerned with individual motivational factors as determinants of the likelihood of performing specific behaviors. The TRA and TPB rest on an underlying assumption that the best predictor of a behavior is intention, which is determined by attitudes toward and social normative perceptions regarding the behavior. The TPB (an extension of the TRA) includes an additional construct, perceived control over performance of the behavior. In recent years we, Fishbein, and colleagues, have expanded the TRA and TPB to include components from other major behavioral theories, and proposed an Integrated Behavioral Model (IBM), also called the Integrative Model (IM).

The TRA and TPB explain a large proportion of the variance in intention and predict a number of different health behaviors and intentions, including smoking, alcohol and substance use, health services utilization, exercise, sun protection, breastfeeding, HIV/sexually transmitted disease (STD) prevention, contraceptive use, mammography and other cancer screening, safety helmet use, nutritional choices, donating blood, and seatbelt use (Conner, Godin, Sheeran, & Germain, 2013; Fishbein & Ajzen, 2010; Jemmott et al., 2011; Montaño, Phillips, & Kasprzyk, 2000; Montaño, Thompson, Taylor, & Mahloch, 1997; Wolff, Nordin, Brun, Berglund, & Kvale, 2011).

KEY POINTS

This chapter will:

- Describe the historical development of the theory of reasoned action (TRA), theory of planned behavior (TPB); and integrated behavioral model (IBM).

- Describe and explain the main constructs in TRA, TPB, and IBM.

- Explain the similarity between these theories' key constructs and constructs from other behavioral theories.

- Describe measurement of the key constructs of TRA, TPB, and IBM.

- Explain how and why elicitation should be conducted to identify and select the content for the model construct measures and the behavior and population studied.

- Illustrate in a cross-cultural application how the IBM can be used as a framework to evaluate and explain why a behavior change intervention to increase condom use was not effective.

- Provide a cross-cultural example to understand circumcision behavior among adult males in Zimbabwe, and to use the findings to design messages for behavior change communications.

- Summarize strengths and limitations of TRA, TPB, and IBM.

Evidence comes from hundreds of studies summarized in meta-analyses and reviews (Albarracín, Johnson, Fishbein, & Muellerleile, 2001; Albarracín et al., 2003, 2005; Albarracín, Kumkale, & Johnson, 2004; Armitage & Conner, 2001; Downs & Hausenblas, 2005; Durantini, Albarracín, Mitchell, Earl, & Gillette, 2006; McEachan, Conner, Taylor, & Lawton, 2011). While the TRA/TPB have been criticized, based on whether correlational results can explain behaviors (Weinstein, 2007), many published interventions show that changing TRA or TPB constructs leads to subsequent changes in behaviors (Albarracín et al., 2003, 2005; Glasman & Albarracín, 2006; Jemmott, 2012; Johnson, Scott-Sheldon, Huedo-Medina, & Carey, 2011; Kamb et al., 1998; Mosleh, Bond, Lee, Kiger, & Campbell, 2013; Rhodes, Stein, Fishbein, Goldstein, & Rotheram-Borus, 2007; Webb & Sheeran, 2006). The TRA and TPB have been used to develop effective behavior change interventions (Fisher, Amico, Fisher, & Harman, 2008; Gastil, 2000; Hardeman et al., 2005; Jemmott, 2012; Jemmott et al., 2011; Mosleh et al., 2013).

Origins and Historical Development

The TRA was developed to better understand relationships between attitudes, intentions, and behaviors (Fishbein, 1967). Many previous studies of these relationships found relatively low correspondence between attitudes and behaviors, and some theorists proposed eliminating attitude as a factor underlying behavior (Abelson, 1972; Wicker, 1969). In work that led to development of the TRA, Fishbein distinguished between attitude toward an object and attitude toward a behavior with respect to that object. Most attitude theorists measured attitude toward an object (such as an attitude toward cancer) in trying to predict a behavior (e.g., mammography). Fishbein demonstrated that attitude toward the behavior (attitude toward mammography) is a much better predictor of that behavior (obtaining mammography) than attitude toward the object (cancer) at which the behavior is directed (Fishbein & Ajzen, 1975). This is known as the principle of compatibility and was clearly described by Ajzen (1985, 2012).

Fishbein and Ajzen (1975, 2010; Ajzen & Fishbein, 1980) defined underlying beliefs (behavioral and normative), intentions, and behaviors and their measurement. They showed that it is critical to have a high degree of correspondence between measures of attitude, norm, perceived control, intention, and behavior in terms of action (e.g., go get), target (e.g., a mammogram), context (e.g., at the breast screening center), and time (e.g., in the next twelve months). A change in any of these factors results in a different behavior being explained. Low correspondence between model construct measures on any of these factors will result in low correlations between TRA/TPB variables (Ajzen, 2012; Fishbein & Ajzen, 2010).

Operationalization of TRA constructs was developed from a long history of attitude measurement theory rooted in the concept that an attitude (toward an object or an action) is determined by expectations or beliefs concerning attributes of the object or action and evaluations of those attributes. This expectancy-value conceptualization has been applied extensively in psychology in many areas, including learning theories, attitude theories, and decision-making theories (Edwards, 1954; Rosenberg, 1956; Rotter, 1954).

In addition to the TRA and TPB, a few other behavioral theories and models are among those most often used to investigate health behaviors (Glanz, Rimer, & Viswanath, 2008), including Social Cognitive Theory (see Chapter Nine), the Health Belief Model (see Chapter Five), the theory of subjective culture (Triandis, 1972), and the Transtheoretical Model (see Chapter Seven). Though many constructs in these theories are similar or complementary, more attention has been paid to their differences than their similarities (Weinstein, 1993). Thus in 1992, the National Institute of Mental Health (NIMH) convened the primary architects of several theories to develop a theoretical framework to integrate their constructs. Consensus was reached concerning behavioral constructs likely to be important in predicting and changing behaviors. These constructs included intentions, skills, anticipated outcomes (positive and negative), social normative pressure, self-image, emotional reaction, self-efficacy, and environmental constraints (Fishbein & Ajzen, 2010).

At the same time, we conducted a longitudinal study of HIV prevention behaviors in which we developed an integrated model that coincided substantially with recommendations from the NIMH theorists' workshop (Kasprzyk, Montaño, & Fishbein, 1998). With increased interest in theory integration, Fishbein and colleagues described an integrative model focused primarily on determinants of behavioral intention (Fishbein, 2008; Fishbein & Ajzen, 2010; Fishbein & Cappella, 2006). In addition, a 2002 Institute of Medicine [IOM] report, *Speaking of Health*, recommended an integrated model for using communication strategies to change health behaviors (IOM, 2002). Based on this work and on our experience over the past two decades, we propose use of the Integrated Behavioral Model (IBM) as a further extension of the TRA and TPB and describe it in this chapter.

Theory of Reasoned Action and Theory of Planned Behavior

An underlying premise of the TRA (Figure 6.1, unshaded boxes) is that the most important determinant of *behavior* is *behavioral intention*. Direct determinants of individuals' behavioral intentions are their *attitudes* toward performing the behavior and *subjective norms* associated with a behavior. TPB adds *perceived control* (Figure 6.1, shaded boxes) over the particular behavior, taking into account situations where one may not have complete volitional control over a behavior.

Attitude is determined by individuals' beliefs about outcomes or attributes of performing the behavior (*behavioral beliefs*), weighted by evaluations of those outcomes or attributes. Thus a person who holds strong beliefs that positively valued outcomes will result from performing the behavior in question will have a positive attitude toward the behavior. Conversely, a person who holds strong beliefs that negatively valued outcomes will result from the behavior will have a negative attitude.

Similarly, a person's subjective norm is determined by his or her *normative beliefs*: that is, whether important referent individuals approve or disapprove of performing the behavior, weighted by the person's motivation to comply with those referents. A person who believes that certain referents think that he or she should perform a behavior and who is motivated to meet their expectations will hold a positive subjective norm. Conversely, a person who believes these referents think that he or she should not perform the behavior will have a negative subjective norm, and a person who is less motivated to comply with those referents will have a relatively neutral subjective norm.

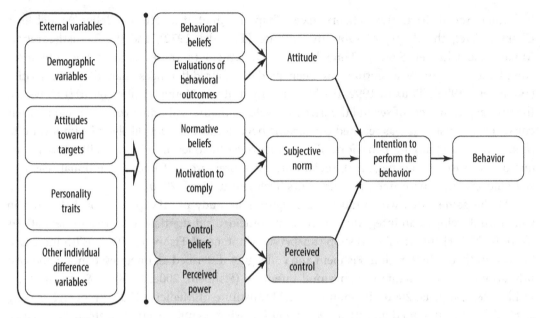

Figure 6.1 Theory of Reasoned Action and Theory of Planned Behavior
Note: The unshaded boxes show the Theory of Reasoned Action; the entire figure shows the Theory of Planned Behavior.

Central to the TRA is the assumption that the most important direct determinant of behavior is behavioral intention. Success of the theory in explaining behaviors depends on the degree to which a particular behavior is under volitional control (that is, individuals can exercise a large degree of control over the behavior). TRA components may be insufficient to predict behaviors in which volitional control is reduced. Thus Ajzen (1991) added *perceived behavioral control* (shaded boxes in Figure 6.1) to the TRA to account for factors outside individual control that may affect intentions and behaviors, forming the Theory of Planned Behavior (TPB). Perceived control is determined by *control beliefs* concerning the presence or absence of facilitators and barriers to behavioral performance, weighted by their perceived power (impact of each control factor to facilitate or inhibit the behavior). Although this may have a superficial resemblance to the HBM's concepts of barriers and facilitators, barriers and facilitators as they are defined in the HBM are more akin to the outcome expectations of the *behavioral beliefs* described above.

Ajzen's inclusion of perceived control was, in part, based on the idea that behavioral performance is determined jointly by motivation (intention) and ability (behavioral control). A person's perception of control over behavioral performance, together with intention, is expected to have a direct effect on behavior, particularly when perceived control is an accurate assessment of actual control over the behavior and when volitional control is not high. The effect of perceived control declines, and intention is a sufficient behavioral predictor in situations in which volitional control over the behavior is high (Madden, Ellen, & Ajzen, 1992). Thus, similar to Triandis's (1980) conceptualization of facilitating conditions, perceived control is expected to moderate the effect of intention on behavior. However, this interaction hypothesis has received very little empirical support (Fishbein & Ajzen, 2010).

The TPB also postulates that perceived control is an independent determinant of behavioral intention, along with attitude toward the behavior and subjective norm. Holding attitude and subjective norm constant, a person's perception of the ease or difficulty of behavioral performance will affect behavioral intention. Relative weights of these three factors in determining intentions should vary for different behaviors and populations. Few studies have operationalized perceived control using the underlying measures of control beliefs and perceived power. Instead, researchers have mostly used the direct measure of perceived control (Ajzen, 2002). Most recently, Fishbein and Ajzen (2010) have argued that perceived behavioral control and self-efficacy, as defined by Bandura (1997), are essentially the same theoretical construct.

The TRA and TPB assume a causal chain that links behavioral beliefs, normative beliefs, and control beliefs to behavioral intentions and behaviors via attitudes, subjective norms, and perceived control. One of the major strengths of the TRA/TPB approach is that hypothesized causal relationships among model components are clearly specified, as are their measurement and computation (Bleakley & Hennessy, 2012; Fishbein & Ajzen, 2010; Hennessy, Bleakley, & Fishbein, 2012). Other factors, including demographic and environmental characteristics, are assumed to operate through model constructs and are not thought to independently contribute to explain the likelihood of performing a behavior.

Measures of TRA and TPB Constructs

TRA and TPB measures can use either 5- or 7-point scales. A person's behavioral beliefs about the likelihood that performance of the behavior will result in certain outcomes are measured on bipolar "unlikely"–"likely" or "disagree"–"agree" scales. Evaluations of each outcome are measured on bipolar "good"–"bad" scales. For example, one outcome of "my quitting smoking" may be that this "will cause me to gain weight." A person's behavioral belief about this outcome is measured by having the individual rate the likelihood that "my quitting smoking will cause me to gain weight." The person's evaluation of this outcome is measured by having the individual rate the degree to which "my gaining weight" is good versus bad. Behavioral belief and evaluation ratings are scored from -3 to $+3$, capturing the psychology of double negatives, where a belief that a behavior will *not* result in a negative outcome contributes positively to the person's attitude.

An *indirect measure* of the person's attitude toward performing the behavior is computed by first multiplying a behavioral belief concerning each outcome by the corresponding outcome evaluation rating, and summing the product scores across all outcomes of the behavior. For example, a person may believe that "quitting smoking" is very unlikely to result in "gaining weight" (belief scored as -3), and may evaluate gaining weight as very bad (evaluation scored as -3), resulting in a belief $\times$ evaluation product score of $+9$. Thus the strong belief that performing the behavior *will not* result in (will avoid) a negatively valued outcome contributes just as positively to the person's attitude as would a strong belief that the action *will* result ($+3$) in a positively valued ($+3$) outcome (product $= +9$). Conversely, a strong belief that the behavior *will not* result (-3) in a positively valued outcome ($+3$) contributes negatively (product $= -9$) to the person's attitude, because performance of the behavior *will not* achieve a highly valued outcome. In the quitting smoking example, beliefs and evaluations of *all* salient outcomes of this behavior enter into the computation of an indirect measure of the person's attitude.

Similarly, a person's normative beliefs about whether each referent thinks he or she should perform the behavior are measured on bipolar scales scored −3 to +3. The person's motivation to comply with each referent is measured on unipolar scales scored 1 to 7. For example, one potential referent with regard to "quitting smoking" might be a person's best friend. The normative belief concerning the best friend is measured by asking the individual to rate the degree to which he or she believes the best friend thinks the individual *should* versus *should not* quit smoking. Motivation to comply is measured by rating *agreement* versus *disagreement* with the statement: "Generally, I want to do what my best friend thinks I should do." An *indirect measure* of the person's subjective norm is computed by multiplying the individual's normative belief about each referent by the individual's motivation to comply with that referent, and then summing the product scores across all referents.

Applications of TPB suggest that control beliefs regarding each factor should be measured on a bipolar likelihood of occurrence scale scored −3 to +3. Perceived power of each factor is measured on a bipolar "easy"–"difficult" scale (Ajzen, 1991, 2006). For example, a person may identify "restaurant smoking restrictions" as a factor affecting his or her perceived behavioral control over quitting smoking. A control belief about this factor is measured by having the individual rate his or her likelihood of encountering "a restaurant smoking restriction." Perceived power is measured by rating the individual's perception of the effect of "restaurant smoking restrictions" in making it *easy* versus *difficult* to quit smoking. These ratings are obtained for all factors identified as facilitating or impeding the behavior. An *indirect measure* of a person's perceived behavioral control is computed by multiplying each control belief by its corresponding perceived power rating, and summing the product scores across all control factors (Ajzen, 2006).

In addition to *indirect measures* computed from behavioral, normative, and control beliefs, it is important to obtain a *direct measure* of each model component. Table 6.1 summarizes the direct and indirect measures of attitudes, subjective norms, and perceived behavioral control. A direct measure of attitude toward performing the behavior is obtained using semantic differential scale items such as "good"–"bad" and "pleasant"–"unpleasant," and summing them. A direct measure of subjective norm uses a single item asking the person to rate "most people important to me think I should" perform the behavior. Ratings are made on bipolar "unlikely"–"likely" or "agree"–"disagree" scales. The direct measure of perceived behavioral control uses semantic differential scale items such as "under my control"–"not under my control" and "easy"–"difficult."

Direct measures are important for two reasons. First, direct measures are usually more strongly associated with intentions and behaviors than indirect measures. The associations between the direct measures and behavioral intention are used to indicate the relative importance of attitude, subjective norm, and perceived control in explaining or predicting a given behavior. It is important to demonstrate these associations before analyzing indirect measures. Second, *indirect measures* should be associated strongly with *direct measures* to ensure that appropriate beliefs were included in the indirect measures and that composite beliefs

Table 6.1   TRA, TPB, and IBM Constructs and Definitions

	Construct	Definition	Measure
	Behavioral intention	Perceived likelihood of performing the behavior	Bipolar unlikely-likely scale; scored −3 to +3
Attitude	**Experiential attitude (affect)**		
	Direct measure	Overall affective evaluation of the behavior	Semantic differential scales: for example, pleasant-unpleasant; enjoyable-unenjoyable
	Indirect measure		
	Behavioral belief	Belief that behavioral performance is associated with certain positive or negative feelings	Bipolar unlikely-likely scale; scored −3 to +3
	Instrumental attitude		
	Direct measure	Overall evaluation of the behavior	Semantic differential scales: for example, good-bad; wise-foolish
	Indirect measure		
	Behavioral belief	Belief that behavioral performance is associated with certain attributes or outcomes	Bipolar unlikely-likely scale; scored −3 to +3
	Evaluation	Value attached to a behavioral outcome or attribute	Bipolar bad-good scale; scored −3 to +3
Perceived Norm	**Subjective (injunctive) norm**		
	Direct measure	Belief about whether most people approve or disapprove of the behavior	Bipolar disagree-agree scale; scored −3 to +3
	Indirect measure		
	Normative belief	Belief about whether each referent approves or disapproves of the behavior	Bipolar disagree-agree scale; scored −3 to +3
	Motivation to comply	Motivation to do what each referent thinks	Unipolar unlikely-likely scale; scored 1 to 7
	Descriptive norm		
	Direct measure	Belief about whether most people perform the behavior	Bipolar disagree-agree scale; scored −3 to +3
	Indirect measure		
	Normative belief	Belief about whether each referent performs the behavior	Bipolar disagree-agree scale; scored −3 to +3

(continued)

Table 6.1   *(Continued)*

	Construct	Definition	Measure
Personal Agency	**Perceived behavioral control**		
	Direct measure	Overall measure of perceived control over the behavior	Semantic differential scales: for example, under my control–not under my control; easy-difficult
	Indirect measure		
	Control belief	Perceived likelihood of occurrence of each facilitating or constraining condition	Unlikely-likely scale; scored −3 to +3 or 1 to 7
	Perceived power	Perceived effect of each condition in making behavioral performance difficult or easy	Bipolar difficult-easy scale; scored −3 to +3
	Self-efficacy		
	Direct measure	Overall measure of ability to perform behavior	Certain I could *not*–certain I could scale for overall behavior; scored −3 to +3 or 1 to 7
	Indirect measure		
	Self-efficacy belief	Perceived ability to overcome each facilitating or constraining condition	Certain I could *not*–certain I could scale; scored −3 to +3 or 1 to 7

Note: TRA and TPB constructs are shaded.

(behavioral, normative, and control) are adequate measures of the respective TRA/TPB constructs. Once this is demonstrated, indirect measures are of most interest for the development of communication-based interventions. Behavioral, normative, and control beliefs help us understand what drives behaviors and provide foci for intervention messaging using multiple communication modes or channels (Fishbein & Cappella, 2006; von Haeften, Fishbein, Kasprzyk, & Montaño, 2001). Identification of the construct that is most closely related to behavioral intention and also the process of deciding which behavioral, normative, and control beliefs should be used to focus intervention messages are illustrated in the theory application example later in the chapter.

Research Designs and Analytic Approaches to Testing the TRA/TPB

A prospective study design is recommended to discern relationships between constructs, with attitude, subjective norm, perceived control, and intention measured at one time point and behavior measured following a time interval. Cross-sectional studies are often used to test the TRA/TPB but may provide poor prediction and understanding of previous behavior because the time order of motivations and behavior cannot be discerned. Regression and structural equation analytic methods are usually used to test relationships in the TRA/TPB. While these analyses are often used in cross-sectional studies, they are best used in longitudinal, prospective study designs to assess causal relationships (Bleakley & Hennessy, 2012; Bryan, Schmiege, & Broaddus, 2007; Rhodes et al., 2007). Relative weights of model constructs are determined empirically for each behavior and population under investigation. These weights provide guidance as to which constructs are most important to target for behavior change efforts. Some behaviors are entirely under attitudinal control (Albarracín et al., 2003), whereas others are under normative control (Albarracín et al., 2004; Durantini et al., 2006) or perceived control (Albarracín et al., 2005). For example, in a study of adults over age forty, colonoscopy intentions were found to be almost completely under normative control, whereas exercise intentions were influenced by both attitudes and perceived control (Fishbein & Cappella, 2006). Similarly, a behavior may be under attitudinal control in one population but under normative control in another population. Our research found that condom use with a main partner is primarily under normative control for female injecting drug users, but is influenced by attitude, norm, and perceived control for females who do not inject drugs (Kenski, Appleyard, von Haeften, Kasprzyk, & Fishbein, 2001; von Haeften & Kenski, 2001). This obviously has implications for message development for communication campaigns. It is a waste of resources to target messages based on attitudes to change behavior when a behavior is mostly under normative control. Once the significant constructs are identified, analyses of specific beliefs underlying those constructs can determine which specific behavioral, normative, or control beliefs are most strongly associated with intention and behavior, providing empirically identified targets for intervention efforts (see the research examples later in the chapter).

Evidence to Support the TRA/TPB

The name Theory of Reasoned Action has often led to the misrepresentation that the focus of this approach is purely on "rational behavior" (St. Lawrence & Fortenberry, 2007). This is far from correct. A fundamental assumption of the TRA is that individuals are *rational actors* who process information, and that underlying reasons determine their motivation to perform a behavior. These reasons, made up of a person's behavioral, normative, and control beliefs, determine his or her attitudes, subjective norms, and perceived control, regardless of whether those beliefs are rational, logical, or correct by some objective standard. (See Fishbein & Ajzen, 2010, for discussion of this aspect of the TRA/TPB.) A strength of the TRA/TPB is that their approach provides a framework for discerning and understanding the reasons or beliefs that motivate a behavior of interest for each particular population of interest.

Recently, the TPB was used successfully to design an intervention applied among severely mentally ill HIV-negative and HIV-positive patients to increase their condom use. One can certainly argue that many mentally ill individuals are not "rational," yet this intervention illustrates that when their own reasons for their behaviors were discerned and used in counseling messages to encourage condom use, these individuals made reasoned decisions and changed their behaviors (Blank & Hennessy, 2012). The TRA and TPB do not specify particular beliefs about behavioral outcomes, normative referents, or control beliefs that should be measured. Relevant behavioral outcomes, referents, and control beliefs should be discerned for each group and behavior and will likely be different for different populations and behaviors. Then interventions can be designed to target and change these beliefs or the value placed on them, thereby affecting attitude, subjective norm, or perceived control and leading to changes in intentions and behaviors.

An Integrated Behavioral Model

As noted previously, we recommend use of an Integrated Behavioral Model that includes constructs from the TRA/TPB and from other influential theories (Figure 6.2). As in the TRA/TPB, the most important determinant of behavior in the IBM is intention to perform the behavior. Without motivation, a person is unlikely to carry out a behavior. Four other components directly affect behavior (Jaccard, Dodge, & Dittus, 2002). Three of these are important in determining whether behavioral intentions can result in behavioral performance. First, even if a person has a strong behavioral intention, that person needs knowledge and skill to carry out the behavior. Second, there should be no or few environmental constraints that make behavioral performance difficult or impossible (Triandis, 1980). Third, behavior should be salient to the person (Becker, 1974). Finally, experience in performing the behavior may make it habitual, so that intention becomes less important in determining behavioral performance for these individuals (Triandis, 1980).

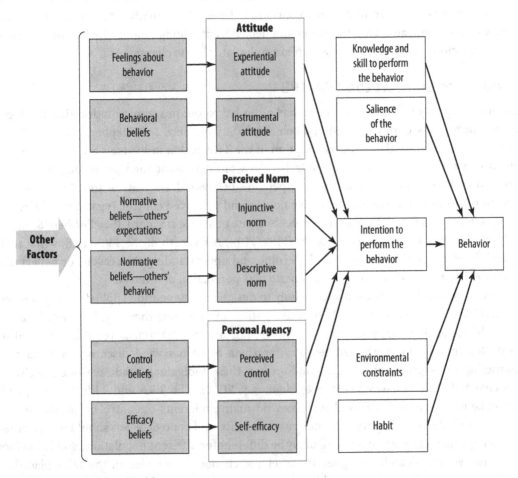

Figure 6.2 Integrated Behavioral Model

Thus a particular behavior is most likely to occur when a person has a strong intention to perform it and the knowledge and skill to do so, no serious environmental constraints prevent behavioral performance, the behavior is salient, and the person has performed the behavior previously. All these components and their interactions are important to consider when designing interventions to promote health behaviors. For example, if a woman has a strong intention to get a mammogram, it is important to ensure that she has sufficient knowledge of her health care system to act on this intention and that no serious environmental constraints, such as lack of transportation or limited clinic hours, may prevent her from getting a mammogram. Increasing behavioral intention is unlikely to change behavior unless skills or environmental constraints are assessed and it is determined that they will not affect behavioral performance. For an action that is carried out between long intervals (a year or more), such as mammography, the behavior must also be made salient, or cued, so that she will remember to carry out her intention. For other behaviors performed more often that may be under habitual control, environmental constraints must be removed to promote performance. Eating high-fat foods and smoking are examples of this behavioral category (Middlestadt, 2012).

A careful analysis should be conducted of the behavior and population being studied to determine which components are likely to be the most important targets for promoting specific behavior changes. Very different strategies may be needed for different behaviors and also for the same behavior in different settings or populations (von Haeften, Fishbein, Kasprzyk, & Montaño, 2000). There is no one-size-fits-all approach.

According to the model, behavioral intention is determined by the three construct categories listed in Table 6.1. The first is attitude toward the behavior. Many theorists have described attitude as composed of affective and cognitive dimensions (Conner et al., 2013; French et al., 2005; Triandis, 1980). Experiential attitude, or affect, is the individual's emotional response to the idea of performing a recommended behavior. Individuals with a strong negative emotional response to the behavior are unlikely to perform it, while those with a strong positive emotional reaction are more likely to engage in it. Instrumental attitude is cognitively based, determined by beliefs about outcomes of behavioral performance, as in the TRA/TPB. Conceptualization of experiential attitude (affect) is different from "mood or arousal," which Fishbein (2007) argued may affect intention indirectly by influencing perceptions of behavioral outcome likelihood or evaluation of outcomes.

Perceived norms reflect the social pressure one feels to perform or not perform a particular behavior. Subjective norm, which is defined within the TRA/TPB as an injunctive norm (normative beliefs about what others think one should do, and motivation to comply), may not fully capture normative influence. Perceptions about what others in one's social or personal networks are doing (descriptive norm) may also be an important part of normative influence (Fishbein & Ajzen, 2010; Rivis & Sheeran, 2003). This construct captures the strong social identity in certain cultures, which according to some theorists is an indicator of normative influence (Bagozzi & Lee, 2002; Triandis, 1980; Triandis, Bontempo, Villareal, Asai, & Lucca, 1988). Both injunctive and descriptive norm components are included in Figure 6.2.

Finally, personal agency, described by Bandura (2006) as bringing one's influence to bear on one's own functioning and environmental events, is proposed as a major factor influencing behavioral intention (Institute of Medicine, 2002). In the IBM, personal agency consists of two constructs, self-efficacy (from Social Cognitive Theory, discussed in Chapter Nine) and perceived control. Perceived control, as described earlier, is determined by one's perception of the degree to which various factors make it *easy* versus *difficult* to carry out the behavior. In contrast, self-efficacy is one's degree of confidence in performing the behavior in the face of various obstacles or challenges, measured by having respondents rate this behavioral confidence on bipolar "certain I could *not*"–"certain I could" scales (see Table 6.1). Although only a few papers have discussed the similarities and differences between these two constructs (Ajzen, 2002; Fishbein, 2007; Fishbein & Ajzen, 2010), our studies suggest the utility of including both measures (Montaño, Kasprzyk, Hamilton, Tshimanga, & Gorn, 2014).

The relative importance of the above three categories of theoretical constructs (attitude, perceived norm, and personal agency) in determining behavioral intention may vary for different behaviors and populations, as described for the TRA/TPB. Thus, to design effective interventions to influence behavioral intentions, it is important to first determine the degree to which intention is influenced by attitude (experiential and instrumental), perceived norm (injunctive and descriptive), and personal agency (self-efficacy and perceived control). Once this is understood for a particular behavior and population, an understanding of the determinants (specific beliefs) of those constructs is essential, as described below.

Instrumental and experiential attitudes, injunctive and descriptive norms, self-efficacy, and perceived control are all functions of underlying beliefs. As seen in Figure 6.2, instrumental attitudes are a function of beliefs about outcomes of performing the behavior, as in the TRA and TPB. In contrast to the TRA and TPB, evaluation of outcomes is not specified in the IBM. Research suggests that for many health behaviors, there is little variance in people's evaluations of behavioral outcomes (von Haeften et al., 2000, 2001; Kasprzyk & Montaño, 2007). If most people agree in their evaluations of the various behavioral outcomes, there is little benefit in measuring them. However, if preliminary study of a behavior indicates individual variation in outcome evaluations, this measure should be assessed.

As in the TRA and TPB, perceived norms are a function of normative beliefs. Again, in contrast to the TRA/TPB, motivation to comply with individuals or groups is not specified in the IBM because, as with outcome evaluations, we have found there is often little variance in these measures. However, if there is variance in motivation to comply, this should also be measured. Perceived control, as in the TPB, is a function of control beliefs about the likelihood of occurrence of various facilitating or constraining conditions, weighted by the perceived effect of those conditions in making behavioral performance easy or difficult. Finally, the stronger one's beliefs that one can perform the behavior despite various specific barriers, the greater one's self-efficacy about carrying out the behavior.

Most important in the application of the IBM as a framework to identify specific belief targets for behavior change interventions is the above conceptualization of the model constructs being determined by specific underlying beliefs. Interventions built on one model construct may have effects that further affect the same or other model constructs. For example, by changing normative beliefs, a person may be sufficiently motivated to engage in the behavior one time. If this is a positive experience, it may result in more positive behavioral beliefs as well as positive emotional feelings about the behavior, or higher perceived self-efficacy, leading to stronger future intention with respect to the behavior.

Finally, as noted in the descriptions of the TRA and TPB, other demographic, personality, and individual difference variables may be associated with behaviors, but their influence is hypothesized to be indirect and to operate via the theoretical constructs. These are considered distal variables. Thus certain demographic groups may be more likely than others to engage in the behavior, because there are demographic differences on the proximal variables. For example, individuals in certain demographic groups may be more likely than those in other demographic groups to hold beliefs about positive outcomes of the behavior, and thus hold more positive attitudes and stronger intention to carry out the behavior. Therefore these variables are shown in Figure 6.2 as external variables, because they are not considered to have a direct effect on intentions or behaviors. It is important to investigate and understand how belief patterns may differ among various groups based on these external variables, since it may be useful to segment populations on such distal variables and to design different interventions for different audience segments if there are clear differences in belief patterns.

The IBM has been used to understand behavioral intention and behavior for condom use and other HIV/STD prevention behaviors (Kasprzyk & Montaño, 2007; Kasprzyk et al., 1998; Kenski et al., 2001; von Haeften et al., 2001). It also served as the theoretical framework for two large multisite intervention studies, the AIDS Community Demonstration Projects (The CDC AIDS Community Demonstration Project Research Group, 1999) and Project Respect (Kamb et al., 1998; Rhodes et al., 2007). The model was used to identify issues to target in these interventions, while the two interventions were delivered in very different ways. The IBM provides a theoretical basis for understanding behavior and identifying specific beliefs to target. Other communication and behavior change theories should be used to guide strategies to change those target beliefs.

Importance of Elicitation Phase in Applying the TRA/TPB/IBM

Often very different behavioral, normative, efficacy, and control beliefs affect intentions to engage in different behaviors. For example, behavioral beliefs about getting a mammogram (such as the belief that it will be painful) are likely to be very different from the relevant behavioral beliefs about using a condom with one's partner (such as the belief that it "will cause my partner to think I don't trust her [or him]"). These relevant underlying beliefs may also be very different for similar behaviors, such as using condoms with one's main partner versus using condoms with a commercial partner (von Haeften et al., 2000). Just as important, the relevant underlying beliefs for a particular behavior may be very different for different populations. For this reason, Fishbein emphasized repeatedly that although an investigator can sit in an office and develop measures of attitudes, perceived norms, self-efficacy, and perceived control, this process may not identify the correct beliefs relevant to the behavior or the population (Fishbein & Ajzen, 2010; Fishbein & Cappella, 2006). One must go to the target population to identify salient behavioral, normative, efficacy, and control beliefs associated with the behavior. A critical step in applying the TRA/TPB/IBM is to conduct open-ended elicitation interviews to identify relevant behavioral outcomes, referents, facilitators, and barriers for each particular behavior and target population under investigation. The formative phase of adapting or designing interventions is an ideal time to conduct these interviews (Craig et al., 2008).

When interviewed, people should be asked to provide four types of information:

- Positive and negative feelings about performing the behavior (experiential attitude or affect)
- Positive and negative attributes or outcomes of performing the behavior (behavioral beliefs)
- Individuals or groups to whom they might listen who are in favor of or opposed to their performing the behavior (normative referents)
- Situational or other facilitators and barriers that make the behavior easy or difficult to perform (control beliefs and self-efficacy)

Table 6.2 provides examples of questions that should be asked systematically of all individuals interviewed. It is important in elicitation interviews to probe both the positive as well as the negative attributes or features of the behavior of interest. Interviews should be conducted with a sample of at least fifteen to twenty individuals from each target group, about half of whom have performed or intend to perform the behavior under investigation and half of whom have not performed it. Ideally, interviews should be continued until "saturation," when no new responses are elicited. The process has been described in detail by Middlestadt and colleagues (Middlestadt, 2012; Middlestadt, Bhattacharyya, Rosenbaum, Fishbein, & Shepherd, 1996).

Table 6.2   Table of Elicitation Questions

Construct	Elicitation Questions
Experiential attitude	How do you feel about the idea of *behavior X*? What do you like/dislike about *behavior X*? What do you enjoy/hate about *behavior X*?
Instrumental attitude	What are the plusses of your doing *behavior X*? (What are some advantages of doing *behavior X*? What are the benefits that might result from doing *behavior X*?)
	What are the minuses of your doing *behavior X*? (What are some disadvantages of doing *behavior X*? What are the negative effects that might result from doing *behavior X*?)
Injunctive norm	Who would support your doing *behavior X*?
	Who would be against your doing *behavior X*?
Descriptive norm	Who can you think of that would do *behavior X*?
	Who can you think of that would not do *behavior X*?
Perceived control	What things make it easy for you to do *behavior X*?
	What things make it hard for you to do *behavior X*?
Self-efficacy	If you want to do *behavior X*, how certain are you that you can?
	What other factors affect your ability to do *behavior X*?

Elicitation interviews are then content analyzed to identify relevant behavioral attributes or outcomes, normative referents, and facilitators and barriers. This information provides questionnaire content, from which TRA/TPB/IBM measures are developed for a defined behavior and population. Measures should capture interviewees' language as much as possible so that questions resonate with the issues raised. A quantitative survey using these measures should be conducted, and analyses carried out to identify the specific beliefs that best explain behavioral intention. A poorly conducted elicitation phase will result in inadequate identification of the relevant issues, poor IBM measures, and thus poor behavioral prediction, ultimately providing inadequate information for the development of effective behavior change interventions.

Although the TRA, TPB, and IBM are sometimes denigrated as being "Western" and not applicable to other cultures (Airhihenbuwa & Obregon, 2000), the elicitation process is what makes the model applicable across cultures. The theoretical constructs in Figure 6.2 are relevant to behaviors across cultures, having been studied in over fifty countries in the developed and developing world (Fishbein & Ajzen, 2010). It is the detailed beliefs underlying the constructs that are specific to the behavior and population being investigated. Failure to elicit these beliefs from the target population, with investigators often measuring beliefs that *they* think should be relevant, is the reason that some investigators have concluded the model is Western and not appropriate cross-culturally. In applying the models, it is critical to investigate and understand the behavior from the perspective of study populations (Middlestadt, 2012).

Application of the IBM to HIV Prevention in Zimbabwe

Here, we provide two examples to show how we applied IBM in a developing world setting to examine cross-cultural applicability of the model. The first is an example of how IBM was applied to evaluate the effect of an intervention to increase condom use with steady partners in Zimbabwe. In this example, we illustrate several important steps in applying the model: (1) using an elicitation phase to identify salient issues, (2) designing a questionnaire to measure model constructs with attention to cultural issues, and (3) conducting analyses to assess whether the intervention influenced model constructs associated with intention and behavior. The second example demonstrates how we applied IBM to design evidence-based intervention messages to motivate men to get circumcised in Zimbabwe, and to evaluate the effect of those messages. This example illustrates additional steps in applying the IBM. including analysis of data to identify targets for intervention, message design, and message testing.

Evaluation of Intervention to Increase Condom Use with Steady Partners

Between 2003 and 2007, we conducted an HIV/STD prevention trial to implement and evaluate the Community Popular Opinion Leader (CPOL) model intervention to increase safe sex behavior among rural residents in Zimbabwe. The intervention taught popular opinion leaders in communities to have conversations with peers about safe sex behavior. Opinion leader training focused on delivery of messages to peers using oneself as an example, emphasized effective conversation skills rather than content of messages, and assumed CPOLs would address relevant issues affecting behaviors. The CPOL intervention is hypothesized to operate via its effects on attitudes, norms, and self-efficacy (Kelly, 2004), though CPOL intervention training does not emphasize these constructs.

Thirty rural communities were randomized to CPOL intervention and comparison sites, with over 5,500 people followed over twenty-four months. All study sites received a basic public health intervention with STD/HIV testing and counseling, treatment for treatable infections, referral for viral infections, and distribution of condoms. At twenty-four months significant decreases in STD incidence and self-reported unprotected sex with casual partners, with *equal* change in both intervention and comparison groups, were found (NIMH Collaborative HIV/STD Prevention Trial Group, 2010). In this example, we describe how IBM was used to evaluate the effect of CPOL and to understand why there was no differential effect between the study arms. The behavioral focus in this example is *using condoms all the time with steady partners in the next three months*. This behavior is specific in terms of action (using), target (condoms), context (all the time with steady partners), and time (next three months).

Elicitation Interviews

Elicitation interviews were conducted as part of formative research to prepare for the trial in thirty-two rural villages. Individual qualitative interviews, structured by IBM components, were conducted in local languages with eight to ten randomly selected people aged eighteen to thirty in each village, half males and half females. Participants were asked to think about using condoms with steady partners, and then to describe feelings and beliefs about outcomes, sources of normative influence, and barriers and facilitators with respect to this behavior. The interviews used questions similar to the ones in Table 6.2. Content analysis of transcribed interviews yielded lists of feelings, behavioral outcomes, normative referents in favor and opposed, and barriers and facilitators with respect to using condoms with steady partners.

Questionnaire Development and Data Collection

These lists from the content analysis were used to construct items to measure each of the key constructs in Figure 6.2, including direct and indirect measures of instrumental attitude, experiential attitude (affect), injunctive norm, perceived control, and self-efficacy. Pilot tests in two rural villages, representing the two main ethnic groups, led to improved clarity of questions and exclusion of some questions. The elicitation and questionnaire design process is described in detail elsewhere (Kasprzyk & Montaño, 2007). The final survey instrument also included sections about several other safe sex behaviors (using condoms with other partners, sticking to one partner, and avoiding commercial sex workers). Surveys were administered to about 185 residents aged eighteen to thirty in each of thirty rural sites in Zimbabwe ($N = 5,546$) through personal interviews; 2,212 respondents who said they had steady partners within the previous year completed the survey section measuring IBM constructs with respect to condom use with steady partners.

IBM Model Testing

Analyses first were conducted to confirm that indirect measures assessed constructs they were designed to measure and that the model constructs explained behavioral intention. Indirect measures of attitude, perceived norm, and self-efficacy were computed first, as the mean of the respective underlying beliefs. Attitude was computed from thirteen behavioral beliefs about using condoms with steady partners, perceived norm from four normative beliefs, and self-efficacy from eleven beliefs concerning certainty of behavioral performance under different conditions. Intention to use condoms all the time with steady partners was explained significantly by attitude, perceived norm, self-efficacy, and perceived control.

Belief Associations with Intention

The next analytic step was to determine which specific behavioral, normative, and efficacy beliefs best explained intention. Table 6.3 shows that all behavioral, normative, and efficacy beliefs were correlated significantly with both behavioral intention and self-reported condom use behavior with steady partners. These findings indicate that CPOLs should have targeted all of these beliefs via interpersonal communication with peers to change intention and behavior. However, CPOLs were not specifically taught to focus on these beliefs in their persuasive messages.

Evaluation of CPOL Intervention Effect

IBM surveys were conducted again at twenty-four months after the intervention to determine impact. As noted, the intervention showed an equal effect on behavioral and biological outcomes (NIMH, 2010). To explain this null result, we examined change in beliefs in the intervention compared to the control group. Mean change scores (24-month minus baseline ratings) for the two study groups are shown in Table 6.3. T-test analyses conducted to determine whether change scores were greater for the intervention group compared to the control group found significantly greater change for only two behavioral beliefs and one efficacy belief.

These results clearly show that the CPOL intervention was not effective in changing beliefs and intentions to a greater degree in the intervention group than in the control group. This suggests that belief, intention, and behavior changes were likely due to other factors, such as condom availability and the STD/HIV counseling and testing provided to all study participants in both study arms. The CPOL intervention did not proactively train CPOLs to target specific beliefs but assumed that beliefs and attitudes would be influenced through CPOLs' learning conversational skills. Findings suggest that the intervention might have been more effective if CPOLs had been trained to deliver messages explicitly targeting the specific beliefs we identified as significantly correlated with intention and behavior.

Design of Evidence-Based Messages to Promote Male Circumcision

Adult male circumcision (MC) reduces HIV incidence among men by up to 60 percent (Auvert et al., 2005; Bailey et al., 2007; Gray et al., 2007). This led the World Health Organization (WHO) and the Joint United Nations Programme on HIV/AIDS (UNAIDS) to recommend

Table 6.3   Behavioral, Normative, and Efficacy Belief Correlations with Steady Partner Condom Use Intention and Behavior, and Mean Belief Change

	Correlation		Mean Belief Change		
	Intention	Behavior	Control	Intervention	Sig.
Behavioral Beliefs					
Make your partner angry.	−.37	−.30	−.42	−.76	n.s.
Show lack of respect for your partner.	−.40	−.32	−.46	−.61	n.s.
Show that you think your partner is unclean/diseased.	−.37	−.37	−.71	−.95	.05
Show that you are unclean/diseased.	−.37	−.32	−.56	−.80	n.s.
Be embarrassing.	−.29	−.23	−.14	−.14	n.s.
Make your partner think you don't love her/him.	−.37	−.30	−.72	−.82	n.s.
Spoil the relationship.	−.36	−.29	−.43	−.38	n.s.
Show your partner you don't trust him/her.	−.38	−.30	−.87	−.81	n.s.
Mean you would get less pleasure.	−.21	−.18	−.70	−.68	n.s.
Make your partner think you are having other partners.	−.39	−.28	−.95	−1.04	n.s.
Be unnecessary, because your steady partner does not have other partners.	−.31	−.21	−.28	−.72	.05
Mean you will not have physical or sexual release.	−.24	−.19	−.34	−.42	n.s.
Encourage promiscuity in your steady partner.	−.29	−.20	−.73	−.75	n.s.
Normative Beliefs					
Your family.	.25	.18	.13	.40	n.s.
Your closest friends.	.29	.22	−.03	.09	n.s.
Radio shows or radio dramas.	.20	.14	−.12	−.09	n.s.
Your partner.	.56	.39	.42	.59	n.s.
Efficacy Beliefs					
How certain are you that you could always use condoms with steady partner if . . .					
You or your steady partner gets carried away and can't wait to have sex?	.57	.34	.11	.31	n.s.
You have been drinking before you have sex?	.52	.34	.36	.46	n.s.
Your steady partner has been drinking before sex?	.53	.36	.17	.34	n.s.
You or your steady partner is using another method of birth control?	.59	.34	.13	.37	n.s.
Your steady partner doesn't want to?	.56	.35	.28	.60	.05
You believe AIDS will affect you?	.43	.24	−.02	.00	n.s.
You or your steady partner has a condom with you?	.57	.36	−.17	.09	n.s.
You or your steady partner knows how to use a condom?	.59	.35	−.12	.03	n.s.
Condoms are available in your community?	.60	.37	−.13	.06	n.s.
You had to talk about it with your steady partner?	.56	.33	−.14	−.03	n.s.
You thought your steady partner had other partners?	.45	.28	−.37	−.14	n.s.

Note: All correlations significant $p < .001$.

that MC be included as part of HIV prevention strategies in countries where HIV is primarily heterosexually transmitted and MC prevalence is low (WHO & UNAIDS, 2007). The Ministry of Health and Child Care (MOHCC) in Zimbabwe has begun the National Male Circumcision Programme, which has a goal to circumcise 80 percent of adult men by 2017. Despite significant investment in MC capacity infrastructure, MC uptake has been much lower than desired. We applied IBM to identify key beliefs that best explain men's levels of motivation to uptake MC, designed persuasive messages to target those beliefs, and conducted a message testing study to assess the effect of the messages on the IBM beliefs targeted.

Elicitation Phase to Identify Salient Issues

The behavioral focus in this example is *getting circumcised if the MOHCC offered circumcision at no cost*. A sample of thirty-three men aged eighteen to thirty, from four urban and rural areas of Zimbabwe (equally divided), participated in interviews designed to elicit specific issues with respect to each IBM construct. Questions elicited (1) positive and negative beliefs, (2) sources of normative influence about getting circumcised, and (3) factors that may make it easier or harder to get circumcised. Content analysis resulted in the identification of thirty-eight positive and negative beliefs, twenty-one sources of normative influence, fourteen facilitators, and fifteen constraints about getting circumcised.

Questionnaire Development

These results were used to design IBM survey measures. All belief items were measured on 5-point bipolar scales. The thirty-eight positive and negative behavioral beliefs about getting circumcised were measured on "disagree"–"agree" scales. Similarly, injunctive and descriptive norm belief questions measured whether each of twenty-one sources of influence would encourage men to get circumcised, and whether each of four types of people would get circumcised. Control beliefs asked men to rate how difficult or easy each of the twenty-nine facilitators or constraints makes it to get circumcised. Efficacy beliefs were measured for each of the fifteen constraints, with respondents rating how certain they were that they could get circumcised if faced with each constraint. Ratings ranged from "extremely certain I could not" to "extremely certain I could." Finally, intention to get circumcised was measured by asking men to rate how strongly they "disagree" or "agree" that they would get an MC if the MOHCC began a national program with MC offered to adult men at no cost. The survey was conducted with 1,085 uncircumcised men aged eighteen to thirty, selected via household-based sampling and equally distributed between two urban and two rural areas in Zimbabwe.

Confirmation of Model Component Determinants of Intention

Internal consistency analyses found high Cronbach's alpha for all IBM constructs. Negative behavioral belief scores were reflected because stronger disagreement with negative beliefs indicates more positive attitudes. Indirect measures of attitude, injunctive and descriptive norm, perceived control, and self-efficacy were computed by taking the mean of the belief items underlying each construct.

Correlation and stepwise regression analyses were used to investigate the association between these five IBM constructs and MC intention. Intention to get circumcised was explained significantly ($R = .71$; $p < .001$) by attitude, injunctive norm, descriptive norm, perceived control, and self-efficacy, suggesting that all five model constructs may be important potential targets for communication interventions to change intention and behavior.

Identification of Beliefs to Change Intention

Conceptualization of IBM constructs as determined by underlying beliefs is most important to identify specific targets for intervention communications. Analyses were carried out to identify specific beliefs underlying IBM constructs that best explained MC motivation, and that would be the best foci for intervention messages. All IBM construct beliefs were significantly correlated with MC intention, except for three behavioral beliefs. Five stepwise regression analyses were carried out with the beliefs underlying each model construct as the independent variables to explain MC intention. Table 6.4 lists beliefs entering each of the regressions.

Final Regression Model

It is not always feasible to address a large number of beliefs in an intervention, and in that case it is important to identify a smaller set of beliefs across IBM components that may be more amenable to mass media communication strategies. Thus a final stepwise regression analysis was conducted to identify beliefs across all five model constructs that were the strongest in explaining MC intention. We included all beliefs found to be significant in the five previous regressions. The last section of Table 6.4 lists the beliefs that entered the final regression model. Fourteen beliefs in total—five behavioral, two injunctive norm, one descriptive norm, three efficacy, and three control beliefs—independently and significantly explained MC intention. Three beliefs related to women, and four were structural/conditional. The two items with the largest beta weights were normative beliefs about friends and brothers, suggesting there is a strong and very personal social network acceptance component to MC intention. Similar analyses conducted with subgroups are important for segmentation purposes when one is building a communication campaign. These results are presented in more detail by Montaño et al. (2014).

Intervention Message Design

We identified a large number of underlying beliefs that were strongly correlated with MC intention (Table 6.4). The next step was to select beliefs that could be changed through persuasive communications, and to design persuasive messages to target these beliefs. These messages could be used in behavior change communication campaigns, either media or interpersonal. We began with the fourteen beliefs in the final model, since these had the strongest independent effects in explaining MC intention.

Development of messages took several steps. We first conducted discussion groups with young men in Zimbabwe, resulting in the development of an initial set of draft messages. Each draft message was coded and message content was mapped to analytic results to verify that content was based on the evidence from the regression results. This resulted in a final set of

Table 6.4   IBM Construct Beliefs Associated with MC Intention

Behavioral Beliefs About Getting Circumcised	r^*	β ($R = .65$)
Will help encourage friends to get circumcised.	.46	.17
Will give you peace of mind.	.44	.15
Is something that you are too old for now.	−.38	−.17
Will give you sense of achievement.	.43	.10
Might not heal properly, cause disfigurement.	−.35	−.07
Will enhance sexual pleasure for you.	.29	.10
Would be against your religion.	−.37	−.09
Will result in a slowdown of HIV in Zimbabwe.	.40	.06
It may get infected and swollen.	−.34	−.06
Will make it easier to have sons circumcised.	.38	.07
Will cause women to shun you.	−.20	.07
Wife/girlfriend may think you will seek pleasure elsewhere.	−.29	−.07
Will protect you from STIs.	.37	.06

Normative Beliefs About Who Would Encourage You to Get Circumcised	r^*	β ($R = .61$)
Your brothers.	.58	.24
Your closest friends.	.52	.16
Your culture.	.50	.16
People in your community.	.47	.11
Your wife.	.59	.07+
Your girlfriend.	.43	

Descriptive Norm Beliefs About Who Would Get Circumcised	r^*	β ($R = .60$)
Your closest friends.	.57	.23
Your brothers.	.56	.17
Most people like you.	.52	.11
Your other male relatives.	.55	.12

Control Beliefs: Facilitators/Barriers to Getting Circumcised	r^*	β ($R = .66$)
Availability of equipment and materials.	.55	.23
People describe MC as painful.	.42	.09
If you don't know how MC prevents HIV.	.33	.10
If local chiefs/village heads support MC.	.52	.13
MC is new, not offered before in community.	.41	.10
If circumcision is not free to you.	.31	.09
If MC available in local (including rural) clinics.	.44	.07
If MC promoted on TV and radio.	.51	.09
If you cannot do it privately, so others know.	.36	.06
If you did not know where to go for MC.	.17	−.06

(continued)

Table 6.4   *(Continued)*

Efficacy Beliefs: How Certain You Can Get Circumcised If . . .	r^*	β (R = .63)
MC is new and has not been offered before in community.	.51	.17
MC is available in local—including rural—clinics.	.49	.24
Your culture is against it.	.50	.17
Your wife/girlfriend is against it.[+]	.49	.11
You cannot have it done privately, so others might know about it.	.43	.08
Worried about whether there are adequate supplies in clinics.	.34	.06

Final Model		
IBM Construct	**Belief**	β (R = .74)
Behavioral beliefs	Will give you peace of mind.	.11
	Something you are too old for now.	−.09
	Will enhance sexual pleasure/enjoyment for you.	.09
	Cause women to shun you and say your penis is different.	.08
	Might not heal properly—cause disfigurement.	−.06
Injunctive norm beliefs	Brothers encourage.	.14
	Wife/girlfriend encourage.	.07
Descriptive norm beliefs	Closest friends.	.14
Efficacy beliefs	If culture is against MC.	.10
	If MC is new—not offered before in community.	.07
	If wife/girlfriend is against MC.	.09
Control beliefs	Availability of equipment and materials. (B)	.13
	The fact that MC is new, not offered before in community.	.06
	If MC available in local (including rural) clinics. (F)	.06

Note: N = 1,085.
$^*p < .001$ for all correlations.
+ = Instances in which, in order to minimize loss of cases due to missing data, responses for wife and girlfriend were combined into a single variable for the regression analysis, as few respondents had both a wife and a girlfriend.

thirty-two messages, each consisting of one- or two-sentence persuasive statements. Finally, we developed posters, as a vehicle to present messages. We selected posters because posters and billboards are a popular method of advertising in Zimbabwe, including in urban and rural areas, and have great community penetration. Billboards are often used in communication campaigns. A total of thirty-two posters were designed by a professional graphic designer with Zimbabwean cultural experience, using complementary photos and messages to promote MC among men.

Message Testing

A message testing study was carried out to obtain reactions to messages and posters, assess recall, and determine whether the messages affected the beliefs they were designed to target. Participants were University of Zimbabwe students aged eighteen to twenty-five, in order to obtain feedback from an articulate group that was part of the MC communication campaign target audience. The thirty-two posters and thirty-two messages were randomized into sixteen sets of eight posters and eight messages, with each poster or message included in four sets. Message testing sessions consisted of sixteen groups of eight to ten students. In the first session, the students completed a questionnaire to measure all IBM beliefs. This was followed by thirty-second exposures to each of eight posters and eight messages. Following each exposure, participants wrote down immediate reactions to and opinions about the poster or message and completed closed-ended rating scales. Three days later, the students returned and were asked to recall each poster and message verbatim, to assess which ones were incorporated into long-term memory. Eight weeks after the first session, the students completed a postexposure IBM survey to assess whether poster and message exposures had affected IBM constructs (attitude, norm, and personal agency) and MC intention. A total of seventy-eight men participated in the message testing study.

Results of Message Testing Study

We computed IBM construct scores with preexposure and eight-week postexposure survey data and conducted t-test analyses to determine whether there were significant changes in the men's measures. There were significant increases in the men's MC intentions, instrumental attitude, and experiential attitude toward getting circumcised eight weeks postexposure. Next, we tested for change in beliefs and feelings underlying the attitude constructs. We found that nine behavioral beliefs and seven experiential attitude feelings showed significant change. The finding that thirty-second exposures to posters and messages designed to target IBM construct beliefs resulted in significant change in targeted beliefs and feelings is important, suggesting that change in underlying beliefs resulted in significant change in instrumental and experiential attitude IBM constructs and significant change in MC intention among men.

These findings indicate that theory-driven, evidence-based message design was effective in changing behavioral motivation. Next, posters and messages should be revised based on students' ratings and recall results and tested with a larger community-based sample to determine whether there is a similar impact on IBM construct beliefs and MC intention. Most important, a communication campaign using these posters and messages should be evaluated to determine whether it leads to an increased likelihood that men will get circumcised.

Use of Findings to Inform Behavior Change Interventions

In summary, these two cross-cultural examples demonstrate the following steps for applying the IBM as a framework to identify specific targets for intervention messaging and to test the effect of messages on targeted beliefs for two different behaviors. They show how to:

1. Specify the behavior in terms of action, target, context, and time.
2. Conduct qualitative interviews with members of study populations to elicit salient behavioral outcomes, affective responses, sources of normative influence, and barriers and facilitators associated with the target behavior. This step is necessary and critical. These salient issues often are different for different behaviors and different target groups.

3. Use elicitation findings to design culturally appropriate survey instruments to measure IBM constructs. Questions were designed to measure beliefs regarding the specific salient issues identified in the elicitation study. Pilot testing ensured question wording and response scale formats were reliable, valid, and culturally appropriate.

4. Confirm that IBM measures explain behavioral intention, and determine which constructs best explain intention and should serve as foci for intervention efforts.

5. Use findings to analyze and identify specific behavioral, normative, efficacy, and control beliefs that are the best targets for persuasive communications in an intervention to strengthen behavioral intention and lead to greater likelihood of behavioral performance.

6. Design communication messages and materials to change specific behavioral, normative, efficacy, and control beliefs that have the strongest explanation of intention and behavior.

7. Evaluate whether messages are effective in changing beliefs they were designed to influence, and whether resultant changes in IBM constructs and behavioral intention occurred.

The TRA, TPB, and IBM are theories to explain behavioral intentions and behaviors and to identify intervention targets. They can be used to design more effective communication strategies to ensure a higher likelihood of changing behaviors. A mixed-methods approach, with *both* qualitative and quantitative components, is crucial. Many communication campaigns using social marketing as a basis stop at the collection of qualitative data. Our research shows that the issues most frequently mentioned in qualitative phases do not differentiate individuals who are motivated from those who are not motivated to engage in a behavior. This means that communication campaigns that focus on these issues may be ineffective in changing behavior.

Further work needs to develop more systematic theories for implementation of communication strategies. The TRA, TPB, and IBM are *not* theories of communication. Available theories of communication are not as clear as the TRA, TPB, and IBM for guiding how best to design messages and to select channels or modes to deliver persuasive messages that target issues identified through application of behavioral theory (Fishbein & Cappella, 2006; Institute of Medicine, 2002).

Value of the TRA, TPB, and IBM Frameworks

Theoretical frameworks help to organize thought about and planning of research, intervention, and analysis. The TRA, TPB, and IBM provide excellent frameworks to conceptualize, measure, and identify factors that affect behaviors. The TRA focuses on cognitive factors (beliefs and values) that determine motivation (behavioral intention). This theory has been very useful in explaining behaviors, particularly behaviors under volitional control. In applying behavioral theories, it is important to reassess them and consider other theory-driven constructs that may enhance explanatory power. The TPB extends the TRA by adding perceived behavioral control, concerned with facilitating or constraining conditions that affect intention and behavior. This is particularly important for behaviors over which people have less volitional control. The IBM includes constructs from both the TPB and TRA and also constructs—including self-efficacy—from other theories of behavior. The IBM was developed through discussions and consensus among major behavioral theorists and has been modified through empirical work over the past decade.

We cannot stress enough the importance of conducting in-depth, open-ended elicitation interviews with audiences who are being studied with the TRA/TPB/IBM and for whom interventions will be designed. Elicitation interviews identify the behavioral outcomes, normative referents, and barriers and facilitators that are relevant to each particular behavior and population under investigation. This ensures that TRA/TPB/IBM measures are empirically grounded. This qualitative research can also serve as a basis for communication campaigns.

The TRA, TPB, and IBM provide frameworks to guide research to empirically identify factors on which intervention efforts should focus. The strength of the approach is its complementary qualitative to quantitative strategy grounded in what target groups believe. Through experience, we have seen that qualitative identification of beliefs is not enough, though this is where formative research associated with social marketing often stops. We have shown how the most often mentioned beliefs in qualitative data collection are not necessarily the ones most likely to drive intentions. Though they may be broadly held and frequently mentioned, they may not affect intentions precisely because they are already held by most of the target group. This is why confirming the predictors of intentions through quantitative data collection and analyses will yield results allowing researchers to target factors that actually affect intentions. This dual-step process creates evidence-based results for all types of communication interventions.

Selection of specific beliefs to change through interventions must be done carefully. Targeting a few beliefs may not be effective if they represent only a small proportion of the total set of beliefs affecting intentions. Similarly, targeting beliefs that constitute a model component not strongly associated with behavioral intention may be ineffective. It is also important to consider the effect of intervention messages on the entire set of beliefs underlying behavior. A communication intervention may change one targeted belief in the desired direction but also adversely affect other important beliefs. Further, intervention development should pay attention to all model components simultaneously. For example, attempting to modify efficacy or control beliefs may be effective only if a person is sufficiently motivated to perform the behavior in the first place. Conversely, changing attitude may not result in behavior change if the person holds strong control or self-efficacy beliefs about conditions that constrain the behavior.

It is important to monitor the effect of interventions on beliefs targeted and on other components of the model. The TRA/TPB/IBM provide a basis for evaluating behavior change interventions because they lead to hypotheses about how an intervention targeting a set of beliefs will affect the model component to which those items belong (e.g., attitude) and thereby affect intention and behavior. The evaluation design should include measures of model components as intermediate outcomes, both before and after intervention, to assess how they are influenced by the intervention and whether change in model components is associated with behavior change. These theories should be applied in conjunction with communication theories to design and deliver behavior change interventions. In this way, the IBM can complement the use of other theories of change, and thereby improve health behavior research and practice.

Summary

In this chapter, we described the Theory of Reasoned Action (TRA), the Theory of Planned Behavior (TPB), and the Integrated Behavioral Model (IBM), and how the IBM emerged from efforts to integrate constructs from the TRA/TPB with constructs from other important theories of behavior. We provided details on how to measure the constructs in these theories. We emphasized that even though the TRA, TPB, and IBM provide a structure for understanding how behavioral, normative, control, and efficacy beliefs determine the respective model constructs and affect behavioral intention, it is essential to elicit the specific content for measures from the study population with respect to the behavior under investigation. Finally, we described two cross-cultural applications of the IBM in Zimbabwe to demonstrate development of IBM measures, analyses to confirm that model constructs explain behavioral intention, analyses to identify specific key beliefs that should be targeted by behavior change interventions, development of intervention messages to target key beliefs underlying IBM constructs, and analyses to determine whether those key beliefs are changed by communication interventions.

References

Abelson, R. P. (1972). Are attitudes necessary? In B. T. King & E. McGinnies (Eds.), *Attitudes, conflict, and social change*. New York: Academic Press.

Airhihenbuwa, C. O., & Obregon, R. (2000). A critical assessment of theories/models used in health communication for HIV/AIDS. *Journal of Health Communication, 5*(Suppl.), 5–15.

Ajzen, I. (1985). From intentions to actions: A theory of planned behavior. In J. Kuhl & J. Beckman (Eds.), *Action-control: From cognition to behavior* (pp. 11–39). New York: Springer.

Ajzen, I. (1991). The theory of planned behavior. *Organizational Behavior and Human Decision Processes, 50*, 179–211.

Ajzen, I. (2002). Perceived behavioral control, self-efficacy, locus of control, and the theory of planned behavior. *Journal of Applied Social Psychology, 32*, 1–20.

Ajzen, I. (2006). *Constructing a theory of planned behavior questionnaire*. Retrieved from http://www.people.umass.edu/aizen/pdf/tpb.measurement.pdf

Ajzen, I. (2012). Martin Fishbein's legacy: The reasoned action approach. *Annals of the American Academy of Political and Social Science, 640*(1), 11–27.

Ajzen, I., & Fishbein, M. (1980). *Understanding attitudes and predicting social behavior*. Englewood Cliffs, NJ: Prentice Hall.

Albarracín, D., Gillette, J. C., Earl, A. N., Glasman, L. R., Durantini, M. R., & Ho, M. H. (2005). A test of major assumptions about behavior change: A comprehensive look at the effects of passive and active HIV-prevention interventions since the beginning of the epidemic. *Psychological Bulletin, 131*(6), 856–897.

Albarracín, D., Johnson, B. T., Fishbein, M., & Muellerleile, P. A. (2001). Theories of reasoned action and planned behavior as models of condom use: A meta-analysis. *Psychological Bulletin, 127*(1), 142–161.

Albarracín, D., Kumkale, G. T., & Johnson, B. T. (2004). Influences of social power and normative support on condom use decision: A research synthesis. *AIDS Care, 16*(6), 700–723.

Albarracín, D., McNatt, P. S., Klein, C. T., Ho, R. M., Mitchell, A. L., & Kumkale, G. T. (2003). Persuasive communications to change actions: An analysis of behavioral and cognitive impact in HIV prevention. *Health Psychology, 22*(2), 166–177.

Armitage, C. J., & Conner, M. (2001). Efficacy of the theory of planned behaviour: A meta-analytic review. *British Journal of Social Psychology, 40*(4), 471–499.

Auvert, B., Taljaard, D., Lagarde, E., Sobngwi-Tambekou, J., Sitta, R., & Puren, A. (2005). Randomized, controlled intervention trial of male circumcision for reduction of HIV infection risk: The ANRS 1265 trial. *PLoS Medicine, 2*(11), e298. doi: 10.1371/journal.pmed.0020298

Bagozzi, R. P., & Lee, K.-H. (2002). Multiple routes for social influence: The role of compliance, internalization, and social identity. *Social Psychology Quarterly, 65*(3), 226–247.

Bailey, R. C., Moses, S., Parker, C. B., Agot, K., Maclean, I., Krieger, J. N., . . . Ndinya-Achla, J. O. (2007). Male circumcision for HIV prevention in young men in Kisumu, Kenya: A randomised controlled trial. *Lancet, 369*(9562), 643–656.

Bandura, A. (1997). *Self efficacy: The exercise of control.* New York: Freeman.

Bandura, A. (2006). Toward a psychology of human agency. *Perspectives on Psychological Science, 1*(2), 164–180.

Becker, M. H. (1974). The health belief model and personal health behavior. *Health Education Monographs, 2,* 324–473.

Blank, M. B., & Hennessy, M. (2012). A reasoned action approach to HIV prevention for persons with serious mental illness. *Annals of the American Academy of Political and Social Science, 640,* 151–173.

Bleakley, A., & Hennessy, M. (2012). The quantitative analysis of reasoned action theory. *Annals of the American Academy of Political and Social Science, 640,* 28–41.

Bryan, A., Schmiege, S. J., & Broaddus, M. R. (2007). Mediational analysis in HIV/AIDS research: Estimating multivariate path analytic models in a structural equation modeling framework. *AIDS and Behavior, 11*(3), 365–383.

The CDC AIDS Community Demonstration Project Research Group. (1999). Community-level HIV intervention in 5 cities: Final outcome data for the CDC AIDS Community Demonstration Projects. *American Journal of Public Health, 89*(3), 336–345.

Conner, M., Godin, G., Sheeran, P., & Germain, M. (2013). Some feelings are more important: Cognitive attitudes, affective attitudes, anticipated affect, and blood donation. *Health Psychology, 32*(3), 264–272.

Craig, P., Dieppe, P., Macintyre, S., Michie, S., Nazareth, I., & Petticrew, M. (2008). Developing and evaluating complex interventions: The new Medical Research Council guidance. *BMJ, 337,* 979–983.

Downs, D. S., & Hausenblas, H. A. (2005). Elicitation studies and the theory of planned behavior: A systematic review of exercise beliefs. *Psychology of Sport and Exercise, 6*(1), 1–31.

Durantini, M. R., Albarracín, D., Mitchell, A. L., Earl, A. N., & Gillette, J. C. (2006). Conceptualizing the influence of social agents of change: A meta-analysis of HIV prevention interventions for different groups. *Psychological Bulletin, 132*(2), 212–248.

Edwards, W. (1954). The theory of decision making. *Psychological Bulletin, 51,* 380–417.

Fishbein, M. (Ed.). (1967). *Readings in attitude theory and measurement.* New York: Wiley.

Fishbein, M. (2007). A reasoned action approach: Some issues, questions, and clarifications. In I. Ajzen, D. Albarracín, & R. Hornik (Eds.), *Prediction and change of health behavior: Applying the reasoned action approach.* Hillsdale, NJ: Erlbaum.

Fishbein, M. (2008). A reasoned action approach to health promotion. *Medical Decision Making*, 28(6), 834–844.

Fishbein, M., & Ajzen I. (1975). *Belief, attitude, intention, and behavior: An introduction to theory and research*. Reading, MA: Addison-Wesley.

Fishbein, M., & Ajzen, I. (2010). Predicting and changing behavior. New York: Psychology Press.

Fishbein, M., & Cappella, J. N. (2006). The role of theory in developing effective health communications. *Journal of Communication*, 56(Suppl. 1), S1–S17.

Fisher, J. D., Amico, K. R., Fisher, W. A., & Harman, J. J. (2008). The information-motivation-behavioral skills model of antiretroviral adherence and its applications. *Current HIV/AIDS Reports*, 5(4), 193–203.

French, D. P., Sutton, S., Hennings, S. J., Mitchell, J., Wareham, N. J., Griffin, S., . . . Kinmonth, A. L. (2005). The importance of affective beliefs and attitudes in the theory of planned behavior: Predicting intention to increase physical activity. *Journal of Applied Social Psychology*, 35(9), 1824–1848.

Gastil, J. (2000). Thinking, drinking, and driving: Application of the theory of reasoned action to DWI prevention. *Journal of Applied Social Psychology*, 30(11), 2217–2232.

Glanz, K., Rimer, B. K., & Viswanath, K. (Eds.). (2008). *Health behavior and health education: Theory, research, and practice* (4th ed.). San Francisco: Jossey-Bass.

Glasman, L. R., & Albarracín, D. (2006). Forming attitudes that predict future behavior: A meta-analysis of the attitude-behavior relation. *Psychological Bulletin*, 132(5), 778–822.

Gray, R. H., Kigozi, G., Serwadda, D., Makumbi, F., Watya, S., Nalugoda, F., . . . Wawer, M. (2007). Male circumcision for HIV prevention in men in Rakai, Uganda: A randomized trial. *Lancet*, 369(9562), 657–666.

Hardeman, W., Sutton, S., Griffin, S., Johnston, M., White, A., Wareham, N. J., & Kinmonth, A. L. (2005). A causal modelling approach to the development of theory-based behaviour change programmes for trial evaluation. *Health Education Research*, 20(6), 676–687.

Hennessy, M., Bleakley, A., & Fishbein, M. (2012). Measurement models for reasoned action theory. *Annals of the American Academy of Political and Social Science*, 640, 42–57.

Institute of Medicine, Committee on Communication for Behavior Change in the 21st Century: Improving the Health of Diverse Populations. (2002). *Speaking of health: Assessing health communication strategies for diverse populations*. Washington, DC: National Academies Press.

Jaccard, J., Dodge, T., & Dittus, P. (2002). Parent-adolescent communication about sex and birth control: A conceptual framework. In S. Feldman & D. A. Rosenthal (Eds.), *Talking sexuality: Parent-adolescent communication* [Special issue]. *New Directions in Child and Adolescent Development*, 97, 9–42.

Jemmott, J. B., III. (2012). The reasoned action approach in HIV risk-reduction strategies for adolescents. *Annals of the American Academy of Political and Social Science*, 640, 150–172.

Jemmott, J. B., III, Jemmott, L. S., O'Leary, A., Ngwane, Z., Icard, L., Bellamy, S., . . . Makiwane, M. B. (2011). Cognitive-behavioural health-promotion intervention increases fruit and vegetable consumption and physical activity among South African adolescents: A cluster-randomised controlled trial. *Psychology & Health*, 26(2), 167–185.

Johnson, B. T., Scott-Sheldon, L.A.J., Huedo-Medina, T. B., & Carey, M. P. (2011). Interventions to reduce sexual risk for HIV in adolescents: A meta-analysis of trials, 1985–2008. *Archives of Pediatrics & Adolescent Medicine*, 165(1), 77–84.

Kamb, M., Fishbein, M., Douglas, J. M., Jr., Rhodes, F., Rogers, J., Bolan, G., . . . Peterman, T. A. (1998). Efficacy of risk-reduction counseling to prevent human immunodeficiency virus and sexually transmitted diseases: A randomized controlled trial. *JAMA*, 280(13), 1161–1167.

Kasprzyk, D., & Montaño, D. E. (2007). Application of an integrated behavioral model to understand HIV prevention behavior of high-risk men in rural Zimbabwe. In I. Ajzen, D. Albarracín, & R. Hornik (Eds.), *Prediction and change of health behavior: Applying the reasoned action approach* (pp.149–172). Hillsdale, NJ: Erlbaum.

Kasprzyk, D., Montaño, D. E., & Fishbein, M. (1998). Application of an integrated behavioral model to predict condom use: A prospective study among high HIV risk groups. *Journal of Applied Social Psychology, 28*(17), 1557–1583.

Kelly, J. A. (2004). Popular opinion leaders and HIV prevention peer education: Resolving discrepant findings, and implications for the development of effective community programmes. *AIDS Care, 16(*2), 139–150.

Kenski, K., Appleyard, J., von Haeften, I., Kasprzyk, D., & Fishbein, M. (2001). Theoretical determinants of condom use intentions for vaginal sex with a regular partner among male and female injecting drug users. *Psychology, Health & Medicine, 6*(2), 179–190.

Madden, T. J., Ellen, P. S., & Ajzen, I. (1992). A comparison of the theory of planned behavior and the theory of reasoned action. *Personality and Social Psychology Bulletin, 18*(1), 3–9.

McEachan, R.R.C., Conner, M., Taylor, N., & Lawton, R. J. (2011). Prospective prediction of health-related behaviors with the theory of planned behavior: A meta-analysis. *Health Psychology Review, 5*(2), 97–144.

Middlestadt, S. E. (2102). Beliefs underlying eating better and moving more: Lessons learned from comparative salient belief elicitations with adults and youths. *Annals of the American Academy of Political and Social Science, 640,* 81–100.

Middlestadt, S. E., Bhattacharyya, K., Rosenbaum, J., Fishbein, M., & Shepherd, M. (1996). The use of theory based semistructured elicitation questionnaires: Formative research for CDC's Prevention Marketing Initiative. *Public Health Reports, 111*(Suppl. 1), 18–27.

Montaño, D. E., Kasprzyk, D., Hamilton, D. T., Tshimanga, M., & Gorn, G. (2014). Evidence-based identification of key beliefs explaining adult male circumcision motivation in Zimbabwe: Targets for behavior change messaging. *AIDS and Behavior, 18*(5), 885–904.

Montaño, D. E., Phillips, W. R., & Kasprzyk, D. (2000). Explaining physician rates of providing flexible sigmoidoscopy. *Cancer Epidemiology, Biomarkers & Prevention, 9*(7), 665–669.

Montaño, D. E., Thompson, B., Taylor, V. M., & Mahloch, J. (1997). Understanding mammography intention and utilization among women in an inner city public hospital clinic. *Preventive Medicine, 26*(6), 817–824.

Mosleh, S. M., Bond, C. M., Lee, A. J., Kiger, A., & Campbell, N. C. (2013). Effectiveness of theory-based invitations to improve attendance at cardiac rehabilitation: A randomized controlled trial. *European Journal of Cardiovascular Nursing, 13*(3), 201–210.

NIMH Collaborative HIV/STD Prevention Trial Group. (2010). Results of the NIMH collaborative HIV/STD prevention trial of a community popular opinion leader intervention. *Journal of Acquired Immune Deficiency Syndromes, 54*(2), 204–214.

Rhodes, F., Stein, J. A., Fishbein, M., Goldstein, R. B., & Rotheram-Borus, M. J. (2007). Using theory to understand how interventions work: Project RESPECT, condom use, and the integrative model. *AIDS and Behavior, 11*(3), 393–407.

Rivis, A., & Sheeran, P. (2003). Descriptive norms as an additional predictor in the theory of planned behaviour: A meta-analysis. *Current Psychology, 22*(3), 218–233.

Rosenberg, M. J. (1956). Cognitive structure and attitudinal affect. *Journal of Abnormal and Social Psychology, 53,* 367–372.

Rotter, J. B. (1954). *Social learning and clinical psychology*. Englewood Cliffs, NJ: Prentice Hall.

St. Lawrence, J. S., & Fortenberry, J. D. (2007). Behavioral interventions for STDs: Theoretical models and intervention methods. In S. O. Aral & J. M. Douglas (Eds.), *Behavioral interventions for prevention and control of sexually transmitted diseases* (pp. 23–59). New York: Springer.

Triandis, H. C. (1972). *The analysis of subjective culture*. New York: Wiley.

Triandis, H. C. (1980). Values, attitudes, and interpersonal behavior. In H. E. Howe & M. Page (Eds.), *Nebraska Symposium on Motivation, 1979* (pp.195–259). Lincoln: University of Nebraska Press.

Triandis, H. C., Bontempo, R., Villareal, M. J., Asai, M., & Lucca, N. (1988). Individualism and collectivism: Cross-cultural perspectives on self-ingroup relationships. *Journal of Personality and Social Psychology, 54*(2), 323–338.

von Haeften, I., Fishbein, M., Kasprzyk, D., & Montaño, D. E. (2000). Acting on one's intentions: Variations in condom use intentions and behaviours as a function of type of partner, gender, ethnicity and risk. *Psychology, Health & Medicine, 5*(2), 163–171.

von Haeften, I., Fishbein, M., Kasprzyk, D., & Montaño, D. (2001). Analyzing data to obtain information to design targeted interventions. *Psychology, Health & Medicine, 6*(2), 151–164.

von Haeften, I., & Kenski, K. (2001). Multi-partnered heterosexual's condom use for vaginal sex with their main partner as a function of attitude, subjective norm, partner norm, perceived behavioural control, and weighted control beliefs. *Psychology, Health & Medicine, 6*(2), 165–178.

Webb, T. L., & Sheeran, P. (2006). Does changing behavioral intentions engender behavior change? A meta-analysis of the experimental evidence. *Psychological Bulletin, 132*(2), 249–268.

Weinstein, N. D. (1993). Testing four competing theories of health-protective behavior. *Health Psychology, 12*(4), 324–333.

Weinstein, N. D. (2007). Misleading tests of health behavior theories. *Annals of Behavioral Medicine, 33*(1), 1–10.

Wicker, A. W. (1969). Attitudes vs. actions: The relationship of verbal and overt behavioral responses to attitude objects. *Journal of Social Issues, 25*, 41–78.

Wolff, K., Nordin, K., Brun, W., Berglund, G., & Kvale, G. (2011). Affective and cognitive attitudes, uncertainty avoidance and intention to obtain genetic testing: An extension of the theory of planned behaviour. *Psychology & Health, 26*(9), 1143–55.

World Health Organization and the Joint United Nations Programme on HIV/AIDS. (2007). *Male circumcision: Global trends and determinants of prevalence, safety and acceptability*. Geneva: WHO/UNAIDS Press.

CHAPTER 7

THE TRANSTHEORETICAL MODEL AND STAGES OF CHANGE

James O. Prochaska
Colleen A. Redding
Kerry E. Evers

KEY POINTS

This chapter will:

- Explain the stages of change and the other core transtheoretical model (TTM) constructs.

- Explore empirical support for and challenges to TTM.

- Describe how TTM interventions can be tailored to the needs of individuals while treating entire populations for smoking cessation.

- Expand on how such TTM interventions can be applied to change multiple health risk behaviors in high-risk populations.

The Transtheoretical Model (TTM) uses stages of change to integrate processes and principles of change across major theories of intervention, hence the term *transtheoretical*. The TTM emerged from a comparative analysis of twenty-five leading theories of psychotherapy, conducted in an effort to integrate a field that had fragmented into more than 300 theories of psychotherapy (Prochaska, 1979). Surprisingly, those theories had much more to say about *why* people change than about *how* they change. They were really theories of behavior, such as theories of personality and psychopathology, rather than theories of behavior change.

We identified ten processes of change that described key ways in which people changed their behaviors. These included consciousness raising, from the Freudian tradition (Freud, 1959); contingency management, from the Skinnerian tradition (Skinner, 1971); and forming helping relationships, from the Rogerian tradition (Rogers, 1951). Next, among smokers and former smokers, we conducted analyses that compared self-changers to people who received professional treatments, since an integrative model of change should reflect how people change on their own as well as with professional guidance. We assessed how frequently each group used each of the ten processes (DiClemente & Prochaska, 1982). Participants used different processes of change at different times in their struggles to quit smoking. These naive subjects taught researchers about a phenomenon that was not then a part of any therapy theories. They revealed that behavior change unfolds through a series of stages (Prochaska & DiClemente, 1983), with different change processes used at different stages. This profound insight changed the course of our research and led to development of the TTM.

From initial studies of smoking, our team and others expanded the stage model to include applications to a broad range of health risks, behaviors, and problems, including alcohol and substance abuse, anxiety and panic disorders, bullying, delinquency, depression, eating disorders and obesity, high-fat diets, HIV/AIDS prevention, use of mammography and other cancer screening, medication compliance, unplanned pregnancy prevention, pregnancy and smoking, radon testing, sedentary lifestyles, sun exposure, and physicians practicing preventive medicine. Over time, researchers across the world have expanded, validated, applied, and challenged core constructs of the TTM (Hall & Rossi, 2008; Noar, Benac, & Harris, 2007; J. O. Prochaska, Wright, & Velicer, 2008).

Core Constructs

Table 7.1 displays the core constructs of the Transtheoretical Model.

Table 7.1   Transtheoretical Model Constructs

Constructs	Description
Stages of change	
Precontemplation	No intention to take action within the next 6 months.
Contemplation	Intends to take action within the next 6 months.
Preparation	Intends to take action within the next 30 days and has taken some behavioral steps in this direction.
Action	Changed overt behavior for less than 6 months.
Maintenance	Changed overt behavior for more than 6 months.
Termination	No temptation to relapse and 100% confidence.
Processes of change	Covert and overt activities used to progress through stages.
Consciousness raising	Increasing awareness about the causes, consequences, and cures for a problem behavior: e.g., nutrition education.
Dramatic relief	Increasing negative or positive emotions (e.g., fear or inspiration) to motivate taking appropriate action: e.g., personal testimonials.
Self-reevaluation	Cognitive and affective reassessment of one's self-image, with or without an unhealthy behavior: e.g., values clarification.
Environmental reevaluation	Cognitive and affective assessment of how the presence or absence of a behavior affects one's social environment, such as the impact of one's smoking on others: e.g., empathy training.
Self-liberation	Belief that one can change and the commitment and recommitment to act on that belief: e.g., New Year's resolutions.
Helping relationships	Caring, trust, openness, and acceptance as well as support from others for healthy behavior change: e.g., a positive social network.

(continued)

Table 7.1 (Continued)

Constructs	Description
Social liberation	Increase in healthy social opportunities or alternatives: e.g., easy access to walking paths.
Counterconditioning	Learning healthier behaviors that can substitute for problem behaviors: e.g., relaxation replacing alcohol.
Stimulus control	Removing cues for unhealthy habits and adding prompts for healthier alternatives: e.g., removing all ashtrays from house and car.
Reinforcement management	Rewarding oneself or being rewarded by others for making progress: e.g., incentives.
Decisional balance	
Pros	Benefits of changing.
Cons	Costs of changing.
Self-efficacy	
Confidence	Confidence that one can engage in the healthy behavior across different challenging situations.
Temptation	A strong urge or desire to engage in the unhealthy behavior across different challenging situations.

Stages of Change

The TTM posits change as a process that unfolds over time, progressing through a series of six stages, although frequently not in a linear manner. In the past, behavior change was often construed as a discrete event, such as quitting smoking, drinking, or overeating. Our understanding about why some people fail to change or require multiple attempts to change came through identification and elaboration of the stages and processes of change.

Precontemplation is the stage in which people do not intend to take action in the near term, usually measured as the next six months. The outcome interval may vary depending on the behavior. People may be in this stage because they are not informed enough about the consequences of their behavior. Or they may have tried to change a number of times and become demoralized about their abilities to change. Both groups tend to avoid reading, talking, or thinking about their behaviors. They often are characterized as resistant, unmotivated, or not ready for health promotion programs. An alternative explanation is that traditional health promotion programs were not ready for such individuals and were not motivated to match their needs.

People in *contemplation* intend to change their behaviors in the next six months. They are more aware of the pros of changing than precontemplators and are also acutely aware of the cons. This balance between the costs and benefits of changing can produce profound ambivalence and keep some people stuck in contemplation, a phenomenon characterized as chronic contemplation or behavioral procrastination. These people are not ready for traditional action-oriented programs that expect participants to take immediate action. If contemplators are pushed into such programs, they are not likely to succeed.

In the *preparation* stage, people intend to take action soon, usually measured as the next month. Typically, they have taken some steps in the past year. They have a plan of action, such as joining a quit smoking health education class, consulting a counselor, talking to their physician, buying a self-help book, or relying on a self-change approach. These are the people who should be recruited for action-oriented programs, such as traditional smoking cessation or weight loss clinics.

People in the *action* stage have made specific overt modifications in their lifestyles within the past six months. Because action is observable, behavior change has often been equated with action. In the TTM, action is only one of six stages. Typically, not all modifications of behavior count as action in this model. In most applications, people have to attain a criterion that scientists and professionals agree is sufficient to reduce risks for disease. For some behaviors, such as cancer screening, the criterion may be getting an effective cancer screening test (e.g., a mammogram, Pap test, or colonoscopy) that can reduce the risk of dying from cancer. For smoking, there now is consensus that the criterion behavior should be total abstinence, since other changes do not necessarily lead to quitting and do not lower risks to zero. (The rise of e-cigarette use may add some new complexity to the definition of appropriate criterion behavior.) It is important to use validated, accepted measures for each behavioral outcome.

People in *maintenance* have made specific, overt modifications in their lifestyles. They are working to prevent relapse, and they do not apply change processes as frequently as people in action. They are less tempted to relapse and increasingly more confident that they can continue their changes. Based on self-efficacy data, it has been estimated that maintenance lasts from six months to about five years, depending on the targeted behavior. Longitudinal data from the 1990 surgeon general's report (U.S. Department of Health and Human Services, 1990) supported this temporal estimate. After twelve months of continuous abstinence, 43 percent of individuals returned to regular smoking. It was not until five years of continuous abstinence that risks for relapse dropped to 7 percent. The time frame can vary for other health behaviors.

People in *termination* report having zero temptation and 100 percent self-efficacy. Whether they are depressed, anxious, bored, lonely, angry, or stressed, they are sure they will not return to their old, unhealthy behaviors. It is as if they had never acquired the behavior in the first place, and their new behavior has become automatic. Examples include adults who buckle their seatbelts as soon as they get in their cars or automatically take their antihypertensive medications at the same time and place each day. In a study of former smokers and alcoholics, we found that fewer than 20 percent of each group had reached the criterion of zero temptation and total self-efficacy (Snow, Prochaska, & Rossi, 1992). The criterion may be too strict or this stage may be an ideal goal for the majority of people. In other areas, like exercise, consistent condom use, and weight control, the realistic goal may be a lifetime of maintenance, since relapse temptations are so prevalent and strong. Termination has received much less research and practical attention than other stages, because it typically takes so long for individuals to reach this stage.

Processes and Principles of Change

Table 7.1 defines the ten processes that have received the most empirical support in research to date, and briefly describes a technique for applying each process. As described above, the processes of change were derived originally from leading theories of psychotherapy and counseling (Prochaska, 1979).

Decisional balance reflects an individual's weighing of the pros and cons of changing. Initially, TTM relied on Janis and Mann's (1977) model of decision making that included four categories of pros (instrumental gains for self and others and approval from self and others) and four categories of cons (instrumental costs to self and others and disapproval from self and others). Over many studies, a simpler two-factor structure was found—pros and cons of changing.

Self-efficacy is the situation-specific confidence that one can cope with high-risk situations (temptations) without relapsing to one's former behaviors. This construct was integrated into the TTM from Bandura's (1982) Social Cognitive Theory. Self-efficacy reflected what we had seen among self-quitters.

Temptation reflects the converse of self-efficacy, the intensity of urges to engage in a specific unhealthy behavior when in difficult situations. Typically, three triggers account for most common types of temptations: negative affect or emotional distress, positive social situations, and craving.

Critical Assumptions

TTM researchers have concentrated on the first five stages of change, the ten processes of change, the pros and cons of changing, self-efficacy, or temptation (the last has received least attention). TTM is also based on critical assumptions about the nature of behavior change and interventions that can best facilitate such change. The following set of assumptions drive theory, research, and practice related to the Transtheoretical Model.

1. *Theories of health behavior change differ from theories of health behavior.* These differences were recognized by five leading behavioral theorists—Albert Bandura, Social Cognitive Theory (Chapter Nine); Marshall Becker, Health Belief Model (Chapter Five); Martin Fishbein, Theory of Reasoned Action (Chapter Six); Frederick Kanfer, self-regulation; and Harry Triandis, interpersonal behavior—in their 1992 report on a National Institute of Mental Health meeting designed to integrate the most important variables from their theories of behavior. They reported on a major alternative: namely, theories of behavior change and the Integrated Behavior Model, and cited TTM as a key example (Fishbein et al., 1992; also see Chapter Six in this text). Examples of differences between theories of behavior and of behavior change are that the former are more concerned with the best predictors of future behaviors, which of course are past behaviors. The latter are more concerned with the best predictors of future behavior change, such as stages of change. Behavioral theories favor variables that account for the most variance in behaviors, whereas behavior change theories favor variables that can control the most behavior change.

2. *No single theory can account for all complexities of behavior change.* A more comprehensive model is most likely to emerge from integration across major theories, hence the name *Transtheoretical*.

3. *Behavior change is a process that unfolds over time through a sequence of stages.*

4. *Stages are stable and open to change, just as health behavior risks are stable and open to change.*

5. *Most at-risk populations are not prepared for action* and will not be served effectively by traditional action-oriented behavior change programs.

6. *Specific processes and principles of change should be emphasized at specific stages.*

Empirical Support for TTM and Challenges

Prochaska, Wright, and Velicer (2008) developed a hierarchy of criteria from leading philosophers of science to evaluate theories of health behavior change and applied it to the TTM from the perspectives of both advocates and critics. The hierarchy was organized around a risky-test philosophy that advocates assessing a theory against increasingly tougher criteria (Meehl, 1978).

Stage Distribution

A low-risk test would be to use constructs, like stages, that are relatively clear and consistent for describing the readiness of populations. To match needs of individuals in entire populations, we should know population stage distributions for specific high-risk behaviors. A series of studies (e.g., Wewers, Stillman, Hartman, & Shopland, 2003) demonstrated that fewer than 20 percent of U.S. smokers were preparing to quit smoking or using other tobacco products. About 40 percent of smokers were in contemplation, and another 40 percent were in precontemplation. In countries without a long history of tobacco control campaigns, stage distributions were quite different. In Germany, about 70 percent of smokers were in precontemplation and about 10 percent of smokers were in preparation (Etter, Perneger, & Ronchi, 1997); in China, more than 70 percent were in precontemplation, and about 5 percent in preparation (Yang et al., 2001). In the United States, in a sample of 20,000 members of an HMO across fifteen health risk behaviors, only a small minority were ready for action (Rossi, 1992b).

Pros and Cons Structure Across Twelve Behaviors

A somewhat riskier test is to use constructs that, like the pros and cons of changing, can be generalized across behaviors. Across studies of twelve behaviors (smoking cessation, quitting cocaine, weight control, dietary fat reduction, safer sex, condom use, exercise acquisition, sunscreen use, radon testing, delinquency reduction, mammography screening, and physicians practicing preventive medicine), a two-factor structure of pros and cons was remarkably stable (J. O. Prochaska et al., 1994).

Integration of Pros and Cons and Stages of Change Across Twelve Health Behaviors

It is much easier to produce a list of theoretical constructs (Table 7.1) than to develop an empirical integration across constructs. For example, stage of change is often equated with TTM, but stage of change is a construct, not a theory. A theory requires systematic relationships between a set of constructs, ideally culminating in mathematical relationships.

For all twelve studies, the cons of changing were higher than the pros for people in precontemplation (J. O. Prochaska et al., 1994), and pros increased from precontemplation to contemplation. For all twelve behaviors, from contemplation to action, the cons of changing were lower in action than contemplation. In eleven of the studies, pros were higher than cons for people in action. These relationships suggest that to progress from precontemplation to contemplation, action, and subsequent stages, the pros of changing should increase. To progress from contemplation, cons should decrease. To move to action, pros should be higher than cons.

Strong and Weak Principles of Progress Across Forty-Eight Behaviors

Attempting to derive mathematical principles for integrating theoretical variables is a still riskier test for a theory, in part because few behavior change theories have generated such principles. In fact, most have not even developed constructs that are subject to such mathematical principles. Across the twelve studies discussed above, we found mathematical relationships between the pros and cons of changing and the progress across the stages (J. O. Prochaska et al., 1994).

The strong principle is PC → A ≈ 1 SD ↑ PROS. Progress from precontemplation (PC) to action (A) involves about a one standard deviation (SD) increase in the pros of changing. On intelligence tests, a 1 SD increase would be 15 points, which is a substantial increase.

Predicting the magnitude of this principle across a much broader range of behaviors and across diverse populations is much more challenging, or riskier, given the error variance that can be generated by so much heterogeneity. Nevertheless, in a recent meta-analysis of forty-eight behaviors and 120 data sets from ten countries, it was predicted that the pros of changing would increase 1 SD. The strong principle was confirmed to the second decimal with the increase being 1.00 SD (Hall & Rossi, 2008).

The weak principle is PC → A ≈ 0.5 SD ↓ CONS. Progress from precontemplation to action involves an ≈0.5 SD decrease in the cons of changing. Evidence from the recent meta-analysis for the weak principle was not as precise: 0.56 SD (Hall & Rossi, 2008). Nevertheless, data on forty-eight behaviors from 120 data sets were integrated in a single graph that supported two mathematical principles.

The practical implications of these principles are that pros of changing must increase about twice as much as cons must decrease for a person to move from one stage to another. Perhaps twice as much emphasis should be placed on raising benefits as on reducing costs or barriers to enact recommended behaviors. For example, if couch potatoes in precontemplation can list only five pros of exercise, then being too busy will be a big barrier to change. But if program participants accept that there can be more than sixty benefits of exercising most days of the week, being too busy may become a smaller barrier.

Processes of Change Across Behaviors

Building TTM based on ten processes originally identified by theorists with incompatible assumptions about humans and their behaviors (such as Freud, Carl Rogers, and Skinner) has been a tough test that TTM has only partially passed. The assumption is that people can apply a common set of change processes across a broad range of behaviors. The higher order measurement structure of the processes (experiential and behavioral) has been replicated across problem behaviors better than specific processes have been (Rossi, 1992a). Typically, support has been found for the set of ten processes across behaviors including smoking, diet, cocaine use, exercise, condom use, and sun exposure. But the measurement structure of processes has not been as consistent as the mathematical relationships between stages and pros and cons of changing. In some studies, fewer processes are found. Occasionally, evidence for one or two additional processes is found. It is also possible that for some behaviors or some people, fewer change processes may be used. With a regular but infrequent behavior like yearly mammograms, fewer processes may be required to progress to long-term maintenance (Rakowski et al., 1998).

Relationships Between Stages and Processes of Change

The discovery of systematic relationships between stages and processes is reflected in the empirical integration shown in Table 7.2 (Prochaska & DiClemente, 1983; J. O. Prochaska, DiClemente, & Norcross, 1992). This integration suggests that, in early stages, people rely upon cognitive, affective, and evaluative processes. In action-oriented stages, people draw more on commitments, conditioning, contingencies, environmental controls, and support for progressing toward maintenance or termination.

The relationships of processes to stages of change have important practical implications. To help people progress from precontemplation to contemplation, processes like consciousness raising and dramatic relief should be used. Encouraging the use of processes such as contingency management and stimulus control in precontemplation would be a theoretical, empirical, and practical mistake. But for people in action, such strategies would reflect optimal matching.

As with the structure of processes, relationships between the processes and stages have not been as consistent as relationships between the stages and the pros and cons of changing. While this may be due in part to the greater complexity of integrating ten processes across five stages, processes of change need more basic research and may be more specific to each problem behavior.

Table 7.2 Processes of Change That Mediate Progression Between Stages of Change

	Precontemplation	Contemplation	Preparation	Action	Maintenance
Processes	Consciousness raising				
	Dramatic relief				
	Environmental reevaluation				
		Self-reevaluation			
			Self-liberation		
				Counterconditioning	
				Helping relationships	
				Reinforcement management	
				Stimulus control	

Note: Social liberation was omitted due to its unclear relationship to the stages.

Applied Studies

Because health behavior change theories should be the basis for applied science, it is not enough to apply tests of generalization, integration, and prediction. Theory-driven interventions should pass risky tests to demonstrate that they can produce important impacts across a variety of problem behaviors, populations, and treatments. Across a diverse body of applied TTM studies, several trends are clear. The most common application, TTM-tailored expert system communications, matches intervention messages to an individual's needs across TTM constructs, based on information about the individuals for whom messages are tailored. For example, people in precontemplation could receive feedback designed to increase the pros of changing.

TTM-related intervention studies cover a range of health behavior topics, including smoking cessation (Aveyard et al., 1999; Dijkstra, Conijn, & De Vries, 2006; Dijkstra, De Vries, & Roijackers, 1999; Hall et al., 2006; Hollis et al., 2005; O'Neill, Gillespie, & Slobin, 2000; J. O. Prochaska, DiClemente, Velicer, & Rossi, 1993; J. O. Prochaska, Velicer, Fava, Rossi, & Tsoh, 2001; J. O. Prochaska, Velicer, Fava, Ruggiero, et al., 2001; Velicer, Prochaska, Fava, Laforge, & Rossi, 1999), diet (Beresford et al., 1997; Brug, Glanz, Van Assema, Kok, & van Breukelen, 1998; Campbell et al., 1994; Glanz et al., 1998; Horwath, 1999), and exercise (Cardinal & Sachs, 1996; Marcus et al., 1998; Rossi et al., 2005). Other randomized controlled trial outcome studies have addressed stress management (Evers et al., 2006), medication adherence (S. S. Johnson, Driskell, Johnson, Dyment, et al., 2006; S. S. Johnson, Driskell, Johnson, Prochaska, et al., 2006), and bullying prevention (J. O. Prochaska, Evers, Prochaska, Van Marter, & Johnson, 2007). The number of applications has grown, from alcohol abuse (Carbonari & DiClemente, 2000; Project MATCH Research Group, 1997), to condom use (CDC AIDS Community Demonstration Projects Research Group [CDC], 1999; Parsons, Huszti, Crudder, Rich, & Mendoza, 2000; Redding, Morokoff, Rossi, & Meier, 2007), domestic violence offenders (Levesque, Driskell, Prochaska, & Prochaska, 2008), organ donation (Robbins et al., 2001), and multiple behavior changes (Gold, Anderson, & Serxner, 2000; Kreuter & Strecher, 1996; Steptoe, Kerry, Rink, & Hilton, 2001).

TTM has been applied in many settings, including primary care (Goldstein et al., 1999; Hollis et al., 2005), homes (Gold et al., 2000), churches (Voorhees et al., 1996), schools (Aveyard et al., 1999), campuses (J. M. Prochaska et al., 2004), communities (CDC, 1999), and worksites (J. O. Prochaska, Butterworth, et al., 2008). While many of these applications have been effective, some have not (e.g., Aveyard et al., 1999).

A recent meta-analysis of tailored print communications found that TTM was the most commonly used theory across a broad range of behaviors (Noar et al., 2007). TTM or stage of change models were used in thirty-five of the fifty-three studies examined. Significantly greater effect sizes were found when tailored communications included the following TTM constructs: stages of change, pros and cons of changing, self-efficacy, and processes of change. In contrast, interventions that included the non-TTM construct of perceived susceptibility had significantly worse outcomes. Tailoring on non-TTM constructs like social norms and behavioral intentions did not produce significantly greater effect sizes.

While each TTM construct (stage, pros and cons, self-efficacy, and processes) produced greater effect sizes when included in tailored communications, what happened when only some constructs were used? Spencer, Pagell, Hallion, and Adams (2002) systematically reviewed twenty-three interventions that used one or more TTM variables for smoking cessation. Most studies used just stage; of these, only about 40 percent produced significant effects. Five used stage plus pros and cons or self-efficacy; 60 percent had significant effects. Another five used all TTM variables; 80 percent found significant effects. This analysis raises the important dissemination question of what it means for practice and applied research to be theory-driven. Most of these studies were variable-driven (e.g., using the stage variable) rather than theory-driven. Future research should determine whether interventions are most effective when a full theory, like TTM, is applied, or whether there are an optimal number of theoretical variables that can produce the same effect sizes.

Challenging Studies

Some researchers have explored alternative ways of formulating stages or have attempted to develop more parsimonious theories that use fewer constructs. These include Herzog, Abrams, Emmons, Linnan, and Shadel (1999); Herzog Abrams, Emmons, and Linnan (2000), and Abrams, Herzog, Emmons, and Linnan (2000). Other research has found that change processes and other TTM variables predict stage progress (e.g., DiClemente et al., 1991; Dijkstra et al., 2006; Evans et al., 2000; J. O. Prochaska, DiClemente, Velicer, Ginpil, & Norcross, 1985; J. O. Prochaska, Velicer, Guadagnoli, Rossi, & DiClemente, 1991; J. O. Prochaska, Velicer, Prochaska, & Johnson, 2004; J. O. Prochaska, Butterworth, et al., 2008; Sun, Prochaska, Velicer, & Laforge, 2007; Velicer, Redding, Sun, & Prochaska, 2007). Evans and colleagues (2000) explained some of the inconsistencies in previous research by demonstrating better predictions over six months versus twelve months, and better predictions using all ten processes of change instead of a subset.

In response to criticism that addiction levels are better predictors of long-term outcomes than stage of change, a series of studies was conducted to determine which types of effects predict long-term outcomes across multiple behaviors. To date, four effects have been found across a variety of health behaviors (Blissmer et al., 2010; Redding et al., 2011). The first is a severity effect in which individuals with less severe behavioral risks at baseline are more likely to have progressed to action or maintenance at the twenty-four-month follow-up for smoking, diet, and sun exposure. This effect includes the level of addiction that Farkas et al. (1996) and Abrams et al. (2000) preferred. The second is a stage effect in which participants in preparation at baseline have better twenty-four-month outcomes for smoking, diet, and sun exposure than those in contemplation; they do better than those in precontemplation. This stage effect is what Farkas et al. (1996) and Abrams et al. (2000) criticized. The third is a treatment effect in which participants in treatment do better at twenty-four months than those randomly assigned to control groups for smoking, diet, and sun exposure. The fourth is an effort effect in which participants in both treatment and control groups who progressed to action and maintenance at twenty-four months were making better efforts with TTM variables like pros and cons, self-efficacy, and processes at baseline. There were no consistent demographic effects across the three behaviors. What these results indicate is that either-or thinking (such as either severity or stage) is not as helpful as a more inclusive approach that seeks to identify the most important effects, whether they are based on TTM or on an addiction or severity model.

Other Stage Models

The TTM is one of many stage models. Here we provide a brief overview of some other stage models of behavior change. The Precaution Adoption Process Model (PAPM) was developed to describe and explain the process by which people adopt precautions against a new risk (Weinstein, 1988). The model was first applied to adoption of precautionary behaviors after new risk warnings were released about high levels of radon in some homes. PAPM specifies seven stages: Stage 1: unaware; Stage 2: aware, but no thought of adopting precautions; Stage 3: thinking but undecided; Stage 4: decided against adopting the precaution; Stage 5: decided to adopt but have not yet acted; Stage 6: acted on their decision to adopt; and Stage 7: for some behaviors, maintenance may be needed.

PAPM asserts that these stages represent qualitatively different patterns of behaviors, beliefs, and experiences, and that factors that produce transitions between stages vary depending on the specific transition being considered (Weinstein & Sandman, 1992; Weinstein, Sandman, & Blalock, 2008). An increase in knowledge is needed to move people from Stage 1 to 2. Belief that the problem is likely (e.g., in one's home) is a powerful factor to move people to Stage 3 to think about making a decision, but does not predict whether people will decide against adopting a precaution (Stage 4) or to adopt it (Stage 5). The decision to act appears to be due to situational factors (e.g., convenience and guidance from public officials) rather than internal motivations. Finally, the influence of peers at decision stages suggests that people sometimes use behaviors and attitudes of others to help them bypass the challenge of reaching decisions on their own.

The Health Action Process Approach (HAPA) was developed by Ralf Schwarzer (2008), one of Europe's leading health psychologists. Five major principles make it distinct. Principle 1 is that the behavior change process is divided into two phases: *motivation*, where people develop their intentions to change, and *volition*, which displays two subphases—individuals who have not yet translated intentions into actions, and those who have. Principle 2 is that individuals can be categorized into three stages: pretenders, intenders, and actors. Principles 3 and 4 state that planning is a key strategy for translating intentions into action. Action planning pertains to the when, where, and how of intended action. Coping planning includes the anticipation of barriers and the design of alternative actions to reach one's goals in spite of barriers. Principle 5 is that the nature of self-efficacy differs from phase to phase: pre-action or task self-efficacy affects one's motivation, coping self-efficacy deals with barriers, and recovery self-efficacy allows rebounding from relapse.

In this approach, interventions should be tailored to different phases, stages, or mindsets. Nonintenders, with the mindset not to act, can benefit most from communications about positive outcome expectancies resulting from changing and the risks associated with not changing. Intenders would benefit most from translating their intentions into actions. Actors may not need treatment except perhaps to prepare for high-risk situations or to develop high self-efficacy to recover from lapses or relapses.

Applications of TTM: Treating Populations of Smokers

Applying TTM to an entire at-risk population, such as smokers, requires a systematic approach that begins with recruiting and retaining a high percentage of the eligible population. The program should help participants progress through the stages of change by applying a process that matches or tailors interventions to the needs of each individual at each stage of change. Such systematic applications can then be evaluated in terms of outcomes by assessing impacts on reducing the prevalence of smoking in the target population.

Continuum of Population Engagement

The architects of health care reform in the United States aimed to transform a fragmented health care system into a population-based system accountable for keeping people as healthy as possible. Health care payers and providers are incentivized to be responsible for the health and well-being of entire populations. One of the most important challenges in health care is how patient or employee populations can be encouraged to participate in evidence-based interventions designed to prevent and manage chronic conditions that produce high costs from health care, disability, and lost productivity. We have organized this population cessation section around the factors we apply at each phase of engagement.

Reach and Recruit

We begin with considering how we can reach and recruit populations, since population smoking cessation requires interventions that reach or recruit high percentages of smokers. In two home-based programs with 5,000 smokers in each study, we reached out either by telephone alone or by personal letters for the first step, followed by telephone calls, if needed, and recruited smokers to stage-matched interventions. We communicated that whether individuals were ready, getting ready, or not ready to quit, our programs could be of help. For each of five stages, interventions included self-help manuals; individualized computer feedback reports based on assessments of pros and cons, processes, self-efficacy, and temptations; and/or counselor protocols based on computer reports. Using proactive recruitment methods and stage-matched communications and interventions resulted in rates for the two programs of 80 percent to 85 percent, respectively (J. O. Prochaska, Velicer, Fava, Rossi, et al., 2001; J. O. Prochaska, Velicer, Fava, Ruggiero, et al., 2001). Such high recruitment rates provide the potential to generate unprecedented impacts with entire populations of smokers.

Population impact has been defined as participation rate multiplied by the rate of efficacy or action (Velicer & DiClemente, 1993). If a program produced 30 percent efficacy (e.g., long-term abstinence) historically, it was judged to be better than a program that produced 25 percent abstinence. A program that generates 30 percent efficacy but only 5 percent participation has an impact of only 1.5 percent (30% × 5%). A program that produces only 25 percent efficacy but has 60 percent participation has an impact of 15 percent. With health promotion programs, the impact on a high-risk population would be ten times greater.

TTM programs shift outcomes from efficacy alone to impact. To achieve high impact, it is necessary to move from reactive recruitment to proactive recruitment, where we reach out to interact with all potential participants, including those not yet ready to change behaviors. This is really the meaning of population-based strategies.

Employers rely increasingly on incentives to maximize employee participation in wellness programs. In many cases, incentives are needed to attract employees into the programs. Once high recruitment rates are achieved, the next challenge is to generate high retention rates, lest many initial participants drop out.

Retain

Psychotherapy and behavior change programs suffer from relatively poor retention rates. One meta-analysis found that across 125 studies, the average retention rate was only about 50 percent (Wierzbicki & Pekarik, 1993). Furthermore, there were few consistent predictors of who would drop out prematurely and who would continue in therapy. In studies on smoking, weight control, substance abuse, and a mixture of mental health problems, stage of change measures proved to be the best predictors of premature termination. In a study of psychotherapy for mental health problems, the pretreatment stage profile of the entire 40 percent who dropped out prematurely, as judged by their therapists, was that of patients in precontemplation. The 20 percent who terminated quickly but appropriately had a profile of patients in action. Pretreatment stage-related measures correctly classified 93 percent of the two groups (Brogan, Prochaska, & Prochaska, 1999).

Historically, the best strategy to promote retention was to match interventions to stage of change. In three smoking cessation studies using matching strategies, smokers in precontemplation were retained at the same high levels as those who started in preparation (J. O. Prochaska et al., 1993; J. O. Prochaska, Velicer, Fava, Rossi, et al., 2001; J. O. Prochaska, Velicer, Fava, Ruggiero, et al., 2001). Increasingly, we have had to include incentives as an important factor to retain individuals in behavior change programs (e.g., J. L. Johnson et al., 2013). With increasing reliance on incentives to engage patient and employee participation, the concern has become how we can transform extrinsic motivation (e.g., money) into intrinsic motivation. A key factor here is to be able to give feedback to participants that they are making progress toward increasing their health and well-being.

Progress

The amount of progress participants make following health promotion programs is directly related to their stage at baseline. Across sixty-six different predictions of progress, smokers starting in contemplation were about two-thirds more successful than those in precontemplation at six, twelve, and eighteen months. Similarly, those in preparation were about two-thirds more successful than those in contemplation at the same follow-ups (J. O. Prochaska, Velicer, Fava, Rossi, et al., 2001). In TTM computer-tailored intervention (CTI) coaching, online and mobile programs, participants can be given feedback that they have advanced a stage and have almost doubled their chances of quitting smoking in the next few months. Coaches (in-person, telephone-based, and virtual) and computer programs also can provide positive feedback for other changes and offer suggestions for alternative pathways when individuals are not making progress.

Behavior change programs should first engage individuals in the treatment process during the recruitment and retention phases. With financial incentives, individuals can go through the motions of completing coaching or computer sessions to earn their extrinsic motivators. In the progress and success phases, individuals must be engaged in the behavior change process.

These results can be used in practice. A reasonable goal for each interaction is to help current smokers to progress one stage. If, over the course of brief coaching, they progress two stages, they will be about 2.66 times more successful at longer-term follow-ups (J. O. Prochaska, Velicer, Fava, Rossi, et al., 2001).

Success

In our first large-scale clinical trial, we compared four treatments: (1) one of the best home-based, action-oriented cessation programs (standardized); (2) stage-matched manuals (individualized); (3) expert system computer reports plus manuals (interactive); and (4) counselors plus computers and manuals (personalized). We randomly assigned by stage 739 smokers to one of the four treatments (J. O. Prochaska et al., 1993).

In the computer condition, participants completed by mail or telephone forty questions that were used as the basis for computer-generated feedback reports. These reports informed participants about their stage of change, the pros and cons of changing, and the use of change processes appropriate to their stages. At baseline, participants were given positive feedback on what they were doing correctly and guidance on which principles and processes they should apply to progress. In two progress reports delivered over the next six months, they also received positive feedback on any improvement they made on any of the variables relevant to progressing. Demoralized and defensive smokers could begin progressing without having to quit and without having to work too hard. Smokers in the contemplation stage could begin taking small steps to decrease severity (like delaying their first cigarette in the morning for an extra thirty minutes or reducing the number of cigarettes they smoke) that would increase their self-efficacy and help them become better prepared for quitting. In the personalized condition, smokers received four proactive counselor calls over the six-month intervention period.

Outcomes for the two self-help manual conditions paralleled each other for twelve months. At eighteen months, the stage-matched manuals moved ahead. This is an example of a *delayed action effect*, which is often observed with stage-matched programs specifically, and others have observed with self-help programs generally (Glynn, Anderson, & Schwarz, 1991). It takes time for participants in early stages to progress to action. Thus some treatment effects, measured by action, will be observed only after considerable delay. It is encouraging to find treatments producing therapeutic effects months and even years after treatment ended.

Computer alone and computer plus counselor conditions paralleled each other for twelve months. Then the effects of the counselor condition flattened out while the computer condition effects increased. Participants in the personalized condition may have become somewhat dependent on the social support and social control of the counselor calling. The last call was after the six-month assessment, and benefits would be observed at twelve months. Termination of counselors could result in no further progress, because of the loss of social support and control. The classic pattern in smoking cessation clinics is rapid relapse as soon as treatment is terminated. Some of this rapid relapse could well be due to the sudden loss of social support or social control provided by the counselors and other participants in the clinic.

Outcomes with Diverse Groups

Testing how interventions succeed with diverse groups that have been understudied and underserved is a riskier test than assessing outcomes in general populations. Outcomes with diverse groups were part of an analysis that combined data from five effectiveness trials in which 2,972 smokers were proactively recruited, and all received the same TTM-tailored interventions plus stage-matched manuals. Intervention produced a consistent 22 percent to 26 percent long-term cessation rate across the five studies, with a mean of about 24 percent (Velicer et al., 2007). There were no significant differences in abstinence rates between females (24.6%) and males (23.6%) or between African Americans (30.2%) and Caucasians (23.9%) or between Hispanics and non-Hispanics. Older smokers (65 and older) had abstinence rates (35.2%) that were 45 percent higher than the mean. College graduates had abstinence rates (30.1%) that were significantly higher than average.

These outcomes from diverse groups receiving TTM-tailored treatments challenge stereotypes that assume some groups are more resistant to change. Access to quality behavior change programs may be the key differentiator.

Benchmarking: A Case Study on Multiple Health Behavior Change

For a theory to be useful, outcomes and lessons learned from randomized clinical trials (RCTs) should generalize to real-world applications. Several characteristics of good research are relevant to evaluation of health behavior theories, including number of replications, magnitude of outcomes, the participation rate, the number of behaviors treated, and the strength of study designs.

We compared results of our MHBC multiple behavior case study to average outcomes for four behaviors (exercise, low-fat diets, fruit and vegetable consumption, and smoking) from a comprehensive review of fifty-three treatment arms of RCTs and case studies of health promotion programs for employees (Soler et al., 2010). These interventions included repeated health risk assessments (HRAs) and at least one additional intervention, and used national criteria for outcomes reflecting progression from at-risk (not at criteria) to not-at-risk (at criteria). These studies generated an average of about 50 percent participation and about 2.75 years of follow-up. We also compared our case study to the averages of our outcomes from twenty-six arms of RCTs applying our best practice TTM CTIs to the same four risk behaviors and to effective stress management and depression prevention (Johnson et al., 2013).

These studies generated an average of about 70 percent participation and average follow-ups comparable those reported in Soler et al. (2010).

Our case study involved a national employer and thirty worksites. The employee population and employees' adult dependents began by being incentivized to complete yearly HRAs and biometric screenings. Employees later had to complete at least one TTM intervention for one behavior per year. These interventions could be either tailored telephonic coaching or online programs. A cohort of 6,544 was tested at baseline and at a follow-up conducted after at least two years.

Figure 7.1 shows that with each of four common risk behaviors, our TTM-based RCTs produced substantially greater outcomes than the averages found in the Soler et al. (2010) body of knowledge. Contrary to our expectations and to predictions from diffusion theory, our case study also outperformed the results from RCTs for each of the four common behaviors and for effective stress management and depression prevention. There may be many explanations for this outcome, including artificial limits on treatment length of programs. In the real world of employers, treatments may not have to end if people still are benefiting.

These important issues aside, Figure 7.1 provides a benchmark that decision makers can use to compare alternative health promotion programs when considering which interventions to provide for their populations. Without the help of such benchmarks, employers could choose average interventions that would produce only a fraction of the impacts of high-performing programs.

The health promotion community can use such benchmarks to compare case studies to identify which programs are average and which are high performing. With many more case studies than RCTs, and with many more interventions and innovations, the field can have a larger and more rapidly growing body of knowledge for benchmarking impacts of programs for different risks with different populations both nationally and internationally.

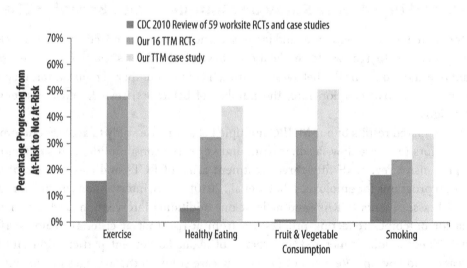

Figure 7.1 Comparative Outcomes of Health Promotion Interventions
Source: Johnson et al., 2013.

These results indicate that TTM-tailored interventions may be producing benchmark impacts on multiple behaviors for disease prevention and multiple domains for enhancing well-being. If these results are replicated, health promotion programs with lower treatment demands could produce benchmark impacts on multiple risk behaviors in entire populations. Such impacts require scientific and professional shifts from:

1. An action paradigm to a stage paradigm
2. A single behavior paradigm to a multiple behavior paradigm
3. Reactive recruitment to proactive recruitment
4. Expecting participants to match the needs of programs to expecting programs to match the needs of participants
5. Clinic-based behavioral health programs to community-based programs that still apply the field's most powerful individualized and interactive intervention strategies to entire populations
6. Limited accessibility to assuring that all individuals have easy accessibility to evidence-based programs, such as free, digitally delivered programs that can be accessed at any time and any place

Limitations

Although the Transtheoretical Model has been applied across at least forty-eight behaviors and populations from many countries, the model has limitations. To date, population trials based on TTM have not produced significant prevention effects in preventing substance abuse among children (see, e.g., Aveyard et al., 1999; Hollis et al., 2005). Unfortunately, little can be concluded from nonsignificant results. For example, Peterson, Kealey, Mann, Marek, and Sarason (2000) reported that sixteen out of seventeen trials failed and suggested that the field should move beyond social influence models. Prevention trials are challenging across theories.

It might be assumed that TTM does not apply very well to children and adolescents. There is a basic question regarding the age at which intentional behavior change begins. But applied studies of bullying prevention in elementary, middle, and high schools produced significant results (J. O. Prochaska et al., 2007). Similarly, early intervention with adolescent smokers using TTM-tailored treatments produced significant abstinence rates at twenty-four months that were almost identical to rates among treated adult smokers (Hollis et al., 2005). This was also true for TTM-tailored interventions targeting sun protective behaviors in adolescents (Norman et al., 2007). One problem is that there has been much more research applying TTM to reducing risks than to preventing risks.

Given the global application of TTM, it will be important to determine the cultures in which TTM can be applied effectively and the cultures for which it may require major adaptations. In basic meta-analysis research on the relationships between stages and pros and cons of changing in a number of countries, there was no significant effect by country (Hall & Rossi, 2008). But this research looked at only ten of the many countries in the world.

Future Research

While research results to date are encouraging, much still needs to be done to advance understanding about the processes of behavior change, effective interventions to achieve population impact, and other issues related to the Transtheoretical Model specifically and to behavior change research more generally. Basic research should be done with other theoretical variables, such as processes of resistance, well-being, and problem severity, to determine whether such variables relate systematically to the stages and predict progress across particular stages.

More research is needed on the structure and integration of processes and stages of change across a broad range of behaviors, such as acquisition behaviors, like exercise, and extinction behaviors, like smoking cessation (Rosen, 2000). It is important to examine what modifications are needed for specific types of behaviors, such as fewer processes perhaps for infrequent behaviors, like mammography screening, or behaviors that may relapse less often, such as sunscreen use.

Because tailored communications represent the most promising interventions for applying TTM, more research needs to compare the effectiveness, cost effectiveness, and impacts of alternative technologies. The Internet is excellent for delivering individualized interactions at low cost, but it cannot produce the high participation rates generated by person-to-person outreach via telephone or primary care practitioners (J. O. Prochaska, Butterworth, et al., 2008; J. O. Prochaska et al., 2004, 2005). One promising approach added tailored texting to best practice, Internet-based CTIs. This enhancement produced an improvement in abstinence of 11 percentage points (44% versus 33%) (Jordan, Evers, Levesque, & Prochaska, 2015).

Our best practice TTM CTIs at the individual and behavioral levels should be applied within multiple level interventions, such as biological (e.g., pharmacological adjuncts) and social (e.g., policy) level interventions. One limitation of most medications is they are designed for individuals prepared to take action. We tried to recruit smokers to a combined nicotine replacement therapy and TTM CTIs, but were not successful in recruiting smokers in precontemplation.

While application of TTM-tailored interventions to diverse populations has been promising, more research should be done to compare alternative modalities for reaching and helping such populations. Perhaps menus of alternative intervention modalities (such as telephone, Internet, neighborhood or church leaders, person-to-person efforts, or community programs) empower diverse populations to best match health-enhancing programs to their needs.

Changing multiple behaviors creates special challenges, including the demands placed on participants and providers. Alternative strategies, beyond the sequential (one at a time) and simultaneous (each treated intensely at the same time) approaches, should be assessed. Integrative approaches are promising. In bullying prevention, multiple behaviors (e.g., hitting, stealing, ostracizing, mean gossiping and labeling, and damaging personal belongings) and multiple roles (bully, victim, and passive bystander) require treatment. In one instance, the available classroom intervention time was only thirty minutes. If behavior change is construct-driven (e.g., by stage or self-efficacy), what is a higher order construct that could integrate all of these more concrete behaviors and roles? In this case, that concept was relating with respect. As indicated earlier, significant and important improvements across roles and behaviors were found for elementary, middle, and high school students (J. O. Prochaska et al., 2007). As with any theory, effective applications may be limited more by our creativity and resources for testing than by the ability of the theory to drive significant research and effective interventions.

The Transtheoretical Model is dynamic, and should be open to modifications and enhancements as more students, scientists, and practitioners apply the stage paradigm to a growing number of theoretical issues, public health problems, and at-risk populations.

Summary

In this chapter, we described the fifteen core constructs of TTM and how these constructs can be integrated across stages of change. Empirical support for the basic constructs of TTM and for applied research was presented, along with conceptual and empirical challenges from critics. Applications of TTM-tailored interventions with entire populations were explored, with examples for the single behavior of smoking and for multiple behaviors. A major theme is that programmatically building and applying core constructs of TTM at the individual level can lead to high-impact programs for enhancing health at the population level.

References

Abrams, D. B., Herzog, T. A., Emmons, K. M., & Linnan, L. (2000). Stages of change versus addiction: A replication and extension. *Nicotine & Tobacco Research, 2*(3), 223–229.

Aveyard, P., Cheng, K. K., Almond, J., Sherratt, E., Lancashire, R., Lawrence, T., . . . Evans, O. (1999). Cluster randomised controlled trial of expert system based on the transtheoretical ("stages of change") model for smoking prevention and cessation in schools. *BMJ, 319*(7215), 948–953.

Bandura, A. (1982). Self-efficacy mechanism in human agency. *American Psychologist, 37*(2), 122–147.

Beresford, S. A., Curry, S. J., Kristal, A. R., Lazovich, D., Feng, Z., & Wagner, E. H. (1997). A dietary intervention in primary care practice: The eating patterns study. *American Journal of Public Health, 87*(4), 610–616.

Blissmer, B., Prochaska, J. O., Velicer, W. F., Redding, C. A., Rossi, J. S., Greene, G. W., . . . Robbins, M. (2010). Common factors predicting long-term changes in multiple health behaviors. *Journal of Health Psychology, 15*(2), 205–214.

Brogan, M. M., Prochaska, J. O., & Prochaska, J. M. (1999). Predicting termination and continuation status in psychotherapy using the transtheoretical model. *Psychotherapy, 36*(2), 105–113.

Brug, J., Glanz, K., Van Assema, P., Kok, G., & van Breukelen, G. J. (1998). The impact of computer-tailored feedback and iterative feedback on fat, fruit, and vegetable intake. *Health Education & Behavior, 25*(4), 517–531.

Campbell, M. K., DeVellis, B. M., Strecher, V. J., Ammerman, A. S., DeVellis, R. F., & Sandler, R. S. (1994). Improving dietary behavior: The effectiveness of tailored messages in primary care settings. *American Journal of Public Health, 84*(5), 783–787.

Carbonari, J. P., & DiClemente, C. C. (2000). Using transtheoretical model profiles to differentiate levels of alcohol abstinence success. *Journal of Consulting and Clinical Psychology, 68*(5), 810–817.

Cardinal, B. J., & Sachs, M. L. (1996). Effects of mail-mediated, stage-matched exercise behavior change strategies on female adults' leisure-time exercise behavior. *Journal of Sports Medicine and Physical Fitness, 36*, 100–107.

CDC AIDS Community Demonstration Projects Research Group. (1999). Community-level HIV intervention in 5 cities: Final outcome data from the CDC AIDS community demonstration projects. *American Journal of Public Health, 89*(3), 336–345.

DiClemente, C. C., & Prochaska, J. O. (1982). Self-change and therapy change of smoking behavior: A comparison of processes of change in cessation and maintenance. *Addictive Behavior, 7*(2), 133–142.

DiClemente, C. C., Prochaska, J. O., Fairhurst, S. K., Velicer, W. F., Velasuez, M. M., & Rossi, J. S. (1991). The process of smoking cessation: An analysis of precontemplation, contemplation, and preparation stages of change. *Journal of Consulting and Clinical Psychology, 59*(2), 295–304.

Dijkstra, A., Conijn, B., & De Vries, H. A. (2006). A match-mismatch test of a stage model of behaviour change in tobacco smoking. *Addiction, 101*(7), 1035–1043.

Dijkstra, A., De Vries, H., & Roijackers, J. (1999). Targeting smokers with low readiness to change with tailored and nontailored self-help materials. *Preventive Medicine, 28*(2), 203–211.

Etter, J. F., Perneger, T. V., & Ronchi, A. (1997). Distributions of smokers by stage: International comparison and association with smoking prevalence. *Preventive Medicine, 26*(4), 580–585.

Evans, J. L., Regan, R. M., Maddock, J. E., Fava, J. L., Velicer, W. F., Rossi, J. S., & Prochaska, J. O. (2000). What predicts stage of change for smoking cessation? *Annals of Behavioral Medicine, 22(S173)*. Poster presented at the Twenty-First Annual Scientific Sessions of the Society of Behavioral Medicine, Nashville, TN.

Evers, K. E., Prochaska, J. O., Johnson, J. L., Mauriello, L. M., Padula, J. A., & Prochaska, J. M. (2006). A randomized clinical trial of a population- and transtheoretical model–based stress-management intervention. *Health Psychology, 25*(4), 521–529.

Farkas, A. J., Pierce, J. P., Zhu, S. H., Rosbrook, B., Gilpin, E. A., Berry, C., & Kaplan, R. M. (1996). Addiction versus stages of change models in predicting smoking cessation. *Addiction, 91*(9), 1271–1280.

Fishbein, M., Bandura, A., Triandis, H. D., Kanfer, F. H., Becker, M. H., Middlestadt, S. E., & Eichler, A. (1992). *Factors influencing behavior and behavior change: Final report—theorist's workshop.* Bethesda, MD: National Institute of Mental Health.

Freud, S. (1959). The question of lay analysis. In J. Strachey (Ed. & Trans.), *The standard edition of the complete psychological works of Sigmund Freud* (Vol. 20, pp. 183–250). London: Hogarth Press.

Glanz, K., Patterson, R. E., Kristal, A. R., Feng, Z., Linnan, L., Heimendinger, J., & Hebert, J. R. (1998). Impact of work site health promotion on stages of dietary change: The Working Well Trial. *Health Education & Behavior, 25*(4), 448–463.

Glynn, T. J., Anderson, D. M., & Schwarz, L. (1991). Tobacco-use reduction among high-risk youth: Recommendations of a National Cancer Institute expert advisory panel. *Preventive Medicine, 20*(2), 279–291.

Gold, D. B., Anderson, D. R., & Serxner, S. A. (2000). Impact of a telephone-based intervention on the reduction of health risks. *American Journal of Health Promotion, 15*(2), 97–106.

Goldstein, M. G., Pinto, B. M., Marcus, B. H., Lynn, H., Jette, A. M., Rakowski, W., . . . Tennstedt, S. (1999). Physician-based physical activity counseling for middle-aged and older adults: A randomized trial. *Annals of Behavioral Medicine, 21*(1), 40–47.

Hall, K. L., & Rossi, J. S. (2008). Meta-analytic examination of the strong and weak principles across 48 health behaviors. *Preventive Medicine, 46*(3), 266–274.

Hall, S. M., Tsoh, J. Y., Prochaska, J. J., Eisendrath, S., Rossi, J. S., Redding, C. A., . . . Gorecki, J. A. (2006). Treatment for cigarette smoking among depressed mental health outpatients: A randomized clinical trial. *American Journal of Public Health, 96*(10), 1808–1814.

Herzog, T. A., Abrams, D. B., Emmons, K. M., & Linnan, L. (2000). Predicting increases in readiness to quit smoking: A prospective analysis using the contemplation ladder. *Psychology & Health, 15*(3), 369–381.

Herzog, T. A., Abrams, D. B., Emmons, K. M., Linnan, L. A., & Shadel, W. G. (1999). Do processes of change predict stage movements? A prospective analysis of the transtheoretical model. *Health Psychology, 18*(4), 369–375.

Hollis, J. F., Polen, M. R., Whitlock, E. P., Lichtenstein, E., Mullooly, J. P., Velicer, W. F., & Redding, C. A. (2005). Teen REACH: Outcomes from a randomized controlled trial of a tobacco reduction program for teens seen in primary medical care. *Pediatrics, 115*(4), 981–989.

Horwath, C. C. (1999). Applying the transtheoretical model to eating behaviour change: Challenges and opportunities. *Nutrition Research Review, 12*(2), 281–317.

Janis, I. L., & Mann, L. (1977). *Decision making: A psychological analysis of conflict, chance and commitment.* London: Cassil & Collier Macmillan.

Johnson, J. L., Prochaska, J. O., Paiva, A. L., Fernandez, A. C., Dewees, S. L., & Prochaska, J. M. (2013). Advancing bodies of evidence for population-based health promotion programs: Randomized controlled trials and case studies. *Population Health Management, 16*(6), 373–380.

Johnson, S. S., Driskell, M. M., Johnson, J. L., Dyment, S. J., Prochaska, J. O., Prochaska, J. M., & Bourne, L. (2006). Transtheoretical model intervention for adherence to lipid-lowering drugs. *Disease Management, 9*(2), 102–114.

Johnson, S. S., Driskell, M. M., Johnson, J. L., Prochaska, J. M., Zwick, W., & Prochaska, J. O. (2006). Efficacy of a transtheoretical model–based expert system for antihypertensive adherence. *Disease Management, 9*(5), 291–301.

Jordan, P. J., Evers, K. E., Levesque, D. A., & Prochaska, J. O. (2015). Tailored texting to enhance a stage-based online tailored program for veterans who smoke: A randomized breakthrough and benchmark trial. Article submitted for review.

Kreuter, M., & Strecher, V. J. (1996). Do tailored behavior change messages enhance the effectiveness of health risk appraisal? Results from a randomized trial. *Health Education Research, 11*, 97–105.

Levesque, D. A., Driskell, M., Prochaska, J. M., & Prochaska, J. O. (2008). Acceptability of a stage-matched expert system intervention for domestic violence offenders. *Violence and Victims, 23*(4), 432–445.

Marcus, B. H., Bock, B. C., Pinto, B. M., Forsyth, L. H., Roberts, M. B., & Traficante, R. M. (1998). Efficacy of an individualized, motivationally-tailored physical activity intervention. *Annals of Behavioral Medicine, 20*(3), 174–180.

Meehl, P. E. (1978). Theoretical risks and tabular asterisks: Sir Karl, Sir Ronald, and the slow progress of soft psychology. *Journal of Consulting and Clinical Psychology, 46*, 806–834.

Noar, S. M., Benac, C., & Harris, M. (2007). Does tailoring matter? Meta-analytic review of tailored print health behavior change interventions. *Psychological Bulletin, 133*(4), 673–693.

Norman, G. J., Adams, M. A., Calfas, K. J., Covin, J., Sallis, J. F., Rossi, J. S., . . . Patrick, K. (2007). A randomized trial of a multicomponent intervention for adolescent sun protection behaviors. *Archives of Pediatrics & Adolescent Medicine, 161*(2), 146–152.

O'Neill, H. K., Gillespie, M. A., & Slobin, K. (2000). Stages of change and smoking cessation: A computer-administered intervention program for young adults. *American Journal of Health Promotion, 15*(2), 93–96.

Parsons, J. T., Huszti, H. C., Crudder, S. O., Rich, L., & Mendoza, J. (2000). Maintenance of safer sexual behaviours: Evaluation of a theory-based intervention for HIV seropositive men with haemophilia and their female partners. *Haemophilia, 6*(3), 181–190.

Peterson, A. V., Jr., Kealey, K. A., Mann, S. L., Marek, P. M., & Sarason, I. G. (2000). Hutchinson Smoking Prevention Project: Long-term randomized trial in school-based tobacco use prevention—results on smoking. *Journal of the National Cancer Institute, 92*(24), 1979–1991.

Prochaska, J. M., Prochaska, J. O., Cohen, F. C., Gomes. S. O., Laforge, R. G., & Eastwood, A. L. (2004). The transtheoretical model of change for multi-level interventions for alcohol abuse on campus. *Journal of Alcohol and Drug Education, 47*(3), 34–50.

Prochaska, J. O. (1979). *Systems of psychotherapy: A transtheoretical analysis.* Homewood, IL: Dorsey Press.

Prochaska, J. O., Butterworth, S., Redding, C. A., Burden, V., Perrin, N., Leo, M., . . . Prochaska, J. M. (2008). Initial efficacy of MI, TTM tailoring and HRI's with multiple behaviors for employee health promotion. *Preventive Medicine, 46*(3), 226–231.

Prochaska, J. O., & DiClemente, C. C. (1983). Stages and processes of self-change of smoking: Toward an integrative model of change. *Journal of Consulting and Clinical Psychology, 51*(3), 390–395.

Prochaska, J. O., DiClemente, C. C., & Norcross, J. C. (1992). In search of how people change: Applications to the addictive behaviors. *American Psychologist, 47*(9), 1102–1114.

Prochaska, J. O., DiClemente, C. C., Velicer, W. F., Ginpil, S., & Norcross, J. C. (1985). Predicting change in smoking status for self-changers. *Addictive Behaviors, 10*(4), 395–406.

Prochaska, J. O., DiClemente, C. C., Velicer, W. F., & Rossi, J. S. (1993). Standardized, individualized, interactive, and personalized self-help programs for smoking cessation. *Health Psychology, 12*(5), 399–405.

Prochaska, J. O., Evers, K. E., Prochaska, J. M., Van Marter, D., & Johnson, J. L. (2007). Efficacy and effectiveness trials: Examples from smoking cessation and bullying prevention. *Journal of Health Psychology, 12*(1), 170–178.

Prochaska, J. O., Velicer, W. F., Fava, J. L., Rossi, J. S., & Tsoh, J. Y. (2001). Evaluating a population-based recruitment approach and a stage-based expert system intervention for smoking. *Addictive Behaviors, 26*(4), 583–602.

Prochaska, J. O., Velicer, W. F., Fava, J. L., Ruggiero, L., Laforge, R. G., Rossi. J. S., . . . Lee, P. A. (2001). Counselor and stimulus control enhancements of a stage-matched expert system intervention for smokers in a managed care setting. *Preventive Medicine, 32*(1), 23–32.

Prochaska, J. O., Velicer, W. F., Guadagnoli, E., Rossi, J. S., & DiClemente, C. C. (1991). Patterns of change: Dynamic typology applied to smoking cessation. *Multivariate Behavioral Research, 26*(1), 83–107.

Prochaska, J. O., Velicer, W. F., Prochaska, J. M., & Johnson, J. L. (2004). Size, consistency, and stability of stage effects for smoking cessation. *Addictive Behaviors, 29*(1), 207–213.

Prochaska, J. O., Velicer, W. F., Redding, C., Rossi, J. S., Goldstein, M., DePue, J., . . . Plummer, B. A. (2005). Stage-based expert systems to guide a population of primary care patients to quit smoking, eat healthier, prevent skin cancer, and receive regular mammograms. *Preventive Medicine, 41*(2), 406–416.

Prochaska, J. O., Velicer, W. F., Rossi, J. S., Goldstein, M. G., Marcus, B. H., Rakowski, W., . . . Rosenbloom, D. (1994). Stages of change and decisional balance for twelve problem behaviors. *Health Psychology, 13*(1), 39–46.

Prochaska, J. O., Wright, J., & Velicer, W. F. (2008). Evaluating theories of health behavior change: A hierarchy of criteria applied to the transtheoretical model. *Applied Psychology: An International Review, 57*(4), 561–588.

Project MATCH Research Group. (1997). Matching alcoholism treatments to client heterogeneity: Project MATCH posttreatment drinking outcomes. *Journal of Studies on Alcohol, 58*(1), 7–29.

Rakowski, W. R., Ehrich, B., Goldstein, M. G., Rimer, B. K., Pearlman, D. N., Clark, M. A., . . . Woolverton, H., III. (1998). Increasing mammography among women aged 40–74 by use of a stage-matched, tailored intervention. *Preventive Medicine, 27*(5), 748–756.

Redding, C. A., Morokoff, P. J., Rossi, J. S., & Meier, K. S. (2007). A TTM-tailored condom use intervention for at-risk women and men. In T. Edgar, S. M. Noar, & V. Freimuth (Eds.), *Communication perspectives on HIV/AIDS for the 21st century*. Hillsdale, NJ: Erlbaum.

Redding, C. A., Prochaska, J. O., Paiva, A., Rossi, J. S., Velicer, W., Blissmer, B. J., . . . Sun, X. (2011). Baseline stage, severity, and effort effects differentiate stable smokers from maintainers and relapsers. *Substance Use and Misuse, 46*(13), 1664–1674.

Robbins, M. L., Levesque, D. A., Redding, C. A., Johnson, J. L., Prochaska, J. O., Rohr, M. S., & Peters, T. G. (2001). Assessing family members' motivational readiness and decision making for consenting to cadaveric organ donation. *Journal of Health Psychology, 6*(5), 523–536.

Rogers, C. (1951). *Client-centered therapy*. Boston: Houghton Mifflin.

Rosen, C. S. (2000). Is the sequencing of change processes by stage consistent across health problems? A meta-analysis. *Health Psychology, 19*(6), 593–604.

Rossi, J. S. (1992a). *Common processes of change across nine problem behaviors*. Paper presented at the 100th meeting of the American Psychological Association, Washington, DC.

Rossi, J. S. (1992b). *Stages of change for 15 health risk behaviors in an HMO population*. Paper presented at the 13th meeting of the Society for Behavioral Medicine, New York.

Rossi, J. S., Clark, P., Greaney, M., Riebe, D., Greene, G., Saunders, S., . . . Nigg, C. (2005). Effectiveness of transtheoretical model–based interventions on exercise and fruit and vegetable consumption in older adults. *Annals of Behavioral Medicine, 29*, S134.

Schwarzer, R. (2008). Modeling health behavior change: How to predict and modify the adoption and maintenance of health behaviors. *Applied Psychology, 57*(1), 1–29.

Skinner, B. F. (1971). *Beyond freedom and dignity*. New York: Bantam/Vintage.

Snow, M. G., Prochaska, J. O., & Rossi, J. S. (1992). Stages of change for smoking cessation among former problem drinkers: A cross-sectional analysis. *Journal of Substance Abuse, 4*(2), 107–116.

Soler, R. E., Leeks, K. D., Razi, S., Hopkins, D. P., Griffith, M., Aten, A., . . . Task Force on Community Preventive Services. (2010). A systematic review of selected interventions for worksite health promotion. *Journal of Preventive Medicine, 38*(Suppl. 2), S237–S262.

Spencer, L., Pagell, F., Hallion, M. E., & Adams, T. B. (2002). Applying the transtheoretical model to tobacco cessation and prevention: A review of the literature. *American Journal of Health Promotion, 17*(1), 7–71.

Steptoe, A., Kerry, S., Rink, E., & Hilton, S. (2001). The impact of behavioral counseling on stages of change in fat intake, physical activity, and cigarette smoking in adults at increased risk of coronary heart disease. *American Journal of Public Health, 91*(2), 265–269.

Sun, X., Prochaska, J. O., Velicer, W. F., & Laforge, R. G. (2007). Transtheoretical principles and processes for quitting smoking: A 24-month comparison of a representative sample of quitters, relapsers, and non-quitters. *Addictive Behaviors, 32*(12), 2707–2726.

U.S. Department of Health and Human Services. (1990). *The health benefits of smoking cessation: A report of the surgeon general*. Rockville, MD: U.S. Department of Health and Human Services, Public Health Service, Centers for Disease Control, Office on Smoking and Health.

Velicer, W. F., & DiClemente, C. C. (1993). Understanding and intervening with the total population of smokers. *Tobacco Control, 2*(2), 95–96.

Velicer, W. F., Prochaska, J. O., Fava, J. L., Laforge, R. G., & Rossi, J. S. (1999). Interactive versus noninteractive interventions and dose-response relationships for stage-matched smoking cessation programs in a managed care setting. *Health Psychology, 18*(1), 21–28.

Velicer, W. F., Redding, C. A., Sun, X., & Prochaska, J. O. (2007). Demographic variables, smoking variables, and outcome across five studies. *Health Psychology, 26*(3), 278–287.

Voorhees, C. C., Stillman, F. A., Swank, R. T., Heagerty, P. J., Levine, D. M., & Becker, D. M. (1996). Heart, body, and soul: Impact of church-based smoking cessation interventions on readiness to quit. *Preventive Medicine, 25*(3), 277–285.

Weinstein, N. D. (1988). The precaution adoption process. *Health Psychology, 7*(4), 355–386.

Weinstein, N. D., & Sandman, P. M. (1992). A model of the precaution adoption process: Evidence from home radon testing. *Health Psychology, 11*(3), 170–180.

Weinstein, N. D., Sandman, P., & Blalock, S. (2008). The precaution adoption model. In K. Glanz, B. K. Rimer, & K. Viswanath (Eds.), *Health behavior and health education: Theory, research, and practice* (4th ed., pp. 123–165). San Francisco: Jossey Bass.

Wewers, M. E., Stillman, F. A., Hartman, A. M., & Shopland, D. R. (2003). Distribution of daily smokers by stage of change: Current Population Survey results. *Preventive Medicine, 36*(6), 710–720.

Wierzbicki, M., & Pekarik, G. A. (1993). A meta-analysis of psychotherapy dropout. *Professional Psychology: Research and Practice, 24*(2), 190–195.

Yang G., Ma, J., Chen, A., Zhang, Y., Samet, J., Taylor, C., & Becker, K. (2001). Smoking cessation in China: Findings from the 1996 national prevalence survey. *Tobacco Control, 10*(2), 170–174.

PART THREE

MODELS OF INTERPERSONAL HEALTH BEHAVIOR

CHAPTER 8

INTRODUCTION TO MODELS OF INTERPERSONAL INFLUENCES ON HEALTH BEHAVIOR

Catherine A. Heaney
K. Viswanath

Humans are social beings, and the power of social connections to influence health is one of the most pervasive, consistent findings in the public health literature. There have been myriad and divergent changes in our social fabric over the last two decades. In his book *Bowling Alone*, political scientist Robert Putnam (2000) documented how participation in many traditional social groups and structures (such as bowling leagues, religious organizations, and parent-teacher associations) has been diminishing. At the same time, there has been exponential growth in the social media and virtual communications as important ways for people to connect (Pew Research Center, 2014).

The mechanisms that link individuals' social contexts with health effects revolve around two important social processes: the provision of social support and the exercise of social influence. A fundamental assumption driving the theories and models in the chapters in Part Three is that the cognitions, affect, and behaviors of individuals are generally shaped by the people with whom they interact. The theories and models covered in Part Three describe these mechanisms and the various points of intervention that can be used to strengthen health behaviors. This chapter provides an introduction to the section, describes defining characteristics of the models, and discusses challenges in developing and evaluating interventions based on these interpersonal theories and models.

Social Cognitive Theory

Social Cognitive Theory (SCT) addresses the classic tension between human agency and the social structure by offering the construct of *reciprocal determinism*, which suggests that human agency and the environment interact and influence each other, leading to individual and social change. As Kelder, Hoelscher, and Perry explain in Chapter Nine, underlying SCT is the proposition that individuals have the capacity to change or even build the environment. By emphasizing the *dynamism in the interactions* among human behavior, personal cognitive factors, and socioenvironmental influences, SCT moves away from an exclusive focus on one level or another, and it has been one of the most influential theories to do so.

The key SCT constructs and the relationships among them are detailed in Chapter Nine, but it is worth noting that many researchers have tested only selected concepts from the model rather than the entire model. Two deserve particular attention: self-efficacy and observational learning or modeling. *Self-efficacy* is one of the most widely used constructs among health behavior theorists and practitioners. Self-efficacy has been applied to many domains of health behavior and has been adopted for use in other theories, such as the Health Belief Model (Chapter Five) and the Theory of Planned Behavior and the Integrated Model of Behavior (Chapter Six). A major appeal of self-efficacy in health behavior stems from the fact that it is a modifiable factor that can be intervened on because sources of self-efficacy include personal experiences, persuasion, and vicarious experiences learned from observing others, or modeling.

The concept of *observational learning* (or *modeling*) is also a rich and potent source of intervention that has been adopted widely. In recent years, modeling and observational learning have been applied in understanding prosocial change: for example, entertainment education has been used to promote condom use (Keller & Brown, 2002) and to avoid negative outcomes such as aggressive behavior after watching violent TV programs (Huesmann, 2007).

Despite the intuitive sense that vicarious learning through media has a powerful influence on knowledge, beliefs, and behaviors, particularly in the context of so-called edutainment, it is difficult to use SCT to empirically test this assumption without isolating other factors that also influence social change. Other theories explain the why and the how: that is, the mechanisms through which narratives may lead to real-world behavior change. For example, *transportation theory* posits that exposure to narratives, whether short public service announcements or longer dramas or serials, transports viewers to a fictional world, making the experience more enjoyable (Green & Brock, 2000). Transportation may encourage consumers of messages to identify with characters, may reduce counterarguments, and may provide vivid exemplars for the real world (Gerbner, Gross, Morgan, & Signorielli, 2002; Green, 2006; Zillmann, 2002), thus leading to behavior change. While the theory of narratives does not replace SCT's hypothesis about observational learning, it offers greater elaboration of how observation may work and delineates mechanisms that lead to behavior change.

Models of Social Support and Health

Holt-Lunstad and Uchino (Chapter Ten) provide a clear conceptualization of social support and summarize the empirical evidence linking support to good health. Here, we highlight a few issues from the chapter. Holt-Lunstad and Uchino point out the important distinction between perceived support and received support. *Perceived support*, or the expectation that others will provide support if it is needed, has been consistently associated with better health. *Received support*, or the actual provision of support by another person, has a more complicated relationship with health. Sometimes received support has a positive association with good health, but at other times it has been linked with adverse effects on health (Uchino, 2009). It has been suggested that the effect of received support is dependent on whether the support receiver perceives the support to be responsive to his or her needs.

In view of strong empirical evidence for the health-promoting power of perceived support, as opposed to received support, it might be worthwhile to explore what interventions to increase behavior-specific perceived support might look like. Rather than training support providers to engage in provider-driven support provision, they might be trained in (1) how to help support recipients articulate the form of support that they think will be most helpful, and (2) how to make sure that those involved in health behavior change believe that support is available to them when they need it. Involving recipients in the planning and development of social support programs will likely increase program acceptability and effectiveness.

Another important issue that Holt-Lunstad and Uchino raise is that social relationships, in addition to being sources of support, can be sources of conflict and stress. Over several decades, studies have shown that social undermining may be more strongly associated with negative affect and behaviors than is social support. Recently, negative social interactions have been related to heightened chronic inflammatory responses that may lead to increased risk of hypertension, coronary heart disease, and diabetes (Chiang, Eisenberger, Seeman, & Taylor, 2012). This is an important arena for further research and intervention.

Lastly, Holt-Lunstad and Uchino raise the intriguing issue, in the randomized trials they describe, of whether support recipients need to be aware of the support that they are receiving in order for it to be health promoting. Research investigating the effects of "invisible support" suggests that it can be effective in helping support recipients cope with stress (Bolger & Amarel, 2007). This may be a fruitful line of research for developing and evaluating effective social support interventions.

Social Networks and Health Behavior

The study of social networks is currently one of the most generative areas of inquiry in the health behavior arena. Social network theory (SNT) focuses on the structure and system-level properties of the web of social relationships within which individuals live. Social network analysis (SNA) provides tools for understanding how social context influences decision-making processes and actions. In Chapter Eleven, Valente defines the important components of SNT and SNA and provides examples of how they inform health behavior interventions.

Social network analysis quantifies the extent to which members of one's social network endorse certain attitudes or engage in specific behaviors. Research suggests that on the one hand, when people are considering how often an unhealthy or risky behavior (such as smoking) is being performed by their peers, they tend to overestimate the prevalence. On the other hand, people tend to underestimate the extent to which healthy behaviors are being performed. SNA provides information necessary for an accurate descriptive norm among network members, thus providing the data needed to influence people's behaviors to become more in line with the accurate—and ideally, healthy—behavioral norm (Berkowitz, 2003).

Another example of how SNA can aid in health behavior change programs is that it can identify maximally effective change agents. Chapter Eleven describes several successful examples of this process. By mapping social networks and analyzing individuals' positions within their networks, those who have many ties to others (i.e., who are highly central network members) and those who bridge between disparate subgroups within a network can be identified and recruited to be change agents for their communities.

A third example of the applicability of social network analysis is its potential to inform decisions about when the introduction of new social ties is likely to be effective in bringing about health behavior change. Social network theory posits that when a high proportion of social network members are very similar to each other, it is likely to be difficult to bring about change among these members (Valente, 2010). Thus, for example, it will be harder for a smoker to quit when embedded in a social network composed of smokers. And network analyses have shown that overweight and obese individuals tend to cluster within networks. In such situations, it will be important as part of any intervention strategy to create new social ties for people attempting to change difficult behaviors. Researchers and practitioners will expand their tool kits for understanding and leveraging social networks with the constructs and methods described in Chapter Eleven.

Stress, Coping Adaptation, and Health Behavior

The experience of stress is pervasive, and its potential adverse effects on health well known. Chapter Twelve explores the influence of physical and social environments on individual cognitions, affect, and behavior. Wethington, Glanz, and Schwartz describe the transactional model of stress and coping, first proposed by Lazarus and Folkman (1984). This model posits that the ways in which individuals experience and handle stress depend on their appraisals of the stressors and the psychological and social resources that they can bring to bear to cope with the stressors. Social support and self-efficacy (see Chapters Ten and Nine) play important roles in stress appraisal processes and in the successful management of stress.

The stress process unfolds over time. Some exposures to stressors persist for long periods of time whereas others are of short duration. The experience of racism, for example, is often persistent over time and across contexts, resulting in profound physiological and psychological changes (Krieger, 2014; Kwate & Goodman, 2015). Conversely, daily hassles might include getting caught in traffic or having an argument, and these types of stressors usually manifest less intense, shorter duration responses. For quite some time, a hypothesis of adaptation (positing that individuals react most strongly when first exposed to stressors but then adapt to them over time so that adverse stress effects diminish) has competed with a hypothesis of accumulation (positing that individuals can successfully cope with stressors when first encountered but then exhaust their ability to cope as exposure to the stressor continues) (Frese & Zapf, 1988). Recent advances in our understanding of the physiological processes underlying the effects of stress on health (McEwen, 2012) have supported the accumulation hypothesis, but the specific nature of the stress may explain why adaptation occurs in some situations and why accumulation is a more prevalent response to certain stressors. In Chapter Twelve, Wethington and colleagues demonstrate how the effect of stress over time continues to be a productive theme of research, with some researchers taking a life-course perspective to understand potential accumulated and delayed effects of stress on health.

Another important line of inquiry into stress and health revolves around the possible role of stress in explaining health disparities based on socioeconomic status (SES) (Lantz, House, Mero, & Williams, 2005). Research is exploring the extent to which people with lower SES are exposed to more stressors and/or are more distressed by exposure to stressors because they do not have the opportunities and resources to cope with them that those of higher SES may have. The idea that tangible social support is an important resource for successful coping remains an exciting and potentially important topic for further research.

Another key lesson in Chapter Twelve is that it is important to match one's coping strategy to the characteristics of the stressor and the context within which it is encountered. Thus individuals should have a wide array of coping strategies available to them and be flexible in their use. Recent research supports the use of such a *shift-and-persist* coping style among people in low-SES contexts (Chen, Miller, Lachman, Gruenewald, & Seeman, 2012). This style involves being able to try different coping strategies in response to stressors while maintaining confidence that ultimately the stressor can be successfully addressed or managed. This research has important implications for stress management interventions across the socioeconomic spectrum.

Interpersonal Communication in Health and Illness

Chapter Thirteen, the last chapter in Part Three, focuses on interpersonal communication within a formal relationship: the relationship between a health care provider and his or her patients. Recently, research in this area has become even more important because of greater availability of health information to the public, the information and communication technology revolution (addressed in Chapter Seventeen), consumer activism, and technological developments that place greater responsibility on patients to make complex health-related decisions.

In Chapter Thirteen, Duggan and Street discuss some of these issues through the lens of relationship-centered health care, with a specific focus on physician-provider communication. They propose that communication between physicians and patients has two goals: accomplishment of tasks and management of relations. In relationship-centered care, patients and physicians engage in communications with no judgment on the part of physicians, potentially leading to greater empathy, solidarity, and mutual respect. Uncertainty management, often considered a key outcome of provider-patient communication, is theorized as being composed of both relational elements and task-driven elements.

The chapter authors bring these different functions together into a theoretical model that depicts how relational and task-driven functions of communication between patients and physicians could potentially influence health outcomes, either directly or indirectly.

Their approach offers some advantages over conventional discussions of physician-patient communication. They go beyond descriptive models of medical encounters to explain the underlying mechanisms between communications and health outcomes and the various theories that could connect them. Also, the functions of clinician-patient communications and the pathways linking the communications to health outcomes are general enough that they could be extended to exploring how other interpersonal communications may affect health. For example, research may focus on how communications with people in close social networks help in managing uncertainty and validating emotions leading to less psychological distress (Brashers, Goldsmith, & Hsieh, 2002).

The approach taken in Chapter Thirteen suggests leverage points where interventions can influence both satisfaction with care and health outcomes. For example, one might focus on training physicians to assess and be sensitive to patients' emotional needs and needs for additional information (Brédart, Bouleuc, & Dolbeault, 2005). While the model is appealing and relevant in contemporary times, rigorous empirical work is necessary to confirm the pathways.

Future Directions

If there is one defining theme of the chapters in this section, it is that the web of relationships in which we are embedded influences how we learn about the world, our emotional responses and our feelings of belonging, the decisions we make, and how we cope with stress. These chapters convey a rich understanding of the influence of interpersonal interactions on health and their underlying mechanisms of action. Even so, some important areas for further research remain. These include matching the best strategy to a given situation; expanding our understanding of the roles of social class, race, and ethnicity; and examining how new communication technologies affect social support, networks, and health behaviors.

While many strategies for strengthening social relationships are available, there is little research to aid in deciding which strategy to use in any given situation. How should a family member or provider choose between a program to encourage healthy role models and one that tries to build new social ties? How can we develop effective interventions that account for the different interpersonal contexts in which health behavior occurs? Interpersonal influences in the context of the workplace differ from those in family or medical contexts. Translation of our understanding of interpersonal influences on health to effective interventions in various contexts remains a work in progress.

The role of social class and of race and ethnicity is another fruitful avenue for inquiry. Socioeconomic position and race and ethnicity influence interpersonal relationships, the support that we receive (or perceive), and the stress that we experience. However, we are only now beginning to develop an understanding of how the accumulation of daily experiences due to racism or classism can affect health. An important question to explore on this issue is what are the effects on interpersonal interactions and health at the intersection of class with race and ethnicity? The combined effect of class and race could be even more devastating to individual health than class or race alone (Williams et al., 2012).

Platforms such as online support groups and social media have created important new opportunities for seeking and offering information and other types of support (Griffiths, Calear, Banfield, & Tam, 2009; Meier, Lyons, Frydman, Forlenza, & Rimer, 2007). However, the role of virtual social interactions and Internet-based exchange of social support is only beginning to be rigorously explored and evaluated. To what extent will computer-mediated relationships prove to be health promoting? Will online communication increase the number of social relationships but reduce the quality or depth of those networks? Or is it creating an entirely new type of support that is enabled by the online domain? Can all the mechanisms introduced in Part Three for enhancing the health-promoting aspects of social relationships take place in a virtual environment? How should virtual interventions be developed to be optimally effective?

Models and theories of interpersonal influences on health behavior stand at the critical juncture where the social environment molds and modifies intraindividual factors such as cognitions, emotions, and health behaviors. A thorough understanding and appreciation of issues at this level will assist in developing more effective interventions and policies to enhance individual and public health.

References

Berkowitz, A. D. (2003). Applications of social norms theory to other health and social justice issues. In W. Perkins (Ed.), *The social norms approach to preventing school and college age substance abuse: A handbook for educators, counselors, and clinicians*. San Francisco: Jossey-Bass.

Bolger, N., & Amarel, D. (2007). Effects of social support visibility on adjustment to stress: Experimental evidence. *Journal of Personality and Social Psychology, 92*, 458–475.

Brashers, D. E., Goldsmith, D. J., & Hsieh, E. (2002). Information seeking and avoiding in health contexts. *Human Communication Research, 28*, 258–271.

Brédart, A., Bouleuc, C., & Dolbeault, S. (2005). Doctor-patient communication and satisfaction with care in oncology. *Current Opinion in Oncology, 17*, 351–354.

Chen, E., Miller, G. E., Lachman, M. E., Gruenewald, T. L., & Seeman, T. E. (2012). Protective factors for adults from low childhood socioeconomic circumstances: The benefits of shift-and-persist for allostatic load. *Psychosomatic Medicine, 74*, 178–186.

Chiang, J. J., Eisenberger, N. I., Seeman, T. E., & Taylor, S. E. (2012). Negative and competitive social interactions are related to heightened proinflammatory cytokine activity. *Proceedings of the National Academy of Sciences, 109*, 1878–1882.

Frese, M., & Zapf, D. (1988). Methodological issues in the study of work stress: Objective vs. subjective measurement of work stress and the question of longitudinal studies. In C. L. Cooper & R. Payne (Eds.), *Causes, coping, and consequences of stress at work*. New York: Wiley.

Gerbner, G., Gross, L., Morgan, M., & Signorielli, N. (2002). Growing up with television: Cultivation processes. In J. Bryant and D. Zillmann (Eds.), *Media effects: Advances in theory and research* (2nd ed., pp. 43–68). Mahwah, NJ: Erlbaum.

Green, M. (2006). Narratives and cancer communication. *Journal of Communication, 56* (Suppl.), S163–S183.

Green, M., & Brock, T. C. (2000). The role of transportation in the persuasiveness of public narratives. *Journal of Personality and Social Psychology, 79*, 701–721.

Griffiths, K. M., Calear, A. L., Banfield, M., & Tam, A. (2009). Systematic review on Internet Support Groups (ISGs) and depression: What is known about depression ISGs? *Journal of Medical Internet Research, 11*, e41.

Huesmann, L. R. (2007). The impact of electronic media violence: Scientific theory and research. *Journal of Adolescent Health, 41*, S6–S13.

Keller, S. N., & Brown, J. D. (2002). Media interventions to promote responsible sexual behavior. *Journal of Sex Research, 39*, 67–72.

Krieger, N. (2014). On the causal interpretation of race. *Epidemiology, 25*, 937.

Kwate, N. O., & Goodman, M. S. (2015). Cross-sectional and longitudinal effects of racism on mental health among residents of black neighborhoods in New York City. *American Journal of Public Health, 105*(4), 711–718.

Lantz, P. M., House, J. S., Mero, R. P., & Williams, D. R. (2005). Stress, life events, and socioeconomic disparities in health: Results from the Americans' Changing Lives Study. *Journal of Health and Social Behavior, 46*, 274–288.

Lazarus, R. S., & Folkman, S. (1984). *Stress, appraisal, and coping*. New York: Springer.

McEwen, B. S. (2012). Brain on stress: How the social environment gets under the skin. *Proceedings of the National Academy of Sciences, 109*(Suppl. 2), 17180–17185.

Meier, A., Lyons, E. J., Frydman, G., Forlenza, M., & Rimer, B. K. (2007). How cancer survivors provide support on cancer-related internet mailing lists. *Journal of Medical Internet Research, 9*(2), e12.

Pew Research Center. (2014). Internet Project January Omnibus Survey, January 23–26, 2014. Retrieved from http://www.pewinternet.org/Commentary/2012/March/Pew-Internet-Social-Networking-full-detail.aspx

Putnam, R. (2000). *Bowling alone: The collapse and revival of American community*. New York: Simon & Schuster.

Uchino, B. (2009). Understanding the links between social support and physical health: A lifespan perspective with emphasis on the separability of perceived and received support. *Perspectives in Psychological Science, 4*, 236–255.

Valente, T. (2010). *Social networks and health: Models, methods, and applications*. New York: Oxford University Press.

Williams, D. R., Kontos, E. Z., Viswanath, K., Haas, J. S., Lathan, C., MacConaill, L., . . . Ayanian, J. Z. (2012). Integrating multiple social statuses in health disparities research: The case of lung cancer. *Health Services Research, 47*, 1255–1277.

Zillmann, D. (2002). Exemplification theory of media influence. In J. Bryant & D. Zillmann (Eds.), *Media effects: Advances in theory and research* (2nd ed., pp. 19–42). Mahwah, NJ: Erlbaum.

CHAPTER 9

HOW INDIVIDUALS, ENVIRONMENTS, AND HEALTH BEHAVIORS INTERACT

Social Cognitive Theory

Steven H. Kelder
Deanna Hoelscher
Cheryl L. Perry

In a famous and influential 1960s experiment known as the Bobo doll study, a group of psychologists and social scientists led by Albert Bandura demonstrated that children learned aggressive behaviors *vicariously* through observation and imitation of other children who aggressively punched a plastic, inflated Bobo clown doll (Bandura, 2010; Bandura, Ross, & Ross, 1961). In these experiments and his interpretation of them, Bandura departed from prevailing models of how people acquired new behaviors that were based on either a conditioned reflex (Pavlov, 1927) or positive or negative reinforcement or punishment (Skinner, 1953). In 1977, Bandura published his groundbreaking text *Social Learning Theory* (Bandura, 1977b) and a landmark article on self-efficacy, a key social learning construct (Bandura, 1977a). Bandura argued that reducing behavior acquisition to a stimulus-response cycle was too simplistic. He proposed instead that behavior is more strongly mediated by cognitive processes that occur through observation of social modeling. The process can occur via the observation of a *social role model*. The memory of this observation will then be used later to inform an individual's response when a similar situation arises. In addition, the memory of the original observation is stronger if the model was an important person (someone of higher status or higher authority—a parent, sibling, opinion leader,

KEY POINTS

This chapter will:

- Define and describe the history and concepts of Social Cognitive Theory (SCT).

- Describe how SCT concepts explain health behaviors and guide intervention design.

- Illustrate the application of key SCT concepts and principles in two case studies: one on childhood obesity in the United States and one on youth smoking prevention in India.

or teacher), or if the event was emotionally charged. In his 1986 book *Social Foundations of Thought and Action*, Bandura renamed Social Learning Theory, calling it Social Cognitive Theory (SCT) in order to emphasize the increasingly important role of observation and cognitive factors in learning, understanding, and predicting behavior.

In Bandura's fully developed SCT model, human behavior is explained in terms of a triadic and dynamic model of causation in which behavior, personal cognitive factors, and socioenvironmental influences all interact, called *reciprocal determinism.* An individual's behavior is uniquely determined by the combination of these factors. SCT has been used to inform, enable, guide, and motivate people to adapt habits that promote health and to reduce habits that impair health (Bandura, 2004). It has also been used to explain the mechanisms of the ways people may learn about risky behaviors: for example, from observing smoking in movies. SCT is one of the most widely applied models of health behavior, and it has been applied to the initiation and achievement of personal and group-level changes, maintenance of behavior changes, and relapse prevention. SCT has been used in a variety of contexts, including clinical settings for self-management of chronic diseases and emotional disorders, as the basis for community health promotion programs, for the social diffusion of health-promoting practices, and in health policy initiatives and environmental change strategies. The SCT model is a valuable public health tool in societal efforts to promote health, particularly among youth, since many behaviors related to acute and chronic disease begin in childhood and early adolescence and continue into adulthood where morbidity and mortality manifest. In fact, the recognition that it is far easier to prevent the initiation of unhealthy behaviors than to change entrenched habits later in life is the foundation for the field of youth health promotion (Bandura 1997, 2006a).

Major Constructs for Social Cognitive Theory

For decades, SCT has helped researchers and practitioners to determine the factors motivating health behaviors and, once those factors are understood, to design health interventions that promote behavior change (Bandura 2004). According to SCT, prediction of behavior and behavior change are regulated by forethought and a personal sense of control (often called *agency*). Cognitive influences on behavior comprise three main factors: *self-efficacy*, *outcome expectations*, and *knowledge*.

Application of SCT to health problems requires an understanding of reciprocal determinism, which involves a dynamic triad of factors: (1) personal cognitive factors, (2) the physical and social environment, and (3) behavioral factors. **Personal cognitive factors** include the individual's ability to self-determine or self-regulate behavior and to reflect upon and analyze experience. This is reflected in three major constructs: confidence to engage in a behavior (*self-efficacy*), ability to foresee the outcomes of given behavior patterns (*outcome expectations*), and level of understanding about enacting a behavior (*knowledge*) (Bandura, 2004). **Socioenvironmental factors** are aspects of the perceived and/or physical environment that promote, permit, or discourage engagement in a particular behavior. These factors include influential role models (*observational learning*), cultural beliefs about the social acceptability and perceived prevalence of a behavior (*normative beliefs*), perceptions of encouragement (*social support*) and facilitation of or impediments to engagement in the health behavior (*opportunities and barriers*). **Behavioral factors** affect health directly. Health behaviors are actions taken by individuals that are *health-enhancing* (leading to improved health) or *health-compromising* (leading to poorer health). Behavioral factors include a person's existing repertoire of health behavior capabilities, or coping skills (*behavioral skills*); their goals to add or modify a behavior (*intentions*); and the rewards or punishments they receive for engaging in a health behavior (*reinforcement*) (Perry, 1999). SCT suggests that prevention of morbidity and mortality—through the development of healthy behaviors and reduction of unhealthy behaviors—can be achieved by modifying these three interacting factors. Table 9.1 defines and illustrates all of these SCT constructs.

Table 9.1   Major Constructs for Social Cognitive Theory

Cognitive influences on behavior: personal abilities for processing information, applying knowledge, and changing preferences.

Construct	Definition	Explanation
Self-efficacy	A person's confidence in his or her ability to perform a behavior that leads to an outcome.	Self-efficacy is a core SCT construct. Confidence is enhanced through mastery experiences, social modeling, verbal persuasion, and practice under stress-free conditions.
Collective efficacy	Belief in the ability of a group of individuals to perform concerted actions to achieve an outcome.	Because people operate individually and collectively, self-efficacy can be both a personal and a social construct. Group efficacy is enhanced by shared goals, communication, teamwork, and prior success.
Outcome expectations	Outcomes arise from actions. Outcome expectations are judgments about the likely consequences of actions.	Outcome expectations, either positive or negative, are a core SCT construct. Expected consequences can be divided into *physical* (e.g., use of condoms protects against STDs), *social* (reactions from others: such as interest, approval, recognition, status), and *self-evaluative* (reactions to one's own behavior based on internal personal standards).
Knowledge	Knowledge is an understanding of the health risks and benefits of different health practices and the information necessary to perform a behavior.	Knowledge of risks and benefits is a precondition for change. Information is also needed to perform certain behaviors; e.g., to cook a healthy meal one needs to know a recipe, where to purchase healthy ingredients, and methods of preparation.

Environmental influences on behavior: physical and social factors in an individual's environment that affect a person's behavior.

Construct	Definition	Explanation
Observational learning	A type of learning in which a person learns new information and behaviors by observing the behaviors of others and the consequences of others' behaviors.	Accomplished by observing an influential role model or peer-leader performing a behavior and achieving an outcome. Methods include observation made in the context of peer-led education, mass media, behavioral journalism, and dramatic performances.
Normative beliefs	Cultural norms and beliefs about the social acceptability and perceived prevalence of a behavior.	Interventions seek to correct normative beliefs (such as adolescents' common misperceptions about how many of their peers smoke cigarettes) through discussions of perceptions versus actual data.
Social support	The perception of encouragement and support a person receives from his or her social network.	Interventions seek to provide informational, instrumental, or emotional support (through, e.g., program flyers, offers to babysit, or a sympathetic conversation) for behavior changes.

(continued)

Table 9.1 *(Continued)*

Construct	Definition	Explanation
Barriers and opportunities	Attributes of the social or physical environment that make behaviors harder or easier to perform.	Interventions seek to facilitate behavior change by increasing opportunities to safely engage in and master the behavior, or by removing impediments to developing the behavior.

Supporting behavioral factors: actions taken by individuals that can be classified as either *health-enhancing* (leading to improved health) or *health-compromising* (leading to poorer health).

Construct	Definition	Explanation
Behavioral skills	The abilities needed to successfully perform a behavior.	Many behaviors require developing a repertoire of specific skills to be successfully enacted. Examples include avoiding high-risk situations, playing a sport, or preparing a healthy meal. Knowledge and skills together comprise what is called *behavioral capability*.
Intentions	The goals of adding new behaviors or modifying existing behaviors, both proximal and distal.	Intentions serve as self-incentives and guides to health behaviors. Attaining specific behaviors is often accomplished by writing or verbalizing goals, setting target dates and activities for skill mastery, and monitoring progress.
Reinforcement and punishment	Behavior can be increased or attenuated through provision or removal of rewards or punishments.	Rewards and punishments can be either tangible (e.g., money, goods, physical ailments, weight gain) or social (e.g., praise, approval, attention, exclusion, or ridicule).

Personal Cognitive Influences on Behavior

Social cognitive theory was developed in the 1970s, during a paradigm shift in psychology when the cognitive influences on behavior came to be seen as crucial to behavior change, in contrast to the previously widely accepted stimulus-response models of behavior change.

Self-Efficacy

Self-efficacy regulates a number of cognitive processes that enhance or impede the development or maintenance of a behavior. It is the unifying and seminal construct of SCT, directly related to the initiation of a behavioral goal, the level of effort expended to develop and master new skills, and how long the effort will be sustained in the face of impediments, setbacks, and failure. Because it is an internal mental process, it is often called *perceived self-efficacy* and is defined by a person's level of confidence in his capability to control his behavior. People with a low level of self-efficacy tend to be pessimistic, less likely to try or maintain a behavior, or apt to avoid certain situations. Conversely, when a person feels a high level of self-efficacy, he is more likely to be confident in his ability to succeed. People tend to select tasks and activities in which they feel competent and avoid those in which they do not. For a discussion of the measurement of self-efficacy, see Betz (2013).

Not surprisingly, behavioral interventions based on SCT include components designed to increase a person's perceived level of *situational self-efficacy*, the confidence to succeed with a specific task. For example, a person may feel very confident in her ability to prepare a healthy meal (self-efficacy for cooking) but have low confidence for eating fewer calories (self-efficacy for controlling food consumption). Because self-efficacy influences individuals' thought patterns and emotional reactions, a person's self-efficacy will influence her persistence to succeed with a task. For example, an objective for an HIV prevention program among low-income, inner-city women may be to increase safe-sex behaviors. By employing an SCT approach, the HIV program designer would first assess (1) the target population's previous experience and knowledge about safe sex; (2) their emotional states regarding safe sex, such as anxiety, stress, and arousal; and (3) their self-efficacy beliefs about managing high-risk situations that might require safe-sex behaviors. This information can be gathered by examining the published literature or by directly querying the target population using focus groups or structured interviews. With this information, the program designer can plan tailored or targeted methods to increase self-efficacy.

Bandura describes a person's formation of self-efficacy through four primary sources: (1) previous mastery experiences, (2) vicarious experience, (3) social persuasion, and (4) emotional arousal (Bandura, 1997). Self-efficacy is strongly influenced by *previous experience* with a particular behavioral task, which in turn is related to a person's likelihood to engage in the behavior again. Through previous experience, a person begins to develop behavioral skills, beliefs about expected outcomes, and a mental representation of his level of self-efficacy for that behavior. Typically, outcomes interpreted by a person as positive will increase self-efficacy; those interpreted as a negative outcome will lower self-efficacy. Arguably, with the exception of behaviors that have calamitous consequences (such as crimes resulting in incarceration) or the application of an effective treatment or intervention, an influential predictor of future behavior is current behavior and the continued mastery of that behavior. Research bears this out, particularly for habitual, health-related behaviors over the short term, such as diet and physical activity (Kelder, Perry, Klepp, & Lytle, 1994), or for addictive behaviors, like tobacco and alcohol use (Rohrbach, Sussman, Dent, & Sun, 2005). As an intervention strategy, active learning strategies that coach a person through incremental steps toward a *mastery experience* should raise self-efficacy and increase the frequency of a healthful behavior. A review of SCT-based interventions designed to increase self-efficacy for leisure-time physical activity found that feedback on past performance, others' performance, and vicarious experience produced the highest levels of self-efficacy (Ashford, Edmunds, & French, 2010).

An important construct that distinguishes SCT from stimulus-response theory is *observational learning.* In addition to forming self-efficacy from personal experience, self-efficacy is also formed through *vicarious experience* by watching the success or failure of other people performing a task. The effect of vicarious experience on self-efficacy is strengthened when the person performing the task is an influential opinion leader or desirable role model. Individuals designing health interventions will often tailor role models by gender, race or ethnicity, culture, or socioeconomic groupings so that the observer will see people similar to herself and will come to believe "if they can do it, I can do it." Although not so influential as personal experience, modeling (particularly through mass media) is a ubiquitous and useful tool for working with people who have little prior experience with the task or for those who lack confidence.

The third method of forming self-efficacy beliefs includes *social persuasion, support,* and *reinforcement.* Social persuasion generally manifests as direct encouragement or discouragement from a socially desirable individual. For instance, the social influences model of youth health promotion relies on credible classroom role models to persuasively transmit social information via small-group discussions and role play (U.S. Department of Health and Human Services [DHHS], 2012). In many youth smoking prevention programs, a crucial element is the recruitment and training of desirable role models who, by virtue of their status in the school, can effectively *persuade* others to recognize the negative consequences of smoking, *support* the social norm that smoking is not desirable, and *reinforce* the advantages of remaining a nonsmoker.

Fourth and finally, a person's self-efficacy is influenced by *emotional arousal*. Strong emotional arousal in response to a task acts as a cue to the person about anticipated failure or success. Negative emotions and anger may generate a state of cognitive confusion and lower self-efficacy, leading to poorer task performance, whereas a positive emotional state creates an optimistic viewpoint and higher performance. Because individuals have the capability to alter their own thinking and feelings, enhanced self-efficacy beliefs can in turn powerfully influence the physiological states themselves. People typically show stronger memory for information related to emotional events and poorer memory for less emotionally charged secondary details (Levine & Edelstein, 2009).

These four factors that influence formation of self-efficacy (previous experience, vicarious experience, social persuasion, and emotional arousal) vary in importance and strength, with self-mastery typically being considered the strongest (Bandura, 1997). For example, the application of self-efficacy for the development of skills has been widely and successfully used in sports (Short & Ross-Stewart, 2008). Ashford et al. (2010) conducted a meta-analysis of methods to change self-efficacy for recreational physical activity and identified vicarious experiences as the strongest predictor. Although self-efficacy is a straightforward concept, manipulation of the four sources of self-efficacy does not always translate into increased self-efficacy. Individuals perceive events, interpret event meanings, and recall memories through their own specific lenses. Bandura (1997) has observed that "people live in psychic environments that are primarily of their own making." Ultimately, the sources of self-efficacy serve first as guidelines for understanding a person's motivation to perform a task, and second, are useful for program planning designed to change self-efficacy and, ultimately, related health behaviors.

Collective Efficacy

The second form of cognitive influence on behavior is *collective efficacy*. There are many circumstances in which individuals do not have control over the social conditions or institutions that affect their lives, and thus cannot achieve their goals by acting on their own (Bandura, 2000). In these circumstances, groups of individuals (e.g., parent groups, neighborhood organizations, schools, and unions) can develop a sense of social cohesion and a willingness to take action for the common good. Similar to an individual's developing belief in his or her personal self-efficacy, a group can build upon its successes and develop shared beliefs in its capability to attain goals and accomplish tasks. Perceived collective efficacy fosters a group's motivational commitment to its missions and resilience to adversity, and serves as a vitalizing influence on performance of objectives. Research suggests that perceived collective efficacy is strongly related to student achievement in schools (Goddard, Hoy, & Hoy, 2004).

Outcome Expectations

Self-efficacy and collective efficacy refer to the confidence, capability, and personal control or agency to engage in and complete a task. *Outcome expectations* refer to a person's expectation about the consequences, either physical or social, of taking action. A *physical outcome expectation* is an understanding of the relationship between a behavior and a health or physical outcome, either positive or negative (e.g., pleasure, pain, or change in disease symptoms). For example, most runners understand that a run will clear their head and make them feel energized (short-term positive consequences) and will reduce their chances of chronic diseases (long-term positive consequence). They may also understand that running carries a risk of knee injury (short-term negative consequence). *Social outcome expectations* are the social responses to behavior change (such as approval, disapproval, power, or applause). Runners might expect approval from their family and friends for taking care of themselves or for looking more fit (a short-term positive consequence). Disapproval can happen if the runner is exercising away from home so much that it interferes with family or social events. A review by Williams, Anderson, and Winett (2005) supports the association between outcome expectations and self-efficacy—specifically, between positive expectations and physical activity in older adults.

Self-Evaluative Outcome Expectations

Bandura describes *self-evaluative outcome expectations* as the anticipated feelings that arise from a comparison between a person's behavior and his or her internal standards (Bandura, 1997). People do things that give them self-satisfaction, pride, joy, or self-worth. Conversely, they refrain from behaviors that elicit feelings of self-censure, sadness, shame, or disgust. Self-evaluative outcomes come from internally held symbolic values attached to behavior. For example, on the one hand, a student may feel *self-satisfaction* when he receives an A in a difficult course if he belongs to a family or peer group that values A-level performance. On the other hand, for a different person, a grade of A may bring *self-censure* because her peer group devalues academic achievement and is quick to ridicule, harass, or ostracize high achievers. The evidence is largely supportive of the theoretical predictions: high personal academic expectations predict subsequent performance, course enrollment, and occupational aspirations (Bandura, 1997).

Knowledge

Bandura (2004) describes knowledge of the health risks and benefits of different health practices as a *precondition for change*. That is, knowledge has an important cognitive influence on behavior but generally is insufficient alone to produce behavior change. For example, Thomas, McLellan, and Perera (2013) reviewed forty years of smoking prevention studies and concluded that information-only smoking prevention programs (knowledge) were not effective, whereas programs that focused on combined social competence and social influences were effective in preventing the onset of smoking. In the design of behavioral health programs, methods that influence knowledge are typically combined with other SCT constructs: self-efficacy, outcome expectations, and development of related skills. The combination of skills and knowledge is often referred to as *behavioral capability* (knowledge of what to do and how to do it).

When designing the knowledge component of a behavior change program, two main approaches are typically employed: (1) use of strategies to describe the health risks and benefits and (2) use of a scaffolding approach in which relevant information is presented in a step-by-step scope and sequence. An example of describing health risk and benefits can be seen in a smoking prevention program. Middle school students are asked to meet in a peer group to brainstorm the consequences of smoking behavior (bad breath, cancer, death) followed by another activity where they prepare a list of why kids their age begin to smoke (to show off, to act mature, because it tastes good). This exercise is designed to elicit socially relevant information from within the student's local social and cultural context. By contrasting knowledge about the pros and the cons of smoking, students are able to refine their own expectations and normative beliefs about smoking (see DHHS, 2012, for detailed examples of youth smoking prevention). An example of scaffolding is a presentation describing the concept of energy balance (nutrition density versus energy expenditure), its relationship to obesity and fitness, and the variety of metabolic health conditions that arise from an energy imbalance.

Environmental Influences on Behavior

Like ecological models (see Chapter Three), Social Cognitive Theory includes factors that describe the influence of environment on behavior. The concept of reciprocal determinism and the prediction of behavior through the interaction of personal, environmental, and behavioral factors imply that neither self-efficacy nor vicarious experiences will ensure behavior change unless the environment supports acquisition of the new behavior (Bandura, 2008). Socioenvironmental factors are aspects of the perceived or physical environment that promote, permit, or discourage engagement in a particular behavior. These factors are *observational learning, normative beliefs, social support,* and *barriers and opportunities.*

Observational Learning

The underpinning of SCT rests on a person's ability to *learn* by observing someone else's behavior and the consequences of that behavior (see the self-efficacy section above). In theory, if you observe a person receiving positive reinforcement for a behavior, then you are more likely to imitate the behavior in anticipation that you too will receive the reinforcement. Likewise, viewing someone receiving negative reinforcement for a behavior should lower your likelihood of performing that behavior. Modeling of positive and negative consequences appears to be effective for young children, as demonstrated in research by Greenhalgh et al. (2009) where (1) children observing a positive reinforcement for eating healthy food were more likely to select the food, (2) children observing negative reinforcement inhibited their consumption of healthy food, and (3) children first exposed to negative reinforcement followed by positive reinforcement remained inhibited even after the positive reinforcement.

Although observational learning is a seemingly simple concept, a number of variables influence the process, including characteristics of the observed person (the role model) and characteristics of the learner. Research supports the premise that when people are presented with a choice, they are more likely to pay attention to role models with characteristics similar to themselves (including their own selves on videotape) and to ignore those with whom they have little in common (Bandura, 1997, 2004). For example, adolescents are more likely to mimic the actions of their peers (or slightly older peers) regarding social behaviors (such as a decision to smoke or drink alcohol) than the actions of adolescents from another culture or social class, their parents, or other adults (DHHS, 2012). Unfortunately, some criminal, deviant, or antisocial behaviors modeled by peer role models are positively rewarded within their peer social context (Gifford-Smith, Dodge, Dishion, & McCord, 2005). Likewise, intervention programs that portray dissimilar models (from outside the peer group) are typically ignored and are neither valued nor learned.

Characteristics of learners also influence opportunities to observe and learn from another's behavior. A person's neighborhood; preference for online, printed, or televised media; family members; and choice of friends determine the behaviors that person is able to observe and learn. Bandura (1986, 2006b, 2008) suggests that four processes influence observational learning: (1) attention, (2) retention, (3) production, and (4) motivation. When viewing a behavior, a person's level of *attention* depends on the internal functional value of the observed behavior. People are less likely to attend to consequences they do not value. Cognitive *retention* can depend on a person's intellectual capacity (such as ability to read or readiness to learn), stage of physical growth and maturity, state of inebriation, or psychological impairment. People are not likely to be influenced by observed events if they do not remember them. An important source of self-efficacy from observational learning also comes from remembering past outcomes from behavior and having the ability to reconstruct past events. *Production* is the level of knowledge, skills, and self-efficacy already possessed (or the level of willingness to learn them) for performing the modeled behavior. The richer the knowledge and repertoire of needed subskills, the easier it is to integrate them into new forms of behavior. *Motivation* is determined by the expected costs and benefits of the observed behavior.

Normative Beliefs

In Social Cognitive Theory, norms influence behavior through two types of outcome expectations: *social consequences* and *self-evaluative consequences*. (Normative beliefs were discussed in Chapter Six in the context of the Theory of Reasoned Action and Theory of Planned Behavior.) Behavior that violates prevailing social norms brings social consequences, whereas behavior that fulfills socially valued norms is approved and rewarded. People can also adopt their own standards of behavior and regulate their actions through their idealized self-concept. They do things that give them self-satisfaction and self-worth and refrain from behaving in ways that bring self-dissatisfaction. Over time, through direct consequences or vicarious learning, an individual learns the dominant norms within a new social environment. Thus the motivation to comply with social norms corresponds to the balance between the expected social consequences (e.g., admiration, rebuke, loss of status) for a given behavior and the individual's internalization of self-evaluative consequences (e.g., confidence, shame, angst). The more one believes that certain behaviors are encouraged or approved by significant role models, and the more one is motivated to comply with those people, the more social pressure one will feel with respect to performing the behavior.

Research supports the importance of normative beliefs in predicting and guiding behavior in direct and meaningful ways (Borsari & Carey, 2003), and this has spurred research aimed at changing health behaviors by changing norms. The rationale for changing normative beliefs is based on two consistent findings: (1) most individuals overestimate the prevalence of many undesirable behaviors, such as tobacco use among peers, and (2) individuals use their perceptions of peer norms as a standard against which to compare their own behaviors. Health interventions based on SCT frequently include components designed to help people understand the social norms in their environment and to correct misperceptions about norms. For example, a common classroom lesson in youth smoking prevention programs is to correct the overestimation of tobacco use norms and to express social disapproval of smoking (DHHS, 2012). In health communication research, social norms marketing campaigns that focus on correcting normative misperceptions and presenting desirable social norms have shown promise in changing behaviors. These campaigns have addressed, for example, youth bullying behaviors (Perkins, Craig, & Perkins, 2011), college drinking (Neighbors, Larimer, & Lewis, 2004), and household energy consumption (Schultz, Nolan, Cialdini, Goldstein, & Griskevicius, 2007).

Social Support

Enlisting and creating social support is important for the maintenance of desired personal change. Broadly defined, social support refers to the process by which interpersonal relationships promote and protect an individual's well-being, particularly when that person is faced with stressful life circumstances (Wills & Ainette, 2012). Social support is generally classified into four categories: (1) emotional support (expressing positive affect, caring, love, and companionship), (2) esteem support (validating beliefs, emotions, and actions), (3) informational support (providing information or advice,), and (4) instrumental support (providing materials or equipment necessary for the behavior). Social support not only aids adherence to a new behavior but also contributes to perceived self-efficacy. Self-efficacy is strengthened through observation, modeling, and activation of social support systems, social networks, and self-help activities. By strengthening interpersonal relationships, influential role models are in a position to display their preferences and approval (or disapproval), and this may alter the observer's self-efficacy and the value of the desired behavior. For example, abstainers from drugs, alcohol, or tobacco need social support when life events overwhelm their self-regulatory capacity. Supportive relationships reduce stress, strengthen self-regulatory efficacy, provide necessary aids to continue abstaining, and enable those struggling with self-control to weather the storm. (Chapter Ten discusses social support in depth.)

Barriers and Opportunities

Personal change would be much easier if there were no *barriers* on the path to success. SCT distinguishes between two classes of barriers: cognitive and environmental (see the discussion in Chapter Five of the Health Belief Model). For example, a person can have low self-efficacy in his ability to overcome the barriers involved with becoming physically active or he may overemphasize the negative outcomes associated with physical activity. But barriers are not solely a cognitive matter; some barriers to healthful living are in the physical environment. Some individuals live where opportunities to engage in healthy behavior and supportive resources don't exist and thus are not available. For example, barriers to physical activity may include high-crime areas, unkempt or nonexistent parks and walking trails, lack of sidewalks, or even packs of wild dogs, as often seen on the Texas-Mexico border. An individual's self-efficacy to succeed and receive positive consequences is balanced against the perceived negative consequences and environmental barriers. Efficacious people are quick to take advantage of opportunities and figure out how to circumvent environmental constraints. Conversely, low-efficacy people focus on barriers or lack of opportunity, can be easily discouraged by impediments, and are less apt to exploit the enabling opportunities provided by social systems (Bandura, 1997, 2000). Sometimes city governments or philanthropists are puzzled when a newly funded environmental improvement such as a bike trail or park is underutilized; the answer may lie in the community members' low self-efficacy for exercise or their anticipated negative outcomes (e.g., sweating or discomfort) to increasing physical activity.

Supporting Behavioral Factors

The term *Social Cognitive Theory* conveys the importance of cognitive factors in the adoption and maintenance of health behaviors. However, SCT builds on elemental behavioral factors of stimulus-response theory that were conceptualized before the importance of cognition was fully understood. These supporting behavioral factors include a person's existing repertoire of health behavioral capabilities (*behavioral skills* and *coping skills*), her goals to add or modify a behavior (*intentions and goal setting*), and the rewards or punishments she receives for engaging in a health behavior (*reinforcement*) (Perry, 1999).

Behavioral Skills

Self-regulation and the effective exercise of control, especially for complex behaviors, often require the development of new behavioral skills. The concept of *behavioral capability* maintains that if a person is to perform a particular behavior he must know the behavior's significance and components (*knowledge*) and know how to perform the behavior (*skills*). The successful performance of a behavior depends on a person's behavioral capability as well as on the cognitive and environmental influences on behavior as described in previous sections. Cognitive representations, often discovered through observational learning, serve as guides for the mastery of skilled behaviors and as internal standards for making corrective adjustment in the achievement of behavioral proficiency. Skills are perfected by repeated corrective adjustments.

Bandura (1997) describes five ways in which behavioral skill acquisition and self-regulation are achieved: (1) self-monitoring, or a person's systematic observation of her own behavior; (2) goal setting, or the identification of incremental and long-term changes; (3) feedback about the quality of performance and how to improve; (4) self-reward, or the provision of tangible and intangible rewards; and (5) self-instruction, or self-critique, before and during performance of a complex behavior. Instruction in the development of self-regulation through guided practice, coaching, self-help, or computer-assisted instruction is a widely used application of SCT (similar to and overlapping with the steps described to increase self-efficacy). This is particularly true in educational settings where important SCT constructs are used to improve academic success: managing distractions, setting goals, self-reflection, managing time, self-efficacy and perceived responsibility for learning, and setting a place for homework completion (Ramdass & Zimmerman, 2011).

Intentions and Goal Setting

Behavioral intentions (as discussed in Chapter Six on the Theory of Planned Behavior) are an indication of an individual's readiness to perform a given behavior, and are assumed to be an important antecedent to behavior (Ajzen, 2002). Behavioral intentions include a person's thoughts and statements about the proximal and distal future (Montaño, Kasprzyk, & Taplin, 1997), such as whether he will ever try a cigarette, eat broccoli, exercise regularly, or use condoms. When these intentions are specific and have a relatively short time frame, they are quite powerful predictors of future behavior (Ajzen, 2002). A meta-analysis of forty-seven experimental tests of the intention-behavior relationship showed that interventions with relatively large changes in subjects' intentions resulted in modest changes in behavior over time (Webb & Sheeran, 2006).

Bandura (1986) argues that intentions operate through two cognitive sources of motivation. One is the capacity for forethought, or people's ability to participate in planning their own futures. The second is goal setting, which sets up internal standards for behavior. Goals are therefore one way of actualizing behavioral intentions in order to achieve behavior changes. As individuals shift to self-management of their health behaviors, setting behavioral goals becomes crucial to behavior change (Bandura, 2005). Goal achievement is enhanced by an individual's high level of self-efficacy and positive outcome expectations for behavior change (Bandura, 2005).

Reinforcement and Punishment

Reinforcement and punishment are two primary constructs in stimulus-response theory and operant conditioning (Skinner, 1953) and refer to the strengthening of a specific behavior due to its repeated association with a stimulus. A *reinforcer* is the stimulus that strengthens the behavior, in contrast to a *punishment*, which is the stimulus that weakens the behavior. According to stimulus-response theory, both reinforcement and punishment can be either positive or negative. *Positive reinforcement* occurs when a stimulus or reward is given to a person after she performs a specific behavior, so that the behavior increases (giving students a dance party after they have eaten a specific number of servings of fruits and vegetables for a week). *Negative reinforcement* occurs when an aversive (unpleasant) stimulus is removed as a result of performing a specific behavior, so that the behavior increases (e.g., the buzzing of a car indicator stops when the passenger fastens the seatbelt). *Positive punishment* is the addition of an aversive (unpleasant) stimulus to decrease a specific *behavior* (giving students time out from the class when they misbehave). *Negative punishment* is the removal of a pleasant stimulus to decrease a behavior or response (not letting students attend a football game if they are tardy too many times). Simply put, reinforcements increase behaviors, whereas punishments decrease behaviors; positive means adding a stimulus in response to a behavior, whereas negative means removing a stimulus in response to a behavior.

A key distinction between stimulus-response theory and SCT lies in outcome expectations. In stimulus-response theory, *primary reinforcers* (e.g., sleeping, breathing, or sustenance) are not conditioned and do not require repeated pairings of behavior (response) and behavioral outcome (stimulus). Secondary reinforcers are conditioned; that is, they acquire power as reinforcers only after repeated pairings, usually with an unconditioned stimulus. A famous example is pairing the sound of a clicker with a treat after a dog performs a desired behavior. The treat serves as a primary unconditioned reinforcement (a tasty food stimulus), and the clicker is paired repeatedly with the treat when the dog returns after hearing the clicker (the desired response). After repeated pairings, the dog becomes conditioned to return to the sound of the clicker, even without a treat. According to SCT, an individual develops his *outcome expectations* for a specific behavior not just through repeated pairings with reinforcements but also through cognitive and environmental influences on behavior. By adding cognition to the stimulus-response process, Bandura provides a more detailed explanation for the origins of outcome expectations and a more complete roadmap to assist in adding and maintaining new behaviors.

Case Studies

In this section, we discuss two case studies that provide examples of SCT applications. The first describes how SCT constructs were used to develop and evaluate an intervention, and the second discusses applying SCT in cultures outside the United States.

Case Study 1: Coordinated Approach to Child Health (CATCH)

The Coordinated Approach to Child Health (CATCH) is a program designed to promote and improve physical activity, healthful food choices, and family environment, and to prevent the onset of tobacco use in elementary school–aged children (Perry et al., 1990). CATCH was originally funded by the National Heart, Lung, and Blood Institute (NHLBI) as the Child and Adolescent Trial for Cardiovascular Health, and was evaluated in one of the largest elementary school–based randomized controlled trials conducted in the United States. Results from the CATCH study showed significant program effects for decreasing fat consumption and increasing physical activity among children and adolescents (Luepker et al., 1996). Follow-up research found that these behavior changes were maintained three years after the program, without further intervention (Nader et al., 1999). The CATCH program was developed using SCT as a guiding theoretical framework, and it has four components: classroom curricula for children, a physical education program, a cafeteria program, and family home materials. Although the original NHLBI program focused on third-grade to fifth-grade children, CATCH has been expanded to include program materials for children in preschool and grades K–8 (Sharma, Chuang, & Hedberg, 2011; Springer et al., 2013), and materials have been updated to include changes in dietary and physical activity recommendations. CATCH was originally developed to prevent risk factors for cardiovascular health, but recent studies have shown an effect on decreasing child obesity and overweight among low-income minority students (Coleman et al., 2005; Hoelscher, Kelder, et al., 2010; Hoelscher, Springer, et al., 2010).

CATCH illustrates *reciprocal determinism* in that it targets cognitive, environmental, and behavioral factors that influence children's health behaviors related to obesity prevention. The major outcome of the original CATCH trial was decreased blood cholesterol levels; to change cholesterol levels, the intervention was developed to change behaviors related to cholesterol levels (e.g., diet and physical activity). SCT constructs that influenced these behaviors were used to develop strategies that guided specific intervention activities. To evaluate the impact of the intervention program, measurements were developed for both the targeted behaviors and SCT constructs. For the constructs used in CATCH, measurement scales were designed with multiple questions assessing the same concept; these scales were then aggregated and the sums were used to evaluate changes in intervention constructs (see Table 9.2).

Table 9.2   Operationalization of Individual-Level SCT Constructs in the CATCH Intervention and Evaluation

Construct	CATCH-Specific Intervention Application and Strategy	Example of Measurement Item	Response Categories	Scale
Behavioral capability	*Dietary knowledge:* children learn to identify foods as GO, SLOW, or WHOA, based on frequency of consumption.	Which food is better for you?	Dichotomous choices (one healthy, one unhealthy)	14-item scale
Intention	*Dietary intentions:* children record their lunches and categorize foods as GO, SLOW, or WHOA, with a goal of a certain number of GO lunches per week.	Which food would you ask for?	Dichotomous choices (one healthy, one unhealthy)	13-item scale
Self-control	*Usual food consumption:* children prepare healthy snacks; children are taught to read labels to avoid foods high in fat.	Which foods do you eat most of the time?	Dichotomous choices (one healthy, one unhealthy)	14-item scale
Environment/ situation	*Social support for physical activity:* parents and children set goals for physical activities for a week; teacher reinforcement during physical education.	One or both of my parents or guardians do exercises with me like running, jogging, dancing or skating.	Dichotomous scored items (yes/no)	11-item positive support scale; 7-item negative support scale
Environment	*Social support for healthy food choices:* teachers reinforce appropriate food choices with group acknowledgment and small prizes; cafeteria workers encourage taste tests of fruits and vegetables.	Who wants you to eat lots of fruits and vegetables? Your parents? Your teachers? Your friends?	Dichotomous scale, with yes/no for each group (parents, teachers, friends)	21-item scale, divided into family, teacher, and friend support (7 items each)
Self-efficacy	*Dietary self-efficacy:* observation of role models achieving dietary goals through CATCH story characters; using foods labeled in cafeteria as GO when choosing lunch or breakfast items.	How sure are you that you can eat cereal instead of a donut?	3-point ordinal scale with "not sure," "a little sure," and "very sure"	16-item scale
Self-efficacy	*Physical activity self-efficacy:* physical education teachers lead classes in which all children can participate and remain active.	How sure are you that you can be physically active 3–5 times a week?	3-point ordinal scale with "not sure," "a little sure," and "very sure"	5-item scale

Behavioral Capability

The CATCH curriculum teaches healthful dietary behaviors by classifying foods as GO (foods that can be consumed every day), SLOW (foods that should be consumed with less frequency), or WHOA (foods that should be served and eaten only occasionally). GO, SLOW, and WHOA is an age-appropriate classification system designed by nutritionists to give children the knowledge to make better food choices. Using the scale developed for the CATCH main trial, an increase in food knowledge was observed (Luepker et al., 1996).

Intentions

In CATCH, dietary intentions were operationalized with a goal-setting activity where children classified the foods in their lunches as GO, SLOW, or WHOA. If they consumed more GO foods than SLOW and WHOA foods, their lunch was classified as GO. Each child set a goal for a certain number of GO lunches per week and tracked his or her own progress. Dietary intentions were shown to improve significantly after the CATCH main trial. The skills used to classify the foods, along with the knowledge necessary to determine which classification was appropriate, illustrate behavioral capability.

Self-Control

Self-control was measured in terms of usual food consumption and operationalized through strategies such as preparation of easy snacks during classroom lessons. New, healthy foods that tasted good were introduced to change outcome expectations about the acceptability of nutritious foods. Goal setting for trying new foods at home was part of the family activities. Usual food consumption of healthier foods was significantly increased in intervention students compared to students in control schools at the end of the CATCH trial.

Social Environment

Social support for both dietary and physical activity behaviors was targeted through use of strategies such as having teachers and parents reinforce consumption of healthy food and physical activity through praise and recognition of children making appropriate choices. In addition, activities within the classroom emphasized setting peer norms for consumption of healthy food and being active as usual behaviors.

Evaluation of social support during the main CATCH trial showed mixed results. At the end of the trial, there were no differences in either positive or negative support for physical activity, although changes in positive support for physical activity were seen in an interim measure during the study. Evaluation of support for dietary behaviors increased in students from intervention schools for combined peer, teacher, and parent support at the end of the trial. When examining support by each group, parent and teacher support increased at interim and final measurement periods, but support by peers was not significant at the final measurement period.

What do these evaluation results mean? It may be that the parts of the CATCH program (classroom curriculum, PE program, and family program) that address social support for physical activity need additional or enhanced strategies to achieve significant results. Physical activity levels of children decrease as they move through middle school, so strategies to promote activity levels might need to be intensified to effect change in these constructs. Evaluation of SCT constructs as in this example shows how results can be used to further modify or enhance interventions to produce more robust effects.

Self-Efficacy

To increase self-efficacy for dietary and physical activity behaviors, strategies such as observational learning were used. In the CATCH curricula, narratives were included that used characters (e.g., Hearty Heart and Dynamite Diet) that served as role models for students. To further increase self-efficacy, students practiced the new skills they learned in safe and supportive environments by choosing healthful foods in the cafeteria or by practicing new activities in physical education (PE) class. Self-efficacy for both dietary and physical activity behaviors increased at interim time points during the study but was not significantly different in students from intervention schools compared to students from control schools at the end of the trial (Edmundson et al., 1996).

As with social support, it appears that that the curricular strategies and environmental changes in CATCH meant to enhance self-efficacy were adequate for children in the third and fourth grades, but might need to be intensified or of longer duration to produce changes in fifth-grade children. Alternately, it might be that the curriculum is appropriate but that it is difficult for preadolescents in fifth grade to counteract the media messages and social influences in the larger community environment (Edmundson et al., 1996).

School Environment

In addition to the cognitive and behavioral support constructs targeted in CATCH, changes in the social and physical environments of schools were also intervention targets. For example, in the Eat Smart school meal program, cafeteria personnel were trained to alter recipes so that the foods served were lower in fat, saturated fat, and sodium but still appetizing. Children learned about which foods were high in fat and sodium from classroom lessons, using the GO, SLOW, and WHOA classifications. When children ate in the cafeteria, the foods were labeled as GO, SLOW, or WHOA, and the children could use these food classifications to practice selecting healthful foods. Selecting and eating the foods provided an outcome expectation that healthful foods could be tasty and fun to eat. This also reinforced the selection of healthful foods and increased self-efficacy. Physical environment changes were measured as a part of the CATCH trial. These variables included assessing the nutrient content of food offered to the children, signage that reinforced norms of healthful eating and activity, and the percentage of PE class time spent in moderate to vigorous physical activity. Environmental variables showed some of the most robust and significant changes during the CATCH trial, and several, especially those in the cafeteria and PE program, were sustained over time (Hoelscher et al., 2004).

Although further evaluation trials of CATCH have been associated with reductions in child obesity (Coleman et al., 2005; Hoelscher, Kelder, et al., 2010; Hoelscher, Springer, et al., 2010), recent work suggests that the onset of child obesity is sensitive to environmental influences and systems outside the school (Institute of Medicine, 2012). In the 2005 El Paso CATCH RCT replication study, Coleman and colleagues applied CATCH as described above in low-income, Hispanic border schools and reported an increase in overweight and obese students in control schools of 11 percent in overweight from third to fifth grade, whereas CATCH intervention schools rose only 1.5 percent (Coleman et al., 2005). This finding stimulated funding and implementation of CATCH district-wide in over one hundred El Paso elementary schools nested within the Paso del Norte community obesity program, which included a mass media campaign, grocery store cooking demonstrations, parent walking clubs, and citywide 5K run/walks. Hoelscher, Kelder, and colleagues (2010) treated the district-wide school (CATCH) plus community environmental intervention as a population-level natural experiment and reported a serial, cross-sectional reduction in fourth-grade overweight and obesity of 7 percent over a four-year period. During this same time period, the prevalence of fourth-grade obesity rose in Texas overall. In the more recent Travis County CATCH experimental study, over one hundred elementary schools were trained in CATCH with three levels of program implementation intensity: (1) training and supplies, (2) training, supplies, and site program facilitation, and (3) training, supplies, facilitation, and community support. In the community environmental condition, local community organizations were invited to participate and support the CATCH schools. Students in schools in the community environmental condition showed a decrease of 8 percentage points in overweight and obesity compared to students in the least intensive condition (Hoelscher, Springer, et al., 2010).

Thus, in the CATCH experience, it appears important to develop intervention programs that include strategies addressing environmental factors both on and off school campuses, as well as addressing the underlying cognitive processes or behavioral factors that support and reinforce the environment, and vice versa.

Case Study 2: Cultural Adaptations of SCT and Project MYTRI

In the early 1970s, an exploration of how SCT might be conceptualized, utilized, adapted, and evaluated in cultural settings outside the United States was tested in North Karelia, Finland (Puska et al., 1985). Key elements in the success of the North Karelia Project included media portrayals of powerful role models, social support for behavior changes, and increased access to services and opportunities for healthy behaviors. The North Karelia Project relied on community input and grassroots organization in planning and implementation in order to ensure that the components of the intervention were culturally appropriate and relevant to the population (Puska et al., 1985).

Further research to examine and use SCT has been ongoing in many developed and less-developed countries outside the United States (Bandura, 2006b). According to Hofstede (1997), cultural differences between countries involve (1) the emphasis on collectivism versus individualism, (2) the degree of disparity or inequality in power, (3) the amount of uncertainty that is acceptable, and (4) the masculinity or femininity of the culture. These differences in culture may change how the key components of SCT manifest in behavior (Oettingen, 1995). For example, social support may be directed more toward an entire group in a collectivist culture, where group accomplishments are reinforced, and more toward personal accomplishment in an individualist culture, where there is more competition between individuals (Oettingen, 1995). Similarly, Klassen (2004) found that for some non-Western cultures, collective efficacy operates in the same way as self-efficacy does for Western cultures in predicting functioning. Thus, in collectivist cultures, the individual sees himself or herself as inextricably linked to others in a defined group, so that individual accomplishment is more like a cog in the wheel of the group, thus *the factors influencing behavior change are also in reference to the behavior of others in the group.* In individualist cultures, one's own accomplishments (and failures) are paramount.

Differences in culture are also considered in health behavior interventions. Interventions may involve serial dramas presented on television and radio (e.g., *telenovelas*) that address social and health problems in a society (Bandura, 2002). These serial dramas utilize social modeling primarily. Not only are the models in the serial dramas believable and attractive to audiences, they engage in situations and environments that engender emotional attachment to the models and the outcomes of their behaviors. Audiences are shown realistic opportunities and barriers to engagement or participation, and the role models show both positive and negative outcomes of the decisions that are made. The dramas conclude with epilogues that address further opportunities in the audience's community to engage in the promoted actions (Bandura, 2002). For example, one drama encouraged residents in Mexico City to sign up for a literacy program, and on the day after the epilogue appeared, delivered by a famous actor, 25,000 people went to the distribution center for literacy primers (Bandura, 2006b).

A key question in adapting SCT in non-U.S. cultural settings, then, is how do the key constructs manifest in a given culture? In tobacco use prevention research in New Delhi and Chennai, India, the components of our intervention model were examined using focus groups and quantitative data to verify the validity and appropriateness of each construct (Perry, Stigler, Arora, & Reddy, 2008; Stigler, Perry, Arora, & Reddy, 2006). The focus groups were conducted in Hindi and English in New Delhi, with 435 sixth- and eighth-grade students who represented government, private, same-sex, and co-ed schools (Mishra et al., 2005), and the results mostly confirmed our SCT-based theoretical model. The model hypothesized that changes in intrapersonal (knowledge, outcome expectations, beliefs, self-efficacy, and skills), environmental (opportunities and social support), and social contextual (norms and role models) factors would result in changes in tobacco use onset and prevalence among young adolescents (Mishra et al., 2005). We explored each of these factors within the lengthy focus groups, finding that the importance of most of these factors among Indian youth was comparable to their importance in our prior U.S. tobacco research (DHHS, 2012). Cultural differences were noted too, however. The students in New Delhi had inadequate information on the harmful effects of smoking and smokeless tobacco, which was not true of students in the United States. In addition, the students in India expressed collective efficacy in wanting to dissuade their peers from using tobacco. The two-year, peer-led, school-based intervention (Project MYTRI) was implemented in thirty-two schools in India with sixth- through ninth-grade students ($n = 12,484$), with schools randomized to intervention and control conditions.

The intervention was purposely designed to creatively change the SCT factors in our model but within the cultural context of urban India, with a particular emphasis on increasing knowledge about the harmful outcomes of tobacco use, promoting new and attractive role models who did not support tobacco use, providing skills training in resisting influences to use tobacco and also in changing policies around tobacco, and organizing the social support of peers, teachers, and family members. Project MYTRI, then, consisted of four primary components aimed at changing the factors in our model: peer-led behavioral curricula over two school years, media for parents and media for the school environment in the form of postcards and posters, and after-school, peer-led activism (Perry, Stigler, Arora, & Reddy, 2009). The intervention had a significant impact on cigarette and *bidi* smoking (a South Asian cigarette, also known as *beedi*), as well as on intentions to use tobacco (Perry et al., 2009). In a subsequent mediation analysis, changes in students' knowledge of the social and health effects, outcome expectations, normative beliefs, and advocacy skills self-efficacy were all associated with reduced intentions to use and actual use of tobacco (Stigler, Perry, Smolenski, Arora, & Reddy, 2011). Project MYTRI demonstrates the importance of understanding cultural nuances associated with the theoretical components of SCT, the relevance of these components in intervention design and measurement, and their power in achieving behavior change with young adolescents in a less-developed country.

Future Directions in SCT

Social cognitive theory provides essential building blocks, or constructs, for understanding the development of human behavior. However, because SCT focuses primarily on individual behavior change, environmental influences are often overlooked or not adequately considered in intervention design. Health promotion and prevention programs often produce short-lived or weak results because they rely too heavily on didactic, knowledge-based strategies and place too little emphasis on the development of *behavioral capability*. It is a straightforward task to deliver health knowledge, but far more difficult to change a person's level of self-efficacy, outcome expectations, social support, or opportunities that require careful planning, resources, and qualified personnel. Thus it is important to consider the constructs associated with SCT, but at multiple levels of the social and physical environment. For example, changes in policies that support the new behaviors could add another dimension that could support behavior change. The depth of SCT could be enhanced by the breadth of the socioecological model (see Chapter Three) if the constructs associated with SCT are considered within the various domains—family, neighborhood, community, school, and so forth—of the socioecological model (Perry, 1999). Particularly relevant to this discussion is the focus on the physical and policy environments that is now emphasized in health promotion efforts. While barriers and opportunities in the physical and policy environment have been incorporated into several studies using SCT as a framework, the effects and interactions among environmental, behavioral, and cognitive factors have not always been explicitly analyzed or explored. Given the recognized differences in the ways SCT constructs manifest with different cultural groups, the careful delineation, tailoring, measurement, and application of these constructs is critical for successful interventions. Measurement issues are also paramount to future research, and the development of reliable and valid measurement tools for SCT constructs that are specific to a variety of behaviors and target groups will be a continuing priority. As Bandura has frequently noted, poorly developed SCT constructs cannot confirm or refute the theory (Bandura, 1999). New types of data collection, such as the repeated measures now possible through smartphone technology or computer-based applications, can provide information and context for SCT constructs and behavioral outcomes on a continuous basis, which can further develop inter-vention effectiveness. When a full-scale evaluation is warranted, a pretest-posttest randomized or quasi-experimental study design offers the strongest evidence to determine the effects of the intervention on behavioral outcomes compared to a controlled condition, and mediation analyses are conducted to confirm constructs responsible for behavior change. Although used sparingly in the past, the increased use of mediation analyses, both quantitative and qualitative, can lead to more efficiency in application of theory and intervention design.

Summary

Social cognitive theory is an action-oriented approach to understanding cognitive, environmen-tal, and behavioral influences on behaviors and to using that understanding in the development and evaluation of theory-based interventions to improve the health status of societies. SCT has broad application across a diverse array of health-enhancing and health-compromising behaviors and has been used successfully in a variety of cultures with a variety of intervention methods. For the beginning interventionist, the application of SCT to behavior change is not necessarily a logical or linear process, and the number of theoretical factors can at times seem overwhelming. In summary, in the application of SCT, a typical first step is to carefully review the SCT-oriented risk factor literature for the selected behavioral outcomes (e.g., goal setting predicting physical activity) and to examine relevant intervention literature to determine the strongest evidence-based combination of intervention components. The second step is often qualitative and quantitative assessment in conjunction with the recipients of the intervention in order to identify the most salient and powerful SCT constructs associated with the tar-geted behavior and to ensure that the constructs are age appropriate and culturally relevant. A third step might be to explain the usefulness of SCT constructs and the tenets of reciprocal determinism to community partners, so that they understand the rationale for the proposed intervention approaches. These preliminary data are then used in the application of SCT constructs to intervention design. In the words of Albert Bandura (2004): "As you venture forth to promote your own health and that of others, may the efficacy force be with you!"

References

Ajzen, I. (2002). Perceived behavioral control, self-efficacy, locus of control, and the theory of planned behavior. *Journal of Applied Social Psychology, 32*(4), 665–683.

Ashford, S., Edmunds, J., & French, D. P. (2010). What is the best way to change self-efficacy to promote lifestyle and recreational physical activity? A systematic review with meta-analysis. *British Journal of Health Psychology, 15*(2), 265–288.

Bandura, A. (1977a). Self-efficacy: Toward a unifying theory of behavioral change. *Psychological Review*, *84*(2), 191–215.

Bandura, A. (1977b). *Social learning theory.* New York: General Learning Press.

Bandura, A. (1986). *Social foundations of thought and action.* Englewood Cliffs, NJ: Prentice Hall.

Bandura, A. (1997). *Self-efficacy: The exercise of control.* New York: Freeman.

Bandura, A. (1999). Moral disengagement in the perpetration of inhumanities. *Personality and Social Psychology Review*, *3*(3), 193–209.

Bandura, A. (2000). Exercise of human agency through collective efficacy. *Current Directions in Psychological Science*, *9*(3), 75–78.

Bandura, A. (2002). Social cognitive theory in cultural context. *Applied Psychology*, *51*(2), 269–290.

Bandura, A. (2004). Health promotion by social cognitive means. *Health Education & Behavior*, *31*(2), 143–164.

Bandura, A. (2005). The primacy of self-regulation in health promotion. *Applied Psychology*, *54*(2), 245–254.

Bandura, A. (2006a). Adolescent development from an agentic perspective. In F. Pajares & T. Urdan (Eds.), *Self-efficacy beliefs of adolescents* (pp. 1–43). Charlotte, NC: Information Age.

Bandura, A. (2006b). On integrating social cognitive and social diffusion theories. In A. Singhal & J. W. Dearing (Eds.), *Communication of innovations: A journey with Ev Rogers* (pp. 111–135). Thousand Oaks, CA: Sage.

Bandura, A. (2008). Social cognitive theory of mass communication. In J. Bryant & M. B. Oliver (Eds.), *Media effects: Advances in theory and research* (3rd ed., pp. 121–153). New York: Routledge.

Bandura, A. (2010, November 9). Bobo doll experiment [video]. Retrieved from http://www.youtube.com/watch?v=xfG55uY2NSU

Bandura, A., Ross, D., & Ross, S. A. (1961). Transmission of aggression through imitation of aggressive models. *Journal of Abnormal and Social Psychology*, *63*(3), 575–582.

Betz, E. (2013). Assessment of self-efficacy. In K. F. Geisinger (Ed.), *APA handbook of testing and assessment in psychology, Vol. 2. Testing and assessment in clinical and counseling psychology* (pp. 379–391). Washington, DC: American Psychological Association.

Borsari, B., & Carey, K. B. (2003). Descriptive and injunctive norms in college drinking: A meta-analytic integration. *Journal of Studies on Alcohol*, *64*(3), 331–341.

Coleman, K. J., Tiller, C. L., Sanchez, J., Heath, E. M., Sy, O., Milliken, G., & Dzewaltowski, D. A. (2005). Prevention of the epidemic increase in child risk of overweight in low-income schools: The El Paso coordinated approach to child health. *Archives of Pediatrics & Adolescent Medicine*, *159*(3), 217–224.

Edmundson, E., Parcel, G. S., Feldman, H. A., Elder, J., Perry, C. L., Johnson, C. C., . . . Webber, L. (1996). The effects of the Child and Adolescent Trial for Cardiovascular Health upon psychosocial determinants of diet and physical activity behavior. *Preventive Medicine*, *25*(4), 442–454.

Gifford-Smith, M., Dodge, K. A., Dishion, T. J., & McCord, J. (2005). Peer influence in children and adolescents: Crossing the bridge from developmental to intervention science. *Journal of Abnormal Child Psychology*, *33*(3), 255–265.

Goddard, R. D., Hoy, W. K., & Hoy, A. W. (2004). Collective efficacy beliefs: Theoretical developments, empirical evidence, and future directions. *Educational Researcher*, *33*(3), 3–13.

Greenhalgh, J., Dowey, A. J., Horne, P. J., Fergus Lowe, C., Griffiths, J. H., & Whitaker, C. J. (2009). Positive and negative peer modelling effects on young children's consumption of novel blue foods. *Appetite*, *52*(3), 646–653.

Hoelscher, D. M., Feldman, H. A., Johnson, C. C., Lytle, L. A., Osganian, S. K., Parcel, G. S., . . . Nader, P. R. (2004). School-based health education programs can be maintained over time: Results from the CATCH institutionalization study. *Preventive Medicine*, *38*(5), 594–606.

Hoelscher, D. M., Kelder, S. H., Pérez, A., Day, R. S., Benoit, J. S., Frankowski, R. F., . . . Lee, E. S. (2010). Changes in the regional prevalence of child obesity in 4th, 8th, and 11th grade students in Texas from 2000–2002 to 2004–2005. *Obesity*, *18*(7), 1360–1368.

Hoelscher, D. M., Springer, A. E., Ranjit, N., Perry, C. L., Evans, A. E., Stigler, M., & Kelder, S. H. (2010). Reductions in child obesity among disadvantaged school children with community involvement: The Travis County CATCH Trial. *Obesity*, *18*(Suppl. 1), S36–S44.

Hofstede, G. (1997). *Cultures and organizations: Software of the mind*. New York: McGraw-Hill.

Institute of Medicine, Committee on Accelerating Progress in Obesity Prevention. (2012). *Accelerating progress in obesity prevention: Solving the weight of the nation*. Washington, DC: National Academies Press.

Kelder, S. H., Perry, C. L., Klepp, K. I., & Lytle, L. L. (1994). Longitudinal tracking of adolescent smoking, physical activity, and food choice behaviors. *American Journal of Public Health*, *84*(7), 1121–1126.

Klassen, R. M. (2004). Optimism and realism: A review of self-efficacy from a cross-cultural perspective. *International Journal of Psychology*, *39*(3), 205–230.

Levine, L. J., & Edelstein, R. S. (2009). Emotion and memory narrowing: A review and goal-relevance approach. *Cognition and Emotion*, *23*(5), 833–875.

Luepker, R. V., Perry, C. L., McKinlay, S. M., Nader, P. R., Parcel, G. S., Stone, E. J., . . . & Smisson, J. (1996). Outcomes of a field trial to improve children's dietary patterns and physical activity: The Child and Adolescent Trial for Cardiovascular Health (CATCH). *JAMA*, *275*(10), 768–776.

Mishra, A., Arora, M., Stigler, M. H., Komro, K. A., Lytle, L. A., Reddy, K. S., & Perry, C. L. (2005). Indian youth speak about tobacco: Results of focus group discussions with school students. *Health Education & Behavior*, *32*(3), 363–379.

Montaño, D. E., Kasprzyk, D., & Taplin, S. (1997). The theory of reasoned action and the theory of planned behavior. In K. Glanz, F. M. Lewis, & B. K. Rimer (Eds.), *Health behavior and health education: Theory, research, and practice* (2nd ed., pp. 85–112). San Francisco: Jossey-Bass.

Nader, P. R., Stone, E. J., Lytle, L. A., Perry, C. L., Osganian, S. K., Kelder, S., . . . Luepker, R. V. (1999). Three-year maintenance of improved diet and physical activity: The CATCH cohort. *Archives of Pediatrics & Adolescent Medicine*, *153*(7), 695–704.

Neighbors, C., Larimer, M., & Lewis, M. (2004). Targeting misperceptions of descriptive drinking norms: Efficacy of a computer-delivered personalized normative feedback intervention. *Journal of Consulting and Clinical Psychology*, *73*, 434–447.

Oettingen, G. (1995). Cross-cultural perspectives on self-efficacy. In A. Bandura (Ed.), *Self-efficacy in changing societies* (pp. 149–176). New York: Cambridge University Press.

Pavlov, I. P. (1927). *Conditioned reflexes*. Oxford, UK: Oxford University Press.

Perkins, H. W., Craig, D. W., & Perkins, J. M. (2011). Using social norms to reduce bullying: A research intervention among adolescents in five middle schools. *Group Processes & Intergroup Relations*, *14*(5), 703–722.

Perry, C. L. (1999). *Creating health behavior change: How to develop community-wide programs for youth*. Thousand Oaks, CA: Sage.

Perry, C. L., Stigler, M. H., Arora, M., & Reddy, K. S. (2008). Prevention in translation: Tobacco use prevention in India. *Health Promotion Practice*, *9*(4), 378–386.

Perry, C. L., Stigler, M. H., Arora, M., & Reddy, K. S. (2009). Preventing tobacco use among young people in India: Project MYTRI. *American Journal of Public Health*, *99*(5), 899–906.

Perry, C. L., Stone, E. J., Parcel, G. S., Ellison, R. C., Nader, P. R., Webber, L. S., & Luepker, R. V. (1990). School-based cardiovascular health promotion: The Child and Adolescent Trial for Cardiovascular Health (CATCH). *Journal of School Health*, *60*, 406–413.

Puska, P., Nissinen, A., Tuomilehto, J., Salonen, J. T., Koskela, K., McAlister, A., . . . Farquhar, J. W. (1985). The community-based strategy to prevent coronary heart disease: Conclusions from the ten years of the North Karelia project. *Annual Review of Public Health*, *6*(1), 147–193.

Ramdass, D., & Zimmerman, B. J. (2011). Developing self-regulation skills: The important role of homework. *Journal of Advanced Academics*, *22*(2), 194–218.

Rohrbach, L. A., Sussman, S., Dent, C. W., & Sun, P. (2005). Tobacco, alcohol, and other drug use among high-risk young people: A five-year longitudinal study from adolescence to emerging adulthood. *Journal of Drug Issues*, *35*(2), 333–356.

Schultz, P. W., Nolan, J. M., Cialdini, R. B., Goldstein, N. J., & Griskevicius, V. (2007). The constructive, destructive, and reconstructive power of social norms. *Psychological Science*, *18*(5), 429–434.

Sharma, S., Chuang, R. J., & Hedberg, A. M. (2011). Pilot-testing CATCH early childhood: A preschool-based healthy nutrition and physical activity program. *American Journal of Health Education*, *42*(1), 12–23.

Short, S., & Ross-Stewart, L. (2008). A review of self-efficacy based interventions. In S. D. Mellallieu & S. Hanton (Eds.), *Advances in applied sport psychology: A review* (pp. 221–280). New York: Routledge.

Skinner, B. F. (1953). *Science and human behavior*. New York: Free Press.

Springer, A. E., Kelder, S. H., Byrd-Williams, C. E., Pasch, K. E., Ranjit, N., Delk, J. E., & Hoelscher, D. M. (2013). Promoting energy-balance behaviors among ethnically diverse adolescents: Overview & baseline findings of the Central Texas CATCH Middle School Project. *Health Education & Behavior*, *40*(5), 559–570.

Stigler, M. H., Perry, C. L., Arora, M., & Reddy, K. S. (2006). Why are urban Indian 6th graders using more tobacco than 8th graders? Findings from Project MYTRI. *Tobacco Control*, *15*(Suppl. 1), i54–i60.

Stigler, M. H., Perry, C. L., Smolenski, D., Arora, M., & Reddy, K. S. (2011). A mediation analysis of a tobacco prevention program for adolescents in India: How did Project MYTRI work? *Health Education & Behavior*, *38*(3), 231–240.

Thomas, R. E., McLellan, J., & Perera, R. (2013). School-based programmes for preventing smoking. *Cochrane Database of Systematic Reviews*, *2013*(4), CD001293.

U.S. Department of Health and Human Services. (2012). *Preventing tobacco use among youth and young adults: A report of the surgeon general*. Atlanta: U.S. Department of Health and Human Services, Centers for Disease Control and Prevention, National Center for Chronic Disease Prevention and Health Promotion, Office on Smoking and Health.

Webb, T. L., & Sheeran, P. (2006). Does changing behavioral intentions engender behavior change? A meta-analysis of the experimental evidence. *Psychological Bulletin*, *132*(2), 249–268.

Williams, D. M., Anderson, E. S., & Winett, R. A. (2005). A review of the outcome expectancy construct in physical activity research. *Annals of Behavioral Medicine*, *29*(1), 70–79.

Wills, T. M., & Ainette, M. G. (2012). Social networks and social support. In A. Baum, T. A. Revenson, & J. Singer (Eds.), *Handbook of health psychology* (pp. 465–492). New York: Psychology Press.

CHAPTER 10

SOCIAL SUPPORT AND HEALTH

Julianne Holt-Lunstad
Bert N. Uchino

There is now robust evidence linking social support to both morbidity and mortality from certain diseases and conditions (Holt-Lunstad, Smith, & Layton, 2010). An understanding of the nature and types of support and of the pathways by which associations with health occur is important for guiding effective interventions. Although many questions remain, theories and evidence suggest that social support is a heterogeneous concept and that there are multiple pathways by which social support may influence mental and physical health. We first provide a review of different conceptualizations of support as well as the evidence linking social support to health outcomes, and then we discuss the major theoretical models linking social support to health. We end by focusing on intervention implications and describing two recent applications of social support to modify health-relevant outcomes.

Definition and Conceptualizations of Social Support

Terms such as *social support*, *social networks*, and *social integration* are often used interchangeably but are distinct concepts. Although the influence of social relationships has been conceptualized and measured in diverse ways, these can be broken down into two broad categories: one examines the structure and the other examines the functions of social relationships (Berkman, Glass, Brissette, & Seeman, 2000; Cohen & Wills, 1985; Uchino, 2006). Generally, these two approaches distinguish the aspects of

KEY POINTS

This chapter will:

- Define social support, including how it is conceptualized and measured.

- Provide a historical background for examining the association between social support and health.

- Provide a theoretical framework for understanding the association between social support and health.

- Briefly review the evidence of protective and potentially deleterious effects of social support.

- Present two examples of social support interventions for promoting health.

social networks and the support that they provide. *Structural* aspects of relationships refer to the extent to which individuals are situated within or integrated into social networks. *Social network* describes connections between individuals and their relationships or network ties (see Chapter Eleven). Measures of social networks typically assess the density, size, or number of social contacts. *Social integration* describes the extent of an individual's participation in a broad range of social relationships, including active engagement in a variety of social activities or relationships and a sense of communality and identification with one's social roles. In contrast, *functional* measures focus on the specific functions served by relationships, and they are measured by actual or perceived availability of support, aid, or resources from these relationships. Thus three major components of social relationships are evaluated consistently: (1) degree of integration in social networks, (2) social interactions that are intended to be supportive (e.g., received social support), and (3) beliefs and perceptions about support availability held by individuals (e.g., perceived social support). The first component, or subconstruct, represents structural aspects of social relationships; the latter two represent functional aspects. Epidemiological studies that have linked social relationships to mortality can be categorized according to the specific measurement approaches described in Table 10.1.

The breadth of these two approaches—structural and functional—has been both a strength and weakness of research on social support and health. On the one hand, a broad approach more adequately describes how aspects of social relationships may influence health and the potential interconnection among these constructs. On the other hand, such an approach makes it difficult to identify what particular aspects of support are related to health outcomes

Table 10.1   Measurement Approaches Used to Assess Social Relationships

Type of Measure	Description
Functional	*Functions provided by or perceived to be available from social relationships*
Received support	Self-reported receipt of emotional, informational, tangible, or belonging support
Perceptions of social support	Perceptions of availability of emotional, informational, tangible, or belonging support if needed
Perception of loneliness	Feelings of isolation, disconnectedness, and not belonging
Structural	*The existence of and interconnections among differing social ties and roles*
Marital status	Married vs. other (never married, divorced, or widowed)
Social networks	Network density or size; number of social contacts
Social integration	Participation in a broad range of social relationships, including active engagement in a variety of social activities or relationships, and a sense of communality and identification with one's social roles
Complex measures of social integration	A single measure that assesses multiple components of social integration, such as marital status, network size, and network participation
Living alone	Living alone vs. living with others
Social isolation	Pervasive lack of social contact or communication, participation in social activities, or confidants
Combined	*Assessment of both structural and functional measures*
Multifaceted measurement	Multiple measures obtained that assess more than one of the above conceptualizations

and through which pathways. It also is challenging to reconcile conflicting evidence when different measures are used to measure social support. In this chapter, we focus primarily on the perspective that social support is the functional aspect of relationship processes when describing specific mechanisms and outcomes.

Functional social support describes the particular functions served by social relationships (Table 10.2). Supportive individuals make available or provide what can be termed *emotional* support (e.g., expressions of caring), *informational* support (e.g., information that might be used to deal with stress), *tangible* support (e.g., direct material aid, also referred to as instrumental, practical, or financial support), and *belonging* support (e.g., having others to engage with in social activities) (Cohen, Mermelstein, Kamarck, & Hoberman, 1985; Cutrona & Russell, 1990). Factor analyses have shown that these support components are distinct lower order processes that, together, make up the higher order concept of social support (Cutrona & Russell, 1990). These functions can also be differentiated in terms of whether social support is perceived or received (Dunkel-Schetter & Skokan, 1990). Perceived support refers to the perception that others will be available to provide support if needed. Received support refers to the actual support provided by others. Perceived support is correlated only moderately with received support, and hence they are distinct constructs (Wills & Shinar, 2000).

There is now a relatively large literature linking social support to health-relevant outcomes, including health behaviors (e.g., smoking cessation), adherence to medical regimens (e.g., medication), development of and the course of specific chronic conditions (e.g., cardiovascular disease), and all-cause mortality (Barth, Schneider, & von Kanel, 2010; DiMatteo, 2004; Holt-Lunstad et al., 2010; Uchino, 2006). Overall, there is good epidemiological evidence that distinct measures of social support are related to positive health outcomes. More specific findings will be described later, but a recent meta-analysis by Holt-Lunstad and colleagues (2010) found that those reporting greater social support (averaged across different measurement approaches utilized in studies) were associated with a 50 percent increased odds of survival relative to those

Table 10.2   Definitions and Examples of Dimensions of Functional Support

Type of Support	Definition	Example
Perceived support	The expectation that others will provide support if needed	You perceive that your friends will be there for you no matter the circumstance.
Received support	The actual provision of support by another	Your friend directly provides you with support to handle an important problem.
Emotional	Expressions of comfort and caring	Someone makes you feel better just because he or she listens to your problems.
Belonging	Shared social activities, sense of social belonging	You have a friend you enjoy simply "hanging out" with.
Tangible*	Provision of material aid	A family member would give you a personal financial loan.
Informational	Provision of advice and guidance	You know a person who can give you trusted advice and guidance on an issue.

*This is also referred to as instrumental support.

lacking social support. They also found that perceived functional support was a significant individual predictor of lower mortality. Received support, however, did not predict mortality rates. These data are consistent with studies finding that perceived support is a more consistent predictor of both mental and physical health outcomes compared to received support (Wills & Shinar, 2000; Uchino, 2009). As will be discussed later, this is a significant theoretical issue as interventions aimed at increasing support often try to increase the receipt of social support without considering whether it responds to the individual's needs or is perceived as supportive.

Historical Perspectives

The study of social relationships and physical health has a long research tradition. One early influence was the renowned French sociologist Émile Durkheim. In his classic analysis of suicide rates across social classes, cultures, religious affiliation, and gender, he argued that suicide rates were closely tied to the social environment (Durkheim, 1951). For instance, egoistic suicide results from an excessive individualism and a lack of integration of the individual into society or family life. As a result, individuals are left to face the challenges of life on their own. Durkheim's analysis was compelling and led to a subsequent focus on more specific aspects of social relationships that were related to health outcomes.

In 1976, two influential reviews were published that emphasized the health relevance of the qualitative aspects of social networks and that gave rise to an emphasis in health psychology on the functional support that social networks may provide. Cobb (1976) defined social support as information from others that one is cared for, loved, esteemed, and part of a mutually supportive network. Cobb then reviewed evidence suggesting that these social support resources were important in dealing with a range of stressful life events, such as pregnancy, hospitalization, and bereavement. Cassell (1976) focused more on the biological processes linking support to health. He argued that social support might best be seen as a protective factor, and he reviewed studies suggesting that such a relationship factor might modify bodily processes (e.g., blood pressure or endocrine activity) in health-relevant ways. These two reviews highlighted the important role that functional social support might play in physical health outcomes.

A few years after these groundbreaking reviews, one of the first population-based longitudinal research studies linking social relationships to mortality was published. Lisa Berkman and Leonard Syme (1979) examined the survey responses of nearly 7,000 residents of Alameda County, California. More specifically, they linked answers to questions about the extent of people's social connections to overall mortality and found that people who had fewer social ties had higher mortality rates. This paper is a classic, because it rules out possible alternative explanations (e.g., results due to poorer initial health status) and provides highly compelling evidence for the link between social relationships and mortality.

While Berkman and Syme (1979) focused on the structure of social relationships, one of the first community-based epidemiological studies linking functional support to health was conducted by Dan Blazer (1982) in a community sample of older adults in Durham County, North Carolina. Even when adjusting for standard control variables, such as physical health status and smoking, analyses showed that perceptions of functional support predicted lower mortality rates. These results also held when accounting for structural measures of social integration, such as those utilized by Berkman and Syme (1979), thereby showing an association between perceptions of support and physical health regardless of the size of one's network.

Finally, in 1988, James House and his colleagues published a paper titled "Social Relationships and Health" in the journal *Science*. The authors examined evidence from the available prospective studies indicating that being socially integrated had an independent protective effect on mortality. They argued that these effects were of similar magnitude to those found for blood pressure, smoking, and physical activity. Due to these authors' careful analysis of well-designed prospective studies, their review stimulated further research on the links between more specific aspects of support and health outcomes.

Theoretical Models

Since the 1970s, there has been growing interest and subsequent systematic research examining the health relevance of social support. General models emerging from this work suggest that social support can be health promoting by influencing both psychological and behavioral processes (Uchino, 2006). For instance, relevant psychological pathways include stress appraisals, and behavioral pathways include health behavior change. These pathways were thought to influence health-relevant biological pathways that ultimately influence either the development or course of physical health problems. An overarching framework that highlights these general pathways but incorporates more specific models (e.g., direct effect, stress-buffering models) is highlighted in Figure 10.1.

As shown in Figure 10.1, functional support can have both a stress-related and a direct effect on health outcomes but via distinct theoretical pathways. The *direct effect pathway* highlights the generally health-enhancing influence of social support. The *stress-buffering pathway*, in

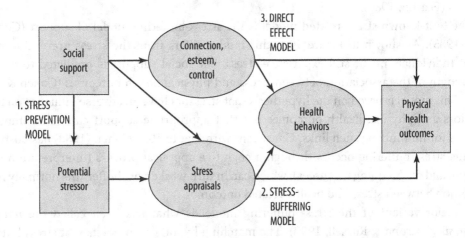

Figure 10.1 Theoretical (Stress Prevention, Stress-Buffering, and Direct Effect) Models and Pathways Linking Social Support to Physical Health Outcomes

comparison, suggests that social support diminishes the negative health effects of stress (Cohen & Wills, 1985). A *stress prevention pathway* is also included, as it was highlighted in an early review by Gore (1981), who pointed to the importance of a stress preventive function of support. As such, the pathways depicted in Figure 10.1 are not necessarily competing perspectives but highlight different contexts and processes by which social support operates (Uchino, 2006). Where they converge is in the "downstream" processes that ultimately link them to health. That is, the final common pathways include health behaviors such as exercise, diet, drug use, and sleep patterns, which in turn can influence health-relevant outcomes. These outcomes range from biological results (e.g., blood pressure) to clinical disease endpoints such as hypertension. The model also suggests that social support can have a direct impact on physical health outcomes.

Social Support as a Buffer for Stress

One of the earliest models of social support in relation to health, the stress prevention model, focused on the possibility that social support might decrease exposure to negative life events (Gore, 1981). As shown in Figure 10.1, this model suggests that social support is beneficial, because network members may provide us with the resources to avoid or reduce our exposure to some types of stressors. There are a number of intriguing pathways by which social support may reduce our exposure to stress. First, social support may influence cognitive processes so that we are less likely to appraise or interpret a situation as threatening or challenging (Cohen, 1988). Second, social support that encourages proactive coping (e.g., informational support on planning for a rainy day) can help individuals make informed decisions that minimize their subsequent exposure to stress (Aspinwall & Taylor, 1997). Finally, adequate social support may decrease exposure to *secondary stressors* (Pearlin, 1989). For instance, stress at work can lead to conflict at home. However, if spousal support reduces the stress of work, it may effectively eliminate potential spillover into marital interactions and reduce exposure to such secondary stressors (Pearlin, 1989).

The best-known stress-related model is the stress-buffering model of support (Cohen & Wills, 1985). As shown in Figure 10.1, this model differs from the stress prevention model in that individuals might still experience stress, but social support is predicted to decrease the strength of the association between stress and physical health outcomes (Cohen & Wills, 1985). This model is based on the hypothesis that stressors have an adverse influence on health behaviors and physical health outcomes but that appropriate support can be an important resource for minimizing such links. Consistent with Figure 10.1, Cohen (1988) has postulated that this stress buffering occurs through a cognitive appraisal process (interpretation of the situation and one's coping resources), which can in turn weaken or "buffer" the normally robust association between stress and health-related outcomes.

A major variant of the stress-buffering model is what has been called the *matching hypothesis* (Cutrona & Russell, 1990). The matching hypothesis predicts that stress buffering is most effective when the type of support matches the needs or challenges of the stressful event. More specifically, it predicts that informational and tangible support should be most effective for controllable events (e.g., preparing for a job interview), whereas emotional and belonging support should be most effective for uncontrollable events (e.g., being laid off from a job) (Cutrona & Russell, 1990). This is one of the few theoretical models that highlight how different functional components of support might be related to outcomes based on the nature of the stressor (e.g., controllability).

Overview of the Direct Effect Model

The direct effect model postulates that social support is effective more generally, regardless of stress levels (Cohen & Wills, 1985). Cohen and Wills's 1985 review found that structural measures of support were more likely to demonstrate direct effects. The direct effect of structural measures was seen as representing the influence of social support on social identity, via direct (e.g., demands from others to behave more healthily) or indirect (e.g., behaving more healthily because relationships add greater life meaning) social control processes (Umberson, 1987). However, there is now evidence that functional support can also have direct effects on outcomes by promoting a sense of connection, self-esteem, and control over life due to knowing that one is cared for and supported by others (Lakey & Orehek, 2011; Thoits, 2011).

Recently, Lakey and Orehek (2011) extended this model by proposing the relational regulation theory (RRT) to account for direct effects of social support on mental health outcomes. According to RRT, everyday interactions (e.g., talking about events of a typical day, gossip, or sports talk) regulate an individual on a daily basis, which may result in positive outcomes like general comfort with the person one is interacting with and a sense of well-being (Lakey & Orehek, 2011). These daily interactions can also serve as the basis for stress buffering or prevention links, as individuals generalize their relationship representations to stressful contexts (i.e., is this person I am comfortable with likely to be supportive during stress?). In fact, these researchers have been able to forecast which relationships might be most beneficial months later, based on analyses of brief (e.g., ten-minute) lab-based general discussions (Veenstra et al., 2011).

Empirical Evidence Supporting the Models

Before we discuss the evidence linking social support to morbidity and mortality, we will focus on other health-relevant links in the models. The stress-buffering model has also been tested in a number of well-controlled laboratory studies. In general, the results of laboratory studies suggest that received support decreases cardiovascular reactivity during acute stress (Thorsteinsson & James, 1999). In these laboratory studies, either a friend or a stranger (the experimenter or a confederate) provides the participant with support while the person is undergoing a standardized stress task (e.g., a speech task). Emotional support is the most common support provided. It matches the needs of the current situation as it is typically viewed as more nurturing and less controlling than either informational or tangible support (Trobst, 2000). In another study focusing on health behaviors, Steptoe, Wardle, Pollard, Canaan, and Davies (1996) found that individuals high in stress and support showed a more healthy behavior profile (e.g., less alcohol consumption) than those who were high in stress and low in support.

There is much less research evaluating links between the other stress-related models and processes in the model. The matching hypothesis has received some support in terms of psychological outcomes (Cutrona & Russell, 1990), but has been infrequently tested in epidemiological and physical health studies. The studies that do exist in the health domain are mixed. For instance, in one study researchers found that only tangible support consistently decreased the association between financial stress and alcohol involvement (Peirce, Frone, Russell, & Cooper, 1996). However, other studies, looking specifically at individuals with low financial resources, have not found tangible support to be the most effective form of support (e.g., Krause, 1997). One problem with this finding is the categorization of job strain as relatively controllable, but in the absence of direct measures of stressor controllability over time, a strong test of the matching hypothesis will be difficult.

The stress prevention model is the least tested of the stress-related models in the health domain despite the fact that existing longitudinal studies are consistent with its basic premise. One longitudinal study of older adults found that individuals with higher social support experienced a lower number of daily hassles over a subsequent eleven-month period (Russell & Cutrona, 1991). In addition, one cross-sectional study of adolescents did find that stress exposure was one downstream mediator of links between parental support and drug abuse (Wills & Cleary, 1996).

The direct effect model suggests that social support should demonstrate direct effects on physical health outcomes. There is strong evidence that perceived social support is directly related to beneficial influences on biological function (Glaser, Kiecolt-Glaser, Bonneau, Malarkey, & Hughes, 1992; Lutgendorf et al., 2005). Consistent with a health behavior link, there is also consistent evidence linking perceived support to better health behaviors, including more exercise, less smoking or alcohol consumption, and better sleep quality (Ailshire & Burgard, 2012; Steptoe et al., 1996; Stewart, Gabriele, & Fisher, 2012). Finally, social support is also associated with better patient cooperation with treatment regimens in chronic disease populations, as shown by a comprehensive meta-analysis (DiMatteo, 2004).

The overall model in Figure 10.1 posits that only part of the link between social support and health is due to health behaviors as shown in prior studies. One recent study reported that the link between social support and cardiovascular disease was mediated by poor sleep in women but not men (Nordin, Knutsson, & Sundbom, 2008). Thus there is both a direct and indirect (through health behaviors) link between social support and physical health, though future studies will have to directly test such association using stronger tests of mediation (Rucker, Preacher, Tormala, & Petty, 2011).

Empirical Evidence of the Health Effects of Social Support

Evidence for the Protective Influence of Social Support

Overall, there is strong evidence for the protective effect of social support on health, with stronger evidence for perceived support than received support (see Uchino's 2009 review). This evidence comes from laboratory, field, and epidemiological studies across morbidity and mortality outcomes. Here, we summarize the evidence for effects of social support on heart disease and the evidence of a protective effect on overall mortality.

Coronary Heart Disease

There is substantial evidence linking low levels of social support to coronary heart disease (CHD), the leading cause of death in most industrialized countries. Barth and colleagues' 2010 systematic review and meta-analysis examined prospective studies that measured both structural and functional social support and cardiovascular outcomes at follow-up. These included studies of CHD etiology, development of CHD in previously healthy individuals, and CHD prognosis, which includes individuals with preexisting CHD (Barth et al., 2010; Lett et al., 2005, 2007). Across multiple studies, there is evidence for the beneficial effect of functional support. However, no significant effect was found for structural measures of support (e.g., living alone). Perceived support was associated negatively with both the development and prognosis of CHD, with stronger effects for prognosis (Berkman, Leo-Summers, & Horwitz, 1992; Brummett et al., 2005; Lett et al., 2007; Woloshin et al., 1997). Social support is also a significant predictor of rehospitalization and lower mortality in heart failure patients (Luttik, Jaarsma, Moser, Sanderman, & van Veldhuisen, 2005).

Mortality

There is now substantial evidence for the protective effect of social connections on risk for mortality from all causes. Some of the first epidemiological evidence was highlighted in the review by House and colleagues (1988). They summarized data from five prospective studies: the Alameda County (Berkman & Syme, 1979), Evans County, Tecumseh, Eastern Finland, and Gothenburg studies. These studies examined large community samples of initially healthy individuals, assessed their involvement with social relationships, and then followed them over several years to determine whether level of social integration predicted who would still be alive. Indeed, the evidence confirmed that those low in social integration had significantly higher age-adjusted mortality risk.

Since that time, the number of studies examining the influence of social relationships (both functional and structural aspects) and mortality has grown exponentially. In a meta-analysis of 148 independent prospective studies with data from 308,849 individuals, followed for an average of 7.5 years, results indicate that individuals with greater social connections (averaged across the different measurement approaches seen in Table 10.1) have a 50 percent greater likelihood of survival compared to those with fewer social connections (Holt-Lunstad et al., 2010). The effect was consistent across gender, age, initial health status, and causes of mortality. This meta-analysis provided evidence of the directional effect of social relationships influencing mortality. Most studies were population based and thus examined initially healthy participants. However, even among those who were ill, greater social connectedness (high in both structural and functional support) was associated with greater odds of survival. Thus, regardless of initial health status, those who were more socially connected lived longer. Most notably, the overall magnitude of the effect of social connections on

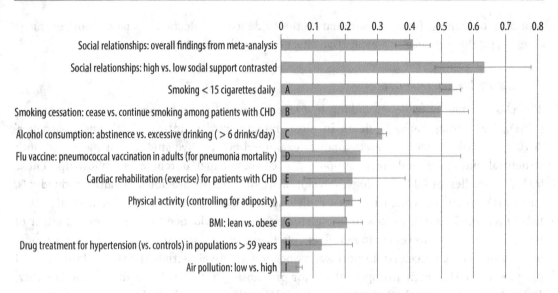

Figure 10.2 Benchmark Data Comparing the Magnitude of Effect of Social Support on Odds of Decreased Mortality Relative to Other Factors

Note: Effect size of zero indicates no effect. The effect sizes were estimated from meta-analyses.

Source: Holt-Lunstad et al., 2010.

risk for mortality was comparable with and in many cases exceeded the effect of many well-established risk factors for mortality. For instance, lacking social connectedness carries a risk equivalent to smoking up to fifteen cigarettes per day, and is greater than that for alcohol abuse, physical inactivity (sedentary lifestyle), obesity, and air pollution, among others (see Figure 10.2).

Across studies, the influence of social relationships was measured in diverse ways, including both functional and structural aspects (Table 10.1). The magnitude of risk reduction differed significantly across type of measurement approach examined. Although both structural (OR = 1.57) and functional measures (OR = 1.46) were significantly associated with greater odds of survival, specific measurement approaches within these broader categorizations varied in their predictive utility. Within functional support measures, perceived support was a significant predictor of longevity (OR = 1.35) whereas received support was not (OR = 1.21). When examining structural measures, living alone (OR = 1.19) was the poorest predictor, and complex measures of social integration were the best predictor (OR = 1.91). Thus assessments that took into account the multidimensional aspects of social relationships were associated with a 91 percent increased odds of survival. Taken altogether, these data suggest that both social networks and the social support they provide are important.

Overall effects of social relationships on mortality may be a conservative estimate. Most studies made adjustments for initial health and other lifestyle risk factors to establish the independent influence of social connections on risk for mortality. However, social relationships are inextricably linked with multiple pathways associated with mortality. For example, excessive alcohol consumption is associated with poor social support; moreover, individuals with positive social relationships engage in fewer risky health behaviors (Jessor, Turbin, & Costa, 1998).

This means they are more likely to exhibit behaviors such as smoking cessation, seatbelt use, adequate sleep, healthy diet, regular exercise, and dental hygiene (Brummett et al., 2006; Fuemmeler et al., 2006). Therefore, these analyses eliminate one of the pathways by which social relationships may influence risk for mortality. The overall effect may also represent a conservative estimate because most studies failed to measure relationship quality. Thus estimates likely include both high- and poor-quality relationships (potential detrimental influences of poor quality relationships are discussed next).

Factors That May Potentially Moderate the Influence of Social Support

Perceived and Received Support

Although social support is generally related to better health, in some circumstances, received support is unrelated or is even linked to negative health outcomes (Holt-Lunstad et al., 2010; Uchino, 2009). Many of the studies reviewed above that found links between social support and physical health are based upon measures of perceived support. In prior work, the concepts of perceived and received support have been used interchangeably, with the assumption that individuals high in perceived support also receive greater support (Dunkel-Schetter & Bennett, 1990; Uchino, 2009). However, measures of perceived and received support are only moderately correlated, and hence seem to represent distinct constructs (Haber, Cohen, Lucas, & Baltes, 2007). Consistent with this possibility, a complicated set of findings emerges throughout these studies when examining measures of received support on health outcomes. For instance, several prospective epidemiological studies examining received support (especially tangible support) found it to be associated with *higher* subsequent mortality rates (Forster & Stoller, 1992; Krause, 1997). This is also consistent with cross-sectional laboratory studies in which receiving support appears to be stress enhancing (e.g., Bolger & Amarel, 2007). Although a simple plausible explanation, based on the concept of support mobilization, is that individuals who are more dependent on receiving support are simply more physically impaired to begin with, these studies do not appear to support this explanation, because most considered the influence of initial health status prospectively (Kaplan et al., 1994).

It has been argued that the links between received support and health might be more contextual. Hence, stressor factors (e.g., match between stressor and support type), provider factors (e.g., relationship quality), and recipient factors (e.g., threats to independence) are important considerations (Bolger & Amarel, 2007; Dunkel-Schetter & Skokan, 1990; Uchino, 2009). All these factors can influence whether or not recipients see received support as responsive, and it has been argued that this is a key factor in the efficacy of received support (Maisel & Gable, 2009). Consistent with this possibility, the Midlife in the United States study (MIDUS) found that only when received support was viewed as unresponsive was it associated with higher mortality rates (Selcuk & Ong, 2013). This is an important issue, and future interventions should consider such issues in designing effective interventions. In fact, it is the component of received tangible support that appears to be most consistently related to higher mortality (Forster & Stoller, 1992; Kaplan et al., 1994).

Relationship Quality

Another important issue is relationship quality. Much of the epidemiological evidence that has established the health relevance of social support did not take the quality of the relationships into account and assumed that all relationships are positive. However, even though our relationships with others may be caring, considerate, and sources of warmth and love, these social relationships can also be demanding, insensitive, and sources of conflict and stress. Although the stress-buffering model suggests that relationships can buffer the negative health effects of stress, it is also possible that some relationships may be sources of stress. Among the few epidemiological studies that examined relationship quality, findings indicate that negativity in social relationships predicts greater risk for mortality (Friedman et al., 1995). For instance, a study that followed 2,264 breast cancer patients for an average of 10.8 years found that while network support is associated with better prognosis, poor quality and burden in family relations was associated with higher risk of all-cause mortality (Kroenke et al., 2013).

Relationship distress may be particularly salient in the context of marriage, given the importance and amount of contact of this particular relationship. Indeed a growing body of research among couples shows that despite the health advantage of marital status, distressed marriages are associated with greater morbidity and risk for mortality (Robles, Slatcher, Trombello, & McGinn, 2013). Relationship distress also has been associated with deleterious health relevant processes, including immune dysregulation and delayed wound healing (Kiecolt-Glaser et al., 2005), high ambulatory blood pressure, and metabolic syndrome (Troxel, Matthews, Gallo, & Kuller, 2005). There is also evidence that unsupportive behavior and partner distress are associated with poorer quality of life among women with breast cancer (Manne, Ostroff, Winkel, Grana, & Fox, 2005).

Likewise, interpersonal stress may be more impactful than other sources of stress. For instance, the Stockholm Female Coronary Risk Study found that after controlling for standard risk factors, marital distress was associated with a nearly a threefold increase in risk of recurrent events, whereas work stress was unrelated (Orth-Gomer et al., 2000).

Technology and Social Support

Within the last decade, advancements in technology have led to dramatic shifts in the way social support is communicated (Griffiths Calear, Banfield, & Tam, 2009; Meier, Lyons, Frydman, Forlenza, & Rimer, 2007; Rimer et al., 2005). Use of the Internet and smartphones is widespread in most developed nations and is now the primary form of communication. Research is now exploring equivalencies between technology-mediated and face-to-face communication and also the potential unique benefits of each approach to social support. There is some evidence to support both potential advantages and disadvantages of online compared to face-to-face support.

Beyond merely connecting individuals at a distance, technology-mediated social support may have a number of potential advantages. For example, those with stigmatized conditions can seek Internet-mediated support that allows them to remain anonymous (Malik & Coulson, 2008); users of online forums can search previous posts for informational and emotional support, thereby reducing the burden for both provider and recipient (Wright & Bell, 2003); and individuals who are able to link up across geographic distances can create support networks around their specific support needs, rather than having to consider simple geographic proximity (Rainie & Wellman, 2012). Overall, these data point to the general utility of communicating informational and emotional support online (Dare & Green, 2011). More recently, evidence has also emerged that participation in the broader social network available online can promote well-being and provide a buffering effect during times of stress (Nicholas et al., 2012). Likewise, there is some evidence to suggest that individuals participate in online support groups to help others (Rimer et al., 2005), thereby increasing provision of support.

We must also acknowledge that technology-communicated social support may be less effective than other forms of support or even have deleterious effects. For instance, there is evidence demonstrating that text messages, despite having similar effects psychologically to talking with someone about a stressful event, do not have similar physiological effects (Seltzer, Prososki, Ziegler, & Pollak, 2012). Similarly, research examining use of the Internet for support after a traumatic event found that despite perceptions of benefit, there was no evidence of an effect on psychological well-being (Vicary & Fraley, 2010). There is also evidence to suggest that the same technology that can facilitate support from others across geographic distance, can also interfere with face-to-face support. For instance, the presence of a mobile phone in social settings may reduce closeness and quality of interactions, interfering with social support (Przybylski & Weinstein, 2013). Of course, there is also the potential for Internet-mediated support to undermine health, given the issues previously discussed for received support. (See Chapter Seventeen for further discussion of the changing media environment in relation to health.) Future research that directly examines the links between perceived and received Internet-mediated support and physical health outcomes will be needed to make this final link.

Taken together, this evidence has a number of important implications for social support interventions. First, we should consider several contextual factors: stress-related factors that may influence efficacy of support, support provider factors and characteristics, and support recipient factors and support desires. Second, the data on relationship quality show that researchers and practitioners must assess both positivity and negativity in the context of social support. Interventions aimed at increasing social support may have unintended detrimental effects if they fail to account for negativity in relationships and the responsivity of the support provided. Likewise, by reducing negativity and increasing responsiveness, interventions may have larger effects than previously estimated. Finally, when designing an intervention utilizing online tools, it should not be assumed that it will be equivalent to face-to-face support.

Health Behavior Applications

Theoretical models linking social support to health highlight the potential role of behavior (e.g., medical cooperation and health behaviors) in linking support to disease outcomes (Uchino, 2006). We approach this by highlighting intervention-based evidence in two examples to illustrate modifiable consequences of social support on health behaviors. First, we summarize the evidence from a randomized clinical trial targeting diabetes peer support to improve glycemic control, and second, we describe an intervention study that demonstrates the potential importance of social support in smoking cessation.

Application 1: Diabetic Control

One way that social support may influence health is through its impact on diabetic control. Diabetes is among the leading causes of death in the United States and many other industrialized countries, and it can involve significant health complications, including heart disease, stroke, high blood pressure, blindness, kidney disease, neuropathy, and amputation (American Diabetes Association, 2015). Glycemic control is important to reduce the risk of these serious health complications; however, this requires significant self-management. Many diabetic individuals have elevated blood glucose levels as a result of poor self-management, despite receiving standard medical treatment.

In an effort to examine the influence of peer support on diabetic control, a randomized trial was developed to compare guided peer support with standard nurse care (Heisler, Vijan, Makki, & Piette, 2010). Participants comprised 244 men with type 2 diabetes and elevated blood glucose levels, defined as hemoglobin A1c (also called HbA1c or A1c) levels higher than 7.5 percent during the previous six months. Participants were identified and recruited from Veterans Affairs (VA) facilities. All participants, regardless of condition, received standard care management advice on managing insulin level; had A1c, blood pressure, and cholesterol levels assessed; and received educational materials. In the intervention group (the peer support condition), patients were paired with an age-matched peer, to encourage both to provide and receive support. Participants assigned to this condition attended a 3-hour group session and were encouraged to call each other once a week, using an automated telephone program, to offer exchange of information, advice, and encouragement. The system recorded the frequency and duration of calls, and prompted reminders if calls were not made within seven days. The control group (nurse care condition) attended a 1.5 hour group session where they were encouraged to ask questions about diabetes self-management and medications and to obtain information about management resources provided by the VA. Each was also encouraged to follow up with the nurse. Both groups were followed for six months, and changes in A1c were assessed to determine whether any significant improvement was achieved.

Results from this randomized trial indicated that those in the peer support intervention group showed significant improvements in glycemic control relative to those in the nurse support only group. The results showed both statistically and clinically significant changes. Follow-up tests were conducted on 212 participants for whom the researchers had complete data at six months to examine potential factors that might explain these findings and the types of patients most strongly impacted (Piette, Resnicow, Choi, & Heisler, 2013). Specifically, the researchers examined perceived diabetic social support and insulin uptake as potential mediators, and they also examined health literacy, diabetes-specific social support, and diabetes-specific distress as potential moderators. Results suggested that the improvement associated with the peer support intervention were primarily mediated by insulin initiation, which accounted for nearly half of the improvement in A1c levels, but not by perceived social support. Additional analyses were conducted to determine if this might depend on whether an individual was actually lacking social support and literacy. These analyses indicated that those with low diabetes-specific social support and low diabetes literacy had heightened improvement in A1c levels compared to the control condition. This is consistent with other work that has shown that social support interventions are particularly, and in some cases only, beneficial among those lacking adequate social support resources within their own network (Cohen, 2004). Although the intervention was associated with significant improvement, a closer examination of the frequency of the calls revealed a range between 2.4 and 0.8 calls per month—far less than one per week as planned. Pairing patients who were strangers to each other, particularly when their interactions were not face to face, might have been uncomfortable, making interaction less likely to be utilized. It should also be noted that this intervention included only male participants. Prior research suggests that females may be more comfortable with both seeking and offering support and more likely to do so (Barbee, Gulley, & Cunningham, 1990); thus it is possible that both provision of support and receipt of support may differ for females. It is possible that this already effective intervention could have been strengthened further by including women and using existing relationships (Cohen, 2004).

Application 2: Support Intervention Aimed at Smoking Cessation

The relationship between smoking and increased mortality has been demonstrated unequivocally (U.S. Department of Health and Human Services, 2004). Smoking cessation is difficult, with high percentages of smokers attempting to quit and very low success rates. Cessation aids such as quit helplines have been demonstrated to be effective, increasing success two- to threefold, yet are underutilized (Patten et al., 2011). Thus the success of quit attempts could be dramatically increased if such resources were used. Given that social support has been correlated with smoking cessation, and many callers to smoking helplines are nonsmokers trying to help a family member or friend quit, utilization of nonsmokers as social support may increase smokers' use of helplines.

In a randomized trial, the efficacy of boosting natural support networks to support the use of an evidence-based helpline was examined (Patten et al., 2011). Nonsmokers interested in helping a friend or family member quit smoking were identified and randomized to the intervention ($n = 267$) or control ($n = 267$) group. Thus the intervention was aimed at support providers and not the smokers. All participants were provided with cessation resources and a study ID number they could share with the smokers they were trying to help. With this study ID, all smokers they were attempting to help, regardless of condition, received the helpline number they could use for up to six months after the intervention and were eligible for free nicotine replacement therapy and counseling regardless of insurance. Participants (i.e., support providers) in the control condition received no further training. Participants assigned to the intervention condition received three training sessions that were aimed at encouraging the smoker to use the helpline and also encouraging any small steps toward quitting. Intervention effectiveness was determined by whether use of the helpline increased as a result of the participants' involvement in the intervention compared to the proportion of people who used the quit helpline among the control group.

Smokers in both groups were more likely to use the quit helpline than smokers not involved in the study; however, smokers linked to the intervention group were twice as likely to use the helpline as smokers associated with the control group. This difference held true across smokers of differing levels of readiness to quit. Supportive behaviors, however, were not a significant mediator of the intervention effect. Thus it is unclear what processes accounted for the intervention effects. Although the study did not limit participation based on gender or relationship to the smoker, the majority of support providers were female (79%) and were spouses or partners of the smokers. Thus it is possible that the intervention may have capitalized on relationships in which there was significant contact and opportunity for social control. The intervention was aimed at having support providers encourage the use of evidence-based tools rather than having them attempt to act as smoking cessation counselors or coaches (which has been unsuccessful in the past). Nonetheless, future research is needed to examine whether this translates to smokers' actual attempts or success at quitting.

Future Directions for Research and Practice

Several conceptual issues need greater attention in future research and interventions. As noted earlier, received support can be associated with negative influences on health if it is not seen as responsive (Selcuk & Ong, 2013). Interventions that seek to mobilize support from either similar peers or family and friends should be sure that support is responsive to individuals in order to provide either direct or stress-related beneficial links to health behaviors and related outcomes (see Figure 10.1).

Quality of relationships is another factor that can influence the responsiveness of support. It has not been considered strongly in prior work. While our relationships with others may be sources of warmth and love, these social relationships can also be sources of conflict and stress, resulting in relationships that have a mix of both positive and negative qualities (i.e., ambivalent relationships). Prior work suggests that such ambivalent ties are related to less effective support provision and greater biological risk for disease (Holt-Lunstad, Uchino, Smith, Olson-Cerny, & Nealey-Moore, 2003; Reblin, Uchino, & Smith, 2010). Besides not providing effective support, such ambivalent ties may be a source of stress in their own right, which may directly affect health (Holt-Lunstad, Uchino, Smith, & Hicks, 2007). Future work should give strong consideration to the quality of relationships, given that it may affect health-relevant support processes.

Future research should also consider social support in the context of a changing social climate. Despite the increases in technology that would presumably foster social connections, people are reporting greater social isolation and loneliness (McPherson, Smith-Lovin, & Brashears, 2006). Given the increase in the extent to which individuals rely on digital communication (in the form of online social networking, texting, etc.), greater attention needs to be paid to the health relevance of online social support. Although this is a burgeoning area of research, there are still important gaps in our understanding. For instance, research must distinguish between social support gained from exclusively online relationships (e.g., online support groups and chat groups) and support from friends. It must identify individual differences (e.g., extraversion or self-esteem) that may contribute to effectiveness (Van Zalk, Branje, Denissen, Van Aken, & Meeus, 2011), and also the factors that enhance and those that detract from face-to-face support. Importantly, we must also recognize that because our epidemiological data collection (reported earlier) began prior to the widespread use of social media tools, it is presently unclear whether online social connections and contact have protective effects on mortality similar to those seen for other forms of social support. Therefore it will be important to examine what pathways may be capitalized on and what pathways may be absent when individuals seek or provide support using online tools.

Summary

There is robust evidence that social support significantly and positively influences health and longevity and can occur through multiple types of support and various pathways. Epidemiological and experimental research suggests that not all aspects of social support are equally effective and that a more nuanced approach to social support is needed. A new generation of research is currently considering the role of technology in interpersonal functioning and utilization of social support, and the implications of that role for public health. Careful attention to these issues is needed in developing effective social support interventions.

References

Ailshire, J. A., & Burgard, S. A. (2012). Family relationships and troubled sleep among US adults: Examining the influences of contact frequency and relationship quality. *Journal of Health and Social Behavior*, *53*(2), 248–262.

American Diabetes Association. (2015). Statistics about diabetes. http://www.diabetes.org/diabetes basics/statistics/?loc=db-slabnav

Aspinwall, L. G., & Taylor, S. E. (1997). A stitch in time: Self-regulation and proactive coping. *Psychological Bulletin*, *121*(3), 417–436.

Barbee, A. P., Gulley, M. R., & Cunningham, M. R. (1990). Support seeking in personal relationships. *Journal of Social and Personal Relationships*, *7*, 531–540.

Barth, J., Schneider, S., & von Kanel, R. (2010). Lack of social support in the etiology and the prognosis of coronary heart disease: A systematic review and meta-analysis. *Psychosomatic Medicine*, *72*(3), 229–238.

Berkman, L. F., Glass, T., Brissette, I., & Seeman, T. E. (2000). From social integration to health: Durkheim in the new millennium. *Social Science & Medicine*, *51*(6), 843–857.

Berkman, L. F., Leo-Summers, L., & Horwitz, R. I. (1992). Emotional support and survival after myocardial infarction: A prospective, population-based study of the elderly. *Annals of Internal Medicine*, *117*(12), 1003–1009.

Berkman, L. F., & Syme, S. L. (1979). Social networks, host resistance, and mortality: A nine-year follow-up study of Alameda County residents. *American Journal of Epidemiology*, *109*(2), 186–204.

Blazer, D. G. (1982). Social support and mortality in an elderly community population. *American Journal of Epidemiology*, *115*(5), 684–694.

Bolger, N., & Amarel, D. (2007). Effects of social support visibility on adjustment to stress: Experimental evidence. *Journal of Personality and Social Psychology, 92*(3), 458–475.

Brummett, B. H., Babyak, M. A., Siegler, I. C., Vitaliano, P. P., Ballard, E. L., Gwyther, L. P., & Williams, R. B. (2006). Associations among perceptions of social support, negative affect, and quality of sleep in caregivers and noncaregivers. *Health Psychology, 25*(2), 220–225.

Brummett, B. H., Mark, D. B., Siegler, I. C., Williams, R. B., Babyak, M. A., Clapp-Channing, N. E., & Barefoot, J. C. (2005). Perceived social support as a predictor of mortality in coronary patients: Effects of smoking, sedentary behavior, and depressive symptoms. *Psychosomatic Medicine, 67*(1), 40–45.

Cassell, J. (1976). The contribution of the social environment to host resistance. *American Journal of Epidemiology, 104*, 107–123.

Cobb, S. (1976). Social support as a moderator of life stress. *Psychosomatic Medicine, 38*, 300–314.

Cohen, S. (1988). Psychosocial models of the role of social support in the etiology of physical disease. *Health Psychology, 7*(3), 269–297.

Cohen, S. (2004). Social relationships and health. *American Psychologist, 59*(8), 676–684.

Cohen, S., Mermelstein, R. J., Kamarck, T., & Hoberman, H. M. (1985). Measuring the functional components of social support. In I. G. Sarason and B. Sarason (Eds.), *Social support: Theory, research and applications* (pp. 73–94). The Hague: Martinus Nijhoff.

Cohen, S., & Wills, T. A. (1985). Stress, social support, and the buffering hypothesis. *Psychological Bulletin, 98*(2), 310–357.

Cutrona, C. E., & Russell, D. W. (1990). Type of social support and specific stress: Towards a theory of optimal matching. In B. R. Sarason, I. G. Sarason, & G. R. Pierce (Eds.), *Social support: An interactional view* (pp. 319–366). New York: Wiley.

Dare, J., & Green, L. (2011). Rethinking social support in women's midlife years: Women's experiences of social support in online environments. *European Journal of Cultural Studies, 14*(5), 473–490.

DiMatteo, M. R. (2004). Social support and patient adherence to medical treatment: A meta-analysis. *Health Psychology, 23*(2), 207–218.

Dunkel-Schetter, C., & Bennett, T. L. (1990). Differentiating the cognitive and behavioral aspects of social support. In B. R. Sarason, I. G. Sarason, & G. R. Pierce (Eds.), *Social support: An interactional view* (pp. 267–296). New York: Wiley.

Dunkel-Schetter, C., & Skokan, L. A. (1990). Determinants of social support provision in personal relationships. *Journal of Social and Personal Relationships, 7*, 437–450.

Durkheim, É. (1951). *Suicide: A study in sociology*. London: Free Press.

Forster, L. E., & Stoller, E. P. (1992). The impact of social support on mortality: A seven-year follow-up of older men and women. *Journal of Applied Gerontology, 11*, 173–186.

Friedman, H. S., Tucker, J. S., Schwartz, J. E., Tomlinson-Keasey, C., Martin, L. R., Wingard, D. L., & Criqui, M. H. (1995). Psychosocial and behavioral predictors of longevity: The aging and death of the "termites." *American Psychologist, 50*(2), 69–78.

Fuemmeler, B. F., Mâsse, L. C., Yaroch, A. L., Resnicow, K., Campbell, M. K., Carr, C., . . . Williams, A. (2006). Psychosocial mediation of fruit and vegetable consumption in the body and soul effectiveness trial. *Health Psychology, 25*(4), 474–483.

Glaser, R., Kiecolt-Glaser, J. K., Bonneau, R., Malarkey, W., & Hughes, J. (1992). Stress-induced modulation of the immune response to recombinant hepatitis B vaccine. *Psychosomatic Medicine, 54*(1), 22–29.

Gore, S. (1981). Stress-buffering functions of social supports: An appraisal and clarification of research models. In B. S. Dohrenwend & B. P. Dohrenwend (Eds.), *Stressful life events and their context* (pp. 202–222). New York: Prodist.

Griffiths, K. M., Calear, A. L., Banfield, M., & Tam, A. (2009). Systematic review on Internet Support Groups (ISGs) and depression (2): What is known about depression ISGs? *Journal of Medical Internet Research, 11*(3), e41.

Haber, M. G., Cohen, J. L., Lucas, T., & Baltes, B. B. (2007). The relationship between self-reported received and perceived social support: A meta-analytic review. *American Journal of Community Psychology, 39*(1–2), 133–144.

Heisler, M., Vijan, S., Makki, F., & Piette, J. (2010). Diabetes control with reciprocal peer support versus nurse care management: A randomized trial. *Annals of Internal Medicine, 153*(8), 507–515.

Holt-Lunstad, J., Smith, T. B., & Layton, J. B. (2010). Social relationships and mortality risk: A meta-analytic review. *PLoS Medicine, 7*(7), e1000316.

Holt-Lunstad, J., Uchino, B. N., Smith, T. W., Olson-Cerny, C., & Nealey-Moore, J. B. (2003). Social relationships and ambulatory blood pressure: Structural and qualitative predictors of cardiovascular function during everyday social interactions. *Health Psychology, 22*(4), 388–397.

Holt-Lunstad, J. L., Uchino, B. N., Smith, T. W., & Hicks, A. (2007). On the importance of relationship quality: The impact of ambivalence in friendships on cardiovascular functioning. *Annals of Behavioral Medicine, 33*(3), 278–290.

House, J. S., Landis, K. R., & Umberson, D. (1988). Social relationships and health. *Science, 241*(4865), 540–545.

Jessor, R., Turbin, M. S., & Costa, F. M. (1998). Protective factors in adolescent health behavior. *Journal of Personality and Social Psychology, 75*(3), 788–800.

Kaplan, G. A., Wilson, T. W., Cohen, R. D., Kauhanen, J., Wu, M., & Salonen, J. T. (1994). Social functioning and overall mortality: Prospective evidence from the Kuopio Ischemic Heart Disease Risk Factor Study. *Epidemiology, 5*(5), 495–500.

Kiecolt-Glaser, J. K., Loving, T. J., Stowell, J. R., Malarkey, W. B., Lemeshow, S., Dickinson, S. L., & Glaser, R. (2005). Hostile marital interactions, proinflammatory cytokine production, and wound healing. *Archives of General Psychiatry, 62*(12), 1377–1384.

Krause, N. (1997). Received support, anticipated support, social class, and mortality. *Research on Aging, 19*(4), 387–422.

Kroenke, C. H., Quesenberry, C., Kwan, M. L., Sweeney, C., Castillo, A., & Caan, B. J. (2013). Social networks, social support, and burden in relationships, and mortality after breast cancer diagnosis in the Life After Breast Cancer Epidemiology (LACE) study. *Breast Cancer Research and Treatment, 137*(1), 261–271.

Lakey, B., & Orehek, E. (2011). Relational regulation theory: A new approach to explain the link between perceived support and mental health. *Psychological Review, 118*(3), 482–495.

Lett, H. S., Blumenthal, J. A., Babyak, M. A., Catellier, D. J., Carney, R. M., Berkman, L. F., . . . Schneiderman, N. (2007). Social support and prognosis in patients at increased psychosocial risk recovering from myocardial infarction. *Health Psychology, 26*(4), 418–427.

Lett, H. S., Blumenthal, J. A., Babyak, M. A., Strauman, T. J., Robins, C., & Sherwood, A. (2005). Social support and coronary heart disease: Epidemiologic evidence and implications for treatment. *Psychosomatic Medicine, 67*, 869–878.

Lutgendorf, S. K., Sood, A. K., Anderson, B., McGinn, S., Maiseri, H., Dao, M., . . . Lubaroff, D. M. (2005). Social support, psychological distress, and natural killer cell activity in ovarian cancer. *Journal of Clinical Oncology, 23*(28), 7105–7113.

Luttik, M. L., Jaarsma, T., Moser, D., Sanderman, R., & van Veldhuisen, D. J. (2005). The importance and impact of social support on outcomes in patients with heart failure: An overview of the literature. *Journal of Cardiovascular Nursing, 20*(3), 162–169.

Maisel, N., & Gable, S. L. (2009). The paradox of received social support: The importance of responsiveness. *Psychological Science, 20*(8), 928–932.

Malik, S. H., & Coulson, N. S. (2008). Computer-mediated infertility support groups: An exploratory study of online experiences. *Patient Education and Counseling, 73*(1), 105–113.

Manne, S. L., Ostroff, J., Winkel, G., Grana, G., & Fox, K. (2005). Partner unsupportive responses, avoidant coping, and distress among women with early stage breast cancer: Patient and partner perspectives. *Health Psychology, 24*(6), 635–641.

McPherson, M., Smith-Lovin, L., & Brashears, M. (2006). Social isolation in America: Changes in core discussion networks over two decades. *American Sociological Review, 71*(3), 353–375.

Meier, A., Lyons, E. J., Frydman, G., Forlenza, M., & Rimer, B. K. (2007). How cancer survivors provide support on cancer-related Internet mailing lists. *Journal of Medical Internet Research, 9*(2), e12.

Nicholas, D. B., Fellner, K. D., Frank, M., Small, M., Hetherington, R., Slater, R., & Daneman, D. (2012). Evaluation of an online education and support intervention for adolescents with diabetes. *Social Work in Health Care, 51*(9), 815–827.

Nordin, M., Knutsson, A., & Sundbom, E. (2008). Is disturbed sleep a mediator in the association between social support and myocardial infarction? *Journal of Health Psychology, 13*(1), 55–64.

Orth-Gomer, K., Wamala, S. P., Horsten, M., Schenck-Gustafsson, K., Schneiderman, N., & Mittleman, M. A. (2000). Marital stress worsens prognosis in women with coronary heart disease: The Stockholm Female Coronary Risk Study. *JAMA, 284*(23), 3008–3014.

Patten, C., Smith, C., Brockman, T., Decker, P., Hughes, C., Nadeau, A., . . . Zhu, S. (2011). Support-person promotion of a smoking quitline: A randomized controlled trial. *American Journal of Preventive Medicine, 41*(1), 17–23.

Pearlin, L. I. (1989). The sociological study of stress. *Journal of Health and Social Behavior, 30*(3), 241–256.

Peirce, R. S., Frone, M. R., Russell, M., & Cooper, M. L. (1996). Financial stress, social support, and alcohol involvement: A longitudinal test of the buffering hypothesis in a general population survey. *Health Psychology, 15*(1), 38–47.

Piette, J., Resnicow, K., Choi, H., & Heisler, M. (2013). A diabetes peer support intervention that improved glycemic control: Mediators and moderators of intervention effectiveness. *Chronic Illness, 9*(4), 258–267.

Przybylski, A. K., & Weinstein, N. (2013). Can you connect with me now? How the presence of mobile communication technology influences face-to-face conversation quality. *Journal of Social and Personal Relationships, 30*(3), 237–246.

Rainie, L., & Wellman, B. (2012). *Networked: The new social operating system.* Cambridge, MA: MIT Press.

Reblin, M., Uchino, B. N., & Smith, T. W. (2010). Provider and recipient factors that may moderate the effectiveness of received support: Examining the effects of relationship quality and expectations for support on behavioral and cardiovascular reactions. *Journal of Behavioral Medicine, 33*(6), 423–431.

Rimer, B. K., Lyons, E .J., Ribisl, K. M., Bowling, J. M., Golin, C. E., Forlenza, M. J., & Meier A. (2005). How new subscribers use cancer-related online mailing lists. *Journal of Medical Internet Research*, 7(3), e32.

Robles, T. F., Slatcher, R. B., Trombello, J. M., & McGinn, M. M. (2013). Marital quality and health: A meta-analytic review. *Psychological Bulletin*, 140(1), 140–187.

Rucker, D. D., Preacher, K. J., Tormala, Z. L., & Petty, R. E. (2011). Mediation analysis in social psychology: Current practices and new recommendations. *Social and Personality Psychology Compass*, 5(6), 359–371.

Russell, D. W., & Cutrona, C. E. (1991). Social support, stress, and depressive symptoms among the elderly: Test of a process model. *Psychology and Aging*, 6(2), 190–201.

Selcuk, E., & Ong, A. D. (2013). Perceived partner responsiveness moderates the association between received emotional support and all-cause mortality. *Health Psychology*, 32(2), 231–235.

Seltzer, L. J., Prososki, A. R., Ziegler, T. E., & Pollak, S. D. (2012). Instant messages vs. speech: Hormones and why we still need to hear each other. *Evolution and Human Behavior*, 33(1), 42–45.

Steptoe, A., Wardle, J., Pollard, T. M., Canaan, L., & Davies, G. J. (1996). Stress, social support and health-related behavior: A study of smoking, alcohol consumption and physical exercise. *Journal of Psychosomatic Research*, 41(2), 171–180.

Stewart, D. W., Gabriele, J. M., & Fisher, E. B. (2012). Directive support, nondirective support, and health behaviors in a community sample. *Journal of Behavioral Medicine*, 35(5), 492–499.

Thoits, P. (2011). Mechanisms linking social ties and support to physical and mental health. *Journal of Health and Social Behavior*, 52(2), 145–161.

Thorsteinsson, E. B., & James, J. E. (1999). A meta-analysis of the effects of experimental manipulations of social support during laboratory stress. *Psychology & Health*, 14(5), 869–886.

Trobst, K. K. (2000). An interpersonal conceptualization and quantification of social support transactions. *Personality and Social Psychology Bulletin*, 26(8), 971–986.

Troxel, W. M., Matthews, K. A., Gallo, L. C., & Kuller, L. H. (2005). Marital quality and occurrence of the metabolic syndrome in women. *Archives of Internal Medicine*, 165(9), 1022–1027.

Uchino, B. (2006). Social support and health: A review of physiological processes potentially underlying links to disease outcomes. *Journal of Behavioral Medicine*, 29(4), 377–387.

Uchino, B. N. (2009). Understanding the links between social support and physical health: A lifespan perspective with emphasis on the separability of perceived and received support. *Perspectives in Psychological Science*, 4(3), 236–255.

Umberson, D. (1987). Family status and health behaviors: Social control as a dimension of social integration. *Journal of Health and Social Behavior*, 28(3), 306–319.

U.S. Department of Health and Human Services. (2004). *The health consequences of smoking: A report of the surgeon general*. Atlanta: U.S. Department of Health and Human Services, Centers for Disease Control and Prevention, National Center for Chronic Disease Prevention and Health Promotion, Office on Smoking and Health.

Van Zalk, M. W., Branje, S. T., Denissen, J., Van Aken, M. G., & Meeus, W. J. (2011). Who benefits from chatting, and why? The roles of extraversion and supportiveness in online chatting and emotional adjustment. *Personality and Social Psychology Bulletin*, 37(9), 1202–1215.

Veenstra, A., Lakey, B., Cohen, J. C., Neely, L. C., Orehek, E., Barry, R., & Abeare, C. A. (2011). Forecasting the specific providers that recipients will perceive as unusually supportive. *Personal Relationships*, 18(4), 677–696.

Vicary, A. M., & Fraley, R. (2010). Student reactions to the shootings at Virginia Tech and Northern Illinois University: Does sharing grief and support over the Internet affect recovery? *Personality and Social Psychology Bulletin, 36*(11), 1555–1563.

Wills, T. A., & Cleary, S. D. (1996). How are social support effects mediated? A test with parental support and adolescent substance use. *Journal of Personality and Social Psychology, 71*(5), 937–952.

Wills, T. A., & Shinar, O. (2000). Measuring perceived and received social support. In S. Cohen, L. Gordon, & B. Gottlieb (Eds.), *Social support measurement and intervention: A guide for health and social scientists* (pp. 86–135). New York: Oxford University Press.

Woloshin, S., Schwartz, L. M., Tosteson, A. N., Chang, C. H., Wright, B., Plohman, J., & Fisher, E. S. (1997). Perceived adequacy of tangible social support and health outcomes in patients with coronary artery disease. *Journal of General Internal Medicine, 12*(10), 613–618.

Wright, K. B., & Bell, S. B., (2003). Health-related support groups on the Internet: Linking empirical findings to social support and computer-mediated communication theory. *Journal of Health Psychology, 8*(1), 39–54.

CHAPTER 11

SOCIAL NETWORKS AND HEALTH BEHAVIOR

Thomas W. Valente

Social networks are important influences on, and outcomes of, many health behaviors. Evidence that friends, family members, colleagues, and other people with whom individuals have relationships act as important conduits for health information, as sources of support, and as determinants (for good or ill) of health behavior has come from many studies and decades of empirical research.

There is debate in the field as to whether social network research constitutes a theory or a method to measure other theoretical constructs. The word *theory* is used when describing the mechanism by which networks influence behavior, and *analysis* (as in *social network analysis*) is used when networks are used as a method to measure or understand constructs used in other theories. *Social network theory* (SNT) stresses the importance of connections or relations for understanding health or other outcomes of individuals (Valente, 2010). SNT is evoked when researchers model outcomes as a function of network processes.

Social network analysis (SNA) is used when network methods are incorporated into other health behavior theories, sometimes as a central component, such as with Diffusion of Innovations theory (Valente, 1995), and sometimes peripherally, as in examining how networks influence normative beliefs. Social network methods have proliferated in many fields of study, including sociology, anthropology, information science, economics, marketing, computer science, physics, ecology, geography, communication, public health, and medicine, to name a few. This rapidly expanding research paradigm shifts the focus of

KEY POINTS

This chapter will:

- Provide a brief review of the history of social network theory (SNT) and social network analysis (SNA).

- Describe and articulate the main components of SNT and SNA.

- Present examples of how SNT is applied to two health behaviors: contraceptive use and adolescent tobacco use.

- Discuss network interventions.

study from the individual to his or her relationships with others (Borgatti, Everett, & Johnson, 2013; Scott, 2008; Valente, 2010; Wasserman & Faust, 1994). These relationships are widely varied, including, for example, friendships among adolescents in schools, intercountry trade among nations, and similarities between book purchases. Relational data are analyzed using models and tools distinct from those traditionally employed by statisticians and epidemiologists, though the approaches are converging (Valente, 2010). Network data typically provide an in-depth view of communities, organizations, settings, and systems, aided by the use of visualization, mathematical algorithms, and computational tools. SNA enables researchers to conduct a mathematical ethnography of the behavior or system(s) being studied. Consequently, network research is simultaneously deceptively simple and maddeningly complex. This chapter focuses on how networks influence health behaviors, and it reviews the many research results to date that show a strong and powerful influence of networks on individual, organizational, community, and system behaviors.

One branch of social network research is social support, which measures the resources individuals have in their social network. These support resources typically are classified as the emotional, cognitive, tangible, and physical support an individual perceives he or she gets from others (see Chapter Ten). Social networks, in contrast, measure relationships such as friendships or other task- or work-oriented relationships (which may or may not provide support) and treats these directional ties themselves as objects of study (Smith & Christakis, 2008). In this chapter, we focus only on social networks.

History of Social Network Analysis and Social Network Theory

Many social scientists employed network research components and the use of mathematics and graph theory in their research prior to 1930 (Freeman, 2004). Most scholars, however, find the beginning of modern social network research in the work of Jacob Moreno, who was one of the first to develop a program of research studying social networks and outcomes, usually among elementary school students, aged six to twelve years (Moreno, 1934). By the 1950s, various research groups had begun to create the field called social network analysis, or *sociometry*. A group dynamics center at the University of Michigan is credited with training scholars on early uses of graph theory to understand social networks. Several noted social psychologists, such as Heider, Cartwright, Homans, and Festinger, as well as many other psychologists, conducted studies on social networks in the workplace and in communities.

Two SNA research communities had emerged by the beginning of the 1960s (Scott, 2008): the Manchester anthropologists (based in Manchester in the United Kingdom) and the Harvard structuralists (centered around sociologist Harrison White). In the mid-1970s, two academic meetings were held in Hawaii in an attempt to bring together the various scholars interested in studying social networks. These meetings culminated in the launch of the International Network for Social Network Analysis (INSNA) and a commitment to hold annual meetings, starting in 1981. The journal *Social Networks* was launched, and a bulletin/journal, *Connections*, was created. INSNA provided a venue that supported the growth of network scholarship, and where social network analysis methods, theories, and applications could be developed. At least two more social network journals have since been created, the *Journal of Social Structure* and *Network Science*.

In the mid- to late 1980s, SNA scholars began to develop a library of social network algorithms for measuring key constructs and a culture of scientific exchange, collegiality, and cooperation. UCINET (Borgatti & Ofem, 2010), a widely used computer program for SNA, was first released in the mid-1980s. The advent of the AIDS epidemic and influx of public health researchers eager to use these tools for investigating important public health issues helped to bolster the viability of the network science community in the early 1990s. Now no longer a nascent community, the network field began to develop more powerful and user-friendly computer tools and programs. The explosive growth of the World Wide Web, the Internet, and computer communications made networks and networking both explicit and ubiquitous. Thus the network field suddenly discovered it was relevant and central to investigations in a number of disparate disciplines.

In the first decade of the twenty-first century, SNT and SNA have been applied to substantive issues in many disciplines. The emergence of *big data* (Lazer et al., 2009) and powerful new computing technologies means that network research is no longer confined to small groups and communities but rather can be applied to whole populations and large, naturally occurring communities. The concept of big data and the refinement of visualization tools for understanding data have made analysis of social networks more feasible and meaningful.

Today, network research is one of the most vibrant and exciting scientific fields in existence, with the potential to contribute substantially to scientific knowledge. These historical developments have enabled SNA researchers to craft specific axioms that have morphed into an identifiable social network theory.

Social Network Theory

Social network theory has three main components: (1) people or actors (organizations, states, collectives, etc.) take actions based on their network environment, (2) a person's position in a network influences his or her behaviors, and (3) networks have structure and these network (or system-level) properties influence system performance. A final component of SNT is that there is a dynamic relationship between the micro and macro levels of network analysis. Another aspect of SNT occurs when theorists develop new concepts, constructs, and algorithms used to study networks primarily as a mathematical or computational enterprise. Throughout this chapter, social networks will be described as relationships among people, but the reader is advised that most statements also apply to networks of organizations, governments, websites, and any other unit that might be studied.

Network Environment

Figure 11.1 displays a social network depicting friendships among students in a sixth-grade classroom (aged 12 years). SNT predicts many things about how and why this network

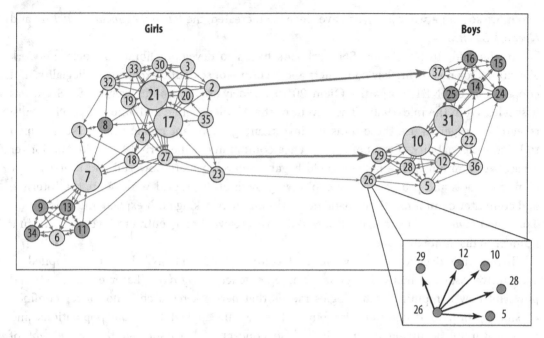

Figure 11.1   Friendship Network: Personal Network of One Student Highlighted
Note: Darker nodes represent smokers and lighter ones nonsmokers.

exists, its structure, and what kinds of processes we can expect to occur among its members. In Figure 11.1, girls are almost exclusively friends with girls and boys with boys; this homophily (see Chapter Sixteen) can extend to health behaviors of interest to scientists. For example, we know that smokers tend to befriend other smokers. Homophily appears in many other adolescent risk behaviors, such as alcohol use, substance abuse, obesity, bullying, and victimization.

This homophily derives from at least two network processes: influence and selection. *Influence* occurs when an individual changes his or her behavior to be the same as his or her network partners. For example, in Figure 11.1, the dark nodes are smokers and the light ones nonsmokers (smoking data are hypothetical here). In Figure 11.1, Person 6 is friends with many smokers; network theory predicts she will likely become a smoker. *Selection* occurs when an individual changes his or her network to make it compatible with his or her behavior. For example, Person 8 is a smoker with nonsmoking friends; thus network theory predicts she will likely become friends with 9, 11, 13, and/or 34 as they are also smokers. It also predicts, however, that Person 8 will be influenced to quit smoking by her present network (Christakis & Fowler, 2007).

Influence and selection effects are environmental in the sense that SNT predicts that individuals are influenced by their immediate social network both in their behaviors and their network choices. The primary network environment is an individual's set of direct ties, as highlighted for Person 26 in Figure 11.1. Network theory has developed many extensions of these environmental or exposure effects, including weighting exposures by (1) tie strength, (2) tie distance (including indirect ties), (3) connectivity to the same third parties, (4) degree of equivalence in network position, (5) centrality of the ties, (6) participation in activities together (e.g., being on the same sports team), or (7) attributes of the networks (girls are more influential than boys). SNT also predicts that individuals vary in the extent to which they are influenced by their personal networks, so that some individuals have low thresholds to action and initiate behaviors when few others in their network do so, whereas others have high thresholds and wait until the majority have engaged in a behavior before they will act (Valente, 1996). Social network theory thus predicts that these network environmental influences are powerful determinants of behavior.

Position in Network

Another core tenet of SNT is that a person's position in a network influences his or her behavior. Several positions have been identified as important: central, bridging, and peripheral. *Central* individuals occupy prominent positions in the network, as indicated by high scores on algorithms that identify important nodes. People can be central if they receive a lot of nominations (*degree centrality*), but also can be central if they occupy strategic positions in the network such that they are, on average, fewer steps from everyone else in the network (*closeness centrality*), or lie on the shortest path connecting other nodes in the network (*betweenness centrality*) (Freeman, 1979). Central individuals learn about new ideas and can have access to information earlier than less central people do. This can be advantageous when the information is valuable, but when the spread of a disease is involved, then being central can be a liability as these individuals are exposed to viruses and bacteria earlier than noncentral members (Christakis & Fowler, 2010). Being central can also make individuals more sensitive to community norms and values, which may either promote or inhibit innovation and/or change.

Bridging individuals, people who connect otherwise disconnected groups, can also be associated with behavior for several reasons (Valente & Fujimoto, 2010): (1) bridging provides access to different subgroups in the network, (2) bridging individuals may be less beholden to the status quo, and (3) bridging individuals are less constrained by their immediate personal network. Granovetter's (1973) influential paper on the strength of weak ties argued that people who are weakly connected often exchange valuable information because they are linked to different people and thus have access to different information. Burt (2005) expanded this argument by showing that individuals whose networks spanned structural holes (gaps in network connectivity) occupied advantageous positions and had better work-related outcomes. Network theory highlights the importance of bridges for linking disparate groups and thus enabling or hindering collective action.

Being peripheral can also influence behaviors. *Peripheral* individuals are free from the social norms in the community or network and so may be less constrained in their behavior and freer to innovate. They might also have more connectivity to other groups and networks, in which case they would be bridges between networks even though peripheral in one. Evidence also exists that being peripheral in a network may be directly associated with health behaviors. For example, adolescents who are isolated in school-based friendship networks are at greater risk for suicidal ideation and suicide attempts (Wyman, Pickering, & Valente, 2013).

Structural or Network Properties

Network theory also makes predictions at the macro, or whole network, level using indicators such as the rates of homophily and reciprocity, and the levels of density, transitivity (clustering), and centralization in the network. In Figure 11.1, homophily is apparent as girls are friends with other girls and boys are friends with boys. There is also homophily in behavior such that smokers are friends with other smokers. SNT predicts this homophily will occur in many networks and that networks with high rates of homophily are more resistant to change.

There is also reciprocity in a network such that a link in any one direction implies a link in both directions. For example, if Bob names John as a friend, John is more likely to name Bob. In Figure 11.1, there are many reciprocated friendships, as indicated by the bidirectional arrows, such as the links between Persons 1 and 7. Interestingly, the boys named as friends by girls did not reciprocate those friendships. SNT argues that all things being equal, high rates of reciprocity are indicative of trusting relationships and a cohesive network.

Transitivity also occurs at higher rates in many networks such that friends of friends become friends. If Sue names Mary and Mary names Beth, then Sue will likely become friends with Beth. In Figure 11.1, Persons 1, 7, and 8 have a transitive triad, but 1, 6, and 7 do not. Clustering is the degree of transitivity in a network, and so highly clustered networks have pockets of dense interconnectivity (Watts, 1999) that accelerate behavior change within clusters but slow it between them.

Figure 11.2 displays networks of the same size ($N = 37$) and density (Density $= 0.14$) yet with different network structures: the empirical data are shown in Figure 11.2a, a random network in 11.2b, a small-world network in 11.2c, and a centralized network in 11.2d. Density is the actual number of links in the network divided by the possible number of links and is expressed as a proportion or percentage (e.g., a network of 4 people has $4 \times 3 = 12$ possible ties, and if 6 of these ties exist then the density is 0.50). A naive view is that dense networks are better than sparse ones as they can generate faster diffusion and increase coordinated action. Empirical evidence, however, suggests that too much density may hinder network performance and that densities below 25 percent may be preferred (Valente, 2010).

As mentioned above, variation in the number of ties each person has means that some people are central and others are peripheral. The overall distribution of these ties is an indication of a network's centralization. Centralized networks, characterized by the extent to which ties are focused around one or a few nodes (also indicated by a high standard deviation in the centrality scores), are thought to be more effective because the central hubs can coordinate activities for the network. Evidence also suggests, however, that centralized networks are less sustainable. There are two reasons why centralized networks are less sustainable: (1) centralized networks have hubs that are very important so their removal has profound consequences, and (2) people are often less satisfied working in centralized networks, where they have little control over or input into decision making.

A final well-known structural property of networks is that they can often be described as having a *small-world* property. That is, the distance between any two people in the network is less than would be expected in a random network of the same size and density (its number

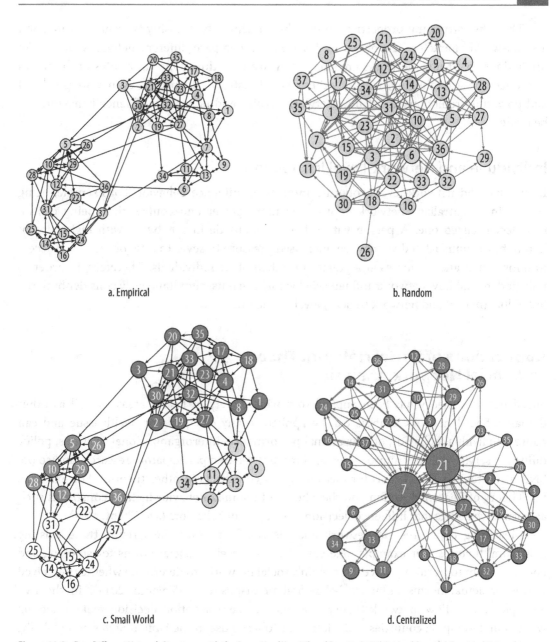

Figure 11.2 Four Different Network Structures with the Same Size (*N* = 37) and Density (14%) Derived from the Empirical Network

Note: Although the networks in Figures 11.1 and 11.2a are the same, the graphs look different because there is no one "correct" way to draw a particular network.

of links). Milgram (1967) conducted the classic small-world study, finding that any two people in the United States chosen at random are separated by six steps: the well-known six degrees of separation. Although there were several major limitations to the study, it was a clever experiment and provided insights into large networks. More recently, computer scientists have been replicating this type of study and finding surprisingly short distances between people regardless of location (Dodds, Muhamad, & Watts, 2003).

These five structural properties—homophily, reciprocity, transitivity, centralization, and a small-world character—enable us to describe and compare different networks, and make predictions about how networks emerge and evolve over time. Once attributes of the nodes are added, the sex, ethnicity, age, and other characteristics of the people, even more profound and powerful predictions about how networks evolve and how they influence behavior, can be made.

Individual- and Network-Level Interaction

Individual- and network-level properties interact to influence behavior. For example, being central in a centralized network affords one more power and control than being central in a decentralized one. A person with a heterophilous tie in a network with high rates of homophily is unusual and so may feel increased pressure to sever that tie or may have access to information and resources at a greater rate than other individuals. Therefore, in order to fully understand how networks influence behavior, one must simultaneously consider both the individual (micro) and network (macro) level of analysis.

Applications of Social Network Theory and Social Network Analysis

Social network theory has been applied to a wide variety of health areas as well as other domains. Social network analysis can be applied to any discipline or health issue and can address individual behavior, organizational performance, interorganizational relations, policy diffusion, service delivery improvements, community-based participatory research, and so on. SNA also provides useful tools for measuring key constructs in other theories. For example, the Theory of Reasoned Action and the Theory of Planned Behavior include constructs such as normative beliefs that influence decisions to engage in behaviors (see Chapter Six).

Measuring exposures via network analysis can help researchers refine these existing behavioral theories. For example, one can identify perceived social norms for smoking and compare them to norms within each person's social networks to determine whether perceived norms or actual norms influence behavioral predispositions (Valente, 2012). In the two examples that follow, network theory is applied to contraception decision making among women in developing countries and adolescent tobacco use in the United States and globally, two important public health issues.

Application 1: Contraception Decision Making in Developing Countries

Many factors influence a couple's desire to have children as well as how many they eventually have. These factors can be classified into supply versus demand factors, or economic versus sociocultural factors, and so on. People know how babies are made of course, but regulating how many children to have has been an evolving concept, one most effectively aided by the use of modern contraceptives. The development, supply, and diffusion of contraceptives are of major public health importance and have generated considerable academic study. Social networks are a frequently cited source of information and influence on contraceptive choices.

An early study applying SNT to understand the adoption and diffusion of contraceptive use was conducted by Rogers (1979) among women in twenty-five Korean villages. Women reported when they had first used a contraceptive method and which ones they had used, in addition to answering questions about their social networks. The authors concluded that women became more likely to adopt contraception as more of their network partners used a method of contraception (Rogers & Kincaid, 1981). The authors also found that a certain contraceptive method, such as the pill, IUD, or condom use, would become widespread in a village and that this method was also the one chosen by the women who received the most nominations as family planning discussion partners (also see Entwisle et al., 1996). In these data, in-degree centrality was associated with behavioral adoption, and in this case there is evidence that perhaps the family planning behavior of the village opinion leaders was imitated by many others. Thus both the network environment and a woman's position in that network influenced the fertility-related behaviors of women in these Korean villages in the 1960s.

Subsequent studies have documented that in many developing countries, women's social networks have influenced their decisions to use contraceptive methods (Bongaarts & Watkins, 1996; Casterline, 2001; Montgomery & Casterline, 1993). Since contraception is not directly observable, information about method use and detailed knowledge about how to get and use contraception must often be transmitted via informal conversations. This social learning thus can be an important influence on the timing of method adoption and on its correct use (Kohler, 1997), and studies have shown that the interconnectedness of these network partners further accelerates behavioral influences (Kohler, Behrman, & Watkins, 2001). Research has shown that women are aware of and use the same method as their friends (Valente, Watkins, Jato, Van der Straten, & Tsitsol, 1997), and that women who report being encouraged to use methods by their friends are more likely to use them (Gayen & Raeside, 2010; Valente et al., 1997).

Many programs have been implemented to accelerate the spread of modern contraceptives, many of which include a mass media or promotional component (Piotrow, Kincaid, Rimon, & Rinehart, 1997). Research has shown that social networks can mediate the effects of these campaigns (Boulay, Storey, & Sood, 2002), and that women lacking social networks of method users will rely on these campaigns to make their adoption decisions (Valente & Saba, 1998). Further, studies have used social network methods to aid promotional programs to improve their effectiveness (Kincaid, 2000; Stoebenau & Valente, 2003).

Application 2: Adolescent Tobacco Use

Despite recent declines in adult smoking prevalence rates in some countries, tobacco use is still a leading cause of morbidity and mortality in the United States and globally. About 88 percent of adult smokers report beginning to smoke during adolescence (U.S. Department of Health and Human Services, 2012). Adolescence is a time when young people form their identities, in part by disassociating from their parents and increasing their identification with peers. Thus adolescent networks can exert strong influences on individual behaviors and social norms, particularly around risk behaviors.

Although many factors are associated with adolescent smoking, peer influence has been identified as a strong correlate and perhaps a cause of smoking initiation (Alexander, Piazza, Mekos, & Valente, 2001; Beal, Ausiello, & Perrin, 2001; Ennett et al., 2008; Fujimoto & Valente, 2012; Hoffman, Sussman, Rohrbach, & Valente, 2006; Kobus, 2003). Research has sought to disentangle this peer influence, primarily by distinguishing between adolescents' perceptions of their peers' smoking and their friends' actual self-reported smoking (Henry, Kobus, & Schoeny, 2011; Ianotti & Bush, 1992; Rice, Donohew, & Clayton, 2003; Valente, Fujimoto, Soto, Ritt-Olson, & Unger, 2012) and by distinguishing between peer influence and peer selection (Ali & Dwyer, 2009; Engels, Knibbe, Drop, & de Haan, 1997; Ennett & Bauman, 1994; Hall & Valente, 2007; Hoffman, Monge, Chou, & Valente, 2007; Kandel, 1978; Mercken, Snijders, Steglich, & de Vries, 2009; Mercken, Snijders, Steglich, Vertiainen, & de Vries, 2010; Valente, 2010). Social influence occurs when a person changes his behavior to be consistent with his network, whereas selection occurs when a person changes his network to be consistent with his behaviors. The latest evidence seems to suggest that homophily in adolescent smoking behavior occurs due in equal parts to influence and selection. In Figure 11.1, influence would occur if Person 6 became a smoker to be consistent with her network environment composed of mostly smokers. In contrast, Person 8 is a smoker surrounded by nonsmoking friends, thus she would feel pressure to either quit smoking or make network changes (selection) so that she becomes friends with other smokers (linking to Persons 9, 11, 13, and/or 34). The stochastic actor behavior model developed by Snijders, van de Bunt, and Steglich (2010) can be used to statistically compare influence and selection processes in the same analyses (but also see Valente et al., 2012).

Some health promotion programs, particularly those designed to reduce risk behaviors, have used the power of adolescent peer relationships. Popular peer opinion leaders were recruited to promote antismoking norms in a large UK trial that showed the use of these popular in-school teens was effective at reducing tobacco use (Hollingworth et al., 2012; Starkey, Audrey, Holliday, Moore, & Campbell, 2009). Valente, Hoffman, Ritt-Olson, Lichtman, and Johnson (2003) used network-defined leader groups to implement tobacco prevention programs in southern California middle schools, which improved the programs' effects on use and mediators of use. The study also showed that the culturally tailored program, which had more interactive elements than a standard, non-peer-led smoking education program, was more effective when implemented in teacher- or network-defined groups that were homophilous (Valente, Unger, Ritt-Olson, Cen, & Johnson, 2006). Thus the effects of the program were dependent on the network context (or environment) of the people who received the intervention.

These two examples (contraceptive adoption and adolescent tobacco use) represent a small fraction of the many applications of social network theory and methods to public health and medicine. Other applications have addressed health policy diffusion (Wipfli, Fujimoto, & Valente, 2010; also see Chapter Sixteen), community-based participatory research (Valente, Fujimoto, Palmer, & Tanjasiri, 2010; also see Chapter Fifteen), interorganizational relationships (Butterfoss, Kegler, & Francisco, 2008; Provan & Milward, 1995), injection drug users (Friedman et al., 1997), physician prescribing behavior (Iyengar, Van den Bulte, & Valente, 2011), and many other areas.

Network Statistics

Although these two applications provide ample evidence for network effects on health behaviors, there is still much work to be done. Estimating network influences can be a challenge because network data are nonindependent. That is, statistical regression approaches typically expect that each unit in the database is independent of (not connected to) every other unit in the data. With network data, this assumption is explicitly violated. The problem is further compounded by the network properties of reciprocity, transitivity, and homophily because they provide alternative explanations for network effects. For example, if the data show that a smoker is more likely to have smoking friends, that doesn't necessarily indicate that the friends' smoking has caused the smoking of the individual. Rather this smoking homophily could be a function of the individual and his or her network being homophilous on ethnicity and of the fact that smoking rates vary by ethnicity (for expanded discussions of inference challenges in networks see Aral, Muchnik, & Sundararajan, 2009).

To address these issues, network statisticians developed several approaches that account for network structure in the estimation of network effects. The critical insight was to make the network the dependent variable, the outcome if you will, and the behavior the independent variable (Wasserman & Faust, 1994; Wasserman & Robins, 2005). The two tools developed using this approach are exponential random graph models (ERGMs), used primarily with cross-sectional data (Robins, Pattison, Kalish, & Lusher, 2007), and stochastic actor-based (SAB) models implemented in RSiena (Simulation Investigation for Empirical Network Analysis), used primarily with longitudinal data (Snijders et al., 2010). Both models are implemented in the open source statistical system R (CRAN).

To estimate an ERGM, the researcher specifies the network and attributes of the nodes in the network and, optionally, attributes of the relationships in the network. For example, the network is a link list of the ID numbers for each relationship and separate fields for the type or strength of the relationship. In a separate file the researcher stores the attributes of the nodes, characteristics such as age, sex, ethnicity, smoking status, and so on. The researcher then specifies a model of the theoretical relationships thought to be contained in the data, such as whether there is reciprocity, transitivity, and homophily on various characteristics. The ERGM software as implemented in statnet or PNet will indicate the magnitude and statistical significance of the effects specified in the model.

Stochastic actor-based models are estimated similarly, though the model specification process is a bit more complicated because the data are longitudinal. The researcher specifies multiple files for the various waves of data, and many more parameters can be estimated. In addition, the researcher specifies both a network evolution component and behavior predictions. The science and theory of social networks has expanded greatly with the development of these tools because they have extended our theoretical thinking about how networks influence health behaviors and how network structure and behaviors coevolve.

Interventions Using Social Network Data

Given that networks have strong and persistent effects on behaviors, many researchers have attempted to use network data to create interventions that improve organizational performance and accelerate diffusion of innovations (Valente, 2012). Valente (2012) proposed that network interventions be classified into four broad strategies (individual identification, segmentation, induction, and alteration), with each strategy having from two to five tactical alternatives (Table 11.1). Many of the tactics have several operational alternatives, giving rise to many network intervention choices. The type of data available, existing behavior prevalence, and type of behavior being promoted, among other things, affect the choice of intervention strategy and tactics. The most frequent network intervention has involved the identification of opinion leaders using SNA.

Network opinion leader interventions consist of using social network data to identify individuals who receive a large number of nominations and using them as change agents or champions. Many field experiments have been conducted using this approach and have demonstrated its effectiveness and efficiency. For example, Lomas and others (Lomas et al., 1991) recruited physicians in two hospitals who were network opinion leaders and recruited them to promote vaginal birth after first C-section, a practice supported by federal guidelines. The study showed an 11.9 percent decrease in C-sections in the experimental hospitals relative

Table 11.1   Network Intervention Choices for Various Theoretical Mechanisms Driving Behavior

Strategy	Tactic	Mechanism
Individual identification (identify individuals to act as change agents)	Leaders	Power
	Bridges	Conflict
	Key players	Cohesion
	Peripherals	Isolation
	Low thresholds	Thresholds
Segmentation (locate subgroups in the network)	Groups	Group identification
	Positions	Structural equivalence
Induction (induce change using the network structure)	Word of mouth	Information diffusion
	Snowball	Hard-to-reach populations
	Outreach	Closure
	Matching	Homophily
Alteration (change the network)	Deleting/adding nodes	Attributes
	Deleting/adding links	Structure
	Rewiring	Structure

to the control ones. In over twenty studies, the approach has been shown to be effective at accelerating practice change (Valente & Pumpuang, 2007; also see Flodgren et al., 2011).

An additional factor that may inform this intervention choice is the mechanism that one believes to be influencing the behavior of study. For example, if power dynamics in an organization are theorized to be important influences on the behavior in question, then an opinion leader intervention may be the most appropriate way to create change. If there is considerable conflict in the organization, perhaps from the merger of different divisions, then perhaps bridging individuals would be the best change agents. At this early stage of network science, there is little evidence to guide intervention choice. Table 11.1 presents a list of network intervention choices linked to the behavioral mechanism that drives the behavior. Future work, however, may lend insight into how understanding theoretical influences on behaviors can be translated into network-appropriate interventions that accelerate behavior change efforts.

Increasingly, communities are being formed on the Internet. Lacking the constraints of geography and time, they enable like-minded people to communicate, share, collaborate, and coordinate on many levels. Several scientists have capitalized on these developments and conducted experiments to determine whether network effects can be replicated online and whether marketers can accelerate diffusion using online networks (Hinz, Skiera, Barrot, & Becker, 2011). The results show that online networks can stimulate behavior changes and that these effects are stronger when coming from close friends (Bond et al., 2012) and when those close friends are connected to each other (Centola, 2010). Although the effect sizes are less than those achieved via face-to-face endorsements, the scale that is achievable substantially magnifies those effects.

Summary

This brief introduction to SNT and SNA has described the many ways that social networks influence behavior and the challenges inherent in estimating these effects. The effects can be simple, such as being more likely to gain weight when exposed to overweight peers, or complex, such as being resistant to adopting radical innovations when occupying a central position in a centralized network. And although social network concepts and diagrams can be quite intuitive, often considerable mathematical and computational methodology undergirds the work. A newcomer to the field may ask, "How do I get started?"

There are many websites, courses, workshops, conferences, and tutorials available to introduce SNA to the novice and provide specialized help to the advanced. A good way to start is with the resources offered by the professional association INSNA (International Network for Social Network Analysis, at www.insna.com), or with UCINET (Windows software for analyzing social network data that is available from Analytic Technologies, at www.analytictech.com). Table 11.2 provides a short list of other valuable websites. A significant barrier to conducting SNA can be the challenge of learning new software programs and platforms. Egocentric and social support studies use standard statistical software such as SAS, SPSS, or STATA for their analyses. Analysis of complete network data, when data are available from all (or most) units

Table 11.2   A Short List of Internet Resources

Resource	Website
Groups	
International Network for Social Network Analysis (INSNA)	www.insna.com
New England Complex Systems Institute	www.necsi.edu/guide
LINKS Center for Social Network Analysis, University of Kentucky	sites.google.com/site/uklinkscenter/home
Mitchell Centre for Social Network Analysis	www.socialsciences.manchester.ac.uk/research/research-centres-and-networks/mitchell-centre
Software	
UCINET	sites.google.com/site/ucinetsoftware/home
R/statnet	statnet.csde.washington.edu
	cran.us.r-project.org
RSiena	www.stats.ox.ac.uk/~snijders/siena/siena_r.htm
Pajek	vlado.fmf.uni-lj.si/pub/networks/pajek
Organizational Risk Analyzer (ORA)	www.casos.cs.cmu.edu/projects/ora
InFlow (by Orgnet; Valdis Krebs)	www.orgnet.com/VKbio.html

in the study, requires use of specialty network software such as UCINET, Pajek, ORA, statnet, and/or SIENA, the latter two being packages in the R platform.

The important takeaway from this chapter is that systems (including human ones) are composed of units that interact and are connected by many and varying relations. These relations have patterns and structures that are increasingly well understood and shown to have profound and enduring influences on health behaviors. Studies and programs that ignore these relations miss out on the opportunity to advance the science of human behavior and, for interventions, potentially fall short of their true capacity to improve outcomes. Social network theory specifies the conditions under which people are likely to be connected and how these individuals influence one another. It also makes similar claims for organizations, states, inanimate objects, and many other things. The application of this theory to other theories and to a vast array of health-related domains promises to improve our understanding of how we can make populations healthier and more productive.

References

Alexander, C., Piazza, M., Mekos, D., & Valente, T. W. (2001). Peers, schools, and adolescent cigarette smoking. *Journal of Adolescent Health*, 29(1), 22–30.

Ali, M. M., & Dwyer, D. S., (2009). Estimating peer effects in adolescent smoking behavior: A longitudinal analysis. *Journal of Adolescent Health*, 45(4), 402–408.

Aral, S., Muchnik, L., & Sundararajan, A. (2009). Distinguishing influence-based contagion from homophily-driven diffusion in dynamic networks. *Proceedings of the National Academy of Sciences*, 106(51), 21544–21549.

Beal, A. C., Ausiello, J., & Perrin, J. M. (2001). Social influences on health-risk behaviors among minority middle school students. *Journal of Adolescent Health, 28*(6), 474–480.

Bond, R. M., Fariss, C. J., Jones, J. J., Kramer, A.D.I., Marlow, C., Settle, J. E., & Fowler, J. H. (2012). A 61-million-person experiment in social influence and political mobilization. *Nature, 489*(7415), 295–298.

Bongaarts, J., & Watkins, S. C. (1996). Social interactions and contemporary fertility transitions. *Population and Development Review, 22*(4), 639–682.

Borgatti, S. P., Everett, M. G., & Johnson, J. C. (2013). *Analyzing social networks.* London: Sage.

Borgatti, S. P., & Ofem, B. (2010). Overview: Social network theory and analysis. In A. J. Daly (Ed.), *The ties of change: Social network theory and application in education* (pp. 17–30). Cambridge, MA: Harvard Press.

Boulay, M., Storey, J. D., & Sood, S. (2002). Indirect exposure to a family planning mass media campaign in Nepal. *Journal of Health Communication, 7*(5), 379–399.

Burt, R. S. (2005). *Brokerage and closure: An introduction to social capital.* New York: Oxford University Press.

Butterfoss, F. D., Kegler, M. C., & Francisco, V. T. (2008). Mobilizing organizations for health enhancement: Theories of organizational and systems change. In K. Glanz, B. K. Rimer, & K. Viswanath (Eds.), *Health education and health behavior: Theory, research, and practice* (4th ed., pp. 335–361). San Francisco: Jossey-Bass.

Casterline, J. B. (Ed.). (2001). *Diffusion processes and fertility transition: Selected perspectives.* Washington, DC: National Academies Press.

Centola, D. (2010). The spread of behavior in an online social network experiment. *Science, 329,* 1194–1197.

Christakis, N. A., & Fowler, J. H. (2007). The spread of obesity in a large social network over 32 years. *New England Journal of Medicine, 357,* 370–379.

Christakis, N. A., & Fowler, J. H. (2010). Social network sensors for early detection of contagious outbreaks. *PLoS ONE, 5*(9), e12948.

Dodds, P. S., Muhamad, R., & Watts, D. J. (2003). An experimental study of search in global social networks. *Science, 301*(5634), 827–829.

Engels, R. C., Knibbe, R. A., Drop, M. J., & de Haan, Y. T. (1997). Homogeneity of cigarette smoking within peer groups: Influence or selection? *Health Education & Behavior, 24*(6), 801–811.

Ennett, S. T., & Bauman, K. E. (1994). The contribution of influence and selection to adolescent peer group homogeneity: The case of adolescent cigarette smoking. *Journal of Personality and Social Psychology, 67*(4), 653–663.

Ennett, S. T., Faris, R., Hipp, J., Foshee, V. A., Bauman, K. E., Hussong, A., & Cai, L. (2008). Peer smoking, other peer attributes, and adolescent cigarette smoking: A social network analysis. *Prevention Science, 9*(2), 88–98.

Entwisle, B., Rindfuss, R. R., Guilkey, D. K., Chamratrithirong, A., Curran, S. R., & Sawangdee, Y. (1996). Community and contraceptive choice in rural Thailand: A case study of Nang Rong. *Demography, 33*(1), 1–11.

Flodgren, G., Parmelli, E., Doumit, G., Gattellari, M., O'Brien, M. A., Grimshaw, J., & Eccles, M. P. (2011). Local opinion leaders: Effects on professional practice and health care outcomes. *Cochrane Database of Systematic Reviews, 2011*(8), CD000125.

Freeman, L. (1979). Centrality in social networks: Conceptual clarification. *Social Networks, 1*, 215–239.

Freeman, L. (2004). *The development of social network analysis: A study in the sociology of science.* Vancouver, BC: Empirical Press.

Friedman, S. R., Neaigus, A., Jose, B., Curtis, R., Goldstein, M., Ildefonso, G., . . . Des Jarlais, D. C. (1997). Sociometric risk networks and risk for HIV infection. *American Journal of Public Health, 87*, 1289–1296.

Fujimoto, K., & Valente, T. W. (2012). Decomposing the components of friendship and friends' influence on adolescent drinking and smoking. *Journal of Adolescent Health, 51*, 136–143.

Gayen, K., & Raeside, R. (2010). Social networks and contraception practice of women in rural Bangladesh. *Social Science & Medicine, 71*, 1584–1592.

Granovetter, M. S. (1973). The strength of weak ties. *American Journal of Sociology, 78*(6), 1360–1380.

Hall, J., & Valente, T. W. (2007). Adolescent smoking networks: The effects of influence and selection on future smoking. *Addictive Behaviors, 32*, 3054–3059.

Henry, D. B., Kobus, K., & Schoeny, M. E. (2011). Accuracy and bias in adolescents' perceptions of friends' substance use. *Psychology of Addictive Behaviors, 25*, 80–89.

Hinz, O., Skiera, B., Barrot, C., & Becker, J. U. (2011). Seeding strategies for viral marketing: An empirical comparison. *Journal of Marketing, 75*(6), 55–71.

Hoffman, B. R., Monge, P., Chou, C. P., & Valente, T. W. (2007). Perceived peer influence and peer selection on adolescent smoking. *Addictive Behaviors, 32*(8), 1546–1554.

Hoffman, B. R., Sussman, S., Rohrbach, L., & Valente, T. W. (2006). Peer influence on adolescent smoking: A theoretical review of the literature. *Substance Use & Misuse, 41*(1), 103–155.

Hollingworth, W., Cohen, D., Hawkins, J., Hughes, R. A., Moore, L.A.R., Holliday, J. C., . . . Campbell, R. (2012). Reducing smoking in adolescents: Cost-effectiveness results from the cluster randomized ASSIST (A Stop Smoking In Schools Trial). *Nicotine and Tobacco Research, 14*(2), 161–168.

Ianotti, R. J., & Bush, P. J. (1992). Perceived vs. actual friends' use of alcohol, cigarettes, marijuana, and cocaine: Which has the most influence? *Journal of Youth and Adolescence, 21*(3), 375–389.

Iyengar, R., Van den Bulte, C., & Valente, T. W. (2011). Opinion leadership and contagion in new product diffusion. *Marketing Science, 30*(2), 195–212.

Kandel, D. (1978). Homophily, selection, and socialization in adolescent friendships. *American Journal of Sociology, 84*(2), 427–436.

Kincaid, D. L. (2000). Social networks, ideation, and contraceptive behavior in Bangladesh: A longitudinal analysis. *Social Science & Medicine, 50*(2), 215–231.

Kobus, K. (2003). Peers and adolescent smoking. *Addiction, 98*(Suppl. 1), 37–55.

Kohler, H. P. (1997). Learning in social networks and contraceptive choice. *Demography, 34*(3), 369–383.

Kohler, H. P., Behrman, J. R., & Watkins, S. C. (2001). The density of social networks and fertility decisions: Evidence from South Nyanza District, Kenya. *Demography, 38*(1), 43–58.

Lazer, D., Pentland, A., Adamic, L., Aral, S., Barabasi, A.-L., Brewer, D., . . . Van Alstyne, M. (2009). Computational social science. *Science, 323*(5915), 721–723.

Lomas, J., Enkin, M., Anderson, G. M., Hanna, W. J., Vayda, E., & Singer, J. (1991). Opinion leaders vs. audit feedback to implement practice guidelines: Delivery after previous cesarean section. *JAMA, 265*(17), 2202–2207.

Mercken, L., Snijders, T.A.B., Steglich, C., & de Vries, H. (2009). Dynamics of adolescent friendship networks and smoking behavior: Social network analyses in six European countries. *Social Science & Medicine, 69*(10), 1506–1514.

Mercken, L., Snijders, T.A.B., Steglich, C., Vertiainen, E., & de Vries, H. (2010). Smoking-based selection and influence in gender-segregated friendship networks: A social network analysis of adolescent smoking. *Addiction, 105*(7), 1280–1289.

Milgram, S. (1967). The small-world problem. *Psychology Today, 2*, 60–67.

Montgomery, M. R., & Casterline, J. B. (1993). The diffusion of fertility control in Taiwan: Evidence from pooled cross-section, time-series models. *Population Studies, 47*(3), 457–479.

Moreno, J. L. (1934). *Who shall survive? A new approach to the problem of human interrelations.* Washington, DC: Nervous and Mental Disease Publishing.

Piotrow, P. T., Kincaid, D. L., Rimon, J. G., & Rinehart, W. (1997). *Health communication: Lessons from family planning and reproductive health.* Westport, CT: Praeger.

Provan, K. G., & Milward, H. B. (1995). A preliminary theory of interorganizational network effectiveness: A comparative study of four community mental health systems. *Administrative Science Quarterly, 40*(1), 1–33.

Rice, R. E., Donohew, L., & Clayton, R. (2003). Peer network, sensation seeking, and drug use among junior and senior high school students. *Connections, 25*(2), 32–58.

Robins, G., Pattison, P., Kalish, Y., & Lusher, D. (2007). An introduction to exponential random graph (p*) models for social networks. *Social Networks, 29*(2), 173–191.

Rogers, E. M. (1979). Network analysis of the diffusion of innovations. In P. W. Holland & H. S. Leinhardt (Eds.), *Perspectives on social network research* (pp. 137–164). New York: Academic Press.

Rogers, E. M., & Kincaid, D. L. (1981). *Communication networks: A new paradigm for research.* New York: Free Press.

Scott, J. (2008). *Network analysis: A handbook* (2nd ed.). Thousand Oaks, CA: Sage.

Smith, K. P., & Christakis, N. (2008). Social networks and health. *Annual Review of Sociology, 34*, 405–429.

Snijders, T.A.B., van de Bunt, G. G., & Steglich, C.E.G. (2010). Introduction to stochastic actor-based models for network dynamics. *Social Networks, 32*(1), 44–60.

Starkey, F., Audrey, S., Holliday, J., Moore, L., & Campbell, R. (2009). Identifying influential young people to undertake effective peer-led health promotion: The example of A Stop Smoking In Schools Trial (ASSIST). *Health Behavior Research, 24*(6), 977–988.

Stoebenau, K., & Valente, T. W. (2003). The role of network analysis in community-based program evaluation: A case study from highland Madagascar. *International Family Planning Perspectives, 29*(4), 167–173.

U.S. Department of Health and Human Services. (2012). *Preventing tobacco use among youth and young adults: A report of the surgeon general.* Atlanta: U.S. Department of Health and Human Services, Centers for Disease Control and Prevention, National Center for Chronic Disease Prevention and Health Promotion, Office on Smoking and Health.

Valente, T. W. (1995). *Network models of the diffusion of innovations.* Cresskill, NJ: Hampton Press.

Valente, T. W. (1996). Social network thresholds in the diffusion of innovations. *Social Networks, 18*, 69–89.

Valente, T. W. (2010). *Social networks and health: Models, methods, and applications.* New York: Oxford University Press.

Valente, T. W. (2012). Network interventions. *Science, 337*(6090), 49–53.

Valente, T. W., & Fujimoto, K. (2010). Bridging: Locating critical connectors in a network. *Social Networks, 32*(3), 212–220.

Valente, T. W., Fujimoto, K., Palmer, P., & Tanjasiri, S. P. (2010). A network assessment of community-based participatory action: Linking communities and universities to reduce cancer disparities. *American Journal of Public Health, 100*(7), 1319–1325.

Valente, T. W., Fujimoto, K., Soto, D., Ritt-Olson, A., & Unger, J. B. (2012). A comparison of peer influence measures as predictors of smoking among predominately Hispanic/Latino high school adolescents. *Journal of Adolescent Health, 52*(3), 358–364.

Valente, T. W., Hoffman, B. R., Ritt-Olson, A., Lichtman, K., & Johnson, C. A. (2003). The effects of a social-network method for group assignment strategies on peer-led tobacco prevention programs in schools. *American Journal of Public Health, 93*(11), 1837–1843.

Valente, T. W., & Pumpuang, P. (2007). Identifying opinion leaders to promote behavior change. *Health Education & Behavior, 34*(6), 881–896.

Valente, T. W., & Saba, W. (1998). Mass media and interpersonal influence in a reproductive health communication campaign in Bolivia. *Communication Research, 25*(1), 96–124.

Valente, T. W., Unger, J., Ritt-Olson, A., Cen, S. Y., & Johnson, A. C. (2006). The interaction of curriculum and implementation method on 1-year smoking outcomes in a school-based prevention program. *Health Education Research, 21*(3), 315–324.

Valente, T. W., Watkins, S., Jato, M. N., Van der Straten, A., & Tsitsol, L. M. (1997). Social network associations with contraceptive use among Cameroonian women in voluntary associations. *Social Science & Medicine, 45*(5), 677–687.

Wasserman, S., & Faust, K. (1994). *Social network analysis: Methods and applications.* New York: Cambridge University Press.

Wasserman, S., & Robins, G. (2005). An introduction to random graphs, dependence graphs, and p*. In P. Carrington, J. Scott, & S. Wasserman (Eds.), *Models and methods in social network analysis.* New York: Cambridge University Press.

Watts, D. (1999). *Small worlds: The dynamics of networks between order and randomness.* Princeton, NJ: Princeton University Press.

Wipfli, H., Fujimoto, K., & Valente, T. W. (2010). Global tobacco control diffusion: The case of the Framework Convention on Tobacco Control. *American Journal of Public Health, 100*(7), 1260–1266.

Wyman, P., Pickering, T., & Valente, T. W. (2013, May). *Network influences on suicide ideation and attempts.* Paper presented at the 34th annual meeting of the International Network for Social Network Analysis, Hamburg, Germany.

CHAPTER 12

STRESS, COPING, AND HEALTH BEHAVIOR

Elaine Wethington
Karen Glanz
Marc D. Schwartz

Understanding stress and coping is essential to health education, health promotion, and disease prevention and management. *Stressors* are demands made by the environment that upset balance or homeostasis, affecting physical and psychological well-being and requiring action to restore equilibrium. *Stress* is the perception that a situation exceeds the psychological, social, or material resources for coping (Cohen, Kessler, & Gordon, 1995). Stress contributes to illness through its direct physiological effects or through indirect effects via maladaptive health behaviors (e.g., smoking or poor eating habits). Stress does not affect all people equally. Some people live through highly threatening experiences yet manage to cope well and do not get ill, whereas others suffer a range of health-related events. Further, many people report experiencing growth and finding positive lessons from stressful experiences (e.g., Park, 2010). Resistance to the negative impacts of stress has been conceptualized as *resilience*, a concept that has become increasingly central to stress research (e.g., Zautra, 2009). The ways in which individuals who are ill or at risk for illness cope with or manage stress, either individually or with support from family, friends, and health care providers, can be important influences on their health outcomes.

Reactions to stressors can promote or inhibit healthful practices and influence individuals' motivation to change or maintain unhealthy habits. Findings related to stress and coping have increasingly been applied to emerging public

KEY POINTS

This chapter will:

- Review major theories and research related to stress, coping and adaptation, resilience, and health.

- Summarize historical concepts of health, stress, and coping, including the Transactional Model of Stress and Coping.

- Discuss theoretical extensions of frameworks of health, stress, and coping/adaptation, including life-course and life-span perspectives on health, resilience, and psychoimmunology and neuroscience.

- Illustrate applications of classic and newly emerging models of health, stress, and coping to the design of interventions to address and reduce health disparities.

health issues in recent years, including preparedness for natural and human-made disasters and recognition of the social costs of health disparities. In response to advances in psychoimmunology, a new synthesis has emerged that focuses on how accumulation of stressful experiences across the individual life course may dysregulate the physiological stress adaptation system and may be mediated by behaviors such as positive coping and use of other resources that promote resilience.

A better understanding of stress-related theory and the empirical literature on stress and coping and their relationships to human physiology may be helpful in developing effective strategies and programs that help individuals to improve their coping and enhance their psychological and physical well-being. The purpose of this chapter is to review and discuss applications of major theories and the research related to stress, adaptation, coping, resilience, and health.

Historical Concepts of Health, Stress, Coping, and Resilience

Conceptualizations of health, stress, coping, and resilience are derived from many disciplines, with the earliest work having been conducted by scientists in the fields of biology and psychophysiology (e.g., Cannon, 1932). Diverse health and behavioral science disciplines, including epidemiology; personality psychology; cognitive, clinical, and social psychology; sociology; and medicine have contributed to our understanding of stress and coping.

Early work on stress focused on physiological reactions to stressors. Cannon (1932) first described the *fight-or-flight* reaction to stress. Hans Selye (1956), the father of modern stress research, extended Cannon's studies with clinical observations and laboratory research. He hypothesized that all living organisms exhibited nonspecific changes in response to stressors, labeling these changes the three-stage *general adaptation syndrome* (GAS). This syndrome consists of an alarm reaction, resistance, and exhaustion (Selye, 1956). Each stage evokes both physiological and behavioral responses. Without curative measures, physical and/or psychological deterioration occurs.

Another influential stream of stress research in the 1960s and 1970s focused on identifying and quantifying potential stressors, or stressful life events. Holmes and Rahe (1967) developed the Social Readjustment Rating Scale (SRRS), a tool to measure stressful life events. Studies showed that people with high scores on the SRRS had more illness episodes than those with low scores. This scale stimulated a substantial body of research that continues to the present day.

Beginning in the 1960s and 1970s, stress was conceptualized as a transaction between the individual and an external stressor in the environment, the impact of which could be attenuated or exacerbated by the individual's appraisals of the threat conveyed by the stressor and of his or her resources available to manage the stressor (Antonovsky, 1979; Lazarus, 1966). The central concept of this transactional model is that different people can appraise identical events or situations differently. Moreover, individual appraisals, rather than objective characteristics, are key determinants of how the event or situation affects behaviors and health status. Some researchers in the field of occupational stress applied the transactional concept to describe occupational stress as resulting from a lack of *fit* between workers' characteristics and the work environment (House, 1974). Transactional theory led to an examination of possible buffering, or moderating, factors, such as social support (Cohen & Wills, 1985; also see Chapter Ten), and of exposure to chronic or recurrent daily stressors as a condition of important life roles.

Work followed on measuring chronic exposure to stressors (Pearlin & Schooler, 1978) and daily event exposure or hassles (Folkman, Lazarus, Dunkel-Schetter, DeLongis, & Gruen, 1986). Chronic stressors are those that persist over time, affect multiple life roles, and erode the personal, social, and material resources needed to cope with stress. Recurring disagreements with a supervisor at work are a chronic stressor that may have an impact on staying in that job. Another example of chronic stress is living with an increased risk of disease or fear of recurrence of cancer. In contrast, daily stressors are small events where the impact is expected to dissipate in a short time but that may arise from persistent chronic stressors, such as work deadlines or waiting for the results of a medical test (Serido, Almeida, & Wethington, 2004). Researchers also began to focus on childhood exposure to stressors, testing the hypothesis that exposure to stressors at critical developmental periods may pose a lifetime risk of poor physical and mental health (e.g., Felitti et al., 1998).

The Felitti et al. (1998) study, using a retrospective design, reported a large number of dose-response relationships between family stressors during childhood (e.g., violence, abuse) on the one hand and subsequent poor health behaviors and the leading causes of death in the United States on the other. Childhood exposures to stress were correlated with adult health risks (e.g., smoking, and physical inactivity), chronic disease (e.g., ischemic heart disease, any cancer, or diabetes), and mental functioning (depression, alcohol use, drug use, or suicide attempts). Although it had a weak design, the study has stimulated stronger prospective research on childhood factors and health.

Concurrent research in biology and epidemiology has shown that some personality dispositions and psychological states (e.g., optimism, conscientiousness, and neuroticism) are linked to coping and disease (see Carver & Connor-Smith, 2010). Chronic stressors and responses to them affect the sympathetic nervous and endocrine systems, thus influencing the progression of health problems including cancer, infectious diseases, and HIV/AIDS (Glaser & Kiecolt-Glaser, 2005).

The increasing focus on chronic stressors and their potential to contribute to negative health impacts has led to new conceptualizations of the stress process. Contemporary research on stress, coping, and adaptation increasingly uses a life-course perspective and longitudinal data to study the long-term health impacts of poverty, accumulating social disadvantage, and associated stressors across the individual's life (e.g., Umberson, Williams, Thomas, Liu, & Thomeer, 2014). At the same time, new mechanistic perspectives have developed in neuroscience and psychoimmunology that elucidate how exposure to chronic stressors may lead to the deterioration of regulatory systems in the body that maintain health (e.g., McEwen, 2012). Models that attempt to integrate biological and social science perspectives on how stress exposure affects development and health across life, including access to resources and coping skills (e.g., Shonkoff, Boyce, & McEwen, 2009), have become more prominent in recent years. Another recent stream of research has reexamined why most people return to normal functioning even after very severe stressors, such as being widowed (e.g., Bonanno, Moskowitz,

Papa, & Folkman, 2005) or experiencing disasters such as the 9/11 terrorist attack in New York City (Bonanno, Galea, Bucciarelli, & Vlahov, 2007). The *resilience* perspective, translated from developmental science, posits that most individuals possess traits or resources that promote recovery after stressor exposure (Luthar, Cicchetti, & Becker, 2000).

There are numerous and important areas of research and theory relating to stress and health. The field has been reenergized in the twenty-first century by new attempts to synthesize life-course, developmental, and resilience perspectives with advances in neuroscience and psychoimmunology.

Transactional Model of Stress and Coping: Overview and Key Constructs

The Transactional Model of Stress and Coping is a classic framework for evaluating processes of coping with stressful events. Stressful experiences are construed as person-environment transactions in which the impact of an external stressor is mediated by the person's appraisal of the stressor and the psychological, social, and material resources at his or her disposal (Lazarus & Folkman, 1984). When faced with a stressor, a person evaluates potential threats or harms (primary appraisal), as well as his or her capacity to alter the situation and manage negative emotional reactions (secondary appraisal). Actual coping efforts, aimed at problem management and emotional regulation, affect outcomes of the coping process (e.g., psychological well-being, functional status, and treatment adherence).

Extensions of coping theory suggest that positive psychological states should also be taken into account. During a stressful period, numerous affect-inducing events occur that may allow the co-occurrence of negative and positive affect during the same period of time. Folkman proposed that a cognitive theory of stress and coping should accommodate positive psychological states (Folkman & Moskowitz, 2000). For example, someone who gives care to a sick loved one may experience a burden, strain, and anxiety. But a caregiver can also find positive meaning in the experience and pride at overcoming challenges (Folkman & Moskowitz, 2000),

Table 12.1 summarizes key concepts, definitions, and applications of the Transactional Model of Stress and Coping and the key extensions discussed in this chapter. Figure 12.1 illustrates interrelationships among these concepts. As shown in the figure, positive psychological states may be the result of meaning-based coping processes and social support, and they can also lead back to appraisal and coping. For more extensive discussions of theoretical underpinnings of the Transactional Model of Stress and Coping and productive extensions, see the work of Lazarus, Folkman, and Moskowitz (Folkman & Moskowitz, 2000; Lazarus & Folkman, 1984).

Primary Appraisal

Primary appraisal is a person's judgment about the significance of an event as stressful, positive, controllable, challenging, benign, and/or irrelevant. For example, health problems usually are

Table 12.1   Transactional Model of Stress and Coping, with Extensions: Definitions and Applications

Concept	Definition	Application
Primary appraisal	Evaluation of the significance of a stressor or threatening event	Perceptions of an event as threatening can cause distress. If an event is perceived as positive, benign, or irrelevant, little negative threat is felt.
Secondary appraisal	Evaluation of the controllability of the stressor and available coping resources	Perceiving the ability to change the situation, manage emotional reactions, and/or cope effectively can lead to successful coping and adaptation.
Coping efforts	Actual strategies used to mediate primary and secondary appraisals	
Problem management	Strategies aimed at changing a stressful situation	Strategies include active coping, problem solving, and seeking information.
Emotional regulation	Strategies aimed at changing the way of thinking or feeling about a stressful situation	Strategies include venting feelings, behavioral avoidance, disengagement, denial, and seeking social support.
Meaning-based coping	Coping processes that produce positive emotions, which in turn sustain the coping process by allowing reenactment of problem- or emotion-focused coping	Processes include positive reappraisal of the stressor, revising goals, drawing on spiritual and religious beliefs, and focusing on positive events.
Outcomes of coping (adaptation)	Emotional well-being, functional status, health behaviors	Coping strategies may result in short- and long-term positive or negative adaptation.
Dispositional coping styles	Generalized ways of behaving that can affect emotional or functional reaction to a stressor; relatively stable across time and situations	
Optimism	Tendency to have generalized positive expectancies for outcomes	Optimists can experience fewer symptoms and/or faster recovery from illness.
Benefit finding	Identification of positive life changes that have resulted from major stressors	Benefit finding may be related to the use of positive reappraisal and active coping.
Information seeking	Use of attentional styles that are vigilant (monitoring) versus those that involve avoidance (blunting)	Monitoring may increase distress and arousal; it may also increase active coping. Blunting may mute excessive worry, but may also reduce adherence.

evaluated initially as threatening, or as negative stressors. Two basic primary appraisals are perceptions of susceptibility to and severity of the threat (similar to the Health Belief Model, discussed in Chapter Five). According to the Transactional Model, appraisals of personal risk and threat severity prompt efforts to cope with the stressors. Those at risk for a disease may be motivated to practice recommended preventive strategies or to obtain care (problem-focused coping) and may seek social support to help with coping (emotion-focused coping). However, heightened perceptions of risk can also generate significant distress—for example, women who perceive themselves to be highly susceptible to ovarian cancer are more prone to experience aversive intrusive thoughts and psychological distress (Schwartz, Lerman, Miller, Daly, & Masny, 1995)—and can also prompt escape-avoidance behaviors (Lazarus & Folkman, 1984).

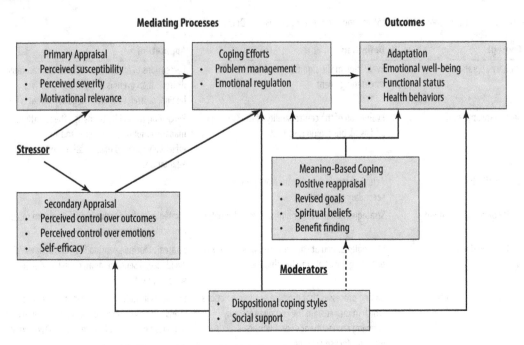

Figure 12.1   Transactional Model of Stress and Coping and Its Major Extensions

Such behaviors may lead an individual to miss opportunities for the disease to be diagnosed when it is still curable or at least treatable.

Primary appraisals also act to minimize the significance of threats, particularly when the threat is ambiguous or uncertain. In experimental studies, Croyle and colleagues (Ditto & Croyle, 1995), employing a test for a fictitious enzyme disorder, showed that those who were informed of "abnormal" test results rated the disorder as less serious and the test itself as less valid than did those who received "normal" test results, as a way to reduce the distress caused by the revelation. However, other studies suggest that minimizing appraisals may also diminish motivation to adopt recommended preventive health behaviors such as dietary restrictions and smoking cessation (Chapman, Wong, & Smith, 1993). Thus the most important aspect of primary appraisals of illness may be whether or not they are generated at all.

Secondary Appraisal

Secondary appraisal is an assessment of coping resources and options in a situation. Examples of secondary appraisals are perceived ability to change the situation, perceived ability to control feelings, and expectations about the effectiveness of one's coping resources.

Positive associations between perceptions of control over illness and psychological adjustment have been observed across a wide variety of diseases. These include cancer (Norton et al., 2005), heart disease (Moser, Riegel, McKinley, Doering, An, & Sheahan, 2007), and HIV/AIDS (Taylor et al., 1992). Moreover, perceived control over illness may improve physical well-being by increasing the likelihood that a person will adopt recommended health behaviors. For example, perceived control over health outcomes is related positively to safe sexual behaviors

(Kok, Hospers, Harterink, & De Zwart, 2007). Beliefs about ability to perform the behaviors necessary to exert control (that is, self-efficacy) play a central role in performance of a variety of health behaviors. Self-efficacy beliefs, one of the central concepts of Social Cognitive Theory, predict success with smoking cessation attempts as well as maintenance of exercise and diet regimens (Bandura, 1997; also see Chapter Nine). Perceived control is also a core construct in the Theory of Planned Behavior (see Chapter Six).

Coping Efforts

According to the Transactional Model, the emotional and functional effects of primary and secondary appraisals are mediated by actual coping strategies (Lazarus & Folkman, 1984). Original formulations of the model conceptualized *coping efforts* along two dimensions: *problem management* and *emotional regulation*. Also referred to as problem-focused coping, problem management strategies are directed at changing the stressful situation. Examples of problem-focused coping are taking action and information seeking. By contrast, emotion-focused coping is directed at changing the way one thinks or feels about a stressful situation. These strategies include seeking social support (although information seeking—enacting social support—may also be classified as problem solving), venting feelings, avoidance, and denial. The Transactional Model predicts that problem-focused coping strategies will be most adaptive for stressors that are changeable, whereas emotion-focused strategies will be most adaptive when the stressors are unchangeable or when the strategies are used in conjunction with problem-focused coping strategies.

Classic empirical studies of coping focused on the extent to which an individual engages versus disengages with the stressor (Carver et al., 1993). When a stressor is perceived as highly threatening and uncontrollable, a person may be more likely to use disengaging coping strategies (Taylor et al., 1992). Examples of disengaging coping strategies are distancing, cognitive avoidance (i.e., trying not to think about a stressor), behavioral avoidance (e.g., cancelling a cancer follow-up test), distraction, and denial. Each of these strategies shifts attention away from the stressor, which may allow individuals to minimize their initial distress by avoiding thoughts and feelings about the stressor (Suls & Fletcher, 1985). Ultimately, however, avoidance or denial may be maladaptive, leading to intrusive thoughts that can generate increased distress over time (Carver et al., 1993; Schwartz et al., 1995) and discouraging healthier coping strategies.

Other common coping responses to health threats are meaning-based strategies to induce positive emotion. These include positive reinterpretation, acceptance, and use of religion and spirituality (Carver et al., 1993; Park, 2010). These processes involve interpretation of a stressful situation in a personally meaningful way.

Several theoretically driven scales have been developed to assess coping efforts. Typically, respondents are asked to answer questions about how they would evaluate and respond to stressful situations. Widely used subscales in the Ways of Coping Inventory (WOC) (Folkman & Lazarus, 1988), the Multidimensional Coping Inventory (Endler & Parker, 1990), and the Coping Orientations to Problems Experienced (COPE) scale (Carver, Scheier, & Weintraub, 1989) address problem-focused coping and emotion-focused coping. For example, the COPE questionnaire uses twelve subscales to measure types of coping strategies: active coping, suppression of competing activities, planning, restraint, social support, positive reframing, religion, acceptance, denial, disengagement, use of humor, and self-distraction (Carver et al., 1993).

Development of coping strategy measurement has continued over time (e.g., Skinner, Edge, Altman, & Sherwood, 2003) in response to empirical and theoretical advances in the field. For example, scales to measure daily use of coping strategies may provide more precise assessments of coping transactions (Stone, Kennedy-Moore, & Neale, 1995) because they address concerns about an individual's retrospective memory bias when recalling how he or she coped. The traditional measures also focus on individual-level coping, although much coping (particularly with health problems) occurs in the context of ongoing social support in dyads, such as support from spouses (Berg & Upchurch, 2007). However, the WOC and the COPE are still used frequently.

The Transactional Model has generated a large body of literature on coping strategies, adjustment to illness, and health behavior (Stanton, Revenson, & Tennen, 2007). In general, these studies provide evidence for the psychological benefits of active coping strategies and acceptance or reappraisal over avoidant or disengaging strategies.

Benefits of more healthy or adaptive coping strategies have also been shown in the literature. For example, use of spirituality has been associated with growth, resilience, and the capacity to derive positive meaning from being an ovarian cancer survivor (Wenzel et al., 2002). However, as discussed next, the effects of specific coping strategies on emotional and functional outcomes of a health threat and the accompanying stress may depend on a person's dispositional coping style and perceptions of support in his or her environment. The literature on the benefits of adaptive coping, the benefits of social support, and dispositional coping styles has informed the translation of resilience models into the stress and coping literature.

Coping Outcomes

Coping outcomes represent a person's adaptation to a stressor, following from appraisal of the situation and resources (primary and secondary appraisal) and influenced by coping efforts. Because a problem or stressor may change over time, outcomes may occur in various time frames. Three main categories of outcomes are emotional well-being, functional status (health status, disease progression, and physiological biomarkers), and health behaviors. These outcomes may also interact with one another. In particular, the hormone cortisol, which is involved in the stress response, has been found to be associated with a variety of health outcomes, including conditions associated with developing heart disease (DeSantis et al., 2012). These recent studies provide support for the premise that stress affects health by affecting the human endocrine, immune, and nervous systems (Glaser & Kiecolt-Glaser, 2005). However, it is important to interpret reported correlations between social and psychological factors and human health and disease cautiously because longitudinal and prospective studies of stress, coping, and health that include physiological data are still relatively uncommon (McEwen, 2012).

Extensions to the Transactional Model

Research on stress and coping and the Transactional Model has been extended greatly by research on coping styles; personality traits such as optimism, benefit finding, and information finding; and social support. Early research in this area (e.g., Antonovsky, 1979) focused on characterizing people who remained relatively healthy while undergoing stressful life experiences because of strong resistance resources (such as social support, as described in Chapter Ten) and a sense of meaningfulness and sense of purpose in their lives. Several studies have found positive associations between a sense of purpose in life and life satisfaction, positive mood states, and happiness (e.g., Gustavsson-Lilius, Julkunen, Keskivaara, & Hietanen, 2007). This research also suggests that purpose in life is negatively associated with depression. In general, these studies suggest that people who endorse a strong purpose in life are likely to experience better emotional well-being.

Research on stress and coping has also been reframed by the translation of related theoretical perspectives from multiple disciplines, brought about by research efforts promoted by the National Institutes of Health to understand and alleviate health disparities related to race and ethnicity (Warnecke et al., 2008). Theoretical integration has been facilitated by application of the life-course and life-span perspectives (Umberson et al., 2014), which emphasize the accumulation of advantages and disadvantages across time in persons, affecting social and material resources as well as emotional development and regulation. It has also been influenced by the *allostatic load* perspective in physiology (McEwen, 2012), which has been applied by many behavioral researchers in examining the physiological impacts of chronic stressors associated with poverty, low socioeconomic status, and race (Schulz et al., 2012). Innovations in the measurement of physiological processes, developed through laboratory research using biomarkers and also through large-scale surveys, have facilitated this research activity, along with the increasing use of longitudinal and prospective research designs in the general population. Sensors and other devices that now can be carried by individuals may add further sensitivity to measuring individuals' responses to stressors.

Coping Styles

In contrast to situation-specific coping efforts, coping styles are conceptualized as stable dispositional characteristics that reflect generalized tendencies to interpret and respond to stress. Coping styles are enduring traits that are believed to drive appraisal and coping efforts (Lazarus, 1993). Individual differences in coping styles can be *moderators* of the impact of stress on coping processes and outcomes but may also have direct effects on the outcomes of stressful situations.

Optimism

Perhaps the most widely studied coping style to date is dispositional optimism, defined as the tendency to have positive rather than negative generalized expectancies for outcomes. These expectancies are relatively stable over time and across situations (Carver & Connor-Smith, 2010). Now-classic studies have demonstrated the direct benefits of optimism on psychological adjustment and quality of life among individuals with a variety of illnesses, including cancer patients (Carver et al., 1993) and HIV-positive men (Taylor et al., 1992). Studies exploring effects of optimism on coping responses are relevant to understanding the Transactional Model, because optimism may affect emotional and behavioral responses to illness. Carver et al. (1993) found that planning and problem solving mediated the beneficial effects of optimism on psychological well-being among early-stage breast cancer patients. Optimism was also related inversely to avoidance, a coping strategy that generated distress in this sample. Among gay men at risk for AIDS, dispositional optimism was associated with perceived lower risk of AIDS, higher perceived control over AIDS, more active coping strategies, less distress, and more risk-reducing health behaviors (Taylor et al., 1992).

Although a recent prospective study examining the association between optimism and lung cancer survival (Schofield et al., 2004) did not confirm the protective effect of optimism, a recent meta-analysis of eighty-three studies (Rasmussen, Scheier, & Greenhouse, 2009) found that optimism is a significant predictor of positive physical health across multiple health outcomes. The largest effect sizes were found for outcomes of subjective, self-reported health rather than more objective functional measures of health. Still, mean estimated effect sizes for optimism were significant even across objective outcomes such as mortality, survival, cardiovascular disease, physiological markers, and immune function. Effect sizes were not significant in studies of pregnancy and in prospective studies of cancer and pain (once baseline levels were taken into account). All findings were adjusted for demographic factors, health status, health risks, and other psychosocial factors.

Benefit Finding

Although much research on positive coping has focused on dispositional characteristics, such as optimism, purpose in life, and sense of coherence (Antonovsky, 1979), more contextual factors are also important, such as finding a benefit in the situation (i.e., identifying positive life changes that have resulted from major stressors; see Helgeson, Reynolds, & Tomich, 2006). Several studies have shown that benefit finding is significantly associated with the use of positive reappraisal and other forms of active coping (e.g., Lechner, Carver, Antoni, Weaver, & Phillips, 2006). Benefit finding has been associated with positive adjustment to a variety of health stressors, such as cardiovascular and other diseases (e.g., Chida & Steptoe, 2008). A caution, however, is that among cancer patients, evidence of benefit finding is more mixed (Lechner et al., 2006).

Information Seeking

Uncertainty of future outcomes can hinder the coping process by making it difficult to appraise the degree of threat associated with a stressor and to choose an effective coping response (Lazarus & Folkman, 1984). Personal health events often evoke uncertainty about outcomes as well as affecting the choice of treatment. Information seeking is frequently used in health care settings to cope with diagnosis and treatment choices (see Chapter Seventeen). There is substantial controversy, however, over whether information seeking is adaptive across situations and people. Those who typically seek information have been called *monitors*, and those who avoid information are called *blunters*. In a review of sixty-three studies that included thirteen interventions, Roussi and Miller (2014) found that although there is substantial evidence that information seeking is related to increased knowledge among patients coping with cancer, there is also evidence that compared to other patients, *high monitors* are less satisfied with the information they receive, appraise the personal threat to be more severe, and demand more from providers. Yet monitoring is beneficial in many situations. When the health threat is shorter-term, such as preparing for a medical test, monitoring can promote active coping (van Zuuren, Grypdonck, Crevits, Vande Walle, & Defloor, 2006).

Individuals differ in the extent to which they seek information beyond their physician's input about a health threat: for example, in the case of cancer (Hesse et al., 2005). Contextual factors, such as community engagement, socioeconomic status, and access to information channels (e.g., new communication media), are also associated with information seeking, in addition to personal styles such as monitoring and blunting. Information seeking is not distributed equally across the population and in fact may contribute to health disparities in treatment and outcomes for conditions such as cancer (Jung, Ramanadhan, & Viswanath, 2013; McCloud, Jung, Gray, & Viswanath, 2013).

Social Support

Social support has been conceptualized in a variety of ways (see Chapter Ten). Some definitions focus on the quantitative and tangible dimensions of support (e.g., number of friendships), whereas others focus on nontangible aspects such as perceived interconnectedness or subjective appraisals of the adequacy of support networks (Cohen, 2004). Substantial evidence shows the direct effects of social support on well-being and health outcomes (e.g., Kroenke, Kubzansky, Schernhammer, Holmes, & Kawachi, 2006). However, evidence also exists for the *stress-buffering* effects of social support (Cohen, 2004). The stress-buffering hypothesis predicts that social support will have stronger positive effects on adjustment and physical well-being when a stressor is present or worsens.

By influencing key processes posited in the Transactional Model, social support can influence how people adapt to stressful events. Availability of confidants could affect a person's primary appraisal of the severity of an illness. Support could also affect secondary appraisal by bolstering beliefs about ability to cope with situations and manage difficult emotions (Cohen & McKay, 1984). A supportive environment can protect against stress by providing opportunities to explore different coping options and to evaluate their effectiveness (Holahan & Moos, 1986).

But just as a supportive environment is related to positive psychosocial and health outcomes, a nonsupportive environment can adversely affect the ability to cope with a health threat (Cohen, 2004). When key social ties actively discourage the disclosure of feelings about a stressor, avoidant coping and adverse psychosocial outcomes can increase. Social support also influences health behaviors and outcomes. Low social support predicts more rapid progression of HIV (Leserman, 2000) and higher mortality among individuals with heart disease and following a heart attack (e.g., Brummett et al., 2005). Recent data from the Nurses' Health Study demonstrated a prospective association between social isolation and both breast cancer and all-cause mortality (Kroenke et al., 2006).

Despite consistent associations between social support and health outcomes in observational studies, application to interventions has proven more difficult. This may be due to the complexity of social support and how it is both given and received. A randomized controlled trial of an intervention designed to improve social support, reduce depression, and reduce mortality among myocardial infarction patients failed to decrease mortality, despite successfully enhancing social support and reducing depression (Berkman et al., 2003). While there is ample evidence to demonstrate a link between low social support and unhealthy behaviors, such as smoking and sedentary lifestyles (Brummett et al., 2005), it remains to be determined whether these behaviors can be improved via social support interventions. In natural settings, ineffective helping, or *negative support* (Cohen, 2004), can promote worse health and health behaviors even when positive behavior is encouraged (e.g., Stephens, Rook, Franks, Kahn, & Iida, 2010). Understanding how dyads cope together as teams, either as effective or ineffective supporters for behavior change, may be a critical and underdeveloped aspect of coping research (Berg & Upchurch, 2007).

Coping and Health Disparities

Health and illness are influenced by both individual and contextual risk and protective factors (Kawachi & Subramanian, 2006), as well as by genetics (Chen & Miller, 2013). Social factors such as racism and discrimination have been conceptualized to have both direct and indirect effects on health and thereby to contribute to health disparities in the population (Warnecke et al., 2008). The Transactional Model predicts that racism and discrimination could affect stress and coping at multiple levels. While racism may indirectly influence health via socioeconomic status (SES), it may also directly affect health by acting as a stressor (Williams, 1999). Laboratory studies have demonstrated that perceived racism is associated with increased cardiovascular reactivity (e.g., Merritt, Bennett, Williams, Edwards, & Sollers, 2006), particularly among African Americans (Lepore et al., 2006), although its association with psychological health is less clear-cut in community studies (e.g., Jackson, Knight, & Rafferty, 2010).

The Transactional Model also predicts that the effects of stress due to racism, low socioeconomic status, and other environmental stressors may be moderated by specific coping styles. One such widely studied coping style is John Henryism, defined as a predisposition to cope actively and persistently with psychosocial and environmental stressors (James, Hartnett, & Kalsbeek, 1983). According to this hypothesis, when coupled with severe constraints—such as low education, low SES, and racism—persistent and highly active coping results in negative health effects (Merritt, Bennett, Williams, Sollers, & Thayer, 2004).

Other perspectives may explain health disparities by race. Young people raised in low-SES circumstances are more likely to acquire common viral infections connected to heart disease and other late-life illnesses early in life (e.g., Helicobacter pylori, cytomegalovirus, herpes simplex virus type 1, and hepatitis B). The accumulation of *viral load* is associated with morbidity and early mortality (e.g., Zajacova, Dowd, & Aiello, 2009).

Stress, Coping, and Human Physiology

The physiological manifestations of stress have long been recognized. Acute stress is characterized by the fight-or-flight response and involves activation of the hypothalamic-pituitary-adrenal (HPA) axis and/or the sympathetic nervous system (SNS) (Glaser & Kiecolt-Glaser, 2005). While acute stress may lead to enhanced or impaired immune function, chronic stress clearly has an adverse impact on immune function (Moynihan, 2003). Ongoing exposure to elevated levels of catecholamines (e.g., epinephrine and norepinephrine), cortisol, and other stress hormones contribute to the immune dysregulation associated with chronic stress (e.g., Glaser & Kiecolt-Glaser, 2005).

McEwen's (2012) biopsychosocial perspective on the stress process, known as allostatic load, outlines an integrative framework to assess the relationship between stressor exposure and health outcomes that has been applied in multiple fields of study and could be translated into interventions to address health disparities (Ganzel, Morris, & Wethington, 2010). An elaboration and update of Selye's GAS, the allostatic load model, describes the physiological impacts of the wear and tear individuals experience when chronic or repeated exposures to stressful circumstances activate a strong physiological response that persists after exposure. The body mobilizes protectively in response to threat, and the responses preserve health. However, long-term chronic activation or overactivation of regulatory systems that secrete glucocorticoids, such as cortisol, affects interacting physical systems (e.g., the HPA axis and the immune system) and may promote stress-related disease. Physiological damage, termed the *allostatic load*, may accumulate because of exposure to stressors across the life course, or perhaps may be embedded in the body as a result of severe stressors during the critical developmental period of childhood.

The allostatic load perspective proposes that there are a series of intermediate physiological effects on interrelated body systems. These effects can be measured using biomarkers that indicate overarousal and inflammation near the time of a severe stressor, impaired immune functioning, and metabolic irregularity associated with chronic and persistent stress. Biomarkers are frequently applied measures of allostatic load that measure cardiovascular functioning, sympathetic nervous and adrenomedullary system functioning, central body obesity, stress hormones, efficiency of glucose metabolism, and risks for atherosclerosis.

The allostatic load framework, however, is controversial, and many of its propositions remain to be tested. Using measures of allostatic load, a study has found that these markers did not mediate the SES-health relationship among middle-aged and older adults; rather obesity and cardiovascular factors mediated the SES-health relationship (Hawkley, Lavelle, Berntson, & Cacioppo, 2011). Competing physiological perspectives suggest that infectious agents such as the cytomegalovirus may compromise the immune system (Pawelec, McElhaney, Aiello, & Derhovanessian, 2012). Gene expression, facilitated by stress and other environmental exposures, may also affect immune function and inflammation (for a review, see Chen & Miller, 2013).

Applications to Current Research

Accumulating research on the emerging models that focus on life-course and life-span development is compelling, even though the evidence (except from animal studies) is primarily observational. Contemporary research focuses not only on stress exposure but also on emotions, attitudes, other risk factors, and access to resources that promote adaptation across the life course and may in turn affect health. In this section, we discuss two examples applying research on the stress process to the understanding of health and health behaviors across the life course. The first example is an observational study using physiological biomarkers. The second example is an intervention that offers a prenatal and infancy nurse home visitation program (for which testing and implementation funding was set aside in the Patient Protection and Affordable Care Act of 2010). If stress exposure in childhood is associated with higher morbidity and earlier mortality, then early intervention that improves access to resources and the ability to cope effectively should have an impact on risk factors associated with the development of chronic disease.

Application 1: Childhood Factors, Coping and Adaptation, and Adult Health

Low SES in childhood and adolescence is a well-established predictor of poor adult health. Despite the strong association found in observational studies, it has remained unclear why some adults raised in low-SES circumstances remain physically healthy (Chen, Miller, Lachman, Gruenewald, & Seeman, 2012). A positive resource for healthy resilience may be learned adaptive coping, which may be amenable to intervention. A recent observational study of a large national sample of middle-aged and older adults (Chen et al., 2012) reported that individuals who were raised in low-SES backgrounds had a lower allostatic load (as measured by a composite of twenty-four stress-related biomarkers) in adulthood if they employed a *shift-and-persist* coping style. This coping style was not associated with allostatic load in high-SES individuals. Shift-and-persist involves adapting to stressors while also maintaining a positive focus on the future. The shift-and-persist style may be a good fit for people in low-SES contexts because direct action against the stressors they tend to experience may not be practical or adaptive (James et al., 1983). The relationship between coping style and allostatic load remained significant after controlling for demographics, objective measures of medical history, smoking, and current SES. The findings suggest that specific coping strategies may be beneficial in some environments but not others.

Application 2: Long-Term Effects of Prenatal and Infancy Nurse Home Visitation

No randomized controlled trials (RCTs) have attempted to mitigate directly the long-term impacts of childhood stress exposure and learned adaptation on adult health outcomes. The Family-Nurse Partnership program, however, was developed over the last thirty years, using RCTs, to reduce the risk of child maltreatment among high-risk mothers by providing education and teaching effective coping skills to mothers. Child maltreatment, which can be conceptualized as a chronic stressor, and which is exacerbated by family and financial stress, is a known risk factor for poorer adult physical and mental health. Eckenrode et al. (2010) examined the effect of this program on the emotional, educational, and behavioral development of nineteen-year-olds whose mothers had participated at the Elmira, New York, trial site. (Other RCTs were conducted in Memphis, Tennessee, and Denver, Colorado.) The trial, based on socioecological and life-course perspectives on health, employed visiting nurses to help improve mothers' health behaviors during pregnancy, to affect children's health by educating mothers about coping with the demands of providing child care, and to help mothers to avoid future financial and other stressors by encouraging them to complete their education, use contraception, and find employment. The direct intervention continued until the child's second birthday. Previous long-term follow-ups on participants in the trial found positive impacts on the mother's welfare use, child maltreatment, child injuries, and criminal behavior, all of which are associated with educational achievement, substance use, pregnancies, and criminal behavior during adulthood, which in turn are associated with health. On the basis of encouraging findings from visitation programs of this kind, funding for increasing the number of nurse home visitation programs was set aside in the Patient Protection and Affordable Care Act of 2010.

Findings from the nineteen-year follow-up study are mixed. The program reduced girls' involvement with crime, but did not have lasting effects on life-course factors that affect health such as use of alcohol and illegal drugs, use of birth control, number of sexual partners, teen pregnancy and childbearing, or completing high school. The intervention did not continue to have an impact on criminal activity or other risk factors among boys. Overall, follow-ups of this RCT suggest that it improved economic well-being and reduced child maltreatment; however, the impact on factors affecting health during adulthood remains to be determined. One possible explanation for the lack of long-term impact from the intervention in comparison to the control may lie in the resilience perspective, which posits that most people eventually overcome the stressors of earlier years.

Research Gaps and Future Directions

Integration of various disciplinary approaches into stress and coping research is proceeding speedily in population and epidemiological studies, and this development should advance our understanding of how social and individual factors may mitigate the impact of stressor exposure on health as well as contribute to understanding major health disparities that have public health impact. A number of major longitudinal cohort data collections in the United States and other countries have incorporated biomarker indicators of allostatic load, particularly among studies of older adults, while others have added biomarkers to assess viral load. (The research reviewed in this chapter suggests that more longitudinal research incorporating biomarkers that covers early childhood, adolescence, and emerging adulthood is also needed.) The Centers for Disease Control and Prevention has developed questions on childhood adverse experiences to include in its Behavioral Risk Factor Surveillance System survey (Anda, Butchart, Felitti, & Brown, 2010). Rapidly changing research technologies that are facilitating the integration of physiological biomarkers into population and epidemiological studies could, in the long run, improve our understanding of stress and coping processes and particularly their relationship to physiological indicators linked to developing or worsening chronic diseases. More intervention studies that include biomarkers of physiological mediators are also needed.

Summary

The theory and research presented in this chapter illustrate the complexities of past research on stress, coping, adaptation, health behavior, and health across the life course. The chapter also illustrates the current translational integration of research from multiple disciplines—including human physiology, neuroscience, social and behavioral science, and public health—as part of the effort to understand the onset and course of chronic disease across life. The outcomes of stress and individual coping processes have emerged as critical to understanding chronic diseases. Individuals' coping processes are likely affected by personality and cognitive factors, embedded physiological response patterns, capacity for resilience, life experiences at least partially determined by socioeconomic and situational factors, individual appraisals of the situation, coping resources, and past coping strategies. Throughout the new integration of theory and research, the core concepts of the Transactional Model of Stress and Coping, with their emphasis on the interaction of person and context, have remained critical to ongoing theoretical development. Effects of the stress and coping processes depend on context (e.g., controllability of the stressor), timing and chronicity of exposure to the stressor (in critical periods such as childhood but also in adult social roles), and each individual's characteristics (e.g., stress responsiveness and resources for resilience).

References

Anda, R. F., Butchart, A., Felitti, V. J., & Brown, D. W. (2010). Building a framework for global surveillance of the public health implications of adverse childhood experiences. *American Journal of Preventive Medicine, 39*(1), 93–98.

Antonovsky, A. (1979). *Health, stress, and coping*. San Francisco: Jossey-Bass.

Bandura, A. (1997). *Self-efficacy: The exercise of control*. New York: Freeman.

Berg, C. A., & Upchurch, R. (2007). A developmental-contextual model of couples coping with chronic illness across the adult life span. *Psychological Bulletin, 133*(6), 920–954.

Berkman, L. F., Blumenthal, J., Burg, M., Carney, R. M., Catellier, D., Cowan, M. J., . . . Schneiderman, N. (2003). Effects of treating depression and low perceived social support on clinical events after myocardial infarction: The Enhancing Recovery in Coronary Heart Disease Patients (ENRICHD) randomized trial. *JAMA, 289*(23), 3106–3116.

Bonanno, G. A., Galea, S., Bucciarelli, A., & Vlahov, D. (2007). What predicts psychological resilience after disaster? The role of demographics, resources, and life stress. *Journal of Consulting and Clinical Psychology, 75*(5), 671–682.

Bonanno, G. A., Moskowitz, J. T., Papa, A., & Folkman, S. (2005). Resilience to loss in bereaved spouses, bereaved parents, and bereaved gay men. *Journal of Personality and Social Psychology, 88*(5), 827–843.

Brummett, B. H., Mark, D. B., Siegler, I. C., Williams, R. B., Babyak, M. A., Clap-Channing, N. E., & Barefoot, J. C. (2005). Perceived social support as a predictor of mortality in coronary patients: Effects of smoking, sedentary behavior, and depressive symptoms. *Psychosomatic Medicine, 67*(1), 40–45.

Cannon, W. B. (1932). *The wisdom of the body.* New York: Norton.

Carver, C. S., & Connor-Smith, J. (2010). Personality and coping. *Annual Review of Psychology, 61,* 679–704.

Carver, C. S., Pozo, C., Harris, S. D., Noriega, V., Scheier, M. F., Robinson, D. S., . . . Clark, K. C. (1993). How coping mediates the effect of optimism on distress: A study of women with early stage breast cancer. *Journal of Personality and Social Psychology, 65*(2), 375–390.

Carver, C. S., Scheier, M. F., & Weintraub, J. K. (1989). Assessing coping strategies: A theoretically based approach. *Journal of Personality and Social Psychology, 56*(2), 267–283.

Chapman, S., Wong, W. L., & Smith, W. (1993). Self-exempting beliefs about smoking and health: Differences between smokers and ex-smokers. *American Journal of Public Health, 83*(2), 215–219.

Chen, E., & Miller, G. E. (2013). Socioeconomic status and health: Mediating and moderating factors. *Annual Review of Clinical Psychology, 9,* 723–749.

Chen, E., Miller, G. E., Lachman, M. E., Gruenewald, T. L., & Seeman, T. E. (2012). Protective factors for adults from low-childhood socioeconomic circumstances: The benefits of shift-and-persist for allostatic load. *Psychosomatic Medicine, 74*(2), 178–186.

Chida, Y., & Steptoe, A., (2008). Positive psychological well-being and mortality: A quantitative review of prospective observational studies. *Psychosomatic Medicine, 70*(7), 741–756.

Cohen, S. (2004). Social relationships and health. *American Psychologist, 59*(8), 676–684.

Cohen, S., Kessler, R. C., & Gordon, L. U. (Eds.). (1995). *Measuring stress: A guide for health and social scientists.* New York: Oxford University Press.

Cohen, S., & McKay, G. (1984). Social support, stress and the buffering hypothesis: A theoretical analysis. In A. Baum, J. E. Singer, & S. E. Taylor (Eds.), *Handbook of psychology and health* (Vol. 4, pp. 253–267). Hillsdale, NJ: Erlbaum.

Cohen, S., & Wills, T. A. (1985). Stress, social support, and the buffering hypothesis. *Psychological Bulletin, 98*(2), 310–357.

DeSantis, A. S., DiezRoux, A. V., Hajat, A., Aiello, A. E., Golden, S. H., Jenny, N. S., . . . Shea, S. (2012). Associations of salivary cortisol levels with inflammatory markers: The Multi-Ethnic Study of Atherosclerosis. *Psychoneuroendocrinology, 37*(7), 1009–1018.

Ditto, P. H., & Croyle, R. T. (1995). Understanding the impact of risk factor test results: Insights from a basic research program. In R. T. Croyle (Ed.), *Psychosocial effects of screening for disease prevention and detection.* New York: Oxford University Press.

Eckenrode, J., Campa, M., Luckey, D. W., Henderson, C. R., Cole, R., Kitzman, H., . . . Olds, D. (2010). Long-term effects of prenatal and infancy nurse home visitation on the life course of youths. *Archives of Pediatrics & Adolescent Medicine, 164*(1), 9–15.

Endler, N., & Parker, J. (1990). Multidimensional assessment of coping: A critical evaluation. *Journal of Personality and Social Psychology, 58*(5), 844–854.

Felitti, V. J., Anda, R. F., Nordenberg D., Williamson, D. F., Spitz, A. M., Edwards, V., . . . Marks, J. S. (1998). Relationship of childhood abuse and household dysfunction to many of the leading causes of death in adults: The Adverse Childhood Experiences (ACE) Study. *American Journal of Preventive Medicine, 14*(4), 245–258.

Folkman, S., & Lazarus, R. S. (1988). *The Ways of Coping Questionnaire*. Palo Alto, CA: Consulting Psychologists Press.

Folkman, S., Lazarus, R., Dunkel-Schetter, C., DeLongis, A., & Gruen, R. (1986). Dynamics of a stressful encounter: Cognitive appraisal, coping, and encounter outcomes. *Journal of Personality and Social Psychology, 50*(5), 992–1003.

Folkman, S., & Moskowitz, J. (2000). Positive affect and the other side of coping. *American Psychologist, 55*(6), 647–654.

Ganzel, B., Morris, P. A., & Wethington, E. (2010). Allostasis and the human brain: Integrating models of stress from the social and life sciences. *Psychological Review, 117*(1), 134–174.

Glaser, R., & Kiecolt-Glaser, J. K. (2005). Stress-induced immune dysfunction: Implications for health. *Nature Reviews: Immunology, 5*(3), 243–251.

Gustavsson-Lilius, M., Julkunen, J., Keskivaara, P., & Hietanen, P. (2007). Sense of coherence and distress in cancer patients and their partners. *Psycho-Oncology, 16*(12), 1100–1110.

Hawkley, L. C., Lavelle, L. A., Berntson, G. G., & Cacioppo, J. T. (2011). Mediators of the relationship between socioeconomic status and allostatic load in the Chicago Health, Aging, and Social Relations Study. *Psychoimmunology, 48*(8), 1134–1145.

Helgeson, V. S., Reynolds, K. A., & Tomich, P. L. (2006). A meta-analytic review of benefit finding and growth. *Journal of Consulting and Clinical Psychology, 74*(5), 797–816.

Hesse, B. W., Nelson, D. E., Kreps, G. L., Croyle, R. T., Arora, N. K., Rimer, B. K., & Viswanath, K. (2005). Trust and sources of health information: The impact of the Internet and its implications for health care providers: Findings from the first Health Information National Trends Survey. *Archives of Internal Medicine, 165*(22), 2618–2624.

Holahan, C. J., & Moos, R. H. (1986). Personality, coping, and family resources in stress resistance: A longitudinal analysis. *Journal of Personality and Social Psychology, 51*(2), 389–395.

Holmes, T. H., & Rahe, R. H. (1967). The Social Readjustment Rating Scale. *Journal of Psychosomatic Research, 11*, 213–218.

House, J. S. (1974). Occupational stress and coronary heart disease: A review and theoretical integration. *Journal of Health and Social Behavior, 15*(1), 12–27.

Jackson, J. S., Knight, K. M., & Rafferty, J. A. (2010). Race and unhealthy behaviors: Chronic stress, the HPA axis, and physical and mental health disparities across the life course. *American Journal of Public Health, 100*(5), 933–939.

James, S., Hartnett, S. A., & Kalsbeek, W. D. (1983). John Henryism and blood pressure among black men. *Journal of Behavioral Medicine, 6*(3), 259–278.

Jung, M., Ramanadhan, S., & Viswanath, K. (2013). Effect of information seeking and avoidance behavior on self-rated health status among cancer survivors. *Patient Education and Counseling, 92*(1), 101–106.

Kawachi, I., & Subramanian, S. V. (2006). Measuring and modeling the social and geographic context of trauma: A multilevel modeling approach. *Journal of Traumatic Stress, 19*(2), 195–203.

Kok, G., Hospers, H. J., Harterink, P., & De Zwart, O. (2007). Social-cognitive determinants of HIV risk-taking intentions among men who date men through the Internet. *AIDS Care, 19*(3), 410–417.

Kroenke, C., Kubzanksy, L. D., Schernhammer, E. S., Holmes, M. D., & Kawachi, I. (2006). Social networks, social support, and survival after breast cancer. *Journal of Clinical Oncology, 24*(7), 1105–1111.

Lazarus, R. S. (1966). *Psychological stress and the coping process*. New York: McGraw-Hill.

Lazarus, R. S. (1993). Coping theory and research: Past, present, and future. *Psychosomatic Medicine*, *55*(3), 234–247.

Lazarus, R. S., & Folkman, S. (1984). *Stress, appraisal, and coping*. New York: Springer.

Lechner, S. C., Carver, C. S., Antoni, M. H., Weaver, K. E., & Phillips, M. (2006). Curvilinear associations between benefit finding and psychosocial adjustment to breast cancer. *Journal of Clinical and Consulting Psychiatry*, *74*(5), 828–840.

Lepore, S. J., Revenson, T. A., Weinberger, S. L., Weston, P., Frisina, P. G., Robertson, R., . . . Cross, W. (2006). Effects of social stressors on cardiovascular reactivity in black and white women. *Annals of Behavioral Medicine*, *31*(2), 120–127.

Leserman, J. (2000). The effects of depression, stressful life events, social support, and coping on the progression of HIV infection. *Current Psychiatry Reports*, *2*(6), 495–502.

Luthar, S. S., Cicchetti, D., & Becker, B. (2000). The construct of resilience: A critical evaluation and guidelines for future work. *Child Development*, *71*(3), 543–562.

McCloud, R. F., Jung, M., Gray, S. W., & Viswanath, K. (2013). Class, race and ethnicity and information avoidance among cancer survivors. *British Journal of Cancer*, *108*(10), 1949–1956.

McEwen, B. S. (2012). Brain on stress: How the social environment gets under the skin. *Proceedings of the National Academy of Sciences*, *109*(Suppl. 2), 17180–17185.

Merritt, M. M., Bennett, G. G., Williams, R. B., Edwards, C. L., & Sollers, J. J., III. (2006). Perceived racism and cardiovascular reactivity and recovery to personally relevant stress. *Health Psychology*, *25*(3), 364–369.

Merritt, M. M., Bennett, G. G., Williams, R. B., Sollers, J. J., III, & Thayer, J. F. (2004). Low educational attainment, John Henryism, and cardiovascular reactivity to and recovery from personally relevant stress. *Psychosomatic Medicine*, *66*(1), 49–55.

Moser, D. K., Riegel, B., McKinley, S., Doering, L. V., An, K., & Sheahan, S. (2007). Impact of anxiety and perceived control on in-hospital complications after acute myocardial infarction. *Psychosomatic Medicine*, *69*(1), 10–16.

Moynihan, J. A. (2003). Mechanisms of stress-induced modulation of immunity. *Brain, Behavior, and Immunity*, *17*(Suppl. 1), S11–S16.

Norton, T. R., Manne, S. L., Rubin, S., Hernandez, E., Carlson, J., Bergman, C., & Rosenblatt, N. (2005). Ovarian cancer patients' psychological distress: The role of physical impairment, perceived unsupportive family and friend behaviors, perceived control, and self-esteem. *Health Psychology*, *24*(2), 143–152.

Park, C. L. (2010). Making sense of the meaning literature: An integrative review of meaning making and its effects on adjustment to stressful life events. *Psychological Bulletin*, *136*(2), 257–301.

Pawelec, G., McElhaney, J. E., Aiello, A. E., & Derhovanessian, E. (2012). The impact of CMV infection on survival in older humans. *Current Opinion in Immunology*, *24*(4), 507–511.

Pearlin, L. I., & Schooler, C. (1978). The structure of coping. *Journal of Health and Social Behavior*, *19*(1), 2–21.

Rasmussen, H., Scheier, M. F., & Greenhouse, J. B. (2009). Optimism and health: A meta-analytic review. *Annals of Behavioral Medicine*, *37*(3), 239–256.

Roussi, P., & Miller, S. M. (2014). Monitoring style of coping with cancer related threats: A review of the literature. *Journal of Behavioral Medicine*, *37*(5), 931–954.

Schofield, P., Ball, D., Smith, J. G., Borland, R., O'Brien, P., Davis, S., . . . Joseph, D. (2004). Optimism and survival in lung carcinoma patients. *Cancer*, *100*(6), 1276–1282.

Schulz, A. J., Mentz, G., Lachance, L., Johnson, J., Gaines, C., & Israel, B. A. (2012). Associations between socioeconomic status and allostatic load: Effects of neighborhood poverty and tests of mediating pathways. *American Journal of Public Health, 102*(9), 1706–1714.

Schwartz, M., Lerman, C., Miller, S. M., Daly, M., & Masny, A. (1995). Coping disposition, perceived risk, and psychological distress among women at increased risk for ovarian cancer. *Health Psychology, 14*(3), 232–235.

Selye, H. (1956). *The stress of life.* New York: McGraw-Hill.

Serido, J., Almeida, D. M., & Wethington, E. (2004). Chronic stressors and daily hassles: Unique and interactive relationships with psychological distress. *Journal of Health and Social Behavior, 45*(1), 17–33.

Shonkoff, J. P., Boyce, W. T., & McEwen, B. S. (2009). Neuroscience, molecular biology, and the childhood roots of health disparities: Building a new framework for health promotion and disease prevention. *JAMA, 301*(21), 2252–2259.

Skinner, E. A., Edge, K., Altman, J., & Sherwood, H. (2003). Searching for the structure of coping: A review and critique of category systems for classifying ways of coping. *Psychological Bulletin, 129*(2), 216–269.

Stanton, A. L., Revenson, T. A., & Tennen, H. (2007). Health psychology: Psychological adjustment to chronic disease. *Annual Review of Psychology, 58*, 565–592.

Stephens, M.A.P., Rook, K. S., Franks, M. M., Khan, C., & Iida, M. (2010). Spouses' use of social control to improve diabetic patients' dietary adherence. *Families, Systems, and Health, 28*(3), 199–208.

Stone, A., Kennedy-Moore, E., & Neale, J. (1995). Association between daily coping and end-of-day mood. *Health Psychology, 14*(4), 341–349.

Suls, J., & Fletcher, B. (1985). The relative efficacy of avoidant and nonavoidant coping strategies: A meta-analysis. *Health Psychology, 4*(3), 249–288.

Taylor, S. E., Kemeny, M. E., Aspinwall, L. G., Schneider, S. G., Rodriguez, R., & Herbert, M. (1992). Optimism, coping, psychological distress, and high-risk sexual behavior among men at risk for acquired immunodeficiency syndrome (AIDS). *Journal of Personality and Social Psychology, 63*(3), 460–473.

Umberson, D., Williams, K., Thomas, P. A., Liu, H., & Thomeer, M. B. (2014). Race, gender, and chains of disadvantage: Childhood adversity, social relationships, and health. *Journal of Health and Social Behavior, 55*(1), 20–38.

van Zuuren, F. J., Grypdonck, M., Crevits, E., Vande Walle, C., & Defloor, T. (2006). The effect of an information brochure on patients undergoing gastrointestinal endoscopy: A randomized controlled study. *Patient Education and Counseling, 64*(1–3), 173–182.

Warnecke, R. B., Oh, A., Breen, N., Gehlert, S., Paskett, E., Tucker, K. L., . . . Hiatt, R. A. (2008). Approaching health disparities from a population perspective: The National Institutes of Health Centers for Population Health and Health Disparities. *American Journal of Public Health, 98*(9), 1608–1615.

Wenzel, L. B., Donnelly, J. P., Fowler, J. M., Hobbal, R., Taylor, T. H., Aziz, N., & Cella, D. (2002). Resilience, reflection, and residual stress in ovarian cancer survivorship. *Psycho-Oncology, 11*(2), 142–153.

Williams, D. R. (1999). Race, socioeconomic status, and health: The added effects of racism and discrimination. *Annals of the New York Academy of Sciences, 896*, 173–188.

Zajacova, A., Dowd, J. B., & Aiello, A. E. (2009). Socioeconomic and race/ethnic patterns in persistent infection burden among U.S. adults. *Journal of Gerontology: Medical Sciences, 64*(2), 272–279.

Zautra, A. J. (2009). Resilience: One part recovery, two parts sustainability. *Journal of Personality, 77*(6), 1935–1943.

CHAPTER 13

INTERPERSONAL COMMUNICATION IN HEALTH AND ILLNESS

Ashley Duggan
Richard L. Street Jr.

Interpersonal communication is a primary source of social influence, a process that is critical for optimizing health behaviors. Interpersonal communication is associated with health outcomes relevant to daily life, including quality of life, illness symptoms, adaptation to illness, disability, and death (Duggan & Thompson, 2011). Social determinants such as education, income, employment, occupation, and place—including type of neighborhood and whether the environment is urban or rural—shape interpersonal communication and health (Ackerson & Viswanath, 2009). Interpersonal, or relational, factors take place in the context of social determinants but occur at a different level of analysis. This chapter describes theory and research on interpersonal communication to illustrate how interpersonal communication behaviors shape relational processes when an individual is dealing with illness, and to illustrate how interpersonal communication behaviors influence health behavior change.

Many behavior change theories focus on behavior change per se. In contrast, interpersonal communication theories are grounded in a fundamental assumption that relationships between people are at the heart of identity and behavior and that expectations regarding behavior are a product of these relationships. Expectations are usually defined implicitly and develop over time. Theories of interpersonal communication explain how communication serves as the manifestation of relational goals.

KEY POINTS

This chapter will:

- Describe the importance of interpersonal communication in health behavior change.

- Outline the pathways through which interpersonal communication may lead to better health outcomes.

- Illustrate how relational and task-oriented communication functions shape theories of health behavior change.

- Review lessons learned from theory and research about interpersonal communication in physician-patient relationships.

- Provide two applications—addressing physical disabilities and chronic pain—to illustrate key concepts and the interplay between relational and task functions of interpersonal communication in shaping health behaviors.

Considering interpersonal communication in the context of health behaviors means recognizing the inherent interconnections among the roles and relationships of health providers, friends, and family members in their attempts to influence health and illness.

Theories of interpersonal communication focus on explaining how relational processes are manifest in behavior. In essence, relational processes involve the expression and interpretation of messages in personal relationships. In the health context, a foundation in interpersonal communication theories allows an understanding of the ways relationships are interconnected with the goals and tasks associated with health behavior change. For example, in physician-patient interactions, a foundation of trust and rapport can promote disclosures about illness behaviors, and a lack of trust and rapport can inhibit these disclosures. Communication in physician-patient interactions also influences decision making and adherence to medical regimens. Trust and rapport may be stronger predictors than biomedical markers of symptoms in predicting the degree of honest disclosure and openness within the physician-patient interaction, as well as subsequent behaviors and health outcomes. Similarly, in families, health behavior change often requires that family members interact around a health issue, and may shift how they relate to each other. Relationships with health providers, family members, and friends can provide support and enhance the chances of behavior change. Relationships can also exacerbate the emotional toll of illness and inhibit behavior change. Because of the breadth of theoretical and practical explanations for communication's influence over health behavior in close relationships, we focus largely on provider-patient behavior in this chapter. (Additional overviews are available in Thompson, Parrott, & Nussbaum, 2011, and Vangelisti, 2013).

Improving health outcomes requires recognizing and attending to both the task functions of health behaviors and the relational functions of attending to human elements, such as emotion, rapport, and fear. In essence, interpersonal communication becomes the manifestation of the interconnection between biomedical or technical information and the complex roles and relationships within which health behaviors are negotiated. Although global interpersonal communication theories are not context-specific, the attributes of the health context shape the application of theories. Interpersonal communication is relevant to behavior change in professional relationships, families, romantic relationships, and friendships. Context attributes should be considered when working to understand health behavior change within any of those contexts.

Because of its explicit connection to health, we focus in this chapter on the physician-patient context, which provides a rich illustration of the interplay between, on the one hand, the professional tasks of treating biomedical symptoms (or lack thereof) and, on the other hand, the relational goals of attending to the whole person and the breadth of the illness experience. We begin by describing relationship-centered health care that assumes a valid provider-patient partnership as the foundation for symptom reduction and behavior change, as well as prevention behaviors such as advice on smoking and physical activity. Yet the tasks of health care also involve a biomedical orientation, and changes in health behavior involve more than a good relationship with health care providers.

In this chapter, we will describe the historical development of concepts of interpersonal communication in health behavior (which embraces but also extends patient-centered health care), delineate the key task-driven functions of provider-patient interactions as parallel processes to relational functions, present evidence for communication predictors of health outcomes, and describe the pathways connecting communication and outcomes. We will also illustrate the key concepts and research by applying them in the contexts of physical disabilities and chronic pain.

Conceptualizing Health Care as Relationship Centered

Data from the National Cancer Institute's Health Information National Trends Survey (HINTS) reveal that physicians remain the most highly trusted source of health information; in contrast, trust in health information from the Internet has decreased over the last decade but the Internet is still a widely used source (Hesse, Moser, & Rutten, 2010). Health information found on the Internet might enhance patient self-efficacy about health care and health behavior, but this issue is quite complicated, given the range of information available, and the ease of searching for it online. Similarly, the organization and the delivery of health care have shifted drastically in the United States over the last two decades, with an explicit aspiration of focusing on achieving patient-centered outcomes in health care (i.e., improved biomedical and psychosocial health in accordance with patient preferences) (Institute of Medicine, 2001).

The foundations of relationship-centered care represent a fundamental shift from the traditional biomedical model of medicine that focused on pathology and physiology of disease, and also from the paternalistic model of Western medicine that saw the provider's role as gathering information and the patient's role as responding to questions. The biopsychosocial model explains illness in a much broader manner than the biomedical model; assumes a *whole person* approach, such that patients come to the interaction as experts in their own life world and illness experience; and also assumes that patient emotions, roles, and experiences are integral to negotiating treatment decisions.

Relationship-centered health care focuses on the primacy of patient autonomy, preferences, and well-being. Thus the model of relationship-centered care conceptually expands patient-centered care to include a philosophy of shared power between health care providers (usually physicians) and patients, and acknowledges the *mutual interplay* in communication between providers, patients, and patients' families (Beach, Inui, & the Relationship-Centered Care Research Network, 2006). Relationship-centered care validates the importance of relational processes, shared decision making, self-awareness, reciprocal processes, difference and diversity, and authentic and responsive participation in provider-patient relationships (Suchman, 2006). Relationship-centered care values the individual characteristics and concerns of patients, acknowledges the importance of affect and emotion, considers reciprocal influence processes, and places moral value on the formation and maintenance of genuine provider-patient relationships (Beach, Inui, et al., 2006).

Research and clinical work explicate the interconnection between a correct biomedical diagnosis and fully exploring the human element of providers' and patients' concerns, understanding, and expectations (Borrell-Carrio, Suchman, & Epstein, 2004). Relationship-centered care assumes that the interaction is co-created, such that the physician comes to a shared understanding of the patient's narrative through negotiated dialogue with the patient. Thus one of the central concerns is removing judgment and developing empathy that allows for care, trust, and openness in establishing solidarity with the patient and respect for his or her humanity (Borrell-Carrio, Suchman, & Epstein, 2004).

Although the concepts of relationship-centered care are philosophically embraced in medical education and practice, models of how relationship-centered care manifest in clinical settings are a work in progress. Medical education should address mindful practice (active awareness), integration of reflection into medical training, and communication skills training as core foundations for teaching relationship-centered care (Frankel, Eddins-Folensbee, & Inui, 2011). The ideals of relationship-centered care were considered radical not so long ago, but now have become a core component of quality recognized by the Institute of Medicine (2001). Nationally standardized evaluations of patient experiences are intended to allow experiences with health care providers to be publicly reported, although patients and medical institutions appear to value different quality criteria. The practical aspects of what it means to be relationship centered are less clear, and organizations struggle with actualizing and implementing the concepts.

Rapid technology developments can shift communication attributes, and technology can alter communication processes (also see Chapter Seventeen). For example, on the one hand, computer use in the exam room can amplify physicians' strong visit organization skills by offering a tool to explicitly address the confidentiality of the electronic medical record and a means of clarifying goals for the visit (Frankel et al., 2005). On the other hand, exam-room computing can also make poor visit organization skills more evident if physicians follow computer screen information instead of responding to patients' concerns and if patients' nonverbal cues are thereby displaced (Frankel et al., 2005). Providers inexperienced in using exam-room computers may be more adversely affected than experienced ones in addressing relational functions, as observed in their spending less time talking with, looking at, and examining the patient (Rouf, Whittle, Lu, & Schwartz, 2007). Use of e-mail in physician-patient communication can increase access, convenience, and timeliness of information exchange, but it can also add difficulty to encounters that would benefit from the sensory-rich relational orientation that interactive face-to-face encounters allow, such as making difficult decisions and breaking bad news (Ye, Rust, Fry-Johnson, & Strothers, 2010). If not used with adequate privacy safeguards, e-mail use can also threaten patient privacy and confidentiality. Use of e-mail varies widely, based on provider preferences, and whether conducting e-mail correspondence is billable time depends on the organization. Videoconferencing may result in interactions as satisfying as face-to-face ones, particularly when face-to-face interactions are limited by geographic access and resources (Agha, Roter, & Schapira, 2009). However, videoconferencing requires addressing potential concerns for patient privacy and trust.

Although the introduction of such technologies has posed unexpected challenges, these technologies have also demonstrated great promise in promoting access to health services, enhanced communications, and health outcomes. Integrating discussion boards and social technologies into clinical care appears to influence health decision making and patient self-care management (Wicks et al., 2012). Moreover, these technologies represent a rapidly moving force, and much will change in the next several years. There is increasing discussion about the potential of connecting patients and health care providers and data to enhance patients' engagement and activation. There is real potential to heighten the integration of patients into their own health and health care.

Once we recognize medical interactions as serving a relational function in addition to attending to the task of addressing symptoms, we are also better equipped to explicate the *meaning* of communication messages. In other words, we need to consider health and illness in a larger context, one that allows us to recognize and respond to the multiple functions of health care encounters. The goal of shaping health behavior poses implications for parallel, even competing, communication functions. Thus we move to a description of the key functions of provider-patient communication.

Key Functions of Provider-Patient Communication

Studies of provider-patient communication (most of which focus on physician providers) employ a variety of measures that range from a focus on observers measuring physicians' and patients' communication behaviors—in terms of, for example, frequency of physician information-giving, number of questions asked by patients, or ratings of degree of communication that is patient centered (Street, Gordon, Ward, Krupat, & Kravitz, 2005)—to patients' perceptions of clinicians' communications (McCormack et al., 2011; Street, 2013). Communication behaviors tied to outcomes are addressed by cross-sectional studies that show a relationship between communication and health behavior, but thorough explanations of the theoretical processes or pathways through which interpersonal communication leads to health outcomes call for further research.

To link interpersonal behaviors to health and behavioral outcomes, researchers must consider the key functions of physician-patient communication that could affect outcomes. These functions include the relational functions of fostering healing relationships and responding to emotions as well as the task-driven functions of making treatment decisions, exchanging information, and enabling (patient) self-management. The additional function of managing uncertainty involves managing uncertainty about treatment (task-driven) and about how illness shapes roles and relationships between patients, providers, and families (relational).

Relational Functions

Fostering Healing Provider-Patient Relationships

The provider-patient relationship can be characterized along two primary dimensions: control and affective orientation to one another (i.e., liking, affiliation, and friendliness). Early models of physician-patient relationships focused prescriptively on the importance of medical expertise in order to legitimize physician control, conceptualizing the health care interaction merely in terms of addressing biomedical concerns. The current model of relationship-centered care assumes that physicians and patients desire a relationship that is characterized by mutual trust, engagement, respect, and agreement on one another's roles in the relationship (Fuertes et al., 2007). Patients' trust is higher when patients perceive physicians as informative, respectful, emotionally supportive, and genuinely interested in the patient's views (Gordon, Street, Sharf, & Souchek, 2006). Similarly, a recent, systematic review of studies, with a specific focus on primary care patients' communication expectations, suggests that patients want their physicians to be friendly, respectful, interested, nonjudgmental, and sensitive, and to treat a patient as a person and as a partner (Deledda, Moretti, Rimondini, & Zimmerman, 2013). Discordance between patient and physician expectations can be subtle, and effective alignment of expectations depends on both parties openly discussing their preferences and the reasons underlying them so that they can establish mutually agreeable norms for the relationship (Epstein, 2006). Note that such discussions are not the norm, and their absence may leave unhealthy outcomes and behaviors unaddressed.

Strong provider-patient relationships are particularly important for patients because of the fear and worry associated with threats to health. Indicators of a strong therapeutic relationship include mutual trust, respect, and emotional support. These alliances are considered thera-peutic, because the quality of physician-patient (and family) relationships can affect health outcomes in two respects. First, strong relationships can directly promote emotional well-being through the patients' feeling known, cared for, and understood (Quirk et al., 2008). Second, strong physician-patient relationships can indirectly improve health through continuity of care, patient satisfaction, and commitment to treatment plans (Fuertes et al., 2007).

Validating and Responding to Emotions

Another important relational function of provider-patient communication is validating and responding to emotions. Patients' emotions indicate their human responses to illness and the challenges of coping. Patients who are diagnosed with or who worry about serious illness experience a range of emotions including fear, sadness, anxiety, frustration, and anger. Such negative emotional states can prompt concerns for health-related quality of life. However, physicians are typically not very effective at uncovering patients' fears and concerns, partly because patients often express their emotions implicitly rather than directly stating how they feel. Providers who miss opportunities to express empathy in response to patients' negative emotions, however, do not completely overlook the issue and sometimes do address the problem underlying the emotion (Hsu et al., 2012).

Physicians can attend to emotion in several ways. Providing clear and understandable disease-specific information may help patients achieve a greater sense of control, a feeling of hope, or better uncertainty management. Validating patients' emotional experiences and encouraging patients to express emotions may help to reduce patient anxiety and depression (Epstein et al., 2007). Behaviors associated with warmth and trust can facilitate information exchange, show interest in the patient, and indicate sensitivity to patient problems and feelings (Arora, 2003). Communication that enhances patient's self-confidence, sense of worth, and hope may confer meaning and motivation that encourages better quality of life despite the disease. In short, physician-patient communication can promote emotional well-being directly by validating patients' feelings, alleviating distress, and facilitating the patient's ability to cope with postconsultation stress, uncertainty, and setbacks, all of which may be associated with patients' physical symptoms.

Task-Driven Functions

Exchanging and Managing Information

Historically, research on physician-patient communication has addressed deficits in information exchange. For example, researchers have focused on patients' lack of health literacy and their dissatisfaction with the amount of information they receive from clinicians (Arora, 2003), and on physicians' lack of understanding of the patient's perspective. Culture, information avoidance, perceived stigma of illness, fear of treatment options, and organizational structures of care can also shape how health information is exchanged and managed (Street, 2013).

A more recent alternative is a process model of information exchange that focuses on the reciprocal efforts of both clinicians and patients to manage information and achieve, even negotiate, a shared understanding of the medical and personal issues underlying the patient's health condition (Kelly et al., 2013). Information exchange is more successful when patients participate actively to garner more and clearer information from physicians (Shepherd et al., 2011), when physicians use partnering and supportive communication to elicit the patient's beliefs and understandings (Street et al., 2005), and when physicians can explain risk and clinical evidence in ways patients understand (Hagerty et al., 2005). The information exchange process is further shaped by information sharing (or lack thereof, including intentional information avoidance) with family members, friends, and other relevant relationships beyond the physician.

Moreover, information is as much "managed" as it is "exchanged." Although patients say they want straightforward information (Quirk et al., 2008), information processing is complicated by individual situations and concerns, such as the emotional salience of some health information (Fallowfield & Jenkins, 2004) and the challenges of communicating health risks (Epstein, Alper, & Quill, 2004). In addition to individual concerns, other factors further complicate the exchange of information, including mismatch in literacy between providers and patients (Street, 2001). On a more positive note, successful information management can increase satisfaction (Puro, Pakarinen, Korttila, & Tallgren, 2013) and can increase the patient's ability to cope with illness (Hagerty et al., 2005).

The relationship of health care information exchange and outcomes involves more than simple recall of information. Achieving a shared understanding can be difficult, because physicians and patients often understand illness through different lenses. Patients' health beliefs are dynamic and complex. When physicians and patients understand one another's respective illness representations, they are in a better position to reconcile differences in viewpoints and come to some agreement on the patient's condition and options for treatment.

Making Treatment Decisions

Effective decision making is one of the most important and complicated aspects of provider-patient communication. Although the decision is about a task-driven decision, social relationships can help with the processing of complex information that otherwise could overwhelm patients' cognitive capacities (Epstein, 2013). Shared decision making addresses treatment options, risks and benefits, patient self-efficacy and preferences, patient expectations and understanding, and a plan for follow-up (Clayman, Makoul, Harper, Koby, & Williams, 2012). Although health care decisions can have profound effects on health outcomes, little is known about what constitutes a quality medical decision. At the very least, a good medical decision is one that the physician and patient mutually agree upon, through a decision process they are satisfied with; one that aligns with the patient's values and with the best available clinical evidence, and one that is feasible to implement (Epstein, 2013; Epstein & Street, 2007). Only recently have researchers tried to incorporate these criteria in developing measures of decision quality (Scholl, Kriston, Dirmaier, Buchholz, & Harter, 2012). Applying these criteria is essential given the importance of the patient-centered approach, particularly in making critical decisions with the active engagement of patients in the process (Barry & Edgman-Levitan, 2012). Also, patients vary greatly in their desire to be involved in medical decision making (Kenealy et al., 2011). Physicians' understanding and accommodation of patients' preferences for involvement is important because patients who believe their actual level of involvement in the consultation is congruent with their preferred level are more satisfied with their care and with the decision made (Lantz et al., 2005).

It is challenging to understand the nature and impact of patients' preferences for involvement, because prior research often fails to distinguish patient preferences for involvement in the process of decision making from the issue of who assumes responsibility for the decision. Many patients want to be actively involved in exchanging information about treatment possibilities and in deliberating on the pros, cons, and value of different treatment options (Elwyn et al., 2013). Yet these same patients may prefer not to assume responsibility for a decision. Thus a shared decision is not inherently a positive outcome of the decision-making process, although active patient participation in information exchange and deliberation is important because it helps physician and patient to achieve a shared understanding of the patient's condition and the best options for treatment. Not involving patients in decision making may also translate into missed opportunities to understand values or to clarify conflicting goals and needs.

Further, clinical evidence supporting particular treatment options may be complicated and even inconsistent. For example, different experts may give conflicting recommendations, forcing patients to choose among different sources of authority. Trust between physicians and patients may enhance decision-making preferences to maximize satisfaction and improve outcomes (Lee & Lin, 2011). Conversely, when physicians and patients cannot achieve a shared understanding of the risks and benefits associated with different treatment possibilities, a lower quality decision may occur, and the patient's choice for treatment may not be fully informed.

Enabling Patient Self-Management

Helping patients to manage their own health is an important but understudied function of communication that promotes individuals managing the symptoms and consequences of living with a chronic condition and of making health behavior changes, including treatment, physical, social, and lifestyle changes (McCorkle et al., 2011). Enabling patients' self-management extends information exchange to include recommendations, instructions, and advocacy. Physicians can enable patients' self-management by providing navigational help, supporting patient autonomy, and providing guidance and advice on better self-care.

Patients with long-term and chronic issues, such as disability and/or pain, must navigate a complex health care system to obtain care. Providing navigational help might include helping patients get follow-up testing, giving directions to specialists' offices, or coordinating care among specialists. Supporting patient autonomy involves bolstering patient self-efficacy and motivating patient control over health. Autonomy-supportive behaviors include exploring patients' ambivalence about taking action, providing alternative options to address goals, and giving patients time to consider choices rather than forcing a premature decision. Providing patients with guidance and advice can also help their self-management. Physicians can do this by giving instructions and recommendations that account for patients' concerns, by using nontechnical language, and by integrating opportunities to listen for whether or not patients understand and remember medical advice. Communication that encourages patients' autonomy and self-management is helpful with regard to lifestyle changes, including smoking cessation, weight loss, medication adherence, and exercise. Similarly, encouraging patient autonomy and self-management can improve success with effective self-management in chronic issues such as controlling blood pressure (Jones, Carson, Bleich, & Cooper, 2012).

Physician-patient communication may empower patients to be active, capable agents in managing their health. With ongoing improvements in detection and treatment, people are living longer with chronic illnesses. Self-management requires attending to a continuum of care, including early detection, diagnosis, treatment, behavior change, and survivorship. One self-management intervention showed decreased pain intensity after teaching patients to manage cancer pain and to communicate with the physician about unmet pain control (Miaskowski et al., 2004). Another intervention reduced symptom severity following use of an interactive, automated telephone response system and after a nurse-assisted symptom management protocol (Sikorskii et al., 2007). A third intervention, among women with early stage breast cancer, indicated significant improvements in mothers' depressed mood, anxiety, and self-confidence, and a significant decrease in children's behavioral problems, following a series of five educational counseling sessions to teach mothers to manage their own emotions, to observe and respond to their child's behavior, and to monitor and reflect on their own self-efficacy (Lewis, Casey, Brandt, Shands, & Zahlis, 2006).

These three interventions are among multiple interventions that address the process through which communication can enhance capacity for agency by empowering patients in clinical environments through active participation and increased control and problem solving about their health conditions. Although information about self-management is inherently oriented to health behavior tasks, co-constructing and navigating the process of patient self-care assumes a relationship characterized by continuity, mutuality, and trust. A recent description of this co-construction in an acupuncture application provides evidence of self-care talk that is initiated by both practitioner and patient and is interwoven with other types of talk (Paterson et al., 2012). Thus task-oriented goals, including self-management, are also inherently connected to relational functions. Promoting patient self-management involves addressing relational components connected to productive interactions and empowerment, as well as goal setting and negotiating a plan for achieving the goals (McCorkle et al., 2011).

Managing Uncertainty

Managing uncertainty involves a task-driven function of making meaning of medical information, also a relational function of navigating unpredictable emotions and also a lack of clarity about how roles and relationships connect to the illness experience. Uncertainty about illness occurs when the details of health situations are ambiguous, complex, unpredictable, or probabilistic, or when people feel insecure in their own state of knowledge or the state of knowledge in general (Babrow, 2001). Managing uncertainty is distinct from other communication functions, because providing information, offering emotional support, and making decisions do not necessarily reduce uncertainty. Uncertainty may be due to a lack of information ("Do I have diabetes?"), too much information ("There are so many options for treatment."), the wrong kind of information, or information that can be interpreted in multiple ways ("Is no change in tumor marker status a positive sign?") (Babrow, 2001). Patients might experience uncertainty about medical treatment at multiple treatment phases. Patient uncertainty about medical disclosure and consent can emerge from language issues, risks and hazards, the nature of the procedure, and the composition and format of the medical disclosure and consent form (Donovan-Kicken, Mackert, Guinn, Tollison, & Breckinridge, 2013).

Patients' experiences of uncertainty exacerbate emotional distress and may leave patients feeling a loss of control. Conversely, uncertainty also may have self-protective value for some patients and families by allowing them to have hope and optimism (Brashers, 2001). Thus uncertainty is best viewed as something to be managed rather than something to be reduced. Health care providers and patients encounter complexity and ambiguity in making decisions about diagnoses and treatment options. And that's especially true for conditions and diseases for which there is no accepted standard of care or for which patients might be offered a choice such as watchful waiting. Furthermore, illness uncertainty is multilayered, and it can exacerbate uncertainty about patients' roles and relationships. For example, questions about disease diagnosis might create uncertainty about financial well-being, about the stability of a romantic relationship, or about the social reactions of others. Challenges of information management, including relational demands (such as coordinating goals of multiple participants) and contextual features (such as cross-cultural interactions) also should be addressed in illness-related uncertainty (Brashers et al., 2003). Managing uncertainty involves understanding and responding to multiple, interrelated uncertainties rather than a single uncertainty.

Communication Predictors of Health Outcomes

Good communication is often associated with improved physical health, more effective chronic disease management, and better health-related quality of life long after the encounter (Arora, 2003). Nearly fifty years of research on provider-patient communication implicates the importance of communication in affecting health outcomes, but theoretical models that explicate key elements of effective communication or that explain *how* and *why* communication predicts health outcomes are sorely lacking (e.g., Street, 2013; World Health Organization, 2003).

Communication processes that predict health outcomes involve elements that occur during provider-patient interactions (e.g., shared decision making, patient self-advocacy, provider expressions of empathy, and mutual responsiveness), immediately after interactions (e.g., satisfaction, intention to follow health recommendations, knowledge), and weeks and months after the interaction (e.g., treatment adherence, self-efficacy, and symptom reduction) (Street, Makoul, Arora, & Epstein, 2009).

Satisfaction Patient satisfaction is influenced strongly by interpersonal processes that require cooperation and coordination between providers and patients (Duggan & Thompson, 2011; Hausman, 2004). Seminal work in this area linked pediatrician communication to mothers' satisfaction (Korsch, Gozzi, & Francis, 1968). Early research documented satisfaction as a valid indicator of both the subjective and objective quality of physicians' medical care. Visit satisfaction has become a focus of health care organizations' and medical schools' communication-training objectives to increase collaborative efforts. Satisfaction is correlated with longer visits, higher rapport, more psychosocial discussion, and fewer indications of physician dominance (Pieterse, van Dulmen, Beemer, Bensing, & Ausems, 2007). Satisfaction is not a static variable, as communication skills training for physicians and for patients can improve a patient's satisfaction with health care (Haskard et al., 2008). Satisfaction measures are also highly skewed toward positive responses, which likely means we have more issues to address than are seen on the surface.

Adherence A large proportion of patients do not follow through with, or adhere to, recommended behavior change or with medical treatment and, in fact, are reported to take only half of their prescribed doses (Nieuwlaat et al., 2014). Conceptualizing communication as a relational process sheds light on patient adherence with recommended treatment and behavior change. Research indicates that patients who perceive that their doctors know them as individuals, rather than just as patients, more consistently follow treatment recommendations and also experience better health (Beach, Keruly, & Moore, 2006). Adherence is also associated with collaboration with providers, with physicians demonstrating more warmth, openness, and interest (Fox et al., 2009) and engaging in more shared decision making with patients (Lakatos, 2009). More broadly, a recent meta-analysis across a body of individual research studies published over a sixty-year period indicates a 19 percent higher risk of nonadherence among patients whose physicians communicate poorly than among patients whose physicians communicate well (Zolnierek & DiMatteo, 2009).

Malpractice Provider communication can predict malpractice claims, again with evidence for relational functions in health care interactions. Instead of actual medical errors predicting litigation, satisfaction with communication is described as moderating the relationship between communication and litigation (Roter, 2006). Communication variables, including tone of voice, were found to most commonly determine medical malpractice lawsuits in an analysis of malpractice research from 1976 to 2003 (Vukmir, 2004). Other research indicates that doctors who are more dominant and less patient centered are most likely to be sued, although gender and ethnic factors moderate this relationship (Wissow, 2004). Similarly, collaboration among health care team members is described as negatively related to malpractice litigation (Hickson & Entman, 2008). Although these studies may be attractive to researchers and clinicians, we recommend interpreting the findings with caution, particularly in light of the correlational nature of the evidence and the major recent changes in organization and delivery of U.S. health care.

Pathways Between Provider-Patient Communication and Health Outcomes

Even with descriptive evidence connecting communication to health outcomes, theoretical explanations are lacking because the reasons *why* elements of clinician-patient interactions are associated with health outcomes are not well understood. As the goal of theory is to explain how and why behaviors predict health outcomes, researchers and practitioners in this area face a lofty challenge in coming years. In part, the lack of a cohesive theoretical framework reflects the reality that any number of cognitive, affective, behavioral, cultural, organizational, and even economic factors can moderate or mediate relationships between communication and subsequent health improvements. Consider two very different examples.

First, clinician-patient communication can help patients understand how to follow complex medication regimens. When they take their medication correctly, patients receive the chemical agents that can treat their diseases and improve their health. Alternately, in a second scenario, clinician-patient communication could affect motivational and cognitive processes underlying health-related behaviors such as stopping smoking, eating a healthy diet, and exercising. These processes might enhance patients' decision-making and problem-solving skills for adopting healthier lifestyles, which in turn could lead to better health. But if patients' social environments do not support these behavior changes, patients may experience barriers in spite of the quality of the clinician-patient encounter. In short, multiple pathways may explain the association between clinician-patient communication and health outcomes in the days, weeks, and months after the encounters.

Figure 13.1 offers a framework for identifying possible theoretical mechanisms that could account for provider-patient communication predicting health outcomes (Street et al., 2009; this framework is also described in the fourth edition of this book [Street & Epstein, 2008]). We have adapted the original model to group the key communication functions into relational and task categories. Provider-patient communication can affect health either directly or indirectly through the mediating effects of proximal outcomes (such as mutual understanding, trust, patient satisfaction, and patient involvement in decisions) and intermediate outcomes (such as changes in patient health behaviors, self-care skills, adherence to treatment, and medical decisions). For example, a physician can decrease emotional distress by providing supportive, empathetic, or confirming responses to patient cues of emotional concerns (Hsu et al., 2012).

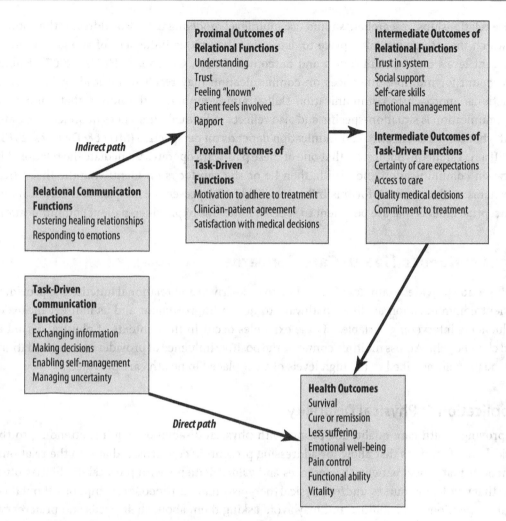

Figure 13.1 Direct and Indirect Pathways from Communication to Health Outcomes

Similarly, a physician can decrease a patient's worry by explaining why an abnormal diagnostic test result is still within the limits of acceptability.

In most situations, a more complex series of mechanisms link communication to health outcomes (Arora, 2003). Provider-patient communication characterized by information exchange perceived as effective and by positive affect can lead to greater patient trust (a proximal outcome) and a greater willingness to commit to treatment (an intermediate outcome), which in turn may affect survival. Patients' participation in encounters can help physicians understand patients' values and discover possible misperceptions about treatment effects. Physicians can then communicate clinical information in a way patients will understand (a proximal outcome) and, together with the patient, negotiate a higher quality decision that matches patients' circumstances (intermediate outcome) and leads to improved health.

Given the complex set of factors affecting physician-patient communication processes, the pathways through which communication achieves desired outcomes, and the moderators of these relationships, researchers should use multilevel modeling that also addresses the context in which the interaction takes place to determine the unique influences of various factors at different levels on communication and outcomes (Street, Gordon, & Haidet, 2007). Failure to account for multiple influences on communication may result in misleading findings. A functional approach to communication skills training embraces the notion that competent communication is situation-specific and also reflects individual differences in preferences, and that what counts as effective communication depends on perspective (Street & De Haes, 2013).

If a researcher hypothesizes that one of these pathways operates to mediate the relationship between communication and health, then he or she can focus on identifying the theoretical mechanisms that account for this influence. Table 13.1 presents examples of theoretical and conceptual models that are pertinent to specific functions of provider-patient communication.

Applications to Health Care Concerns

This section provides examples of attending to task-driven and relational functions of provider-patient communication as direct pathways to health improvement and as indirect means of influencing intervening variables. These examples occur in the contexts of physical disability and chronic pain. Across multiple contexts, the positive influence of provider recommendations can be partially ascribed to the high levels of trust placed in health care providers.

Application 1: Physical Disability

Improving health care quality for people with physical disabilities requires attending to the task-driven functions that allow for addressing presenting concerns and also to the relational functions that reflect patients' preferences and values. Patients with physical disabilities often find that physicians, nurses, and/or physical therapists make erroneous assumptions about their goals, aspirations, and abilities and may avoid asking them about their needs and preferences (Iezzoni, 2006). About fifty million Americans, spanning all ages, have some disability (Centers for Disease Control and Prevention, National Center for Health Statistics [CDC, NCHS], 2010), and they often encounter general practitioners as their first contact for health promotion and treatment and for social support. Individuals with disabilities are especially vulnerable to adverse health care experiences, ranging from short visits in which to address complex issues to sensory and cognitive communication barriers to limited financial resources to physically inaccessible care sites (CDC, NCHS, 2010).

Rather than working forward by measuring provider-patient communication features and then testing whether they lead to desired outcomes, Street (2013) recommends working *backward* by first identifying the outcome of interest and the mechanism for improved health and then modeling a pathway through which communication and proximal outcomes can be measured. Although this is a long-accepted approach in health education, the inherent disconnects among communication functions in provider-patient interactions means health outcomes may not be the primary goal, especially if the health goal is in conflict with a relational goal. Much of the literature on provider-patient interactions provides rich qualitative

Table 13.1   Representative Models of Patient-Centered Communication Functions

Communication Function	Theoretical or Conceptual Models	Key Theme
Relational communication function		
Fostering healing relationships	Four types of physician-patient relationships (Roter & Hall, 1992)	Paternalism: high physician control, low patient control. Mutuality: high physician and patient control. Default: low physician and patient control. Consumerism: low physician control, high patient control.
	Model of relational topoi (Burgoon, Buller, Hale, & deTurck, 1984)	Identifies 12 dimensions of relational communication: dominance-submission, intimacy, affection-hostility, involvement, inclusion-exclusion, trust, depth, emotional arousal, composure, similarity, formality, and task-social orientation.
Responding to emotions	Model of relational topoi (Burgoon et al., 1984)	Identifies 4 dimensions of relational communication that focus on emotional communication: intimacy, affection-hostility, emotional arousal, and composure.
	Model of empathic understanding (Squier, 1990)	Posits that empathic understanding is a function of perspective-taking skill and emotional reactivity and that better understanding of a patient's health problems will be achieved through self-disclosure, open communication, and better labeling of feelings and sensations.
Task-driven communication function		
Exchanging and managing information	Cognitive model (Ley, 1988)	Hypothesizes that (1) patient understanding of medical information enhances memory, (2) memory and understanding increase patient satisfaction, and (3) satisfaction increases compliance.
Making treatment decisions	Linguistic model of patient participation in care (Street, 2001)	Posits that patient participation in consultations, including decision-making processes, is a function of predisposing factors (e.g., motivation, beliefs about patient involvement), enabling factors (e.g., knowledge, communication skills), and provider behavior (e.g., partnership building).
	Integrative model of shared decision making (Makoul & Clayman, 2006)	Identifies 9 degrees of *sharedness* in medical decision making: doctor alone, doctor-led and patient acknowledgment, doctor-led and patient agreement, doctor-led and patient views or opinions, shared equally, patient-led and doctor's views or opinions, patient-led and doctor agreement, patient-led and doctor acknowledgment, patient alone.

(continued)

Table 13.1   (Continued)

Communication Function	Theoretical or Conceptual Models	Key Theme
Enabling patient self-management	Self-determination theory (Ryan & Deci, 2000)	Posits that human behavior is driven to meet three basic needs—competence, autonomy, and relatedness.
	Transtheoretical Model (Prochaska & Velicer, 1997)	Posits that behavior change is on a continuum ranging from precontemplation to contemplation, preparation, action, maintenance, and termination.
	Integrated Behavioral Model (Fishbein & Cappella, 2006)	Posits that health behavior is a function of attitudes, social norms, and self-efficacy, which emanate from behavioral, normative, and control beliefs.
	Self-management chronic care model (McCorkle et al., 2011)	Identifies a cycle for patient agency: patient-provider partnerships, productive interactions, mutually defined care plan, goal setting, self-management interventions, and goal attainment.
Managing uncertainty	Mishel's uncertainty theory (Mishel, 1999)	Posits that uncertainty is experienced when aspects of the illness, treatment, and recovery are perceived as inconsistent, random, complex, and unpredictable.
	Problematic integration theory (Babrow, 2001)	Posits that discrepancies between the likelihood of certain events and the value of those events create four kinds of problematic cognitive states: divergence (difference between what is desired and what is likely), ambiguity (uncertainty about the likelihood of an event), ambivalence (uncertainty about the value of an event), and impossibility (certainty that an event will not happen).
	Uncertainty management theory (Brashers, 2001)	Posits that the management of uncertainty involves multiple options ranging from efforts to reduce the uncertainty (e.g., to alleviate anxiety) to efforts to maintain or create uncertainty (e.g., to have hope).

descriptions that allow an understanding of the ways in which the particular illness context shapes communication pathways and outcomes.

For example, Duggan, Bradshaw, and Altman (2010) videotaped standardized patient educators with physical disabilities. (Standardized patient educators are individuals who play the roles of patients in order to provide a consistent learning experience for medical students around a particular health context.) These standardized patient educators had mobility restrictions (they used a wheelchair or crutches) and presented an initial concern with shoulder pain. The medical students were told that the patient should be diagnosed with shoulder tendonitis, which is an overuse injury; the students were supposed to connect the repetitive motion of using a wheelchair or crutches for mobility with the shoulder tendonitis. In attending to the pain issue, the provider's direct path includes the task-driven function of making decisions about pain control, which can include negotiations about resting the shoulder and taking ibuprofen. The patient with this disability might indicate that he or she is worried about resting the shoulder, which could indicate that functional ability and vitality are additional important outcomes to address. Probing further, the provider might find that the patient expresses fear that resting the shoulder will make him or her more reliant on others for mobility, thus limiting independence. Functional ability is connected to enabling self-management and responding to emotion, or may be modeled indirectly through rapport and trust to involve the patient in a quality decision that includes physical therapy. Communicating about the latter might involve attending to concerns about getting to and from the physical therapist's office (access to care). Additional indirect pathways might include addressing the motion necessary for the patient's daily work and for activities of daily living (including such things as transferring to and from a wheelchair). The person with the disability might also be concerned about being seen as a care recipient. Able-bodied health care providers in encounters with people with disabilities may build trust, rapport, and satisfaction by responding to the many individual features of the person, rather than assuming the limitation is central to the identity of the person (Duggan, Robinson, & Thompson, 2012).

A thorough response to a person with a disability whose presenting concern is shoulder tendonitis includes both the relational functions and the task-driven functions and attends to the subtleties of disclosure. For example, in this study, medical students who reciprocated patient language for naming the disability and acknowledged the patient's expertise in the disability could foster a healing relationship. Responsiveness to the patient's subtle cues about worry that the shoulder pain could interfere with intimacy could validate his or her fears in this area (Duggan et al., 2010). We describe these contexts to illustrate the complexity of the multiple facets to be considered and also to illustrate how multiple functions in context constitute a necessary set of considerations for theory building.

Application 2: Chronic Pain

Pain is one of the most pervasive problems in primary care. Pain affects more Americans than diabetes, heart disease, and cancer combined, and results in increased health care costs, rehabilitation costs, lost worker productivity, and emotional and financial burdens for patients and their families. Unrelieved pain can result in longer hospital stays, increased rates of rehospitalization, increased outpatient visits, and decreased ability to function fully, leading to lost income and insurance coverage (Institute of Medicine, 2011). The common types of pain include low back pain, severe headache or migraine pain, neck pain, shoulder pain, knee pain, and hip pain; most people in chronic pain have multiple sites of pain (Institute of Medicine, 2011). Pain shapes quality of life, decreasing people's overall enjoyment of life, increasing their feelings of depression, and often resulting in difficulty concentrating, low energy, and inability to sleep well (Institute of Medicine, 2011). Addressing both task functions and relational functions involves fostering a healing relationship that allows for trust that encompasses full and honest disclosure. Again working backward, addressing the health outcome of pain control might involve the physician changing the patient's pain management regimen. One possibility would be having patients communicate more openly about their pain-related concerns and questions, which in turn could be the direct result of an intervention designed to increase patient activation (Street, 2013). Trust in the system could be improved through an indirect path by making the patient feeling known, which could involve validating and managing emotions by uncovering patients' fears and concerns, which may include fear and sadness about the possibility that the pain will not go away. Another potential indirect pathway involves recognizing the sources of pain that may be measured not as biomedical markers but instead in terms of their connections to the related *lifeworld* (i.e., mood, appetite, sleep, concentration). Thus commitment to treatment could be, again, mediated by feeling known, and best addressed by fostering a relationship with the patient and enabling self-management to address the lifeworld.

A lay-administered tailored education and coaching intervention aimed at reducing pain misconceptions and enhancing self-efficacy for communicating with physicians tested the effectiveness of these principles (Kravitz et al., 2011). The tailored education and coaching intervention was associated with increased pain communication self-efficacy after the intervention, as well as reductions in pain misconceptions. Two weeks after the intervention, the tailored education and coaching group showed improvements in pain-related impairment, but not in pain severity, compared to the control group that received usual care (Kravitz et al., 2011).

Consistent with overall descriptions of the reciprocal influence of physicians, patients, and family members, the relatively small benefit derived from this intervention and other psycho-educational programs suggests that patient- and family-centered programs alone are insufficient to produce robust, sustained improvements in pain outcomes. Multilevel interventions are likely to be more effective but are also more costly. Identifying patient subgroups that have the greatest need and are most likely to benefit and targeting interventions to groups with the highest need could increase the health benefits for vulnerable populations.

Directions for Future Research

The conceptual framework offered in this chapter has important implications for future research on provider-patient communication. Although we focused our analysis on lessons learned from the provider-patient context, other interpersonal contexts, such as social influence within families, social support within friendships, and shared decision making within romantic relationships, provide similarly rich and robust areas of consideration for multiple and competing communication functions. As illustrated in this chapter in the examples of provider-patient communication, understanding theoretical processes for health behavior change requires in-depth consideration of the communication functions of interpersonal relationships. Family relationships bring a whole host of attributes that shape the development and application of health behavior change theories. Close relationships, friendships, and everyday interpersonal encounters all pose their own sets of attributes that shape the interactions and the receptivity and progression of health behavior change. Like the provider-patient context, other interpersonal interactions are at their core concerned with the development and maintenance of roles and relationships, such that multiple communication functions must be considered in order to make sense of health behavior change.

As mentioned at the outset, researchers should be guided by or develop theoretical models linking the communication process to health outcomes. We have identified key relational and task-driven communication functions as well as potential pathways to improved health. To test the importance of these functions along particular pathways, researchers should develop measures that tap into these key processes. Longitudinal studies are needed to track outcomes, following the interactions and events that occur along the pathways that can affect communication-outcome relationships. Studies of patients' experiences over time may best be completed using designs of physicians nested within patients, the opposite of the traditional "patient-nested-within-clinician" design used in most physician-patient communication studies. Longitudinal studies are rare, likely due to their expense and complexity, but are greatly needed.

Similarly, health care interactions are inherently tied to roles and relationships outside provider-patient encounters. Efforts to change health behavior ideally should address and explain the host of variables found both within these encounters and in everyday life. Future research should consider contexts and extrinsic moderators of communication-outcome associations. This means accounting for multiple layers of organizational, political, geographic, and media contexts that can affect provider-patient communication (Street, 2003). While any number of contextual elements may influence health care, three particularly important aspects of context are the family and social environment, the media environment, and the health care system. For example, family and friends can either reinforce or undermine decisions reached by physicians and patients, and thus affect adherence and health behaviors. Even the best medical decision, in terms of physician-patient agreement and the clinical evidence, may be for naught if family and friends fail to support it. Family members' presence during clinical encounters can facilitate the provider-patient interaction or can interfere with that communication, thus shaping communication functions. Media coverage of a health issue can influence patients' beliefs and expectations, especially when the media reach a large audience. Finally, the media environment, and the Internet in particular, offers extensive resources for health-related information and social support. Patients may benefit, at least in theory, from this information by understanding their conditions and treatment expectations better and participating more effectively in medical interactions (Hesse et al., 2010; Street, 2003). Patients also may receive information and support through online support groups, including those that are disease-specific. However, both lay support groups and other Internet-based information sources may vary in their scientific accuracy and present challenges for patients as they try to identify the most accurate and useful information for their needs.

Summary

Models of provider-patient communication should be simple enough to be understandable and to guide empirical research yet complex enough to approximate clinical reality. We have proposed a model of pathways linking provider-patient communication to health outcomes, and we have identified six communication functions that are key to promoting improved health outcomes: establishing and maintaining the physician-patient relationship, exchanging and managing information, validating and responding to emotions, managing uncertainty, making treatment decisions, and enabling patient self-management. The pathways through which effective communication leads to better health outcomes include improved patient knowledge and shared understanding, improved access to care, improved therapeutic alliances among health professionals and patients or their families, improved management of negative emotions, stronger family and social support, improved quality of medical decisions, and improved patient agency.

Studies of moderators of the relationship between communication and proximal, intermediate, and health and societal outcomes suggest that relationship factors should be studied in greater depth. Furthermore, underlying and modifiable moderating factors may affect communication-outcome relationships. These factors include health literacy, social distance between physician and patient, physician attitudes toward patients, and physician (or other provider) and patient preferences for their roles in the interaction, as well as a number of extrinsic moderators embedded in the context of medical encounters. Future research should use more theoretically, methodologically, and ecologically sound research designs to better understand linkages between good provider-patient communication and improved health.

References

Ackerson, L. K., & Viswanath, K. (2009). The social context of interpersonal communication and health. *Journal of Health Communication, 14*(Suppl. 1), 5–17.

Agha, Z., Roter, D. L., & Schapira, R. M. (2009). An evaluation of patient-physician communication style during telemedicine consultations. *Journal of Medical Internet Research, 11*(3), e36.

Arora, N. K. (2003). Interacting with cancer patients: The significance of physicians' communication behavior. *Social Science & Medicine, 57*(5), 791–806.

Babrow, A. S. (2001). Uncertainty, value, communication, and problematic integration. *Journal of Communication, 51*(3), 553–573.

Barry, M. J., & Edgman-Levitan, S. (2012). Shared decision making—pinnacle of patient-centered care. *New England Journal of Medicine, 366*(9), 780–781.

Beach, M. C., Inui, T., & the Relationship-Centered Care Research Network. (2006). Relationship-centered care: A constructive reframing. *Journal of General Internal Medicine, 21*(Suppl. 1), S3–S8.

Beach, M. C., Keruly, J., & Moore, R. D. (2006). Is the quality of the patient-provider relationship associated with better adherence and improved health outcomes for patients with HIV? *Journal of General Internal Medicine, 21*(6), 661–665.

Borrell-Carrio, F., Suchman, A. L., & Epstein, R. M. (2004). The biopsychosocial model 25 years later: Principles, practice, and scientific inquiry. *Annals of Family Medicine, 2*(6), 576–582.

Brashers, D. E. (2001). Communication and uncertainty management. *Journal of Communication, 51*(3), 477–497.

Brashers, D. E., Neidig, J. L., Russell, J. A., Cardillo, L. W., Haas, S. M., Dobbs, L. K., . . . Nemeth, S. (2003). The medical, personal, and social causes of uncertainty in HIV illness. *Issues in Mental Health Nursing, 24*(5), 497–522.

Burgoon, J. K., Buller, D. B., Hale, J. L., & deTurck, M. A. (1984). Relational messages associated with nonverbal behaviors. *Human Communication Research*, *10*(3), 351–378.

Centers for Disease Control and Prevention, National Center for Health Statistics. (2010). *DATA 2010*. Hyattsville, MD: Author. Retrieved from http://wonder.cdc.gov/data2010/focus.htm

Clayman, M. L., Makoul, G., Harper, M. M., Koby, D. G., & Williams, A. R. (2012). Development of a shared decision making coding system for analysis of patient-healthcare provider encounters. *Patient Education and Counseling*, *88*(3), 367–372.

Deledda, G., Moretti, F., Rimondini, M., & Zimmerman, C. (2013). How patients want their doctor to communicate: A literature review on primary care patients' perspective. *Patient Education and Counseling*, *90*(3), 297–306.

Donovan-Kicken, E., Mackert, M., Guinn, T. D., Tollison, A. C., & Breckinridge, B. (2013). Sources of patient uncertainty when reviewing medical disclosure and consent documentation. *Patient Education and Counseling*, *90*(2), 254–260.

Duggan, A. P., Bradshaw, Y. S., & Altman, W. (2010). How do I ask about your disability? An examination of interpersonal communication processes between medical students and patients with disabilities. *Journal of Health Communication*, *15*(3), 334–350.

Duggan, A. P., Robinson, J. D., & Thompson, T. L. (2012). Understanding disability as an intergroup encounter. In H. Giles (Ed.), *The handbook of intergroup communication* (pp. 250–263). New York: Routledge.

Duggan, A. P., & Thompson, T. L. (2011). Provider-patient communication and health outcomes. In T. L. Thompson, R. L. Parrott, & J. Nussbaum (Eds.), *The handbook of health communication* (2nd ed., pp. 414–427). New York: Routledge.

Elwyn, G., Lloyd, A., Joseph-Williams, N., Cording, E., Thomson, E., Durand, M., & Edwards, A. (2013). Options grids: Shared decision making made easier. *Patient Education and Counseling*, *90*(2), 207–212.

Epstein, R. M. (2006). Making communication research matter: What do patients notice, what do patients want, and what do patients need? *Patient Education and Counseling*, *60*(3), 272–278.

Epstein, R. M. (2013). Whole mind and shared mind in clinical decision-making. *Patient Education and Counseling*, *90*(2), 200–206.

Epstein, R. M., Alper, B. S., & Quill, T. E. (2004). Communicating evidence for participatory decision making. *JAMA*, *291*(19), 2359–2366.

Epstein, R. M., Shields, C. G., Franks, P., Meldrum, S. C., Feldman, M., & Kravitz, R. L. (2007). Exploring and validating patient concerns: Relation to prescribing for depression. *Annals of Family Medicine*, *5*(1), 21–28.

Epstein, R. M., & Street, R. L., Jr. (2007). *Patient-centered communication in cancer care: Promoting healing and reducing suffering*. Bethesda, MD: National Cancer Institute.

Fallowfield, L., & Jenkins, V. (2004). Communicating sad, bad, and difficult news in medicine. *Lancet*, *363*(9405), 312–319.

Fishbein, M., & Cappella, J. N. (2006). The role of theory in developing effective health communications. *Journal of Communication*, *56*, S1–S17.

Fox, S. A., Heritage, J., Stockdale, S. E., Asch, S. M., Duan, N., & Reise, S. P. (2009). Cancer screening adherence: Does physician-patient communication matter? *Patient Education and Counseling*, *75*(2), 178–184.

Frankel, R., Altschuler, A., George, S., Kinsman, J., Jimison, H., Robertson, N. R., & Hsu, J. (2005). Effects of exam-room computing on clinician-patient communication: A longitudinal qualitative study. *Journal of General Internal Medicine, 20*(8), 677–682.

Frankel, R. M., Eddins-Folensbee, F., & Inui, T. S. (2011). Crossing the patient-centered divide: Transforming health care quality through enhanced faculty development. *Academic Medicine, 86*(4), 445–452.

Fuertes, J. N., Mislowack, A., Bennett, J., Paul, L., Gilbert, T. C., Fontan, G., & Boylan, L. S. (2007). The physician-patient working alliance. *Patient Education and Counseling, 66*(1), 29–36.

Gordon, H. S., Street, R. L., Jr., Sharf, B. F., & Souchek, J. (2006). Racial differences in doctors' information-giving and patients' participation. *Cancer, 107*(6), 1313–1320.

Hagerty, R. G., Butow, P. N., Ellis, P. M., Lobb, E. A., Pendlebury, S. C., Leighl, N., . . . Tattersall, M.H.N. (2005). Communicating with realism and hope: Incurable cancer patients' views on the disclosure of prognosis. *Journal of Clinical Oncology, 23*(6), 1278–1288.

Haskard, K. B., Williams, S. L., DiMatteo, R. M., Rosenthal, R., White, M. K., & Goldstein, M. G. (2008). Physician and patient communication training in primary care: Effects on participation and satisfaction. *Health Psychology, 27*(5), 513–522.

Hausman, A. (2004). Modeling the patient-physician service encounter: Improving patient outcomes. *Journal of the Academy of Marketing Science, 32*(4), 403–417.

Hesse, B. W., Moser, R. P., & Rutten, L. J. (2010). Survey of physicians and electronic health information. *New England Journal of Medicine, 362*(9), 859–861.

Hickson, G. B., & Entman, S. S. (2008). Physician behavior and litigation risk: Evidence and opportunity. *Clinical Obstetrics & Gynecology, 51*(4), 688–699.

Hsu, I., Korthuis, P. T., Sharp, V., Cohn, J., Moore, R. D., & Beach, M. C. (2012). Providing support to patients in emotional encounters: A new perspective on missed empathetic opportunities. *Patient Education and Counseling, 88*(3), 436–442.

Iezzoni, L. I. (2006). Make no assumptions: Communication between persons with disabilities and clinicians. *Assistive Technology, 18*(2), 212–219.

Institute of Medicine. (2001). *Crossing the quality chasm: A new health system for the 21st century.* Washington, DC: National Academies Press.

Institute of Medicine. (2011). *Relieving pain in America: A blueprint for transforming prevention, care, education, and research.* Washington, DC: National Academies Press.

Jones, D. E., Carson, K. A., Bleich, S. N., & Cooper, L. A. (2012). Patient trust in physicians and adoption of lifestyle behaviors to control high blood pressure. *Patient Education and Counseling, 89*(1), 57–62.

Kelly, K. M., Ajmera, M., Bhattacharjee, S., Vohra, R., Hobbs, G., Chaudhary, L., . . . Agnese, D. (2013). Perception of cancer recurrence risk: More information is better. *Patient Education and Counseling, 90*(3), 361–366.

Kenealy, T., Goodyear-Smith, F., Wells, S., Arroll, B., Jackson, R., & Horsburgh, M. (2011). Patient preference for autonomy: Does it change as risk rises? *Family Practice, 28*(5), 541–544.

Korsch, B. M., Gozzi, E. K., & Francis, V. (1968). Gaps in doctor-patient communication. *Pediatrics, 42*(5), 855–871.

Kravitz, R. L., Tancredi, D. J., Grennan T., Kalauokalani, D., Street, R. L., Jr., Slee, C. K., . . . Franks, P. (2011). Cancer health empowerment for living without pain (Ca-HELP): Effects of a tailored education and coaching intervention on pain and impairment. *Pain, 152*(7), 1572–1582.

Lakatos, P. L. (2009). Prevalence, predictors, and clinical consequences of medical adherence in IBD: How to improve it? *World Journal of Gastroenterology, 15*(34), 4234–4239.

Lantz, P. M., Janz, N. K., Fagerlin, A., Schwartz, K., Liu, L., Lakhani, I., . . . Katz, S. J. (2005). Satisfaction with surgery outcomes and the decision process in a population-based sample of women with breast cancer. *Health Services Research, 40*(3), 745–767.

Lee, Y., & Lin, J. L. (2011). How much does trust really matter? A study of the longitudinal effects of trust and decision-making preferences on diabetic patient outcomes. *Patient Education and Counseling, 85*(3), 406–412.

Lewis, F. M., Casey, S. M., Brandt, P. A., Shands, M. E., & Zahlis, E. H. (2006). The enhancing connections program: Pilot study of a cognitive-behavioral intervention for mothers and children affected by breast cancer. *Psycho-Oncology, 15*(6), 486–497.

Ley, P. (1988). *Communicating with patients: Improving communication, satisfaction, and compliance.* London: Croom Helm.

Makoul, G., & Clayman, M. L. (2006). An integrative model of shared decision making in medical encounters. *Patient Education and Counseling, 60*(3), 301–312.

McCorkle, R., Ercolano, E., Lazenby, M., Shulman-Green, D., Shilling, L. S., Lorig, K., & Wagner, E. H. (2011). Self-management: Enabling and empowering patients living with cancer as a chronic illness. *CA: A Cancer Journal for Clinicians, 61*(1), 50–62.

McCormack, L. A., Treiman, K., Rupert, D., Williams-Piehota, P., Nadler, E., Arora, N. K., . . . Street, R. L., Jr. (2011). Measuring patient-centered communication in cancer care: A literature review and the development of a systematic approach. *Social Science & Medicine, 72*(7), 1085–1095.

Miaskowski, C., Dodd, M., West, C., Schumacher, K., Paul, S. M., Tripathy, D., & Koo, P. (2004). Randomized clinical trial of the effectiveness of a self-care intervention to improve cancer pain management. *Journal of Clinical Oncology, 22*(9), 1713–1720.

Mishel, M. H. (1999). Uncertainty in chronic illness. *Annual Review of Nursing Research, 17*, 269–294.

Nieuwlaat, R., Wilczynski, N., Navarro, T., Hobson, N., Jeffery, R., Keepanasseril, A., . . . Haynes, R. B. (2014, November 20). Interventions for enhancing medication adherence. *Cochrane Database of Systematic Reviews, 2014*(11), CD000011.

Paterson, C., Evans, M., Bertschinger, R., Chapman, R., Norton, R., & Robinson, J. (2012). Communication about self-care in traditional acupuncture consultations: The co-construction of individualized support and advice. *Patient Education and Counseling, 89*(3), 467–475.

Pieterse, A. H., van Dulmen, A. M., Beemer, F. A., Bensing, J. M., & Ausems, M. G. (2007). Cancer genetic counseling: Communication and counselees' post-visit satisfaction, cognitions, anxiety, and needs fulfillment. *Journal of Genetic Counseling, 16*(1), 85–96.

Prochaska, J. O., & Velicer, W. F. (1997). The transtheoretical model of health behavior change. *American Journal of Health Promotion, 12*(1), 38–48.

Puro, H., Pakarinen, P., Korttila, K., & Tallgren, M. (2013). Verbal information about anesthesia before scheduled surgery—content and patient satisfaction. *Patient Education and Counseling, 90*(3), 367–371.

Quirk, M., Mazor, K., Haley, H. L., Philbin, M., Fischer, M., Sullivan, K., & Hatem, D. (2008). How patients perceive a doctor's caring attitude. *Patient Education and Counseling, 72*(3), 359–366.

Roter, D. (2006). The patient-physician relationship and its implications for malpractice litigation. *Journal of Health Care Law and Policy, 9*(2), 304–314.

Roter, D., & Hall, J. A. (1992). *Doctors talking to patients/patients talking to doctors: Improving communication in medical visits*. Westport, CT: Auburn House.

Rouf, E., Whittle, J., Lu, N., & Schwartz, M. D. (2007). Computers in the exam room: Differences in physician-patient interaction may be due to physician experience. *Journal of General Internal Medicine, 22*(1), 43–48.

Ryan, R. M., & Deci, E. L. (2000). Self-determination theory and the facilitation of intrinsic motivation, social development, and well-being. *American Psychologist, 55*(1), 68–78.

Scholl, I., Kriston, L, Dirmaier, J., Buchholz, A., & Harter, M. (2012). Development and psychometric properties of the shared decision making questionnaire (SDM-Q-Doc). *Patient Education and Counseling, 88*(2), 284–290.

Shepherd, H. L., Barratt, A., Trevena, L. J., McGeechan, K., Carey, K., Epstein, R. M., . . . Tattersall, M.H.N. (2011). Three questions that patients can ask to improve the quality of information physicians give about treatment options: A cross-over trial. *Patient Education and Counseling, 84*(3), 379–385.

Sikorskii, A., Given, C. W., Given, B., Jeon, S., Decker, V., Decker, D., . . . McCorkle, R. (2007). Symptom management for cancer patients: A trial comparing two multimodal interventions. *Journal of Pain Symptom Management, 34*(3), 253–264.

Squier, R. S. (1990). A model of empathic understanding and adherence to treatment regimens in practitioner-patient relationships. *Social Science & Medicine, 30*(3), 325–329.

Street, R. L., Jr. (2001). Active patients as powerful communicators. In W. P. Robinson & H. Giles (Eds.), *The new handbook of language and social psychology* (pp. 541–560). New York: Wiley.

Street, R. L., Jr. (2003). Mediated consumer-provider communication in cancer care: The empowering potential of new technologies. *Patient Education and Counseling, 50*(1), 99–104.

Street, R. L., Jr. (2013). How clinician-patient communication contributes to health improvement: Modeling pathways from talk to outcome. *Patient Education and Counseling, 92*(3), 286–291.

Street, R. L., Jr., & De Haes, H. C. (2013). Designing a curriculum for communication skills training from a theory and evidence-based perspective. *Patient Education and Counseling, 93*(1), 27–33.

Street, R. L., Jr., & Epstein, R. M. (2008). Key interpersonal functions and health outcomes: Lessons from theory and research on clinician-patient communication. In K. Glanz, B. K. Rimer, & K. Viswanath (Eds.), *Health behavior and health education: Theory, research, and practice* (4th ed., pp. 237–269). San Francisco: Jossey-Bass.

Street, R. L., Jr., Gordon, H., & Haidet, P. (2007). Physicians' communication and perceptions of patients: Is it how they look, how they talk, or is it just the doctor? *Social Science & Medicine, 65*(3), 586–598.

Street, R. L., Jr., Gordon, H. S., Ward, M. M., Krupat, E., & Kravitz, R. L. (2005). Patient participation in medical consultations: Why some patients are more involved than others. *Medical Care, 43*(10), 960–969.

Street, R. L., Jr., Makoul, G., Arora, N. K., & Epstein, R. M. (2009). How does communication heal? Pathways linking clinician-patient communication to health outcomes. *Patient Education and Counseling, 74*(3), 295–301.

Suchman, A. L. (2006). A new theoretical foundation for relationship-centered care: Complex responsive processes of relating. *Journal of General Internal Medicine, 21*(Suppl. 1), S40–S44.

Thompson, T. L., Parrott, R. L., & Nussbaum, J. (Eds.). (2011). *The Routledge handbook of health communication* (2nd ed.). New York: Routledge.

Vangelisti, A. (Ed.). (2013). *The Routledge handbook of family communication*. New York: Routledge.

Vukmir, R. B. (2004). Medical malpractice: Managing the risk. *Medicine and Law, 23*(3), 495–513.

Wicks, P., Keininger, D. L., Massagli, M. P., de la Loge, C., Brownstein, C., Isojärvi, J., & Heywood, J. (2012). Perceived benefits of sharing health data between people with epilepsy on an online platform. *Epilepsy and Behavior, 23*(1), 16–23.

Wissow, L. S. (2004). Patient communication and malpractice: Where are we now? *Patient Education & Counseling, 52*(1), 3–5.

World Health Organization. (2003). *Adherence to long-term therapies: Evidence for action.* Geneva: Author.

Ye, J., Rust, G., Fry-Johnson, Y., & Strothers, H. (2010). E-mail in patient-provider communication: A systematic review. *Patient Education and Counseling, 80*(2), 266–273.

Zolnierek, K., & DiMatteo, R. (2009). Physician communication and patient adherence to treatment: A meta-analysis. *Medical Care, 47*(8), 826–834.

PART FOUR

COMMUNITY AND GROUP MODELS OF HEALTH BEHAVIOR CHANGE

CHAPTER 14

INTRODUCTION TO COMMUNITY AND GROUP MODELS OF HEALTH BEHAVIOR CHANGE

Karen Glanz
Alice Ammerman

An understanding of the functioning of groups, organizations, large social institutions, and communities is vital to health enhancement. Designing health behavior and policy, systems, and environmental (PSE) change initiatives to benefit communities and populations is at the heart of a public health orientation (Brownson, Haire-Joshu, & Luke, 2006; Glanz & Bishop 2010; Smedley & Syme, 2000). The collective well-being of communities can be fostered by creating structures and policies that support healthy lifestyles, by reducing or eliminating health constraints in the social and physical environments, and by communication through a range of media. All these approaches require an understanding of how social systems operate, how change occurs within and among communities and organizations, and how ideas and information spread, including through the Internet and social media.

The chapters in Part Four present three theoretically informed approaches to creating and supporting health behavior change through groups, organizations, communities, and social systems. The aim of these chapters is to demonstrate the utility and promise of a variety of theories and frameworks in health behavior and health behavior change.

In Chapter Fifteen, Wallerstein and colleagues provide an up-to-date overview of principles and methods of community engagement for health improvement, including community organization and community building, coalitions and partnerships, and community-based participatory research (CBPR). They discuss the concept of community and the main theoretical and conceptual bases of community engagement, processes, and models for community organization and building for health. They also discuss measurement and evaluation issues and describe a case study of community organizing and capacity building, coalition building, and CBPR with immigrant restaurant workers in San Francisco's Chinatown.

In Chapter Sixteen, Brownson and coauthors address implementation, dissemination, and diffusion of public health interventions as an approach to enhancing the longer-term impact of community and group interventions. They focus on the importance of and strategies for the implementation and dissemination of evidence-based interventions to improve health. This chapter provides key terminology for a rapidly evolving area of inquiry and practice, and describes two models—Diffusion of Innovations and the Consolidated Framework for Implementation Research (CFIR)—in detail. This chapter gives examples of applications of these models and illustrates components that cut across individual, organizational, and societal levels of context, analysis, and intervention.

In Chapter Seventeen, Viswanath, Finnegan, and Gollust focus on communication and health behavior in a rapidly changing media environment. Their chapter characterizes the major features of the communication revolution and its implications for health communication and health behavior; reviews major theories and hypotheses in health communication; and discusses how developments in information and communication technologies are changing the way we conceptualize audiences, media organizations, and media effects. These authors illustrate these concepts and issues with two applications: mHealth interventions that use mobile phone strategies, and interventions that employ risk communication to encourage HPV vaccine uptake. They also examine the potential ways in which new media have the potential both to narrow and to widen health disparities.

Perspectives on Community, Group, and Organizational Interventions

The central theme of the chapters in Part Four is that we must understand, predict, and know how to influence the social systems and structures that provide the context for health behaviors. We need models that help those who lead change efforts and/or study them to be more effective in their efforts to create healthier institutions and communities. The importance of social networks, change within and among systems, organizational processes, and communication channels is apparent across each of the chapters, and each of these raises new concepts and considerations as technology advances, the political environment changes, and researchers and practitioners emphasize scaling up and dissemination to maximize impact while preventing or reducing health disparities.

Each chapter in this section of the book addresses a broad perspective, approach, or type of strategy, rather than a single theory. The chapter authors then describe, synthesize, and apply key theories, frameworks, and models that have been found useful for addressing the core issues of their subject. It is notable that the theories and models focus attention on interpersonal, community or organizational, and policy or environmental levels of action, as well as the individual level, as applicable.

The three chapters in this section bring long-standing approaches together with new concepts and strategies to understand health behaviors and facilitate positive changes. In Chapter Fifteen, Wallerstein and coauthors collect the ideas found in models of community organization and community building under the umbrella of *community engagement*. These newer models emphasize longer-term community assets and capacity building rather than being solely problem driven. They are not simply community-based but are also community-driven. While this is not a new concept (Minkler, 2000), it is updated in a broader context in this chapter.

Wallerstein and colleagues define empowerment, critical consciousness, community capacity, and social capital, and describe how leadership development is a strategy for building community capacity to address multiple health-related concerns. Chapter Fifteen also discusses methods in issue selection, including dialogical problem solving, strategic action planning, and photovoice. The Internet has emerged as a major force in community building, making possible new modes of data collection, disseminating tools for organizing, creating new linkages within disenfranchised communities, and connecting geographically dispersed advocates and activists. In Chapter Sixteen, Brownson and others analyze major concepts within implementation; dissemination and diffusion of innovations; and implications for bridging the gap between health promotion research, policy, and practice. They describe how growing expectations among funders and public health organizations for scaling up evidence-based interventions (EBIs) shine light on the need for implementation and dissemination science and on the importance of blending of individual, organizational, and systems change. These authors examine diffusion as a multilevel change process, which underscores the need to understand organizational context and culture.

In Chapter Seventeen, Viswanath, Finnegan, and Gollust discuss how developments in information and communication technologies are changing the way we conceptualize audiences, media organizations, and media effects. They examine the intersection of two major technology revolutions—biomedical and communication. Four characteristics of the communication revolution that have profound implications for health communication are discussed: (1) the multiplication of platforms for information dissemination, (2) the decentralization of compiling and distributing "health information," (3) the sheer volume of health information available, and (4) the potential exacerbation of the *digital divide* and communication inequalities. These features cut across a range of considerations about mass media: their differential impact on high- and low-socioeconomic status populations, their application in social action and advocacy, the impact of media on people's worldviews, and communication regarding health risks, especially those risks with broad public health implications.

Because each chapter in this section draws on multiple theoretical traditions that contribute to important areas of health behavior and health education, rather than presenting single or unified theories, it offers much for readers to digest. This synthesis focuses on similarities among models, draws their common themes, and critiques their usefulness for research and practice in health behavior and public health.

Multiple Levels of Influence and Action

A central premise of this book is that improvements in health require both an understanding of the multilevel determinants of health behavior and a range of change strategies at the individual, interpersonal, and macro levels. The view that societal-level changes and supportive environments are necessary to address major health problems successfully *and* to maintain individual-level behavior change is now widely endorsed (Brownson et al., 2006; Glanz & Bishop, 2010). The chapters in this section clearly exemplify a multilevel perspective, which builds on intrapersonal and interpersonal theories to explain or affect community change.

The applications described in the three chapters in this section each illustrate how multiple levels of influence interact and require attention to improve conditions and health. The example of the immigrant restaurant workers in Chinatown in Chapter Fifteen begins with a problem of discrimination and harm due to wage theft, which was well documented and then leveraged to pass an ordinance in San Francisco to benefit individual workers. The changes benefiting individual workers, however, came from the community policy and had to be implemented through organizations (the restaurants) (Gaydos et al., 2011). The example of the Pool Cool skin cancer prevention dissemination trial in Chapter Sixteen illustrates how enhanced strategies for implementation or dissemination can simultaneously target individuals, organizations, and environments (Glanz, Escoffery, Elliott, & Nehl, 2014). The MobileMums intervention used mobile phones and text messages to deliver an efficacious intervention rooted in Social Cognitive Theory (Chapter Nine) to new mothers across a broad geographic area (Fjeldsoe, Miller, & Marshall, 2012).

An important message at the heart of these chapters is that the broader, community- or organizational-level models and concepts are not intended to stand alone, at the expense of neglecting the individuals who make up the groups, organizations, and communities (Kegler & Glanz, 2008). Important concepts and issues related to organizational change (Butterfoss, Kegler, & Francisco, 2008) are integrated into Chapter Fifteen in relation to coalitions and partnerships, and into Chapter Sixteen with respect to organizational adoption of evidence-based interventions. Even though macrolevel theories are invaluable for understanding the complex environments in which behavior takes place, creating change in these environments still often requires identifying and targeting individual change agents, such as news gatekeepers, politicians, or school superintendents. In other words, understanding individual behavior remains integral even when the proximal behavior targeted is not health but, for example, an organizational policy. It is collectives of *individuals* who create organizational structures; provide leadership in communities; choose to participate—or not participate—in coalitions; and make decisions about local, state, and federal policies and priorities. Also, it is premature to assume that policy development, social action, and environmental change are sufficient for behavior change across various health topics and populations.

Adoption of Models from Outside the Health Field

The histories of the various frameworks and models discussed in these three chapters reveal that they did not emerge within the field of health, medicine, or public health. Concepts and principles of community engagement and community organization come from social work (Chapter Fifteen). Implementation, dissemination, and Diffusion of Innovations models grew from efforts to spread the use of hybrid seed corn in Iowa (seed that can be non-GMO or GMO in today's agricultural world) (Chapter Sixteen). The core concepts described in the chapter concerning communication and media come from psychology, social psychology, and sociology (Chapter Seventeen).

The adaptation of these models to address health behavior has brought challenges in measurement and research design. Wallerstein and colleagues point to progress in the development of measures of process and outcomes for community engagement and CBPR, but acknowledge that uptake has not been rapid. The CFIR, a framework meant to unify key constructs from many implementation science frameworks (Damschroder et al., 2009), is in the early stages of developing measures to assess its core constructs and domains (Chapter Sixteen).

Research designs to test active strategies for community engagement, implementation and dissemination, and media communication present shared challenges. First, the foundations for such intervention strategies are usually complex, and when they embrace multiple levels (individual; interpersonal; and group, organizational, or community), they present challenges to those conducting rigorous research and evaluation. However, as Brownson and colleagues illustrate in Chapter Sixteen, there have been cluster-randomized, controlled trials of efficacious intervention strategies conducted at schools, churches, worksites, and swimming pools. Trials of mass media communication can take place in randomized media markets. But it is not always feasible (e.g., due to the cost) to undertake such ambitious research—leaving practitioners and researchers challenged with optimizing the assessment of process indicators and intermediate outcomes. No doubt, there will continue to be debates about whether it is necessary to assess individual behavior or health outcomes in large, multiorganization and/or multicommunity interventions, or whether endpoints of adoption and implementation of EBIs are sufficient to conclude that positive impacts have occurred.

Future Directions

Although all three chapters in this section describe trends and the emergence of new research and public health concerns, none makes these points in a more emphatic and dramatic manner than the chapter that addresses communication and health behavior in a changing media environment (Chapter Seventeen). The multiplication of communication platforms, increased grassroots participation, the pace of change, and the persistence of communication inequalities are daunting for public health experts and health behavior researchers. In the months immediately after that chapter was written, the Ebola epidemic in West Africa and beyond brought risk communication into politics, communities, and health care systems at an unprecedented pace. The federal communication approach, relying on "facts, not fear" (www.cdc.gov/vhf/ebola/resources/index.html), is mediated by political forces and the social context of risk. This example of the complexity of communication about health foreshadows challenges that health behavior experts will confront.

An understanding of theory, research, and practice in communities, systems, and organizations will be increasingly critical to wide improvement of health in the future. Part Four of *Health Behavior: Theory, Research, and Practice* provides a diverse set of frameworks and applications for consideration of both researchers and practitioners. Readers should invest time and energy in digesting the complexity of these issues, models, and frameworks.

References

Brownson, R. C., Haire-Joshu, D., & Luke, D. A. (2006). Shaping the context of health: A review of environmental and policy approaches in the prevention of chronic diseases. *Annual Review of Public Health, 27*, 341–370.

Butterfoss, F. D., Kegler, M. C., & Francisco, V. T. (2008). Mobilizing organizations for health promotion: Theories of organizational change. In K. Glanz, B. K. Rimer, & K. Viswanath (Eds.), *Health behavior and health education: Theory, research, and practice* (4th ed., pp. 336–361). San Francisco: Jossey-Bass.

Damschroder, L. J., Aron, D. C., Keith, R. E., Kirsh, S. R., Alexander, J. A., & Lowery, J. C. (2009). Fostering implementation of health services research findings into practice: A consolidated framework for advancing implementation science. *Implementation Science, 4*, 50.

Fjeldsoe, B. S., Miller, Y. D., & Marshall, A. L. (2012). Social cognitive mediators of the effect of the MobileMums intervention on physical activity. *Health Psychology, 32*(7), 729–738.

Gaydos, M., Bhatia, R., Morales, A., Lee, P. T., Liu, S. S., Chang, C., . . . Minkler, M. (2011). Promoting health equity and safety in San Francisco's Chinatown restaurants: Findings and lessons learned from a pilot observational survey. *Public Health Reports, 126*(Suppl. 3), 62–69.

Glanz, K., & Bishop, D. (2010). The role of behavioral science theory in development and implementation of public health interventions. *Annual Review of Public Health, 31*, 399–418.

Glanz, K., Escoffery, C., Elliott, T., & Nehl, E. (2014, December 18). Randomized trial of two dissemination strategies for a skin cancer prevention program in aquatic settings. *American Journal of Public Health*, e1–e9.

Kegler, M., & Glanz, K. (2008). Perspectives on group, organization, and community interventions. In K. Glanz, B. K. Rimer, & K. Viswanath (Eds.), *Health behavior and health education: Theory, research, and practice* (4th ed., pp. 389–403). San Francisco: Jossey-Bass.

Minkler, M. (2000). Using participatory action research to build Healthy Communities. *Public Health Reports, 115*, 191–197.

Smedley, B. D., & Syme, S. L. (Eds.). (2000). *Promoting health: Intervention strategies from social and behavioral research*. Washington, DC: National Academies Press.

CHAPTER 15

IMPROVING HEALTH THROUGH COMMUNITY ENGAGEMENT, COMMUNITY ORGANIZATION, AND COMMUNITY BUILDING

Nina Wallerstein
Meredith Minkler
Lori Carter-Edwards
Magdalena Avila
Victoria Sánchez

The concept of community engagement, viewed through its multiple lenses, is rooted in social justice and community change processes. In the 1997 Centers for Disease Control and Prevention (CDC) publication *Principles of Community Engagement, community engagement* was defined as "the *process* of working collaboratively with groups of people who are affiliated by geographic proximity, special interests, or similar situations with respect to issues affecting their well-being" (CDC, 1997, p. 9). The term has gained traction in recent years, especially with the growth of the Clinical and Translational Science Awards program (www.ctsacentral.org), and draws from three major, often overlapping fields and their histories: community organization and community building, coalitions and partnerships, and community-based participatory research.

Community organizing is defined as the process by which community groups are helped to identify common problems or change targets, mobilize resources, and develop and implement strategies to reach their collective goals. Though it is different from the general sentiment of *community engagement*, it also incorporates conflict

KEY POINTS

This chapter will:

- Provide a brief history of community engagement, incorporating community organization and community building, coalitions and partnerships, and community-based participatory research (CBPR).

- Examine the concept of community for informing community engagement.

- Explore key concepts and principles of community engagement.

- Present models of community organization and building, coalitions, and CBPR, as a backdrop to community engagement.

- Present a case study application of community engagement that integrates community organizing and building, coalition building, and CBPR.

- Discuss measurement and evaluation issues.

and confrontation strategies as well as collaborative ones (Minkler & Wallerstein, 2012). The related concept of *community building* is less a strategic approach than an orientation to community that engages and collectively *builds* capacity in the process (Walter & Hyde, 2012). Community organization and community building practice include, as their base, principles of social action and social justice.

Coalitions and partnerships, formed as people and organizations work together to solve problems, are increasingly common (Butterfoss, 2007), and provide a fundamental base for community engagement. *Community-based participatory research* (CBPR) and *community-engaged research* (CEnR) add a research focus, with a grounding in partner relationships among community, academic, and/or agency stakeholders that characterizes the entire research process. In public health contexts, CBPR has at its core a collective, shared focus on overcoming social and health inequities through community members partnering with researchers and organizational representatives and building on community strengths and priorities to apply research for the goals of social change (Israel, Eng, Schulz, & Parker, 2012; Minkler, Wallerstein, & Wilson, 2008).

This chapter will introduce concepts and methods of community engagement, broadening and building on earlier work on community organization and community building (Minkler et al., 2008) and emphasizing the range and effectiveness of community partnerships. After examining the concept of community, we then turn to the history of community engagement, the concepts and principles of engagement, and a discussion of diverse models from complementary literatures. We present one illustrative application of concepts and models, and conclude with a discussion of measurement issues in assessing engagement effectiveness.

The Concept of Community

Although typically thought of in geographic terms, communities may also be based on shared interests or characteristics, such as race or ethnicity, sexual orientation, or occupation. Communities have been defined variously as (1) *functional spatial units* meeting basic needs for sustenance, (2) *units of patterned social interaction*, (3) *symbolic units of collective identity*, and/or social units where people come together politically to make change (Minkler et al., 2008).

Several key perspectives are relevant to understanding the concept of community. The *ecological systems perspective* (see Chapter Three for a discussion of ecological models) is particularly useful in the study of autonomous geographic communities, focusing on population characteristics, such as size, density, and heterogeneity; the physical environment; the social organization of the community; and the technological forces affecting it. Therefore, "for the community to function well, each part has to carry out its role in relation to the whole organism" (Clinical and Translational Science Awards [CTSA] Consortium, Community Engagement Key Function Committee, & Task Force on the Principles of Community Engagement, 2011, p. 5).

In contrast, the *social systems perspective*, classically articulated by Warren (1963), focuses primarily on formal and informal organizations that operate dynamically within a given community, exploring the interactions of community subsystems, both horizontally, within the community, and vertically, as they relate to other systems of power. The social systems perspective further suggests that getting to know the networks through which a community's members, organizations, and leaders interact is imperative to further strengthening that community and working better with it (CTSA Consortium et al., 2011; Minkler & Wallerstein, 2012).

Clearly, a person's perspective on community influences his or her view of the community engagement process. Community development specialists often have focused on *geographic communities*. In contrast, proponents of a broader social action approach (Alinsky, 1972) have encouraged organizing around *issues*, such as public housing and unemployment, recognizing the tremendous impact of those larger socioeconomic issues on local communities.

Yet other perspectives also influence our ways of thinking about and approaching community (Gutiérrez & Lewis, 2012). Chavez, Minkler, Wallerstein, and Spencer (2010), for example, have emphasized the importance of a *cultural/historical perspective*, noting that an appreciation of the unique characteristics and histories of communities of color should be a major consideration. Cornell West (1993) has argued that in African American communities market exploitation led to a shattering of religious and civic organizations that had historically buffered these communities from hopelessness. He calls for community change through recreating a sense of agency and political resistance based on "subversive memory—the best of one's past without romantic nostalgia" (West, 1993, p. 19). Likewise, in American Indian communities today there is a burgeoning cultural renewal movement that embraces organizing and healing from intergenerational historical traumas that were wrought by the dominant society (Walters, Beltran, Huh, & Evans-Campbell, 2011). A view of community with this perspective would support building on social networks and strengths, emphasizing self-determination and empowerment (Chavez et al., 2010; Gutiérrez & Lewis, 2012).

Of growing importance is the *virtual perspective*, which recognizes that individuals increasingly rely on "computer-mediated communications to access information, meet people and make decisions that affect their lives" (Kozinets, 2002; CTSA Consortium et al., 2011). Facebook alone now has more than a billion registered users, and if a nation, would be the third most populous in the world (Statistic Brain, 2015). With the unprecedented ease and frequency of forming new relationships, these virtual communities cannot be ignored (Bazell & Wong, 2012; Kanter & Fine, 2010). Online groups that both build and support communities (e.g., of people with disabilities, LGBT youth, or Asian Pacific Islanders who have Hepatitis B, or other groups of people who share identities, interests, or often-stigmatizing conditions) are growing in both size and sophistication (Bazell & Wong, 2012).

Finally, an often-overlooked perspective highlighted in the community engagement literature is the *individual perspective*. This view posits that individuals define their community membership(s) with multiple or intersecting identities that go beyond the single definition of community upon which researchers and community engagement practitioners tend to rely (CTSA Consortium et al., 2011). For people who are seeking community engagement, understanding how individuals and communities view themselves through multiple lenses is critical for effective practice.

Histories of Community Engagement

Community engagement draws from many histories. The term *community organization* was coined in the late 1800s by American social workers who coordinated services, such as settlement houses, for newly arrived immigrants and the poor (Garvin & Cox, 2001). While a more complete discussion of community organizing history can be found elsewhere (see Minkler & Wallerstein, 2012), some important milestones in this history are the post-Reconstruction period in which African Americans organized to salvage newly won rights, the Populist agrarian movement, and the labor movement of the 1930s and1940s (Garvin & Cox, 2001). Originally a consensus model, by the 1950s, with labor struggles gaining attention, community organizing began to stress confrontation and conflict strategies for social change (Alinsky, 1972). Since the 1950s, strategies and tactics of community organization increasingly have been applied to achieve broader social change objectives: for example, by the civil rights, women's rights, gay rights, and disability rights movements and even by the New Right in its organizing to ban abortions and gay marriage. From the mid-1990s on, groups across the political spectrum have built online communities, organizing support on a mass scale (Smith, 2011).

A complementary history grounds community engagement in the *participation* strategies of the World Health Organization (WHO), whose 1948 Constitution stated that "informed opinion and active cooperation on the part of the public are of the utmost importance" in improving health. This constitution was followed by other key documents emphasizing participation. In 1978, the Declaration of Alma-Ata, signed at the International Conference on Primary Health Care, convened by WHO and UNICEF, advocated primary health care for all, with a call for participation by community members in the planning and implementation of their health care (www.who.int/publications/almaata_declaration_en.pdf). A decade later, the Ottawa Charter for Health Promotion, signed at the First International Conference on Health Promotion, also convened by WHO, advocated community action as one of five priorities (www.who.int/healthpromotion/conferences/previous/ottawa/en). This human rights approach, emphasized in later health promotion conferences (Fawcett et al., 2010) and by the WHO Commission on Social Determinants (WHO, 2015), envisions health equity through empowerment and participation by all (Wallerstein, Mendes, Minkler, & Akerman, 2011).

In the United States, community participation terminology was embraced in the 1960s, with John F. Kennedy's New Frontier and Lyndon Johnson's War on Poverty supporting federal mandates for "maximum feasible participation," including the *community health center* movement (Geiger, 2005). The Centers for Disease Control and Prevention (CDC) has long embraced participatory planning and program initiatives, with such programs and publications as the Planned Approach to Community Health, the Prevention Research Centers, the REACH initiative for racial and ethnic equity; the first edition of *Principles of Community Engagement*; and recently the Community Transformation Grants (www.cdc.gov/communitytransformation). In 1995, the National Institute of Environmental Health Sciences initiated sustained funding across multiple institutes for community-based participatory research.

In a new, major National Institutes of Health (NIH) initiative that supports community engagement, the Community Engagement Key Functions Committee of the NIH's Clinical and Translational Science Awards (CTSA) consortium has made inroads in community-engaged approaches within academic medical institutions and primary health systems (Carter-Edwards et al., 2013; Westfall et al., 2012). The CTSAs initially were developed to accelerate translation of academic medical research to clinical applications and to maximize improvement in individual and population health. With the first CTSAs funded in 2006, today there are sixty awards across thirty states and the District of Columbia, and they are coordinated through the NIH's new National Center for Advancing Translational Sciences (NCATS) (www.ncats.nih.gov/research/cts/ctsa/about/about.html).

While CTSAs initially were not required to engage communities in their efforts, many did, and community engagement has evolved to become an integral component of the CTSA program, as community efforts have bolstered translational medical and community-based research activities (Katz et al., 2011). The CTSA consortium's Community Engagement Key Function Committee seeks to, among other things, implement a broad plan of community and practice engagement to ultimately "enhance the health of communities and the nation" (CTSA Strategic Goal 4). The 2010 signing of the Affordable Care Act (ACA) into law is strengthening this paradigm shift so that national priorities are focusing much more on prevention; on community, stakeholder, and patient participation; and on systemwide coordinated health care (Selby, Beal, & Frank, 2012; www.pcori.org).

In practice, community engagement efforts are still developing. The revised *Principles of Community Engagement* (CTSA Consortium et al., 2011) offers a continuum of engagement as a framework to guide efforts; it begins with minimal community outreach on one end of the spectrum and moves through consultation and collaboration to a shared leadership approach. Progress at the individual CTSA level has been incremental and varied, as some academic medical institutions have integrated lay community members and organizations as partners in the research decision-making process, while others have relationships but not bidirectional research relationships with community organizations and health systems, and still others are just learning how to identify their community partners. These differences reflect the need for a common understanding and appreciation across CTSAs of principles of community engagement, not only by investigators but also by their infrastructure leadership. Furthermore, there is very little research on the prevalence of community engagement in research, particularly in clinical and translational studies funded by the NIH (Hood, Brewer, Jackson, & Wewers, 2010). However, the institutionalization of community engagement is slowly getting under way.

The Institute of Medicine's 2013 report on the CTSA program, commissioned by the National Institutes of Health in response to a congressional request, provides seven high-level recommendations, one of which involves community engagement, which also is one of the three cross-cutting domains in the report (Institute of Medicine [IOM], 2013, p. 116). The sixth recommendation, *to ensure community engagement in all phases of research*, states that the NCATS and the CTSA program should define community engagement broadly; ensure active and substantive community stakeholder participation throughout the research and leadership process; define and clearly communicate community engagement goals, expectations, and best practices; and explore opportunities and incentives to engage a more diverse community (IOM, 2013, p. 127).

The IOM committee defines a *community* as all stakeholders in the clinical and translational research process, people who "seek and provide health care in community, academic, and private settings, as well as individuals and organizations working in communities to improve the health and well-being of local populations" (IOM, 2013, p. 116). This definition offers a fairly broad view of population health, but it remains largely a clinical perspective, with its implied emphasis on health care within multiple settings. It is different from a public health approach, where social determinants and other environmental and policy conditions are recognized as key socioecological contributors to population health and well-being. Both of these approaches to community engagement are necessary for full research translation.

Because community engagement is new to many researchers, barriers persist, including lack of understanding about the benefits of community engagement and the presence of some academic cultures that discount partnership building. From the community perspective, there may be issues of mistrust owing to histories of manipulation or disrespect, or lack of adequate funding to compensate and provide training for community partners.

There are programs at the NIH that can help serve as models for the CTSAs. The National Cancer Institute's Community Networks Program Centers, which seek to improve access to beneficial cancer interventions and treatments in communities in order to reduce health disparities, provide communities with the resources they need using a community-based participatory research approach (www.cancer.gov/aboutnci/organization/crchd/disparities research/cnpc). The National Institute on Minority Health and Health Disparities sponsors Research Centers in Minority Institutions and Centers of Excellence to Reduce Health Disparities that provide ongoing collaborations with the CTSAs. Across the country, established CBPR partnerships have created successful models as well.

While the inclusion of all stakeholders is important for the successful streamlining of the research process, it is critical that lay community members, those traditionally not a part of the decision-making process, be fully engaged. Increasingly, research teams have come to see the value of the *bridging* social capital function of partners—whether they are university staff or key community members who are part of advisory committees—who have connections to or come from the community where the research is taking place. The people who best perform this bridging function often have the capacity to work across institutional and racial or ethnic cultures and across power relationships to promote greater equality of participation among diverse stakeholders (Muhammad et al., 2014).

Although clinical and public health approaches to community engagement have increased, community engagement is still a contested concept with differing definitions, perceptions, and understandings. Arnstein's classic Ladder of Citizen Participation (Arnstein, 1969) and the newer public health ladder (Morgan & Lifshay, 2006) wisely underline the potential for manipulation, and remind those of us in the academy about the importance of self-reflection regarding our own actions in our efforts to promote successful community engagement.

In sum, community engagement today is viewed primarily as a consensus-building orientation. The possibility of moving from outreach to the shared leadership and partnered CBPR end of the continuum depends on embracing the concepts and principles of empowerment, inclusivity, collaborative action, and health equity, which were also hallmarks of the early community organization traditions.

Community Engagement Concepts and Principles

Concepts and principles of community engagement have guided public health professionals and community leaders with a science base as well as with core values and practical strategies for engaging the public in decision making and social action. Not merely technical or prescriptive processes, these concepts and principles place respect and integrity at the forefront of work with communities. Dorothy Nyswander's (1956) well-known axiom "start where the people are" centered the field of health education in community engagement, making that engagement one of the field's most fundamental principles. During the development of contributing fields, various field-specific sets of principles have been developed, such as the principles of community organizing (Alinsky, 1972), of environmental justice (*Principles of Environmental Justice*, 1991), and of bidirectional community engagement (CTSA Consortium et al., 2011), and for community-engaged research, we have the now classic principles of CBPR (Israel, Schulz, Parker, & Becker, 1998) and principles for CBPR with indigenous peoples (Walters et al., 2009). Each of these sets of principles upholds a natural process of working with community, whether in research or practice, and can be applied to partnerships across the community engagement continuum.

This chapter brings together four overarching concepts, with principles embedded in each concept (see Table 15.1): (1) community capacity, with principles of recognizing the community as a unit of identity and building on community strengths; (2) empowerment and critical consciousness, with principles of promoting co-learning and cultural humility, involving cyclical and iterative processes, and integrating knowledge and action, and a new principle of practicing collaborative mentorship that honors diversity; (3) participation and relevance, with principles of facilitating equitable involvement of all partners in practice and research and undertaking long-term commitment; and (4) recognition of inequities as the major target of change.

Community Capacity

Community capacity is defined as "the characteristics of communities that affect their ability to identify, mobilize, and address social and public health problems" (Goodman et al., 1998, p. 259). These characteristics have multiple dimensions: active participation, leadership, rich support networks, skills and resources, critical reflection, sense of community, understanding of history, articulation of values, and access to power (Goodman et al., 1998).

Underlying community capacity, and the related concepts of community competence, social capital, and community empowerment, is the principle of community as a unit of identity. This involves relationships based on commonalities, and which can hold the greatest

Table 15.1　Key Concepts and Principles in Community Engagement

Key Concepts	Key Definition	Principles	Application
Community capacity	Community characteristics affecting a community's ability to identify problems and then to mobilize and address them.	Community is a unit of identity. Capacity builds on community strengths.	Community members actively participate in identifying and solving their problems and become better able to address future problems collaboratively.
Empowerment	A social action process for people to gain mastery over their lives and the lives of their communities.	Promote co-learning. Integrate knowledge and action.	Community members expand their power or challenge power structures to create desired changes.
Critical consciousness	A consciousness based on praxis: the cycle of reflection and action toward social change.	Involve cyclical and iterative processes. Practice collaborative mentorship that honors diversity and cultural humility.	People are engaged in listening and dialogue and also in action that links root causes and community actions.
Participation and relevance	Community organizing should "start where the people are" and engage community members as equals in their own priorities.	Facilitate equitable involvement of all partners in all stages of practice and research. Undertake long-term commitment. Ensure cultural relevance.	Community members create their own agenda based on felt needs, shared power, and awareness of resources.
Health equity	The opportunity for all to obtain their full health potential regardless of social position or socially determined circumstance.	Address inequitable conditions that create health disparities. Identify social determinants of health.	Resources are allocated to community-, policy-, and system-level changes that challenge inequitable conditions that cause ill health.

potential for being a "community as the unit of solution" (Steckler, Dawson, Israel, & Eng, 1993). Although a community may benefit from academic or health professional skills and resources that exist outside its community of identity, building on community strengths (a second principle), through involving community organizations and leaders, can enhance the connections of those with shared interests (Minkler & Wallerstein, 2012; Israel et al., 1998).

Social networks, the webs of relationships in which people are embedded, and social supports, the tangible and intangible resources they give and receive through these networks, are important for capacity building (also see Chapter Eleven). Strengthening natural helpers or leaders, found through social networks, is key to building capacity and effectiveness. As Gutiérrez and Lewis (2012) suggest, leadership development may be especially important in communities of color, given that outreach efforts often treat such communities as targets, rather than as active participants in change.

Empowerment and Critical Consciousness

Empowerment and critical consciousness are deeply embedded within community engagement. While *empowerment* has been justifiably criticized as a catchall term in social science

(Rappaport, 1984), it remains a central tenet of community organization, community building, and community engagement. Broadly defined, empowerment is a social action process by which individuals, communities, and organizations gain mastery over their lives in the context of changing their social and political environment to improve equity and quality of life (Rappaport, 1984; Wallerstein, 2006). As a theory and a methodology, community empowerment involves both processes and outcomes, and has a focus on transforming power relations for individuals, the organizations of which they are a part, and the community social structure itself. For individuals, psychological empowerment addresses their perceived control, critical consciousness, political efficacy, and participation in change (Peterson et al., 2006). Organizational empowerment incorporates advocacy processes as well as organizational effectiveness in policy change (Laverack, 2007). Community empowerment outcomes include an increased sense of community, or sense of belonging to and identification with a group or geographic area; community capacity; and actual changes in policies, transformed conditions, or increased resources, all of which can contribute to reducing health inequities (Wallerstein, 2006).

Empowerment involves multiple principles. Promoting co-learning emphasizes the reciprocal exchange of skills, knowledge, and capacity among all involved, recognizing that all bring diverse skills, expertise, and experiences to partnership processes (Israel et al., 1998). The process of engagement is a dialectic exchange that challenges and transforms knowledge, promotes critical consciousness (Freire, 1970), and advances the collective power of partnership.

Co-learning, along with the principle of involving cyclical and iterative processes, builds from the dialogical approach of Paulo Freire (1970), with its accent on praxis, the cycle of reflection and action that involves listening, critical dialogue, and action based on reflection, and then cycling back to listening (Wallerstein & Auerbach, 2004). Many would argue that co-learning and empowerment are not possible without the principle of cultural humility, defined as an openness to others' cultures and an ability to reflect on and to seek to redress our own positions of power in relation to community partners (Chavez et al., 2010).

The principle of integrating knowledge and action is aimed at balancing evidence-based knowledge with practice- and community-based knowledge in a bidirectional process that creates action to produce community benefit. Community members provide knowledge informed by their cultural and social contexts; practitioners and researchers bring various skill sets (e.g., for planning, evaluation, and research) and evidence-based approaches to the collective table (Andrews et al., 2012). By engaging community knowledge, the potential for program sustainability and policy actions based on community priorities grows.

An emerging principle of collaborative mentorship honors diversity and emphasizes the exchange of knowledge and experience that fosters co-learning and mentoring among all partners. Mentorship becomes multidimensional and nonhierarchical and shows respect for multiple sources of knowledge. Rather than accepting the traditional view of senior professionals mentoring students, junior staff, or community members, collaborative mentorship suggests the importance of using multiple types of mentoring—top-down, bottom-up, and peer mentoring—an approach that recognizes epistemological diversity and the value of listening deeply, enabling respect for the perspectives and values of each partner (Duran et al., 2012).

Participation and Relevance

The concepts of participation and relevance represent the core value of starting "where the people are" (Nyswander, 1956) and working with communities in ways that acknowledge mutual strengths and the skills of community partners. This implies the principle of involving community in all stages of engagement, from naming the problem and planning for change to implementing and evaluating plans and strategies. Within this principle is the recognition that change is not time bound but requires long-term commitment to tackle "wicked," that is, intractable and multilayered, social and health problems.

One of the most important steps in community engagement involves effectively differentiating between problems that are troubling and issues the community feels strongly about (Staples, 2004). Various methods may be used to help a community group obtain the data needed to document issues while ensuring those issues' relevance. Face-to-face data collection processes include focus groups, door-to-door surveys, and interviews, which also can be useful in assessing felt needs and increasing a sense of participation (Duran et al., 2012). Freire's (1970) dialogical, problem-posing methodology has proven especially helpful for engaging participants in identifying themes that elicit social and emotional involvement, followed by social action and reflection (Wallerstein & Auerbach, 2004).

Photovoice is an approach that emphasizes community strengths along with issue selection (Catalani & Minkler, 2010; Wang & Pies, 2008). Researchers or practitioners provide cameras and skills training to community residents who then use the cameras to convey their own images of their community, including community assets and problems. Photovoice is often used with problem-posing questions. Participants work together to select the pictures that best capture their collective wisdom, and use these to tell their stories and to stimulate change through local organizing and institutional- and policy-level action.

The Internet can be used to facilitate participation and ensure relevance when assessing community needs and strengths, building community, and conducting advocacy (Bazell & Wong, 2012). Two initiatives in Indian country highlight the capacity for Internet tools to inspire, educate, and connect communities that are dispersed and often geographically isolated. Just Move it (JMI) (www.justmoveit.org/jmi), a program initiated by the Health Promotion/Disease Prevention program of the Indian Health Service, and now also an initiative of the Healthy Native Communities Partnership (HNCP) and the Assembly of First Nations in Canada, has a goal of promoting physical activity among one million indigenous people. JMI's website offers health promotion staff and community members opportunities to promote their events, share success stories, and document their achievements.

Similarly, the Healthy Native Communities Fellowship (HNCF), (www.hncpartners.org /HNCP/Fellowship.html), with an organizational trajectory similar to JMI's, has provided nine years of leadership training to strengthen teams of Fellows as change agents for promoting health and wellness within their communities and across regions. Since 2005, 119 teams and 299 Fellows from all twelve Indian Health Service areas have participated. An interactive "Fellow Space" has been used in between weeklong trainings to facilitate blogging by Fellows, teams, and alumni in order to maintain connections, share achievements, receive educational materials, and promote strategic thinking and planning across teams.

In one of the largest shared spaces for educational materials on community organization and planning for health, Steve Fawcett and his colleagues created the Community Tool Box (ctb.ku.edu), close to 9,000 pages in length, which is organized around core competencies, ranging from community assessment, to coalition development, policy advocacy, and evaluation. As part of an international Pan American Health Organization collaboration, the Community Tool Box is being translated into Spanish, with plans for a Portuguese translation as well. While there are still significant barriers to Internet access for poor and rural communities, promising efforts to close the digital divide are underway, with groups like ZeroDivide (www.zerodivide.org) and the Digital Divide Network (www.digitaldivide.net) providing searchable geographic sites for local technology programs and resources and in other ways attempting to reach and assist those who remain unconnected (Bazell & Wong, 2012). Underscoring all these methods is the fact that they are useful only to the extent that they enable the discovery of the real issues of concern to each community.

Recognition of Inequities

With firm evidence of social and health disparities among racial and ethnic minorities and other vulnerable populations, public health practitioners and researchers have increased efforts to eliminate health and social inequities. The focus on disparities and inequities is not new to community organizing; however, it has gained momentum through the building of the evidence base for these social and structural inequities (Brennan Ramirez, Baker, & Metzler, 2008; Wallerstein, Yen, & Syme, 2011). There are persistent challenges to addressing key determinants such as institutionalized racism, discrimination, or differences in educational resources and opportunities, however. Capacity-building partnerships that start where the people are; view knowledge and skills not as a hierarchy but as multileveled and multiple-sourced; and make community participation, knowledge, and power relevant from a strengths-based perspective, rather than a deficit perspective, can help to promote equity. By embracing these concepts and principles, community engagement can build the trust and community mobilization needed to make a difference in community lives and health.

Community Organization and Community-Building Models

Although community organization and community building are frequently treated as though they were a single model of practice, several typologies have been developed. The best known is the work of renowned community organization theorist Jack Rothman (2007) and consists of three distinct but overlapping models of practice. Originally described as locality development, social planning, and social action, the language and sophistication of these three models have subsequently been broadened (Rothman, 2007).

Community capacity development stresses cooperation as an organizing approach, with building group identity and problem solving as key goals. This revised nomenclature avoids the narrower geographic focus implied by *locality development* and strongly incorporates community building. *Social planning and policy* stresses the use of data and rational-empirical problem solving, while also making room for participatory planning and policy development, in keeping with the spirit of true community organization; whereas the earlier term, *social planning*, generally offered by professionals was more limited. Finally, *social advocacy*, like its predecessor, *social action*, emphasizes the use of pressure tactics, including confrontation, to help bring about concrete changes to redress power imbalances, but is more in keeping with the social change tactics and strategies being used in the early twenty-first century (Rothman, 2007). These include both neighborhood actions and far larger efforts, often aided by the Internet, to foster national and even global change programs, such as efforts to address refugee relief and climate change.

Rothman originally presented the models as three ideal types, but with mixing among them, either at the outset or over time. His later work elaborated on mixed forms, highlighting a *predominant mode* and two other *composite models* (Rothman, 2007). Feminist community organizing, for example, may combine the goals of social advocacy organizing with methods that are consistent with community capacity development (Hyde, 2005; Rothman, 2007). Similarly, the Healthy Heartlands Initiative being implemented across five Midwestern states combines faith-based community capacity *development, planning,* and *policy* (or "setting the table with technical experts") with social advocacy that engages legislators and other key players in promoting racial and health equity (Blackwell et al., 2012).

Although not a strategic model per se, Walter and Hyde's (2012) community-building approach places the *community*, rather than the *community organizer*, at the center of practice. Partially emphasizing self-help, this perspective extends beyond community development, which is often externally driven and may implicitly accept the status quo, and focuses instead on creating healthy and more equal power relations (Hyde, 2005; Walter & Hyde, 2012). Though it includes many steps from traditional organizing (e.g., clarifying a community's purpose and building a power base), it puts the heaviest accent on community leadership and empowerment, rather than merely "community betterment" (Wolff, 2010). McKnight's (1987) notion of community regeneration has at its heart enabling people to contribute their gifts, which represent the building blocks a community can use to care for its members. Finally, a macro-conception of community building also emphasizes regional economic development and federal and state policy-level reinvestment in local communities as critical (Blackwell & Colmenar, 2000).

Feminists and scholars of color also point to particulars of organizing within their communities (Gutiérrez & Lewis, 2012; Rivera & Erlich, 1995). As Hyde (2005) points out, feminist organizing need not address "quintessentially feminist issues" such as gender violence or pay equity; rather it's the empowering aspects that make an organizing effort feminist. Organizing by and with people of color focuses attention on the centrality of cultural, historical, racial or ethnic, and/or linguistic identities. It is also important to acknowledge conflict as a necessary part of cross-cultural work (Gutiérrez & Lewis, 2012), and for some theorists, it is important to limit primary levels of involvement to organizers who share racial or ethnic and other identifiers with communities (Rivera & Erlich, 1995).

In sum, several models of community organization and community building have emerged within the last two decades to complement earlier organizing approaches. In Figure 15.1, we integrate models, presenting a typology that incorporates both needs- and strengths-based approaches. Along the needs-based axis, *community development,*

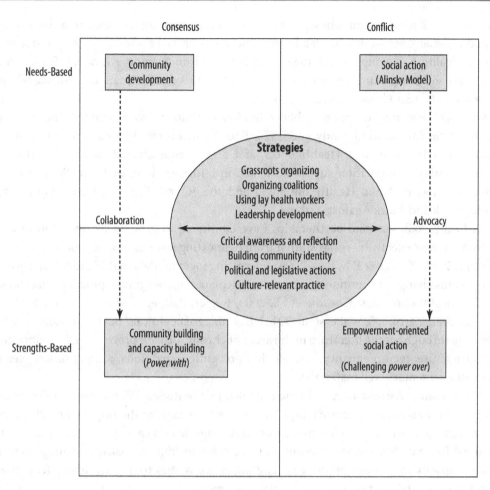

Figure 15.1 Community Organization and Community-Building Typology

as primarily a consensus model, is contrasted with Alinsky's *social action* conflict-based model. The newer strength-based models contrast community capacity building with an empowerment-oriented social action approach. When we look at primary strategies, we see that consensus approaches, whether needs- or strengths-based, primarily use collaboration strategies, whereas conflict approaches use advocacy and ally building to support advocacy efforts. Several concepts span these two strengths-based approaches, such as community competence, leadership development, and the multiple perspectives on gaining power. Much organizing uses combinations of strategies at different times during an organizing campaign and the community engagement process.

Coalition and Partnership-Building Models

Coalitions represent intentional processes of community engagement of individuals and organizations, ranging from formation to institutionalization of coalition infrastructures through sharing resources and streamlining efforts (Butterfoss, 2007; Minkler & Wallerstein, 2012).

Coalitions work within communities of identity to build community capacity by encouraging community members to develop leadership and research skills within the social and health context. Coalitions can mobilize change at any level (Nelson, Salmon, Altman, & Sprigg, 2012), and are dynamic, requiring continued negotiation to achieve or maintain the balance of power and privilege (CTSA Consortium et al., 2011).

Over the last two decades, publicly funded coalitions have included the American Stop Smoking Intervention Study (ASSIST), Racial and Ethnic Approaches to Community Health (REACH), Steps to a Healthier US, and diverse substance abuse and healthy community coalitions. Foundation-supported coalition initiatives have included W. K. Kellogg's Community-Based Public Health Initiative, and the Robert Wood Johnson Foundation's Fighting Back and Allies Against Asthma.

As health coalitions and partnerships have continued to grow in number and diversity, research on their effectiveness has shifted from delineating structures and processes (Granner & Sharpe, 2004; Zakocs & Edwards, 2006) to creating logic models that identify intermediate-term systems change in community capacities, participation, programs, practices, and policies linked to health outcomes (Cheadle et al., 2003; Kegler, Painter, Twiss, Aronson, & Norton, 2009; Sanchez, Carrillo, & Wallerstein, 2011). Examples of coalitions' health impacts have been increasing throughout the literature in the areas of chronic disease prevention, immunizations, substance abuse, teen pregnancy, and alcohol prevention coalitions, among others (see this book's supplementary web materials).

Allies Against Asthma (AAA), funded in 2000 by the Robert Wood Johnson Foundation, illustrates how community partnerships have come to recognize the importance of targeting systems change (AAA, 2011). Community organizations, health care agencies, and universities partnered in seven low-income communities of color to improve asthma management and to build capacity for sustainability by developing active venues to inform, advocate, exchange information, and take action to make substantive changes.

Although grantees were required to employ a community coalition model, each coalition determined key strategies and implementation methods that aligned with community culture, practices, and resources (Clark et al., 2010). Because AAA coalitions recognized the influence of social determinants, each coalition incorporated a multilevel approach in its change strategies to influence both individual and systems changes (Clark et al., 2010). The seven coalitions achieved eighty-nine policy and system changes, ranging from changes in inter- and intra-institutional practice to new statewide legislation, as well as better health outcomes, such as reduced symptoms and improved health care utilization (AAA, 2011).

Community-Based Participatory Research (CBPR)

In the past two decades, community-based participatory research (CBPR), and complementary community-engaged research, practice-based research networks (PBRNs), tribally driven research, and other collaborative research networks have become recognized as instrumental to the reduction of health disparities, through building community capacity, diversifying the research workforce, recognizing the importance of cultural and implementation contexts within diverse communities, and increasing the external validity of research findings. Falling on the end of the continuum of shared leadership or community-driven research, CBPR has a history of supporting bidirectional learning, allowing researchers to combine scientific knowledge with community expertise in the cultural and social contexts of the health issue and potential solutions that may work locally (Andrews et al., 2012). With engaged and equitable partnerships, CBPR has contributed to decreasing local health inequities and building capacity for social change (Cargo & Mercer, 2008; Israel et al., 2012; Minkler et al., 2008).

As with coalition evaluation, CBPR evaluation has been evolving from the publication of partnership processes to reporting on multiple intermediate systems change outcomes. These include often hard-won new health policies, sustainable and culturally centered community programs, and increased research and other community capacities, as well as evidence of improved health outcomes. (Evaluation is discussed further later in this chapter; also see this book's web resources.)

One example is the faith-based Bronx Health REACH partnership, a collaboration of the Institute for Family Health, black and Latino churches, and community-based organizations, among other groups. The partnership has braided its CDC, NIH, and other funding sources to tackle social determinants of health from a community-building, community organization, and CBPR perspective (Bronx Health Reach, 2010–2015). With an early focus on capacity building, it has adopted the community-building strategy of identifying pastors and lay church leaders who are willing to join the growing coalition (up to forty-seven churches from the original seven), which has the goal of creating multilevel interventions. These interventions include promoting healthier foods at church functions, sponsoring nutrition education and fitness activities, creating new health ministries with volunteer nurses and other health professionals in the congregation to sustain wellness efforts, and supporting pastors in integrating health messages into their sermons.

Bronx Health REACH has adopted community organization advocacy strategies to challenge New York City schools to adopt low-fat milk, a policy focus that has had them coming up against the dairy industry lobby. Partnership members have also confronted the two-tier medical system, a type of medical apartheid that results in unequal access to specialty care for their congregants who are either uninsured or on Medicaid on the one hand and the congregants with private insurance on the other hand, a disparity that disproportionately affects people of color. With NIH CBPR funding, they have adapted an evidence-based diabetes curriculum, using their culturally centered, faith-based model, to promote diabetes self-care and management. With commitment to CBPR principles, academic researchers involved in this project have located decision making within a community research committee that oversees Bronx Health REACH's faith-based initiative to codevelop and sustain the research methodology.

Application of Community Engagement: Immigrant Restaurant Workers in San Francisco's Chinatown

This extended application of community engagement showcases the models and principles of community organizing and building, coalition building, and community-based participatory research.

The cultural center of San Francisco's Chinese immigrant community, Chinatown is a dynamic neighborhood and international tourist attraction. For the roughly one-third of its residents who are employed in restaurants, however, Chinatown also means high rates of work-related illness and injury, including not only traditional problems such as cuts, burns, and on-the-job stress but also social and economic problems such as wage theft. A particular concern for low-wage immigrant workers, *wage theft* includes payment of wages below the minimum, delayed payment or denial of back wages, no paid sick leave or overtime pay, and confiscation of tip money (Bernhardt et al., 2009).

The Chinese Progressive Association (CPA) had been organizing around worker issues for over thirty years when it formed a CBPR partnership in 2007 to study restaurant worker health and safety in a coalition with the University of California, Berkeley, School of Public Health and its Labor Occupational Health Program (LOHP); the San Francisco Department of Public Health; and the University of California, San Francisco, Division of Occupational and Environmental Medicine. Six Chinese restaurant workers provided on-the-ground expertise to the research and were a focal point for CPA's efforts to develop leaders for its campaign to address working conditions.

Prior to the research, many hours of partnership meetings were held to reflect on the varying needs, strengths, and visions of different partners, the goals of the partnership, and the adaptations needed to better bridge the needs, strengths, visions, and goals (Chang et al., 2013). Worker partners engaged in an eight-week training using Freirean popular education activities and co-learning dialogue and critical reflection (Freire, 1970; Wallerstein & Auerbach, 2004), with follow-up weekly or biweekly sessions that underscored the importance of workers' insider perspectives, and taught participatory research skills, such as survey design and human subjects protection, as well as strategies to ensure workers' rights and health and safety. Concurrently with their CBPR participation, the worker partners were involved in ongoing CPA organizing activities.

The Chinatown immigrant restaurant workers study included focus groups with restaurant workers, a detailed survey of working conditions and health among 433 Chinatown restaurant workers, creation of an observational checklist that the health department used to collect data on working conditions in 106 of the 108 restaurants, and an evaluation of the partnership (Chang, Salvatore, Lee, Liu, & Minkler, 2012; Gaydos et al., 2011).

Worker partners and the CPA helped tailor both the survey and the checklist to be culturally and linguistically appropriate, with appropriate items of local relevance.

Study findings showed that 50 percent of the workers surveyed reported they did not receive the minimum wage, 17 percent were not paid on time, and 76 percent of those who worked more than forty hours a week were not paid overtime (CPA, 2010). The health department's checklist findings indicated multiple preventable hazards, including lack of posting of required minimum wage and other labor laws (65%) (Chang et al., 2012; CPA, 2010; Gaydos et al., 2011). Initial data analysis was conducted by two academic partners, and findings were quickly made available in accessible formats to worker partners, who participated in six data interpretation workshops. As they learned to speak the language of data analysis, they provided many insights into the data not originally apparent to other academic and agency partners (Chang et al., 2012; CPA, 2010).

A key step in translating the research into action was the CPA's drafting and launch of *Check, Please!*, a comprehensive report issued in three languages that summarized study findings and also discussed how these findings reflected broader trends for low-wage workers citywide and nationally. The report contained recommendations for action and featured a low-wage worker bill of rights, developed by the San Francisco Progressive Workers Alliance (PWA), a new coalition founded by CPA and other local worker organizations. The large press conference that launched *Check, Please!* drew close to two hundred people, including almost twenty reporters from mainstream and ethnic media and several city supervisors. Worker partners played a prominent role in this event, presenting research findings, and telling their own stories to put a human face on the data (the press conference may be viewed at www.youtube.com/watch?v=96dQzjKXFoE).

Following the launch event, the CPA, its worker partners, the PWA, and city supervisors worked together to develop the San Francisco Wage Theft Prevention Ordinance, which was unanimously passed and signed into law in 2011, making San Francisco the first U.S. municipality after Miami to have a wage theft ordinance. To ensure that the new legislation had teeth, several members of the Chinatown project then participated in an implementation task force that met monthly in city hall and saw some real enforcement victories. In February 2013, the city collected the largest wage theft settlement in the city's history (over $525,000) from a Chinatown pastry shop that had paid its employees just $4 an hour for working eleven hours a day, six days a week. Programs that could help incentivize the high-road employers, those who comply with labor laws and maintain healthy and safe working conditions, are also being explored, and the CPA and its partners continue to work on a citywide approach to address all low-wage worker communities (Gaydos et al., 2011).

Although community organizing and CBPR are heavily focused on engaging participants in studying and taking action to change their reality, an equally strong emphasis is placed on personal and collective transformation. In this case, worker partners reported less fear of engaging with new people and "talking to strangers," a greater sense of "courage" and confidence, owning issues and solutions through sharing of their own stories and experiences, and moving into the leadership of the CPA (Chang et al., 2012). In sum, the combination of Freirean popular education, community organizing, working in a coalition, and community-based participatory research increased workers' empowerment and community partners' organizational capacity and visibility, and helped secure passage and enforcement of anti–wage theft legislation. In this project, the participatory research activities were foundational to taking action for change, and the results were evident in the new policy legislation, enforcement of the new policy, and related sequelae. The project also is helping to improve the health of Chinese immigrant workers and of low-wage workers across the city.

Measurement and Evaluation Issues

A challenge for community engagement, community organization and community building, and community-based participatory research has been the difficulty of adequately addressing evaluation processes and outcomes, partially due to funding constraints, the lack of knowledge about how to build meaningful evaluation into community engagement efforts, and the difficulty of determining appropriate outcomes. The continually evolving nature of community engagement, the complex and dynamic contexts in which it occurs, and the fact that these projects often seek change on multiple levels make many traditional evaluative approaches inadequate (Craig et al., 2008; Fetterman & Wandersman, 2005; Glasgow, 2013). The focus of standard evaluation approaches on distal health or social indicators may miss the shorter-term system impacts with which community engagement and organizing is concerned. Although many characteristics of successful community collaborations have been identified, such as shared vision, leadership, skills in building alliances across differences, and a focus on process and not merely tasks (Butterfoss, 2007; Chavez et al., 2010; Lasker & Weiss, 2003; Wolff, 2010), much remains to be assessed.

A growing number of new tools and resources are available for those interested in evaluating community organizing, capacity, coalitions, and engagement. Key among them are Foster and Louie's (2010) summary of tools for measuring community organizing, Butterfoss and Kegler's (2009) comprehensive community action model for understanding coalitions, Wolff's book *The Power of Collaborative Solutions* (2010), and the increasingly used, web-based Partnership Self-Assessment Tool (at www.nccmt.ca/uploads/registry/PSA%20Tool%20Questionnaire.pdf) (see also Lempa, Goodman, Rice, & Becker, 2008; Mattessich, Murray-Close, & Monsey, 2001; Zakocs & Edwards, 2006).

Both newer and time-tested approaches to measuring community empowerment and multilevel perceived control (Peterson et al., 2006; Wallerstein, 2006), civic engagement, and social capital are increasingly being seen as critical. Despite advances in measurement, however, there are limits to scales. For example, self-report measures of individuals cannot capture the full picture of organization- and community-level processes over time. Qualitative approaches are needed to enhance understanding of the context, dynamics of change, and outcomes such as transformed conditions, new policies, participation, and political voice.

Finally, CBPR instruments and measures offer promise for partnership evaluation (Israel et al., 2012), with the development of CBPR logic models (Hicks et al., 2012; Schulz, Israel, & Lantz, 2003) and with new CBPR metrics and measures from a current NIH mixed methods study of CBPR partnerships nationwide (Sandoval et al., 2012). A new community-engaged research infrastructure model within academic health centers presents potential categories for evaluation of university and community capacities (Eder, Carter-Edwards, Hurd, Rumala, & Wallerstein, 2013). Core constructs of partnership synergy (Jagosh et al., 2012; Khodyakov et al., 2011) and trust—measured with one of the earliest tools from the CDC's Prevention Research Centers (CDC, 2012; Lucero & Wallerstein, 2013)—are being seen as critical overarching elements of community engagement, social network formation, and partnership functioning.

Summary

The growing pivotal role of community engagement in health education, public health, social work, medicine, and community-engaged and participatory research reflects this approach's time-tested effectiveness and its fit with the most fundamental principles of these fields. Community engagement, as a whole, stresses strengths-based approaches, relevance or starting "where the people are," and the importance of creating environments in which individuals and communities can become empowered as they increase their capacity to solve problems and demand their human rights to fair and equitable conditions that support health. While community engagement has shifted mostly to a collaborative, capacity-building approach, the social action traditions of community organizing are still critical in advocacy that challenges health-damaging policies and conditions that continue to create health inequities. Employing the full range of practices of honoring diversity and addressing inequities demands time and resources and also intellectual and emotional commitments that are strongly embedded within the key concepts and principles discussed in this chapter.

Whether engaged in pure community-driven organizing and engagement around issues the community identifies or borrowing skills from community organizing, community-building practice, and coalition partnerships, professionals and researchers can challenge themselves to examine their own cultural humility and dynamics of power in order to understand the complexities of working in partnership toward the goals of community ownership and empowerment. In sum, community engagement and organizing bring essential strategies to a wide variety of community and organizational settings and may hold particular relevance in the changing sociopolitical climate of the twenty-first century.

References

Alinsky, S. D. (1972). *Rules for radicals: A pragmatic primer for realistic radicals.* New York: Vintage.

Allies Against Asthma. (2011). [Organization website.] cmcd.sph.umich.edu/Allies-Against-Asthma.html

Andrews, J. O., Cox, M. J., Newman, S. D., Gillenwater, G., Warner, G., Winkler, J. A., . . . Slaughter, S. (2012). Training partnership dyads for community-based participatory research: Strategies and lessons learned from the Community Engaged Scholars Program. *Health Promotion Practice, 14*(4), 524–533.

Arnstein, S. R. (1969). A ladder of citizen participation. *Journal of the American Institute of Planners, 35*(4), 216–224.

Bazell, N., & Wong, A. (2012). Creating an online strategy to enhance effective community building and organizing. In M. Minkler (Ed.), *Community organizing and community building for health and welfare* (3rd ed., pp. 269–287). New Brunswick, NJ: Rutgers University Press.

Bernhardt, A., Milkman, R., Theodore, N., Heckathorn, D., Auer, M., DeFilippis, J., . . . Spiller, M. (2009). *Broken laws, unprotected workers: Violations of employment and labor laws in America's cities.* New York: National Employment Law Project.

Blackwell, A. G., & Colmenar, R. (2000). Community-building: From local wisdom to public policy. *Public Health Reports, 115*, 161–166.

Blackwell, A. G., Thompson, M., Freudenberg, N., Ayers, J., Schrantz, D., & Minkler, M. (2012). Using community organizing and community building to influence public policy. In M. Minkler (Ed.), *Community organizing and community building for health and welfare* (3rd ed., pp. 371–385). New Brunswick, NJ: Rutgers University Press.

Brennan Ramirez, L. K., Baker, E. A., & Metzler, M. (2008). *Promoting health equity: A resource to help communities address social determinants of health.* Atlanta: Centers for Disease Control and Prevention.

Bronx Health Reach. (2010–2015). [Organization website.] http://www.bronxhealthreach.org

Butterfoss, F. D. (2007). *Coalitions and partnerships in community health.* San Francisco: Jossey-Bass.

Butterfoss F. D., & Kegler, M. C. (2009). Toward a comprehensive understanding of community coalitions: Moving from practice to theory. In R. DiClemente, L. Crosby, & M. C. Kegler (Eds.), *Emerging theories in health promotion practice and research* (pp. 1157–1193). San Francisco: Jossey-Bass.

Cargo, M., & Mercer, S. L. (2008). The value and challenges of participatory research: Strengthening its practice. *Annual Review of Public Health, 29,* 325–350.

Carter-Edwards, L., Cook, J., McDonald, M. A., Weaver, S. M., Chukwuka, K., & Eder, M. (2013). Report on CTSA consortium use of the community engagement consulting service. *Clinical and Translational Science, 6*(1), 34–39.

Catalani, C., & Minkler, M. (2010). Photovoice: A review of the literature in health and public health. *Health Education & Behavior, 37*(3), 424–451.

Centers for Disease Control and Prevention. (1997). *Principles of community engagement.* Atlanta: CDC, Public Health Practice Program Office. Retrieved from http://www.cdc.gov/phppo/pce

Centers for Disease Control and Prevention. (2012). PRC Partnership Trust Tool. Retrieved from http://www.cdc.gov/prc/program-material/partnership-trust-tools.htm

Chang, C., Salvatore, A., Lee, P. T., Liu, S. S., & Minkler, M. (2012). Popular education, research and community organizing with immigrant restaurant workers in San Francisco's Chinatown: A case study. In M. Minkler (Ed.), *Community organizing and community building for health and welfare* (3rd ed., pp. 246–264). New Brunswick, NJ: Rutgers University Press.

Chang, C., Salvatore, A. L., Lee, P. T., Liu, S. S., Tom, A. T., Morales, A., . . . Minkler, M. (2013). Adapting to context in community-based participatory research: Participatory starting points in a Chinese immigrant worker community. *American Journal of Community Psychology, 51*(3–4), 480–491.

Chavez, V., Minkler, M., Wallerstein, N., & Spencer, M. (2010). Community organizing for health and social justice. In L. Cohen, V. Chavez, & S. Chehimi (Eds.), *Prevention is primary: Strategies for community well-being* (2nd ed., pp. 87–112). San Francisco: Jossey-Bass.

Cheadle, A., Beery, W. L., Greenwald, H. P., Nelson, G. D., Pearson, D., & Senter, S. (2003). Evaluating the California Wellness Foundation's Health Improvement Initiative: A logic model approach. *Health Promotion Practice, 4*(2), 146–156.

Chinese Progressive Association. (2010). *Check, please! Health and working conditions in San Francisco Chinatown restaurants.* San Francisco: Author. Retrieved from www.cpasf.org

Clark, N., Lachance, L., Doctor, L. J., Gilmore, L., Kelly, C., Krieger, J., . . . Wilkin, M. (2010). Policy and system change and community coalitions: Outcomes from Allies Against Asthma. *American Journal of Public Health, 100*(5), 904–912.

Clinical and Translational Science Awards Consortium, Community Engagement Key Function Committee, & Task Force on the Principles of Community Engagement. (2011). *Principles of community engagement* (2nd ed.). Washington, DC: Department of Health and Human Services, National Institutes of Health, Centers for Disease Control and Prevention, Agency for Toxic Substances and Disease Registry, Clinical and Translational Science Awards.

Craig, P., Dieppe, P., Macintyre, S., Michie, S., Nazareth, I., & Petticrew, M. (2008). Developing and evaluating complex interventions: The new Medical Research Council guidance. *BMJ, 337,* a1655. Retrieved from http://www.ncbi.nlm.nih.gov/pmc/articles/PMC2769032

Duran, B., Wallerstein, N., Minkler, M., Foley, K., Avila, M., & Belone, L. (2012). Initiating and maintaining partnerships. In B. A. Israel, E. Eng, A. J. Schulz, & E. A. Parker (Eds.), *Methods for community-based participatory research for health* (2nd ed., pp. 43–68). San Francisco: Jossey-Bass.

Eder, M., Carter-Edwards, L., Hurd, T. C., Rumala, B. B., & Wallerstein, N. (2013). A logic model for community engagement within the Clinical and Translational Science Awards consortium: Can we measure what we model? *Academic Medicine, 88*(9), 1430–1436.

Fawcett, S., Abeykoon, P., Arora, M., Dobe, M., Galloway-Gilliam, L., Liburd, L., & Munodawafa, D. (2010). Constructing an action agenda for community empowerment at the 7th Global Conference on Health Promotion in Nairobi. *Global Health Promotion, 17*(4), 52–56.

Fetterman, D., & Wandersman, A. (Eds.). (2005). *Empowerment evaluation principles in practice.* Thousand Oaks, CA: Sage.

Foster, C. C., & Louie, J. (2010). *Grassroots action and learning for social change: Evaluating community organizing.* Washington, DC: Center for Evaluation Innovation. Retrieved from http://www.innonet.org/client_docs/File/center_pubs/evaluating_community_organizing.pdf

Freire, P. (1970). *Pedagogy of the oppressed.* New York: Seabury Press.

Garvin, C. D., & Cox, F. M. (2001). A history of community organizing since the Civil War with special reference to oppressed communities. In J. Rothman, J. L. Erlich, & J. E. Tropman (Eds.), *Strategies of community intervention* (6th ed., pp. 65–100). Itasca, IL: Peacock.

Gaydos, M., Bhatia, R., Morales, A., Lee, P. T., Chang, C., Salvatore, A., . . . Minkler, M. (2011). Promoting health equity and safety in San Francisco's Chinatown restaurants: Findings and lessons learned from a pilot observational survey. *Public Health Reports, 126*(Suppl. 3), 62–69.

Geiger, J. (2005). The first community health centers: Model of enduring value. *Journal of Ambulatory Care Management, 28*(4), 313–332.

Glasgow, R. (2013). What does it mean to be pragmatic? Pragmatic methods, measures, and models to facilitate research translation. *Health Education & Behavior, 40*, 257–265.

Goodman, R. M., Speers, M., McLeroy, K., Fawcett, S., Kegler, M., Parker, E., . . . Wallerstein, N. (1998). Identifying and defining the dimensions of community capacity to provide a basis for measurement. *Health Education & Behavior, 25*(3), 258–278.

Granner, M. L., & Sharpe, P. A. (2004). Evaluating community coalition characteristics and functioning: A summary of measurement tools. *Health Education Research, 19*(5), 514–532.

Gutiérrez, L. M., & Lewis, E. A. (2012). Education, participation, and capacity building in community organizing with women of colour. In M. Minkler (Ed.), *Community organizing and community building for health and welfare* (3rd ed.). New Brunswick, NJ: Rutgers University Press.

Hicks, S., Duran, B., Wallerstein, N., Avila, M., Belone, L., Lucero, J., . . . Hat, E. W. (2012). Evaluating community-based participatory research to improve community-partnered science and community health. *Progress in Community Health Partnerships: Research, Education, and Action, 6*(3), 289–299.

Hood, N. E., Brewer, T., Jackson, R., & Wewers, M. E. (2010). Survey of community engagement in NIH-funded research. *Clinical and Translational Science, 3*(1), 19–22.

Hyde, C. A. (2005). Feminist community practice. In M. Weil (Ed.), *Handbook of community practice* (pp. 360–371). Thousand Oaks, CA: Sage.

Institute of Medicine. (2013). *The CTSA program at NIH: Opportunities for advancing clinical and translational research.* Washington, DC: National Academies Press.

Israel, B. A., Eng, E., Schulz, A. J., & Parker, E. A. (Eds.). (2012). *Methods for community-based participatory research for health* (2nd ed.). San Francisco: Jossey-Bass.

Israel, B. A., Schulz, A. J., Parker, E. A., & Becker, A. B. (1998). Review of community-based research: Assessing partnership approaches to improve public health. *Annual Review of Public Health, 19*, 173–202.

Jagosh, J., Macaulay, A. C., Pluye, P., Salsberg, J., Bush, P. L., Henderson, J., . . . Greenhalgh, T. (2012). Uncovering the benefits of participatory research: Implications of a realist review for health research and practice. *Milbank Quarterly*, *90*(2), 311–346.

Kanter, B., & Fine, A. H. (2010). *The networked nonprofit: Connecting with social media to drive change.* San Francisco: Jossey-Bass.

Katz, J. M., Rosas, S. R., Siskind, R. L., Campbell, D., Gondwe, D., Munroe, D., . . . Schouten, J. T. (2011). Community-research partnerships at NIAID HIV/AIDS clinical trial sites: Insights for evaluation and enhancement. *Progress in Community Health Partnerships: Research, Education, and Action*, *6*(3), 311–320.

Kegler, M. C., Painter, J. E., Twiss, J. M., Aronson, R. E., & Norton, B. (2009). Evaluation findings on community participation in the California Healthy Cities and Communities program. *Health Promotion International*, *24*(4), 300–310.

Khodyakov, D., Stockdale, S., Jones, F., Ohito, E., Jones, A., Lizaola, L., & Mango, J. (2011). The effect of community engagement in research on perceived outcomes of partnered mental health services projects in an NIH-funded center. *Society and Mental Health*, *1*(3), 185–199.

Kozinets, R. V. (2002). The field behind the screen: Using netnography for marketing research in online communities. *Journal of Marketing Research*, *39*, 61–72.

Lasker, R. D., & Weiss, E. S. (2003). Creating partnership synergy: The critical role of community stakeholders. *Journal of Health and Human Services Administration*, *26*(1), 119–139.

Laverack, G. (2007). *Health promotion practice: Building empowered communities.* London: McGraw-Hill.

Lempa, M., Goodman, R. M., Rice, J., & Becker, A. B. (2008). Development of scales measuring the capacity of community-based initiatives. *Health Education & Behavior*, *35*(3), 298–315.

Lucero, J. E., & Wallerstein, N. (2013). Trust in community–academic research partnerships: Increasing the consciousness of conflict and trust development. In S. Ting-Toomey & J. Oetzel (Eds.), *Sage handbook of conflict communication* (2nd ed., pp. 537–563). Thousand Oaks, CA: Sage.

Mattessich, P. W., Murray-Close, M., & Monsey, B. R. (2001). *Collaboration: What makes it work* (2nd ed.). St. Paul, MN: Wilder Publishing Center, Amherst H. Wilder Foundation.

McKnight, J. (1987). Regenerating community. *Social Policy*, *17*(3), 54–58.

Minkler, M., & Wallerstein, N. (2012). Improving health through community organizing and community building. In M. Minkler (Ed.), *Community organizing and community building for health and welfare* (3rd ed., pp. 37–58). New Brunswick, NJ: Rutgers University Press.

Minkler, M., Wallerstein, N., & Wilson, N. (2008). Improving health through community organizing and community building. In K. Glanz, B. K. Rimer, & F. M. Lewis (Eds.), *Health behavior and health education: Theory, research, and practice* (4th ed., pp. 287–312). San Francisco: Jossey-Bass.

Morgan, M. A., & Lifshay, J. (2006). *Community engagement in public health.* Retrieved from http://www.barhii.org/resources/downloads/community_engagement.pdf

Muhammad, M., Wallerstein, N., Sussman, A., Avila, M., Belone, L., & Duran, B. (2014). Reflections on researcher identity and power: The impact of positionality on community based participatory research (CBPR) processes and outcomes. *Critical Sociology*. doi:10.1177/0896920513516025

Nelson, G. M., Salmon, M. A., Altman, H. K., & Sprigg, P. E. (2012). Organizing communities around care transitions: The community connections experience. *North Carolina Medical Journal*, *73*(1), 41–44.

Nyswander, D. B. (1956). Education for health: Some principles and their application. *Health Education Monographs*, *14*, 65–70.

Peterson, N. A., Lowe, J. B., Hughey, J., Reid, R. J., Zimmerman, M. A., & Speer, P. W. (2006). Measuring the intrapersonal component of psychological empowerment: Confirmatory factor analysis of the sociopolitical control scale. *American Journal of Community Psychology, 38*(3–4), 287–297.

Principles of Environmental Justice. (1991). Retrieved from http://www.ejnet.org/ej/principles.html

Rappaport, J. (1984). Studies in empowerment: Introduction to the issue. *Prevention in Human Services, 3*(2–3), 1–7.

Rivera, F., & Erlich, J. (1995). An option assessment framework for organizing in emerging minority communities. In J. E. Tropman, J. L. Erlich, & J. Rothman (Eds.), *Tactics and techniques of community intervention* (3rd ed., pp. 198–213). Itasca, IL: Peacock.

Rothman, J. (2007). Multi modes of intervention at the macro level. *Journal of Community Practice, 15*(4), 11–40.

Sanchez, V., Carrillo, C., & Wallerstein, N. (2011). From the ground up: Building a participatory evaluation model. *Journal of Progress in Community Health Partnerships: Research, Education, and Action, 5*(1), 45–52.

Sandoval, J., Lucero, J., Oetzel, J., Avila, M., Belone, L., Mau, M., . . . Wallerstein, N. (2012). Process and outcome constructs for evaluating community-based participatory research projects: A matrix of existing measures. *Health Education Research, 27*(4), 680–690.

Schulz, A., Israel, B. A., & Lantz, P. (2003). Instrument for evaluating dimensions of group dynamics within community-based participatory research partnerships. *Evaluation and Program Planning, 26*(3), 249–262.

Selby, J. V., Beal, A. C., & Frank, L. (2012). The Patient-Centered Outcomes Research Institute (PCORI) national priorities for research and initial research agenda. *JAMA, 307*(15), 1583–1584.

Smith, A. (2011). *The Internet and Campaign 2010.* Washington, DC: Pew Internet & American Life Project. Retrieved from http://pewinternet.org/Reports/2011/The-Internet-and-Campaign-2010.aspx

Staples, L. (2004). *Roots to power: A manual for grassroots organizing* (2nd ed.). Westport CT: Praeger.

Statistic Brain. (2015). Facebook statistics. Retrieved from www.statisticbrain.com/facebook-statistics

Steckler, A. B., Dawson, L., Israel, B. A., & Eng, E. (1993). Community health development: An overview of the works of Guy W. Steuart. *Health Education Quarterly*, Suppl. 1, S3–S20.

Wallerstein, N. (2006). *What is the evidence on effectiveness of empowerment to improve health?* (Health Evidence Network report). Copenhagen: World Health Organization. Retrieved from http://www.euro.who.int/__data/assets/pdf_file/0010/74656/E88086.pdf

Wallerstein, N., & Auerbach, E. (2004). *Problem-posing at work: Popular educators guide* (2nd ed.). Edmonton: Grass Roots Press.

Wallerstein, N., Mendes, R., Minkler, M., & Akerman, M. (2011). Reclaiming the social in community movements: Perspectives from the USA and Brazil/South America: 25 years after Ottawa. *Health Promotion International, 26*(Suppl. 2), ii226–ii236.

Wallerstein, N., Yen, I., & Syme, L. (2011). Integrating social epidemiology and community-engaged interventions to improve health equity. *American Journal of Public Health, 101*(5), 822–830.

Walter, C. L., & Hyde, C. A. (2012). Building practice: An expanded conceptual framework. In M. Minkler (Ed.), *Community organizing and community building for health and welfare* (3rd ed., pp. 78–93). New Brunswick, NJ: Rutgers University Press.

Walters, K. L., Beltran, R. E., Huh, D., & Evans-Campbell, T. (2011). Dis-placement and dis-ease: Land, place and health among American Indians and Alaska Natives. In L. M. Burton, S. P. Kemp, M. C. Leung, S. A. Matthews, & D. T. Takeuchi (Eds.), *Communities, neighborhoods, and health: Expanding the boundaries of place* (pp. 163–199). New York: Springer.

Walters, K. L., Stately, A., Evans-Campbell, T., Simoni, J. M., Duran, B., Schultz, K., . . . Guerrero, D. (2009). Indigenist collaborative research efforts in Native American communities. In A. R. Stiffman (Ed.), *Field survival guide* (pp. 146–173). Oxford, UK: Oxford University Press.

Wang, C., & Pies, C. (2008). Using photovoice for participatory assessment and issue selection: Lessons from a family, maternal, and child health department. In M. Minkler & N. Wallerstein (Eds.), *Community-based participatory research for health* (2nd ed., pp. 183–198). San Francisco: Jossey-Bass.

Warren, R. (1963). *The community in America*. Chicago: Rand McNally.

West, C. (1993). *Race matters*. Boston: Beacon Press.

Westfall, J. M., Ingram, B., Navarro, D., Magee, D., Niebauer, L., Zittleman, L., . . . Pace, W. (2012). Engaging communities in education and research: PBRNs, AHEC, and CTSA. *Clinical and Translational Science, 5*(3), 250–258.

Wolff, T. (2010). *The power of collaborative solutions: Six principles and effective tools for building healthy communities*. San Francisco: Jossey-Bass.

World Health Organization. (2015). *Social determinants of health*. Retrieved from www.who.int/social_determinants/thecommission/en/index.html

Zakocs, R., & Edwards, E. (2006). What explains community coalition effectiveness? A review of the literature. *American Journal of Preventive Medicine, 30*(4), 351–361.

CHAPTER 16

IMPLEMENTATION, DISSEMINATION, AND DIFFUSION OF PUBLIC HEALTH INTERVENTIONS

Ross C. Brownson
Rachel G. Tabak
Katherine A. Stamatakis
Karen Glanz

The gap between the discovery of new research findings and their application in public health, health care, and policy settings is vast (Green, Ottoson, Garcia, & Hiatt, 2009; Institute of Medicine, 2001). To bridge this gap, effective dissemination and implementation (D&I) of evidence-based interventions (EBIs) in public health and health care are critical to improving health (Glasgow et al., 2012). D&I involve the active spreading of EBIs to specific audiences, using planned strategies, in specified settings. Research from clinical and public health settings suggests that EBIs are not being disseminated effectively (Green et al., 2009). For example, only 55 percent of overall health care received by adults in twelve U.S. metropolitan areas was based on what is recommended in the scientific literature (McGlynn et al., 2003). Further, in a survey of U.S. public health departments, an estimated 58 percent of programs and policies were reported as evidence-based (Dreisinger et al., 2008).

Major reports have noted this substantial gap between research and practice in health and medicine, and have drawn attention to the fact that the failure to use available

KEY POINTS

This chapter will:

- Provide an overview of key terminology for dissemination and implementation research and practice.

- Provide an overview of the importance of theoretical models in dissemination and implementation research.

- Describe two models (Diffusion of Innovations and the Consolidated Framework for Implementation Research) and their key constructs in detail.

- Describe two applications in detail, and use them to illustrate some of the key concepts and features of the models.

- Identify challenges and opportunities for the field that should help to shape future inquiry.

This chapter is a product of Prevention Research Center and was supported by Cooperative Agreement Number U48/DP001903 from the Centers for Disease Control and Prevention and grant number R01CA92505 from the National Cancer Institute at the National Institutes of Health. The findings and conclusions in this chapter are those of the authors and do not necessarily represent the official position of the Centers for Disease Control and Prevention or the National Cancer Institute.

research findings is both costly and harmful to society (Institute of Medicine, 2001). As Kerner, Rimer, and Emmons (2005) have noted: "Efforts to move effective preventive strategies into widespread use too often have been unsystematic, uncoordinated, and insufficiently capitalized, and little is known about the best strategies to facilitate active dissemination and rapid implementation of evidence-based practices" (p. 443). The research-practice gap exists across all fields of medical and public health practice as well as in other fields as diverse as education, engineering, music, psychology, business, and agriculture (Green et al., 2009; Rogers, 2003). It is estimated that the lives of six million children could be saved each year if twenty-three proven interventions were implemented in forty-two countries (Bryce et al., 2005). Even for interventions such as tobacco control, where there has been a compelling evidence base for several decades, implementation of effective interventions remains inadequate in most developed countries and even poorer in many developing countries (Davis, Wakefield, Amos, & Gupta, 2007). On a global basis, the World Health Organization Framework Convention on Tobacco Control (FCTC) is one of the most rapidly embraced treaties in the history of the United Nations. In studying its effects among forty-one countries that implemented at least one FCTC policy between 2007 and 2010, it was estimated that almost 7.4 million smoking attributable deaths will be averted (Levy, Ellis, Mays, & Huang, 2013). If progress in these forty-one countries was extended globally, tens of millions of smoking attributable deaths would be averted (Levy et al., 2013).

Research on the uptake of EBIs has now taught us several important lessons: (1) D&I generally do not occur spontaneously and naturally, even when interventions are effective and seem appealing (Glasgow, Marcus, Bull, & Wilson, 2004); (2) theory and frameworks (models) are useful for guiding D&I (Tabak, Khoong, Chambers, & Brownson, 2012); (3) passive approaches to D&I are largely ineffective (Lehoux, Denis, Tailliez, & Hivon, 2005); (4) stakeholder involvement in research and evaluation processes is likely to enhance D&I (Minkler & Salvatore, 2012); (5) D&I should be targeted to specific audiences (Lomas, 1993); and (6) at the agency level (e.g., health departments and CBOs), D&I approaches should be time efficient; consistent with organizational climate, culture, and resources; and within the skills of staff members (Jacobs, Dodson, Baker, Deshpande, & Brownson, 2010).

Many D&I ideas originated in thinking about diffusion of innovations. The French judge Gabriel Tarde described diffusion concepts in his book *The Laws of Imitation* (Tarde, 1903). Tarde took note of new slang and clothing among people coming before the bench, which led him to propose the S-curve of diffusion (Figure 16.1) and the importance of opinion leaders in promulgating innovations. His observations were the foundation for the social system perspective on diffusion as the mechanism by which societies change and progress (Dearing, 2008). Around the same time, a German political philosopher, Georg Simmel, wrote about how individual thought and action were structured by interpersonal relationships (Wolff, 1950). Simmel described a web of group affiliations and was among the first to argue the importance of social ties and networks. His work set the stage for later efforts that described the role of social networks in the diffusion of innovations (Dearing, 2008; also see Chapter Eleven). In the United States, the seminal event in diffusion was publication of a 1943 report on the diffusion of hybrid seed corn in two Iowa communities (Ryan & Gross, 1943). This article stimulated diffusion practice and research and provided a key set of tools for agriculture extension agents (Dearing & Kee, 2012).

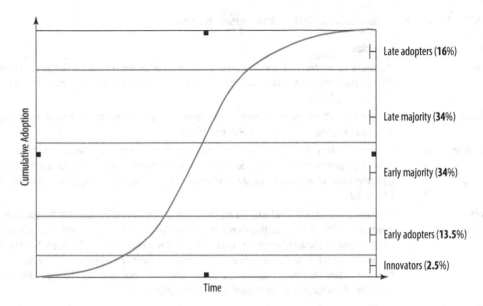

Figure 16.1 S-Shaped Diffusion Curve

Key Terminology

One challenging aspect of D&I research and practice is the lack of standardized terminology. Ciliska et al. (2005) have noted that closing the gap between knowledge generation and use of that knowledge in decision making for practice and policy is hampered by diverse terms and inconsistent definitions of terms. This chapter uses terminology developed primarily in the United States, with several examples showing comparable definitions from other countries (especially the United Kingdom, Canada, and Australia). It uses the broad umbrella term of *dissemination and implementation* to represent the wide scope of translational research, including diffusion research. An illustration of the complexity in the lexicon is that Graham and colleagues identified twenty-nine distinct terms referring to the same aspect of the D&I (or knowledge translation) process when they examined the terminology used by thirty-three applied research funding agencies in nine countries (Graham et al., 2006). Full glossaries on D&I research are available elsewhere (Rabin & Brownson, 2012). In Table 16.1, we provide a list of core definitions (excerpted in part from Rabin and Brownson, 2012). Many of these definitions originated in fields other than health. The definitions listed are those now applied to health and most widely accepted (Rabin, Brownson, Haire-Joshu, Kreuter, & Weaver, 2008).

Theories and Models

As described elsewhere in this text, there is substantial evidence that the use of theories and frameworks sometimes, although not always, enhances the effectiveness of interventions by helping to focus them on the essential processes of behavior change, which can be complex (Bartholomew, Parcel, Kok, & Gottlieb, 2001; Glanz & Bishop, 2010). Because there is considerable overlap in the terminology, for simplicity, this chapter uses the term *models* to cover both theories and frameworks. A recent review identified sixty-one models for D&I

Table 16.1   Selected Terms in Dissemination and Implementation Research and Practice

Term	Definition
Diffusion	The passive, untargeted, unplanned, and uncontrolled spread of new interventions. Diffusion is part of the diffusion-dissemination-implementation continuum, and it is the least focused and intense approach (Lomas, 1993; MacLean, 1996).
Dissemination	An active approach of spreading evidence-based interventions to the target audience via determined channels using planned strategies (Lomas, 1993; MacLean, 1996).
Dissemination research	The systematic study of processes and factors that leads to widespread use of an evidence-based intervention by the target population. Its focus is to identify the methods that best enhance the uptake and utilization of the intervention (Johnson, Green, Frankish, MacLean, & Stachenko, 1996; Sussman, Valente, Rohrbach, Skara, & Pentz, 2006).
Evidence-based interventions	The most common objects of D&I activities in public health and health care. These are interventions with proven efficacy and effectiveness; they should be defined broadly and may include programs, practices, processes, policies, and guidelines (Rabin, Brownson, Kerner, & Glasgow, 2006). In D&I research, we often encounter complex interventions (e.g., interventions using community-wide education) where the description of core intervention components and their relationships involves multiple settings, audiences, and approaches (Greenhalgh et al., 2004; Hawe, Shiell, & Riley, 2004).
Implementation	The process of putting to use or integrating evidence-based interventions within a setting (e.g., a school or worksite) (National Institutes of Health, 2013).
Implementation research	The study of the processes and factors associated with successful integration of evidence-based interventions within a particular setting (e.g., a worksite or school) (National Institutes of Health, 2013).
Implementation science	A broad term that includes the development and application of common principles, models, and designs to study and promote the uptake of evidence-based practices and policies. Implementation science covers an array of activities including building the science of D&I, developing academic-practice partnerships, understanding organizational behavior, and building capacity via focused training programs.
Innovation	An idea, practice, or object that is perceived as new by an individual or other unit of adoption (Rogers, 2003)
Knowledge translation	The term used by the Canadian Institutes of Health Research to denote a dynamic and iterative process that includes synthesis, dissemination, exchange, and ethically sound application of knowledge (Canadian Institutes of Health Research, 2013). Knowledge translation occurs within a complex social system of interactions between researchers and knowledge users and with the purpose of improving population health, providing more effective health services and products, and strengthening the health care system.

research (Tabak et al., 2012). Several of the common models are presented in Table 16.2. This table also includes studies that provide empirical evidence for the models as well as the number of times the models have been cited in the literature, along with their key constructs. The diversity of available models is reflected in the table. Empirical evidence was available for most of the reviewed models; however, it was not always in the form of rigorous, longitudinal use of the model to guide D&I projects (Helfrich et al., 2010).

Diffusion of Innovations: Theory and Practice

As shown in Table 16.2, the most frequently cited model is Diffusion of Innovations (Rogers, 2003). As noted previously, the underpinnings of the Diffusion of Innovations model have been present for over a century. Most of its tenets were developed by rural sociologists who studied the spread of farming innovations in the Midwest. The early studies of agricultural practices often were linked with extension services for funding and in understanding the role of change agents (extension agents) (Dearing, 2008). Diffusion concepts that largely originated

Table 16.2   Examples of Models: Number of Citations, Selected Constructs, and Evaluation Studies

Model Name	Times Cited[a]	Selected Key Constructs	Original Publication Cited	Selected Evaluation Papers
Diffusion of Innovations	51,102[b]	Relative advantage Compatibility Observability Trialability	Rogers, 2003	Deschesnes, Trudeau, & Kebe, 2010; Glanz et al., 2005; Rogers, 2003; Shively et al., 1997; Wiecha et al., 2004
Policy streams	10,428[c]	Process streams Problem recognition stream Policy stream Political stream	Kingdon, 2003	Craig, Felix, Walker, & Phillips, 2010
Conceptual Model for the Diffusion of Innovations in Service Organizations	1,949	Fuzzy boundaries Observability Nature of knowledge required (tacit or explicit) Dedicated time or resources Incentives and mandates Assimilation Decision making developed to frontline teams	Greenhalgh et al., 2004	Deschesnes et al., 2010
RE-AIM	1,107	Reach your intended target population Effectiveness or efficacy Adoption by target settings or institutions Implementation, consistency of delivery of intervention Maintenance of intervention effects in individuals and settings over time	Glasgow, Vogt, & Boles, 1999	Brug, Tak, & Te Velde, 2011; De Meij et al., 2010; Glasgow, Nelson, Strycker, & King, 2006; Van Acker, De Bourdeaudhuij, De Cocker, Klesges, & Cardon, 2011; RE-AIM publications, 2015
Active Implementation Framework	1,448	Staff selection Preservice and inservice training Ongoing consultation and coaching Staff and program evaluation Facilitative administrative support	Fixsen & Mental, 2005	Casado et al., 2008
Implementation Effectiveness Model	1,089	Climate for implementation Innovation values—fit Incentives and disincentives Absence of obstacles Implementation effectiveness Strategies accuracy of innovation adoption	Klein & Sorra, 1996	Dong, Neufeld, & Higgins, 2008; Holahan, Aronson, Jurkat, & Schoorman, 2004; Osei-Bryson, Dong, & Ngwenyama, 2008
Sticky knowledge	5,863[d]	Stickiness—initiation Implementation Ramp-up, integration Causal ambiguity Unproven knowledge Arduous relationship	Elwyn, Taubert, & Kowalczuk, 2007; Szulanski, 1996	Szulanski, 2000

(continued)

Table 16.2   (*Continued*)

Model Name	Times Cited[a]	Selected Key Constructs	Original Publication Cited	Selected Evaluation Papers
Precede–Proceed Model	597	Predispose Reinforce Enable	Green & Kreuter, 2005	Howat, Jones, Hall, Cross, & Stevenson, 1997; Macaulay et al., 1997; *Published Applications of the PRECEDE Model*, 2015.
Consolidated Framework for Implementation Research	339	Characteristics of the intervention Inner setting Outer setting Characteristics of individuals Implementation process	Damschroder et al., 2009	Damschroder et al., 2011; Damschroder & Lowery, 2013; Gordon et al., 2011; Williams et al., 2011
Promoting Action on Research Implementation in Health Services (PARIHS)	810	Evidence Context Facilitation	Kitson, Harvey, & McCormack, 1998; Kitson et al., 2008; Rycroft-Malone, 2004	Cummings, Estabrooks, Midodzi, Wallin, & Hayduk, 2007; Ellis, Howard, Larson, & Robertson, 2005; Helfrich et al., 2010; Helfrich, Li, Sharp, & Sales, 2009; Sharp, Pineros, Hsu, Starks, & Sales, 2004
Availability, Responsiveness & Continuity (ARC)	139	3 levels (community, organization, individual) 4 phases of development (problem identification, direction setting, implementation, stabilization) 10 intervention components: e.g., personal relationships, network development, team building	Glisson & Schoenwald, 2005; Glisson et al., 2010	Glisson, Dukes, & Green, 2006; Glisson et al., 2010

[a] In most cases, the value shows the number of times a model was cited based on the earliest reference to the model; this value serves as an imperfect proxy for use of the model in research studies. In some cases, exceptions were made to this rule, based on the judgment of the authors. These citation numbers were acquired on November 9, 2013.

[b] This is the number of citations of the fourth edition (1995) (the first that appears in Google Scholar), as it is older than the edition that is also cited (Rogers, 2003, 5th edition).

[c] This is the number of citations of the second edition (2003).

[d] Citation numbers for both the Elwyn et al., 2007 (33 citations), and Szulanski, 1996 (5,830 citations); references are provided because these two discussions are sufficiently different that having the citation numbers for both may be useful.

in agriculture have spread to other fields, including health, business, communication, and education (Dearing & Kee, 2012; Rogers, 2003). Many of the current properties of diffusion were formalized by the late Everett M. Rogers, who was trained as a rural sociologist, in his classic text *Diffusion of Innovations* (Rogers, 1962), now in its fifth edition (Rogers, 2003).

Key Components of the Theory

A key premise of Diffusion of Innovations is that some innovations diffuse quickly and widely, following a classic S-curve (Figure 16.1). Other innovations are adopted but subsequently abandoned. Also, innovations are adopted by different individuals and then spread at different rates in subgroups of individuals. The innovators, individuals who seek novelty, are only a small proportion of the overall population. A subset of early adopters comprises the opinion leaders who contribute greatly to the spread of innovations.

Diffusion of Innovations was one of the first attempts to specify the adoption process through a stage-ordered model of awareness, persuasion, decision, implementation, and confirmation (Rogers, 2003).

- *Awareness* occurs when an individual or organizational unit is exposed to an innovation (in health, often—but not always—in the form of an EBI) and gains an understanding of how it functions and how it helps to solve a problem.

- *Persuasion* is the process by which an individual or organizational unit forms a favorable or unfavorable attitude toward an innovation.

- *Decision* is the early stage of adoption, when an individual or organizational unit engages in activities that lead to a choice to adopt or reject an innovation.

- *Implementation* occurs when an individual or organizational unit puts an innovation to use; this typically involves overt behavior change.

- *Confirmation* is the process by which an individual or organizational unit seeks reinforcement of a decision already made. As a result of this process, the individual or organization may make full use of an innovation or choose not to adopt the practice. This concept is similar to the notion of maintenance or sustainability that is present in many other models (Tabak et al., 2012).

How Diffusion of Innovations Is Operationalized

Diffusion of Innovations was developed more than fifty years ago, and the model's underlying constructs and contributions to public health and health care are now vast and complex. At least five operational components of diffusion theory have been summarized (Dearing, 2009; Dearing & Kee, 2012; Haider & Kreps, 2004):

1. Specific properties of innovations affect the rate and extent of adoption, as summarized in Table 16.3.

2. Properties of adopters affect diffusion, especially degree of innovativeness.

3. The social system affects diffusion, especially the structure of the system, its local informal opinion leaders, and potential adopters' perception of social pressure to adopt.

4. External change agents, individuals who influence clients' innovation stage, may secure adoption by showing beneficial effects or may slow diffusion by revealing undesirable effects.

5. A favorable communication relationship between the change agent and clients (defined broadly) is needed to speed diffusion.

Empirical Evidence Supporting the Theory

Diffusion of Innovations has been cited more than 50,000 times over the past fifty years (Table 16.2). Several recent reviews (Green et al., 2009; Greenhalgh et al., 2004, 2005; Haider &

Table 16.3   Diffusion of Innovations: Concepts, Definitions, and Applications to Public Health and Health Care Delivery

Key Innovation Concepts	Definition	Application
Cost	Perceived cost of adopting and implementing innovation	How much time and effort are required to learn to use the innovation and routinize its use? How long does recouping of costs take?
Relative advantage (effectiveness)	The extent to which the innovation works better than that which it will displace	Does a gain in performance outweigh the downsides of cost? Do different stakeholders agree on the superiority of the innovation?
Simplicity	The degree to which the innovation is easy to understand	How easy is it for adopters/implementers to understand an innovative evidence-based program, and/or does the program require a steep learning curve and much training before actual implementation?
Compatibility	The fit of the innovation with the intended audience in order to accomplish desired goal(s)	How much/little will an evidence-based program disrupt the existing routine and/or workflow of the adopting/implementing organization?
Observability	The extent to which outcomes can be seen and measured	To what extent and/or how quickly will the results of an evidence-based program become visible to an implementing organization, its clients, funders, and peer organizations?
Trialability	The extent to which the innovation can be tried before the adopter commits to full adoption	Can an evidence-based program be implemented as a pilot project without much investment and be abandoned without incurring much sunk cost?

Source: Adapted from Dearing & Kee, 2012; Oldenburg & Glanz, 2008; and Rogers, 2003.

Kreps, 2004) have helped to quantify the evidence in support of the theory. These summaries point to the frequency of use, types of use, and qualitative contributions of Diffusion of Innovations theory. Perhaps the most comprehensive review of diffusion theory is found in the interdisciplinary evidence review of 495 sources (a mix of empirical and nonempirical studies) conducted by Greenhalgh and colleagues (Greenhalgh et al., 2004, 2005). One simple way of tracking the impact of diffusion theory is through analysis of publications that use Diffusion of Innovations as a central focus. In conducting their analysis, Greenhalgh et al. (2005) found a peak in diffusion publications for medical education and nursing in 1996 and 1997, with the largest number of articles in the nursing literature. Since then, the frequency of diffusion articles in nursing has dropped considerably, whereas application of diffusion theory in evidence-based medicine and guideline implementation has increased.

Synthesis of the evidence on diffusion theory across four major disciplines (rural sociology, medical sociology, communication, and marketing) largely reinforces the effectiveness and important roles of the attributes displayed in Table 16.3. While much of the relevant literature can be found in public health and medicine, Greenhalgh and colleagues' review extends the uses and usefulness of Diffusion of Innovations to the organizational and management literature (Greenhalgh et al., 2004) and provides some important insights. First, organizational innovativeness is primarily influenced by structural determinants (e.g., internal division of labor and specialization in the organization). Second, the spread of innovations within and across organizations is strongly influenced by interorganizational norms. Third, organizations that strongly support on-the-job learning are often more effective than others in spreading innovations, due to their values and goals of supporting the creation and sharing of new knowledge. Fourth, innovative organizations are often those in which new stories can be told that capture and support the idea of *communities of practice* (i.e., groups that share a common purpose and interact regularly to improve their practice). And fifth, organizations are complex, and effective diffusion addresses this complexity while maintaining the organization's ability to adapt to change.

As these principles are refined, they can be incorporated into more recent health behavior and public health research, in which applications of diffusion models are noteworthy in their focus on *active* dissemination with pre- to postmeasurement of effects (Oldenburg & Glanz, 2008). This is in contrast to the well-established diffusion research emphasis on cross-sectional survey research to explain how innovations spread (Rogers, 2003). In the physical activity field, the SPARK (Sports, Play, and Active Recreation for Kids) and CATCH (Coordinated Approach to Child Health) programs for school-based physical education have been disseminated widely, and some of the core constructs of Diffusion of Innovations have been used to describe D&I efforts (Owen, Glanz, Sallis, & Kelder, 2006). In the cancer control field (and described in more detail later), the Pool Cool sun-safety program for aquatic settings is an example of a health behavior change program that has progressed from an efficacy trial to a D&I trial (Glanz, Steffen, Elliott, & O'Riordan, 2005). Body and Soul, a nutrition intervention conducted through African American churches to increase individuals' fruit and vegetable intake, was disseminated broadly through a partnership of the American Cancer Society, the Centers for Disease Control and Prevention (CDC), and the National Cancer Institute, and was rigorously evaluated (Campbell, Resnicow, Carr, Wang, & Williams, 2007). It was particularly important that major organizations with responsibility for cancer control collaborated in creating and testing the dissemination version of this effective nutrition program. Such collaboration and investment in dissemination is unusual. In HIV/AIDS efforts, Diffusion of Innovations has been used extensively in the development, implementation, and wide diffusion of programs in both developed and developing countries (Bertrand, 2004).

Several limitations of Diffusion of Innovations have been identified (Greenhalgh et al., 2004; Oldenburg & Glanz, 2008). These include a major focus on individual innovation and adopters (perhaps downplaying systems effects), too little focus on nonadoption processes, an inherent pro-innovation bias, a focus on individuals that may lead to a perception of "blaming the victim," too great a focus on fixed personality traits, a failure to account for socioeconomic position in the use of new technologies, and a lack of transferability of diffusion research principles from one setting or context to others. D&I generally are focused on transfer of EBIs, whereas Diffusion of Innovations theory may relate to innovations that are or are not evidence based. In fact, in some settings, the rapid spread of unproven, even harmful, medical treatments and preventive strategies is of great concern.

Application of Diffusion of Innovations: The Pool Cool Skin Cancer Prevention Program

Pool Cool is a multicomponent skin cancer prevention program for use in swimming pool settings that was evaluated for its impact on sun-protection habits and swimming pool environments (Glanz, Geller, Shigaki, Maddock, & Isnec, 2002). The intervention included staff training; sun-safety lessons; interactive activities; provision of sunscreen, shade, and signage; and promotion of sun-safe environments. The program was intended for children five to ten years of age (primarily those taking swimming lessons), their parents, and lifeguards and aquatic instructors. A cluster randomized trial at twenty-eight swimming pools in Hawaii and Massachusetts tested the efficacy of the program compared with an attention-matched injury prevention control program. Results showed significant changes in children's use of shade and sunscreen, overall sun-protection habits, and number of sunburns, and improvements in parents' hat use, sun-protection habits, and reported sun-protection policies and environments.

The Pool Cool Diffusion Trial applied principles of Diffusion of Innovations theory to evaluate the effects of two strategies for dissemination of the Pool Cool skin cancer prevention program in over four hundred swimming pools across the United States and in Okinawa on (1) program implementation, maintenance, and sustainability; (2) improvements in organizational and environmental supports for sun protection at swimming pools; and (3) sun-protection habits and sunburns among children. The research also aimed to identify organizational predictors of these outcomes (Glanz et al., 2005). In the four-year dissemination trial (fieldwork occurred from 2003 to 2006), swimming pools were the main organizational-level unit of study and the unit of measurement for organizational-level diffusion outcomes. Field coordinators throughout the program regions were linkage agents for the program, and clusters of pools affiliated with each field coordinator were the main unit of randomization and intervention for the trial. Lifeguards and aquatic instructors were the potential mediators of program effects on children (Rabin et al., 2010). Children aged five to ten years taking swimming lessons at participating pools were the primary audience for the Pool Cool intervention, with their parents being a secondary audience.

The D&I trial used an experimental design in which all participating swimming pools received an intervention package. Half the pools received additional strategies and resources to increase program implementation. Both the basic and enhanced group pools were given the main components of Pool Cool, including the field coordinator training program and the program provided at swimming pools. In addition, the enhanced group pool sites received additional sun-safety resources for distribution, more ready-made environmental intervention resources, including a set of sun signs, and additional target goals and rewards for documenting high levels of implementation.

The study approach and interventions were grounded in three models: Social Cognitive Theory, Diffusion of Innovations, and theories of organizational change. Key constructs were derived from each of these theories, applied to the intervention, and then measured accordingly at each of the appropriate levels. Results of independent process evaluations at one and two years demonstrated very good implementation and maintenance in a sample of 120 pools

Table 16.4   Key Challenges and Lessons from the Pool Cool Diffusion Trial

Key Concept	Background and Lesson
Study design	• Clustering occurred at differing levels in the efficacy trial and in the diffusion trial (pool level vs. the field coordinator level).
	• The diffusion study design was more feasible in a variety of locations and more cost efficient.
Program implementation	• Study data showed that Pool Cool implementation increased from year 1 to year 2.
	• To support implementation, diffusion trials should be designed for dissemination with a strong process evaluation.
Participation and response rates	• Participant attrition is often a challenge in a diffusion trial.
	• Significant reminders and incentives need to be built into the study to support adequate response rates.
Measurement issues	• Measurement across stages of implementation, maintenance, and sustainability is complex.
	• Self-reported measures may be biased, though an ancillary validity study found good to excellent validity for self-reports of the main behavioral outcomes.
	• Nested reliability and validity studies may be necessary to develop both self-reported and objective measures.

each year. Also, according to the early process evaluation, there were few differences in implementation between the two conditions during the first two years (Escoffery, Glanz, & Elliott, 2008). Some important challenges and lessons from the trial are shown in Table 16.4.

The main results of the study at the organizational level evaluated effects of the two strategies (basic vs. enhanced) for D&I of the Pool Cool skin cancer prevention program on (1) program implementation, maintenance, and sustainability, and (2) improvements in organizational and environmental supports for sun protection at swimming pools. Although both treatment groups improved their implementation of the program over three summers of participation, pools in the enhanced condition had significantly greater overall maintenance of the program than those in the basic group. Further, while both groups revealed improved sun-safety policies and environments, pools in the enhanced condition established and maintained significantly greater sun-safety policies over time (Glanz, Escoffery, Elliott, & Nehl, 2014). Pool Cool demonstrated that more intensive, theory-driven dissemination strategies can have a significant effect on program implementation and maintenance and on health-promoting environmental and policy changes.

To implement, disseminate, and evaluate the program, the project team had to build effective relationships with professional organizations and recreation sites at national, regional, and local levels. This was achieved by participating in aquatics and recreation conferences, developing career opportunities, encouraging local media coverage of program activities (Hall, Dubruiel, Elliott, & Glanz, 2009), and providing resources for conducting the program after research participation concluded (Hall, Escoffery, Nehl, & Glanz, 2010).

Consolidated Framework for Implementation Research

The Consolidated Framework for Implementation Research (CFIR) was created in 2009 to address a gap in implementation research, with support from the U.S. Department of Veterans Affairs (VA), the Veterans Health Administration, and the VA's Health Services Research & Development Service and its Diabetes Quality Enhancement Research Initiative (QUERI) in Ann Arbor, Michigan (Damschroder, 2010). The CFIR was designed to embrace, consolidate, and unify key constructs from the multitude of implementation theories and frameworks into one model that contained the most important constructs and used consistent terminology (Damschroder et al., 2009). Development of the CFIR was based on a literature review of published models (including Diffusion of Innovations) that identified constructs evaluated for strength of conceptual or empirical support for influence on implementation, consistency in definitions, alignment with the development team's own findings, and potential for measurement. Then the constructs were combined across models; redundancies were removed, and constructs that conflated underlying concepts were dissected.

Key Components of the Framework

CFIR is composed of five major domains, each with related constructs: *intervention characteristics* (8 constructs: e.g., intervention source; relative advantage), *outer setting* (4 constructs: e.g., cosmopolitanism, external policies and incentives), *inner setting* (12 constructs: e.g., networks and communications, culture), *characteristics of individuals involved* (5 constructs: e.g., knowledge and beliefs about the intervention, individual identification with organization), and *process of implementation* (8 constructs: e.g., planning, engaging). The five domains along with their definitions and applications are displayed in Table 16.5.

Table 16.5   Consolidated Framework for Implementation Research Domains: Definitions and Applications to Implementation Research

Domain	Definition	Application
Intervention characteristics	Key attributes of interventions, those that influence the success of implementation	Can the intervention be adapted to our local setting? Will this intervention be better than an alternative?
Outer setting	Economic, political, and social context within which an organization resides	To what extent is the implementing organization networked with external organizations? Is implementation of the intervention mandated by an external authority?
Inner setting	Features of structural, political, and cultural contexts inside the organization	Is the setting in which the intervention is being implemented receptive to change?
Characteristics of individuals involved	Characteristics of the individuals involved with the intervention and/or implementation process	What are the attitudes toward the intervention of the individuals responsible for the intervention process?
Process of implementation	Steps to an active change process aimed at achieving individual- and organizational-level use of the intervention as designed	Who should be involved in implementation, and how can they become engaged in the process?

How the Framework Is Operationalized

As with other models, CFIR is operationalized primarily through measurement. Quantitative measures have not yet been developed for each construct. However, constructs in the model were chosen explicitly for their potential to be operationalized and measured. Resources are available online, with examples of interview guides and guidance for qualitative coding (cfirguide.org). Measures have been developed for several of CFIR's constructs—notably, the structural characteristics of the inner setting and the characteristics of individuals. As measures become available, they will be posted on the CFIR technical assistance website. Another way that the CFIR can be operationalized is through its application in other models. The CFIR provides a set of constructs that can guide researchers using models with, for example, formative and maintenance phases. Additionally, CFIR can be used for the organization and synthesis of research findings across time and across studies.

Empirical Evidence Supporting the Model

Empirical evidence supporting the model is found in several research studies. An investigation into implementation of the MOVE! Program in VA medical centers, led by Damschroder, found that key organizational factors at local centers were strongly associated with successful implementation (Damschroder, Goodrich, Robinson, Fletcher, & Lowery, 2011; Damschroder & Lowery, 2013). Studies in the areas of addiction treatment (Gordon et al., 2011) and alcohol screening (Williams et al., 2011) have found relationships between barriers, facilitators, and programs to address inner setting implementation factors and implementation.

Application of CFIR: Substance Use Disorder Treatment

Continuing care following substance use disorder treatment extends beyond a brief episode of acute care and is associated with improved outcomes. While the initial stage of treatment is intensive, continuing care includes treatments such as individual, telephone, and group therapy; brief checkups; and mutual help meetings. Evidence-based interventions for continuing care have been developed, but patient participation is low, and some practices lacking adequate evidence are widely used; a passive approach to dissemination has been hypothesized as a cause of this discrepancy. Though attempts have been made to use typical implementation efforts (e.g., manuals and workshops for clinicians), these have not been effective, and efforts in the contexts of clinical trials are typically not sustained (Lash, Timko, Curran, McKay, & Burden, 2011).

To bridge the gap between research and practice, Lash et al. (2011) reviewed the literature on implementation of EBIs. Their review focused specifically on two EBIs (McKay, 2005)—continuing treatment and monitoring, and mutual help group participation following treatment—and was guided by the CFIR. The primary aim was to assess the current barriers to use of EBIs and to provide recommendations on how to overcome identified barriers (Lash et al., 2011).

Implementation research identified in the review was mapped onto the CFIR domains and constructs. The research came primarily from three types of studies: (1) efficacy/effectiveness trials with patient-level information related to implementation, (2) effectiveness studies with process data on implementation, and (3) trials evaluating implementation. Using this diverse set of studies, the authors abstracted relevant information on implementation, even in the absence of a robust set of direct implementation trials. Current research about continuing care implementation, organized according to the CFIR, was used to provide recommendations for researchers and practitioners in each of the five major domains. Also identified were specific research gaps within each domain. For example, in the intervention domain, the authors determined that the strengths of the intervention were quality of the evidence base and adaptability of the intervention. However, use of the intervention was deterred by its complexity. Furthermore, implementation was made difficult by the lack of information on the advantage of various EBIs relative to each other, the cost effectiveness of each EBI, and the determination of core versus adaptable components of each EBI.

Additional Core Concepts and Areas of Future Research

Four specific areas of D&I research warrant attention in this section to enable readers to better understand the uptake of effective programs and policies. First, the growth of implementation science is briefly described. The second topic involves the timely opportunities in community and public health settings that may lead to stronger linkages between researchers and practitioners. The third area focuses on the concept of designing for dissemination (discussed briefly in the Pool Cool case description earlier), in which dissemination is considered early in the development of programs and policies. The fourth area is the further conceptual and empirical development of methods and measures for D&I research.

Growth of the Field of Implementation Science

The growth of the scientific field of implementation science (defined in Table 16.1) has accelerated greatly over the past decade (Chambers, 2012). In health care settings, the origins of implementation science can be traced to Archibald Cochrane's landmark text *Effectiveness and Efficiency* (Cochrane, 1972) and the subsequent development of the Cochrane Collaboration. For population health, an important milestone involves the Centers for Disease Control and Prevention's development of *The Guide to Community Preventive Services* (a systematic review that summarizes what is known about the effectiveness and cost effectiveness of population-based interventions to promote health; prevent disease, injury, disability and premature death; and also reduce exposure to environmental hazards) (Zaza, Briss, & Harris, 2005). *The Guide to Community Preventive Services* provides a menu of effective EBIs for dissemination and implementation. A growing literature, inherently transdisciplinary, addresses the science and practice of D&I (Brownson, Colditz, & Proctor, 2012). To document these advances in the field, there are now scientific journals dedicated to D&I research (e.g., *Implementation Science* and *Translational Behavioral Medicine*). The U.S. National Institutes of Health (NIH) released its first program announcement on D&I research in 2002, and there is now a study section (a panel to review grants) within NIH dedicated to D&I research.

Challenges and Opportunities in Community and Public Health Settings

The concept of evidence-based public health (EBPH) is central to D&I efforts. EBPH has been defined as the integration of science-based interventions with community preferences to improve population health (Kohatsu, Robinson, & Torner, 2004). This definition can be extended beyond structured interventions to include processes within organizational settings that are associated with performance measures (e.g., workforce development, organizational climate and culture, and leadership) (Brownson, Allen, Duggan, Stamatakis, & Erwin, 2012).

The great variety of community and public health settings offers challenges as well as opportunities for studying and promoting the uptake of EBIs. Even within the public health infrastructure, a system of backbone organizations that provides some centralization of public health authority in states and communities across the United States, the uptake of EBIs varies by setting and level of focus. For example, one study examined the uptake of *The Guide to Community Preventive Services*. In a survey of state and local public health practitioners, only 30 percent of local practitioners had heard of *The Guide to Community Preventive Services*. In state-level agencies, 90 percent had heard of the community guide, but few reported making changes to existing programs (20%) or new programs (35%) on the basis of the guide's recommendations (Brownson et al., 2007). Some barriers to EBPH identified in the literature are lack of time, inadequate funding, absence of cultural and managerial support (especially the absence of incentives), an inconsistent understanding of the definition of *evidence*, perceived lack of institutional priority for EBPH, and not conducting research activities to inform program adoption and implementation (Brownson, Baker, Leet, Gillespie, & True, 2011). Despite such barriers, a variety of online analytic tools and resources are freely available and these tools can facilitate evidence-based practice in public health across the globe (see Appendix 16.1 in the supplementary web materials for this chapter).

Even though there are many challenges, current trends in public health offer opportunities to increase dissemination and implementation of EBIs. First, in public health there is a current movement toward voluntary accreditation and, closely related, continuous quality improvement. In the fall of 2012, the national public health accreditation program was rolled out, and the first round of accredited health departments was recently announced (Public Health Accreditation Board, 2011). This opportunity for studying the effects of accreditation is an example of the ability to generate *practice-based evidence*—evidence that has been developed in the real world, rather than in highly controlled research conditions, and that can be more relevant and actionable (Green, 2008). In another recent development, the Institute of Medicine published a series of three reports on public health, focusing on needed reforms in measurement, law, and financing (Committee on Public Health Strategies to Improve Health, 2010, 2011, 2012). As part of this effort, a minimum set of public health functions was redefined, based in part on an essential services framework previously described (Committee on Public Health Strategies to Improve Health, 2012). Finally, implementation of the Affordable Care Act is opening new opportunities and requirements around integrating public health and health care (Shaffer, 2013). For example, the recent U.S. Internal Revenue Service requirement that nonprofit hospitals conduct community health assessments in partnership with state and/or local public health agencies unlocks new possibilities for cross-sector collaboration, incorporating population-based prevention measures across the spectrum of health care interventions.

Designing for Dissemination

Designing for dissemination is defined as "an active process that helps to ensure that public health interventions, often evaluated by researchers, are developed in ways that match well with adopters' needs, assets, and time frames" (Brownson, Jacobs, Tabak, Hoehner, & Stamatakis, 2013). A recent study of public health researchers in the United States found considerable room for improvement in designing for dissemination (Brownson et al., 2013). About half of the respondents (53%) had a person or team in their unit dedicated to dissemination. Seventeen percent of all respondents used a model to plan their dissemination activities. One-third of respondents (34%) always or usually involved stakeholders in the research process.

The difficulty in designing for dissemination is due in part to differing priorities between researchers and practitioners (Colditz, Emmons, Viswanath, & Kerner, 2008). For researchers, partly because of funding, recognition, and other issues, priority is often on discovery (not application) of new knowledge; whereas for practitioners and policymakers, the focus is often on practical ways to apply these discoveries to their settings, often with some adaptation for local relevance (Kreuter & Bernhardt, 2009). The chasm between researchers and practitioners was illustrated in a workshop on designing for dissemination sponsored by the National Cancer Institute (2002). In this workshop, all participants acknowledged the importance of dissemination. Researchers reported that their role was to identify effective interventions but that they were not responsible for dissemination of research findings. Similarly, practitioners did not believe they were responsible for dissemination. Unfortunately, when no one believes it is his or her job to disseminate, the activity often falls through the cracks or sinks to a low priority in already overstressed organizations.

Specific actions based on the growing body of literature (Brownson et al., 2013; Glasgow & Emmons, 2007; Lehoux et al., 2005; Owen, Goode, Fjeldsoe, Sugiyama, & Eakin, 2012; Tabak et al., 2012) could improve designing for dissemination across levels of system, process, and production (Table 16.6).

Methods and Measures for D&I Research

A public health and quality improvement adage is "What gets measured, gets done" (Thacker, 2007). Successful progress of D&I science will require the development of practical measures of outcomes that are both reliable and valid. These enable empirical testing of the success of D&I efforts. While researchers have built many excellent surveillance systems for measuring long-term (*downstream*) change (e.g., in terms of behavioral risk factors, mortality, and cancer incidence), most of these are only partially useful for D&I research, where a greater focus is needed on *upstream* factors (e.g., health-promoting public policies) (McKinlay, 1998). Few available measures have been designed to focus on D&I research at the population level. Moreover, most measures focus on distal outcomes, such as change in health status, which

Table 16.6   Designing for Dissemination Principles

Domain	Subdomain	Sample Actions
System	Shift research funder priorities and processes.	• Make dissemination (e.g., a dissemination plan) a scorable part of funding announcements. • Include stakeholders in the grant review process. • Provide rapid funding for practice-based research with high dissemination potential. • Provide supplemental funding for dissemination.
	Shift researcher incentives and opportunities.	• Provide academic incentives and credit, including impacts on promotion and tenure decisions (provide prototype promotion/tenure policies). • Hire faculty with practice experience. • Provide opportunities for faculty to spend time in practice settings. • Conduct trainings to improve dissemination, implementation, evaluation, and translation.
	Develop new measures and tools.	• Identify measures for evaluating dissemination efforts. • Maintain systems for tracking the measures. • Develop tools for designing for dissemination.
	Develop new reporting standards.	• Develop standards for reporting research that focus more fully on dissemination. • Promote new dissemination and implementation reporting standards.
	Identify infrastructure requirements.	• Identify people required for dissemination and evaluation. • Identify system requirements (e.g., information technology, media).
Processes	Involve stakeholders as early in the process as possible.	• Engage stakeholders as advisors and collaborators. • Engage stakeholders in the research process.
	Engage key stakeholders (receptors) for research through audience research.	• Identify gaps in research, relevance of methods and messages. • Ensure stakeholders represent potential adopter organizations. • Identify opinion leaders for uptake. • Identify barriers to dissemination. • Identify success and failure stories.
	Identify models for dissemination efforts.	• Review existing frameworks for applicable constructs. • Pilot-test measures for assessing model constructs among key stakeholders. • Develop models for dissemination actions that are context relevant.
	Identify the appropriate means of delivering the message.	• Identify the optimal disseminator (usually *not* the researcher). • Link the researcher and practice and policy specialists with the disseminator. • Identify channels for dissemination/mode of knowledge transfer.

(*continued*)

Table 16.6   *(Continued)*

Domain	Subdomain	Sample Actions
Products	Identify the appropriate message.	• For interventions, document evidence of effectiveness, cost of implementation, and cost effectiveness. • For etiologic research, address risk communication. • Document evidence of disseminability and ease of use.
	Develop summaries of research in user-friendly, nonacademic formats (tailor to audience).	• Develop issue briefs, policy briefs, and case studies. • Identify potential roles for social media (e.g., Twitter, Facebook). • Deliver presentations to stakeholders.

Source: Brownson et al., 2013.

are often beyond the remit of projects. Proximal measures of D&I processes and outcomes are sorely needed. As new measures are developed (or existing metrics adapted), some key considerations include (1) refining core constructs of D&I models; (2) determining how to measure and operationalize core constructs of D&I models; (3) identifying which outcomes should be tracked, and how long it will take to show progress; (4) deciding how implementation fidelity and adaptation can best be measured across a broad range of D&I studies; (5) deciding how to determine criterion validity (how a measures compares with some "gold standard"); (6) identifying how best to measure moderating factors across a range of settings (e.g., schools, worksites); and (7) learning how common, practical, measures can be developed and shared so researchers are not constantly reinventing measures.

Summary

This chapter has highlighted a sample of the many rich areas for dissemination and implementation research and practice, in many cases building upon the Diffusion of Innovations model. Perhaps the most important practical lesson arising from diffusion research has been the importance of achieving a good fit among the attributes of an innovation, the adopting individual or organization, and the environment or context within which the process takes place.

The concepts of D&I research have been defined more fully over the past decade (Brownson, Colditz, et al., 2012) and will continue to evolve as new approaches are developed and new health challenges arise. There is an increasing emphasis on the need to implement multicomponent and multilevel programs to address a diverse range of health behavior issues, such as tobacco use, HIV/AIDS, obesity, and mental health. If outcomes from decades of public health and health behavior intervention research are to be translated into major health improvements, we must better understand and act upon factors that support or inhibit the uptake of effective programs and policies.

References

Bartholomew, L. K., Parcel, G. S., Kok, G., & Gottlieb, N. H. (2001). *Intervention Mapping: Designing theory- and evidence-based health promotion programs*. Mountain View, CA: Mayfield.

Bertrand, J. T. (2004). Diffusion of innovations and HIV/AIDS. *Journal of Health Communication, 9*(Suppl. 1), 113–121.

Brownson, R. C., Allen, P., Duggan, K., Stamatakis, K. A., & Erwin, P. C. (2012). Fostering more-effective public health by identifying administrative evidence-based practices: A review of the literature. *American Journal of Preventive Medicine, 43*(3), 309–319.

Brownson, R. C., Baker, E. A., Leet, T. L., Gillespie, K. N., & True, W. R. (2011). *Evidence-based public health* (2nd ed.). New York: Oxford University Press.

Brownson, R. C., Ballew, P., Brown, K. L., Elliott, M. B., Haire-Joshu, D., Heath, G. W., & Kreuter, M. W. (2007). The effect of disseminating evidence-based interventions that promote physical activity to health departments. *American Journal of Public Health, 97*(10), 1900–1907.

Brownson, R. C., Colditz, G. A., & Proctor, E. K. (Eds.). (2012). *Dissemination and implementation research in health: Translating science to practice.* New York: Oxford University Press.

Brownson, R. C., Jacobs, J. A., Tabak, R. G., Hoehner, C. M., & Stamatakis, K. A. (2013). Designing for dissemination among public health researchers: Findings from a national survey in the United States. *American Journal of Public Health, 103*(9), 1696–1699.

Brug, J., Tak, N. I., & Te Velde, S. J. (2011). Evaluation of nationwide health promotion campaigns in The Netherlands: An exploration of practices, wishes and opportunities. *Health Promotion International, 26*(2), 244–254.

Bryce, J., Black, R. E., Walker, N., Bhutta, Z. A., Lawn, J. E., & Steketee, R. W. (2005). Can the world afford to save the lives of 6 million children each year? *Lancet, 365*(9478), 2193–2200.

Campbell, M. K., Resnicow, K., Carr, C., Wang, T., & Williams, A. (2007). Process evaluation of an effective church-based diet intervention: Body & soul. *Health Education & Behavior, 34*(6), 864–880.

Canadian Institutes of Health Research. (2013). More about knowledge translation at CIHR. Retrieved from http://www.cihr-irsc.gc.ca/e/39033.html

Casado, B. L., Quijano, L. M., Stanley, M. A., Cully, J. A., Steinberg, E. H., & Wilson, N. L. (2008). Healthy IDEAS: Implementation of a depression program through community-based case management. *Gerontologist, 48*(6), 828.

Chambers, D. (2012). Foreword. In R. C. Brownson, G. A. Colditz, & E. K. Proctor (Eds.), *Dissemination and implementation research in health: Translating science to practice* (pp. vii–x). New York: Oxford University Press.

Ciliska, D., Robinson, P., Armour, T., Ellis, P., Brouwers, M., Gauld, M., . . . Raina, P. (2005). Diffusion and dissemination of evidence-based dietary strategies for the prevention of cancer. *Nutrition Journal, 4*, 13.

Cochrane, A. (1972). *Effectiveness and efficiency: Random reflections on health services.* London: Nuffield Provincial Hospital Trust.

Colditz, G. A., Emmons, K. M., Viswanath, K., & Kerner, J. F. (2008). Translating science to practice: Community and academic perspectives. *Journal of Public Health Management and Practice, 14*(2), 144–149.

Committee on Public Health Strategies to Improve Health. (2010). *For the public's health: The role of measurement in action and accountability.* Washington, DC: National Academies Press.

Committee on Public Health Strategies to Improve Health. (2011). *For the public's health: Revitalizing law and policy to meet new challenges.* Washington, DC: National Academies Press.

Committee on Public Health Strategies to Improve Health. (2012). *For the public's health: Investing in a healthier future.* Washington, DC: National Academies Press.

Craig, R. L., Felix, H. C., Walker, J. F., & Phillips, M. M. (2010). Public health professionals as policy entrepreneurs: Arkansas's childhood obesity policy experience. *American Journal of Public Health, 100*(11), 2047–2052.

Cummings, G. G., Estabrooks, C. A., Midodzi, W. K., Wallin, L., & Hayduk, L. (2007). Influence of organizational characteristics and context on research utilization. *Nursing Research, 56*(4), S24.

Damschroder, L. (2010). *Consolidated framework for implementation research (CFIR)*. Retrieved from www.cfirguide.org

Damschroder, L. J., Aron, D. C., Keith, R. E., Kirsh, S. R., Alexander, J. A., & Lowery, J. C. (2009). Fostering implementation of health services research findings into practice: A consolidated framework for advancing implementation science. *Implementation Science, 4*, 50.

Damschroder, L. J., Goodrich, D. E., Robinson, C. H., Fletcher, C. E., & Lowery, J. C. (2011). A systematic exploration of differences in contextual factors related to implementing the MOVE! weight management program in VA: A mixed methods study. *BMC Health Services Research, 11*, 248.

Damschroder, L. J., & Lowery, J. C. (2013). Evaluation of a large-scale weight management program using the consolidated framework for implementation research (CFIR). *Implementation Science, 8*, 51.

Davis, R. M., Wakefield, M., Amos, A., & Gupta, P. C. (2007). The hitchhiker's guide to tobacco control: A global assessment of harms, remedies, and controversies. *Annual Review of Public Health, 28*, 171–194.

De Meij, J.S.B., Chinapaw, M.J.M., Kremers, S.P.J., Van der Wal, M. F., Jurg, M. E., & Van Mechelen, W. (2010). Promoting physical activity in children: The stepwise development of the primary school-based JUMP-in intervention applying the RE-AIM evaluation framework. *British Journal of Sports Medicine, 44*(12), 879–887.

Dearing, J. W. (2008). Evolution of diffusion and dissemination theory. *Journal of Public Health Management and Practice, 14*(2), 99–108.

Dearing, J. W. (2009). Applying diffusion of innovation theory to intervention development. *Research on Social Work Practice, 19*(5), 503–518.

Dearing, J. W., & Kee, K. F. (2012). Historical roots of dissemination and implementation science. In R. C. Brownson, G. A. Colditz, & E. K. Proctor (Eds.), *Dissemination and implementation research in health: Translating science to practice* (pp. 55–71). New York: Oxford University Press.

Deschesnes, M., Trudeau, F., & Kebe, M. (2010). Factors influencing the adoption of a health promoting school approach in the province of Quebec, Canada. *Health Education Research, 25*(3), 438–450.

Dong, L., Neufeld, D. J., & Higgins, C. (2008). Testing Klein and Sorra's innovation implementation model: An empirical examination. *Journal of Engineering and Technology Management, 25*(4), 237–255.

Dreisinger, M., Leet, T. L., Baker, E. A., Gillespie, K. N., Haas, B., & Brownson, R. C. (2008). Improving the public health workforce: Evaluation of a training course to enhance evidence-based decision making. *Journal of Public Health Management and Practice, 14*(2), 138–143.

Ellis, I., Howard, P., Larson, A., & Robertson, J. (2005). From workshop to work practice: An exploration of context and facilitation in the development of evidence-based practice. *Worldviews on Evidence-Based Nursing, 2*(2), 84–93.

Elwyn, G., Taubert, M., & Kowalczuk, J. (2007). Sticky knowledge: A possible model for investigating implementation in healthcare contexts. *Implementation Science, 2*, 44.

Escoffery, C., Glanz, K., & Elliott, T. (2008). Process evaluation of the Pool Cool Diffusion Trial for skin cancer prevention across 2 years. *Health Education Research, 23*(4), 732–743.

Fixsen, D. L., & Mental, L.P.F. (2005). *Implementation research: A synthesis of the literature.* Tampa: University of South Florida, National Implementation Research Network.

Glanz, K., & Bishop, D. B. (2010). The role of behavioral science theory in development and implementation of public health interventions. *Annual Review of Public Health, 31,* 399–418.

Glanz, K., Escoffery, C., Elliott, T., & Nehl, E. (2014, December 18). Randomized trial of two dissemination strategies for a skin cancer prevention program in aquatic settings. *American Journal of Public Health,* e1–e9. doi:10.2105/AJPH.2014.302224

Glanz, K., Geller, A. C., Shigaki, D., Maddock, J. E., & Isnec, M. R. (2002). A randomized trial of skin cancer prevention in aquatics settings: The Pool Cool program. *Health Psychology, 21*(6), 579–587.

Glanz, K., Steffen, A., Elliott, T., & O'Riordan, D. (2005). Diffusion of an effective skin cancer prevention program: Design, theoretical foundations, and first-year implementation. *Health Psychology, 24*(5), 477–487.

Glasgow, R. E., & Emmons, K. M. (2007). How can we increase translation of research into practice? Types of evidence needed. *Annual Review of Public Health, 28,* 413–433.

Glasgow, R. E., Marcus, A. C., Bull, S. S., & Wilson, K. M. (2004). Disseminating effective cancer screening interventions. *Cancer, 101*(Suppl. 5), 1239–1250.

Glasgow, R. E., Nelson, C. C., Strycker, L. A., & King, D. K. (2006). Using RE-AIM metrics to evaluate diabetes self-management support interventions. *American Journal of Preventive Medicine, 30*(1), 67–73.

Glasgow, R. E., Vinson, C., Chambers, D., Khoury, M. J., Kaplan, R. M., & Hunter, C. (2012). National Institutes of Health approaches to dissemination and implementation science: Current and future directions. *American Journal of Public Health, 102*(7), 1274–1281.

Glasgow, R. E., Vogt, T. M., & Boles, S. M. (1999). Evaluating the public health impact of health promotion interventions: The RE-AIM framework. *American Journal of Public Health, 89*(9), 1322–1327.

Glisson, C., Dukes, D., & Green, P. (2006). The effects of the ARC organizational intervention on caseworker turnover, climate, and culture in children's service systems. *Child Abuse & Neglect, 30*(8), 855–880.

Glisson, C., & Schoenwald, S. K. (2005). The ARC organizational and community intervention strategy for implementing evidence-based children's mental health treatments. *Mental Health Service Research, 7*(4), 243–259.

Glisson, C., Schoenwald, S. K., Hemmelgarn, A., Green, P., Dukes, D., Armstrong, K. S., & Chapman, J. E. (2010). Randomized trial of MST and ARC in a two-level evidence-based treatment implementation strategy. *Journal of Consulting and Clinical Psychology, 78*(4), 537–550.

Gordon, A. J., Kavanagh, G., Krumm, M., Ramgopal, R., Paidisetty, S., Aghevli, M., . . . Liberto, J. (2011). Facilitators and barriers in implementing buprenorphine in the Veterans Health Administration. *Psychology of Addictive Behaviors, 25*(2), 215–224.

Graham, I. D., Logan, J., Harrison, M. B., Straus, S. E., Tetroe, J., Caswell, W., & Robinson, N. (2006). Lost in knowledge translation: Time for a map? *Journal of Continuing Education in the Health Professions, 26*(1), 13–24.

Green, L. W. (2008). Making research relevant: If it is an evidence-based practice, where's the practice-based evidence? *Family Practice, 25*(Suppl. 1), i20–i24.

Green, L. W., & Kreuter, M. W. (2005). *Health promotion planning: An educational and ecological approach* (4th ed.). New York: McGraw-Hill.

Green, L. W., Ottoson, J. M., Garcia, C., & Hiatt, R. A. (2009). Diffusion theory, and knowledge dissemination, utilization, and integration in public health. *Annual Review of Public Health, 30*, 151–74.

Greenhalgh, T., Robert, G., Macfarlane, F., Bate, P., & Kyriakidou, O. (2004). Diffusion of innovations in service organizations: Systematic review and recommendations. *Milbank Quarterly, 82*(4), 581–629.

Greenhalgh, T., Robert, G., Macfarlane, F., Bate, P., Kyriakidou, O., & Peacock, R. (2005). Storylines of research in diffusion of innovation: A meta-narrative approach to systematic review. *Social Science & Medicine, 61*(2), 417–430.

Haider, M., & Kreps, G. L. (2004). Forty years of diffusion of innovations: Utility and value in public health. *Journal of Health Communication, 9*(Suppl. 1), 3–11.

Hall, D., Dubruiel, N., Elliott, T., & Glanz, K. (2009). Linking agents' activities and communication patterns in a study of the dissemination of an effective skin cancer prevention program. *Journal of Public Health Management and Practice, 15*(5), 409–415.

Hall, D. M., Escoffery, C., Nehl, E., & Glanz, K. (2010). Spontaneous diffusion of an effective skin cancer prevention program through web-based access to program materials. *Preventing Chronic Disease, 7*(6), A125.

Hawe, P., Shiell, A., & Riley, T. (2004). Complex interventions: How "out of control" can a randomised controlled trial be? *BMJ, 328*(7455), 1561–1563.

Helfrich, C. D., Damschroder, L. J., Hagedorn, H. J., Daggett, G. S., Sahay, A., Ritchie, M., . . . Stetler, C. B. (2010). A critical synthesis of literature on the Promoting Action on Research Implementation in Health Services (PARIHS) framework. *Implementation Science, 5*(1), 82.

Helfrich, C. D., Li, Y. F., Sharp, N. D., & Sales, A. E. (2009). Organizational Readiness to Change Assessment (ORCA): Development of an instrument based on the Promoting Action on Research in Health Services (PARIHS) framework. *Implementation Science, 4*, 38.

Holahan, P. J., Aronson, Z. H., Jurkat, M. P., & Schoorman, F. D. (2004). Implementing computer technology: A multiorganizational test of Klein and Sorra's model. *Journal of Engineering and Technology Management, 21*(1–2), 31–50.

Howat, P., Jones, S., Hall, M., Cross, D., & Stevenson, M. (1997). The PRECEDE-PROCEED model: Application to planning a child pedestrian injury prevention program. *Injury Prevention, 3*(4), 282–287.

Institute of Medicine. (2001). *Crossing the quality chasm: A new health system for the 21st century.* Washington, DC: National Academies Press.

Jacobs, J. A., Dodson, E. A., Baker, E. A., Deshpande, A. D., & Brownson, R. C. (2010). Barriers to evidence-based decision making in public health: A national survey of chronic disease practitioners. *Public Health Reports, 125*(5), 736–742.

Johnson, J. L., Green, L. W., Frankish, C. J., MacLean, D. R., & Stachenko, S. (1996). A dissemination research agenda to strengthen health promotion and disease prevention. *Canadian Journal of Public Health, 87*(Suppl. 2), S5–S10.

Kerner, J., Rimer, B., & Emmons, K. (2005). Introduction to the special section on dissemination: Dissemination research and research dissemination: How can we close the gap? *Health Psychology, 24*(5), 443–446.

Kingdon, J. W. (2003). *Agendas, alternatives, and public policies* (2nd ed.). New York: Addison-Wesley.

Kitson, A., Harvey, G., & McCormack, B. (1998). Enabling the implementation of evidence based practice: A conceptual framework. *Quality in Health Care, 7*(3), 149.

Kitson, A. L., Rycroft-Malone, J., Harvey, G., McCormack, B., Seers, K., & Titchen, A. (2008). Evaluating the successful implementation of evidence into practice using the PARiHS framework: Theoretical and practical challenges. *Implementation Science, 3,* 1.

Klein, K. J., & Sorra, J. S. (1996). The challenge of innovation implementation. *Academy of Management Review, 21,* 1055–1080.

Kohatsu, N. D., Robinson, J. G., & Torner, J. C. (2004). Evidence-based public health: An evolving concept. *American Journal of Preventive Medicine, 27*(5), 417–421.

Kreuter, M. W., & Bernhardt, J. M. (2009). Reframing the dissemination challenge: A marketing and distribution perspective. *American Journal of Public Health, 99*(12), 2123–2127.

Lash, S. J., Timko, C., Curran, G. M., McKay, J. R., & Burden, J. L. (2011). Implementation of evidence-based substance use disorder continuing care interventions. *Psychology of Addictive Behaviors, 25*(2), 238–251.

Lehoux, P., Denis, J. L., Tailliez, S., & Hivon, M. (2005). Dissemination of health technology assessments: Identifying the visions guiding an evolving policy innovation in Canada. *Journal of Health Politics, Policy and Law, 30*(4), 603–641.

Levy, D. T., Ellis, J. A., Mays, D., & Huang, A. T. (2013). Smoking-related deaths averted due to three years of policy progress. *Bulletin of the World Health Organization, 91*(7), 509–518.

Lomas, J. (1993). Diffusion, dissemination, and implementation: Who should do what? *Annals of the New York Academy of Sciences, 703,* 226–235.

Macaulay, A. C., Paradis, G., Potvin, L., Cross, E. J., Saad-Haddad, C., McComber, A., . . . Rivard, M. (1997). The Kahnawake Schools Diabetes Prevention Project: Intervention, evaluation, and baseline results of a diabetes primary prevention program with a native community in Canada. *Preventive Medicine, 26*(6), 779–790.

MacLean, D. R. (1996). Positioning dissemination in public health policy. *Canadian Journal of Public Health, 87*(Suppl. 2), S40–S43.

McGlynn, E. A., Asch, S. M., Adams, J., Keesey, J., Hicks, J., DeCristofaro, A., & Kerr, E.A. (2003). The quality of health care delivered to adults in the United States. *New England Journal of Medicine, 348*(26), 2635–2645.

McKay, J. R. (2005). Is there a case for extended interventions for alcohol and drug use disorders? *Addiction, 100*(11), 1594–1610.

McKinlay, J. B. (1998). Paradigmatic obstacles to improving the health of populations—implications for health policy. *Salud Pública de México, 40*(4), 369–379.

Minkler, M., & Salvatore, A. (2012). Participatory approaches for study design and analysis in dissemination and implementation research. In R. C. Brownson, G. A. Colditz, & E. K. Proctor (Eds.), *Dissemination and implementation research in health: Translating science to practice* (pp. 192–212). New York: Oxford University Press.

National Cancer Institute. (2002). *Designing for dissemination: Conference summary report.* Washington, DC: Author.

National Institutes of Health. (2013). *Dissemination and implementation research in health* (R01). Retrieved from http://grants.nih.gov/grants/guide/PA-files/PAR-13-055.html

Oldenburg, B., & Glanz, K. (2008). Diffusion of innovations. In K. Glanz, B. Rimer, & K. Viswanath (Eds.), *Health behavior and health education: Theory, research, and practice* (4th ed., pp. 313–334). San Francisco: Jossey-Bass.

Osei-Bryson, K. M., Dong, L., & Ngwenyama, O. (2008). Exploring managerial factors affecting ERP implementation: An investigation of the Klein-Sorra model using regression splines. *Information Systems Journal, 18*(5), 499–527.

Owen, N., Glanz, K., Sallis, J. F., & Kelder, S. H. (2006). Evidence-based approaches to dissemination and diffusion of physical activity interventions. *American Journal of Preventive Medicine, 31*(Suppl. 4), S35–S44.

Owen, N., Goode, A., Fjeldsoe, B., Sugiyama, T., & Eakin, E. (2012). Designing for the dissemination of environmental and policy initiatives and programs for high-risk groups. In R. C. Brownson, G. A. Colditz, & E. K. Proctor (Eds.), *Dissemination and implementation research in health: Translating science to practice* (pp. 114–127). New York: Oxford University Press.

Public Health Accreditation Board. (2011). *Public health accreditation board standards: An overview.* Alexandria, VA: Author.

Published applications of the PRECEDE model. (2015). [Bibliography.] Retrieved from http://lgreen.net /precede%20apps/preapps-NEW.htm

Rabin, B. A., & Brownson, R. C. (2012). Developing the terminology for dissemination and implementation research. In R. C. Brownson, G. A. Colditz, & E. K. Proctor (Eds.), *Dissemination and implementation research in health: Translating science to practice* (pp. 23–51). New York: Oxford University Press.

Rabin, B. A., Brownson, R. C., Haire-Joshu, D., Kreuter, M. W., & Weaver, N. L. (2008). A glossary for dissemination and implementation research in health. *Journal of Public Health Management and Practice, 14*(2), 117–123.

Rabin, B. A., Brownson, R. C., Kerner, J. F., & Glasgow, R. E. (2006). Methodologic challenges in disseminating evidence-based interventions to promote physical activity. *American Journal of Preventive Medicine, 31*(Suppl. 4), S24–S34.

Rabin, B. A., Nehl, E., Elliott, T., Deshpande, A. D., Brownson, R. C., & Glanz, K. (2010). Individual and setting level predictors of the implementation of a skin cancer prevention program: A multilevel analysis. *Implementation Science, 5*, 40.

RE-AIM publications. (2015). [Bibliography.] Retrieved from http://www.re-aim.hnfe.vt.edu /publications/index.html

Rogers, E. M. (1962). *Diffusion of innovations.* New York: Free Press.

Rogers, E. M. (2003). *Diffusion of innovations* (5th ed.). New York: Free Press.

Ryan, B., & Gross, N. (1943). The diffusion of hybrid seed corn in two Iowa communities. *Rural Sociology, 8*(1), 15–24.

Rycroft-Malone, J. (2004). The PARIHS framework—a framework for guiding the implementation of evidence-based practice. *Journal of Nursing Care Quality, 19*(4), 297–304.

Shaffer, E. R. (2013). The Affordable Care Act: The value of systemic disruption. *American Journal of Public Health, 103*(6), 969–972.

Sharp, N. D., Pineros, S. L., Hsu, C., Starks, H., & Sales, A. E. (2004). A qualitative study to identify barriers and facilitators to implementation of pilot interventions in the Veterans Health Administration (VHA) Northwest Network. *Worldviews on Evidence-Based Nursing, 1*(2), 129–139.

Shively, M., Riegel, B., Waterhouse, D., Burns, D., Templin, K., & Thomason, T. (1997). Testing a community level research utilization intervention. *Applied Nursing Research, 10*(3), 121–127.

Sussman, S., Valente, T. W., Rohrbach, L. A., Skara, S., & Pentz, M. A. (2006). Translation in the health professions: Converting science into action. *Evaluation and the Health Professions, 29*(1), 7–32.

Szulanski, G. (1996). Exploring internal stickiness: Impediments to the transfer of best practice within the firm. *Strategic Management Journal, 17*, 27–43.

Szulanski, G. (2000). The process of knowledge transfer: A diachronic analysis of stickiness. *Organizational behavior and human decision processes, 82*(1), 9–27.

Tabak, R. G., Khoong, E. C., Chambers, D. A., & Brownson, R. C. (2012). Bridging research and practice: Models for dissemination and implementation research. *American Journal of Preventive Medicine, 43*(3), 337–350.

Tarde, G. (1903). *The laws of imitation.* New York: Henry Holt.

Thacker, S. B. (2007). Public health surveillance and the prevention of injuries in sports: What gets measured gets done. *Journal of Athletic Training, 42*(2), 171–172.

Van Acker, R., De Bourdeaudhuij, I., De Cocker, K., Klesges, L., & Cardon, G. (2011). The impact of disseminating the whole-community project "10,000 Steps": A RE-AIM analysis. *BMC Public Health, 11*(1), 3.

Wiecha, J. L., El Ayadi, A. M., Fuemmeler, B. F., Carter, J. E., Handler, S., Johnson, S., . . . Gortmaker, S. L. (2004). Diffusion of an integrated health education program in an urban school system: Planet Health. *Journal of Pediatric Psychology, 29*(6), 467–474.

Williams, E. C., Johnson, M. L., Lapham, G. T., Caldeiro, R. M., Chew, L., Fletcher, G. S., . . . Bradley, K. A. (2011). Strategies to implement alcohol screening and brief intervention in primary care settings: A structured literature review. *Psychology of Addictive Behaviors, 25*(2), 206–214.

Wolff, K. (1950). *The sociology of Georg Simmel.* Glencoe, IL: Free Press.

Zaza, S., Briss, P. A., & Harris, K. W. (Eds.). (2005). *The guide to community preventive services: What works to promote health?* New York: Oxford University Press.

CHAPTER 17

COMMUNICATION AND HEALTH BEHAVIOR IN A CHANGING MEDIA ENVIRONMENT

K. Viswanath
John R. Finnegan Jr.
Sarah Gollust

The intersection of two major revolutions—the communication revolution and the biomedical revolution (Neuman, 1999; Viswanath, 2005)—magnified by developments in our computational capacity to analyze big data, is changing the landscape of consumer health in the twenty-first century. Developments in information and communication technologies are being felt more personally than ever before in our lives, affecting the way we work, play, learn, and communicate. We have moved from the analog world of relative information scarcity to the digital world of information superabundance. The rapid acceleration of technological change has dramatically lowered the costs of communication, permitting just about anyone with a mobile device or a tablet or laptop computer to assume a role as part of the global news, opinion, and information network.

The biomedical revolution, propelled by the same forces, has given rise to new technologies in genetics, genomics, proteomics, and health informatics, which has led to an extreme proliferation of health information about individuals and communities. Informatics is looking at how information and communication technologies are used to gather, process, and share material for surveillance, prevention, and decision making in public health. The sheer volume and speed of digital information often challenges our capacity to generate understanding, meaning, and certainty.

KEY POINTS

This chapter will:

- Characterize the major features of the communication revolution and its implications for health communication and health behavior.

- Review major theories and hypotheses in health communication.

- Discuss how developments in information and communication technologies (ICTs) are changing the way we conceptualize audiences, media organizations, and media effects on health.

- Discuss two applications of communication and health behavior theories for changing health behaviors.

Several characteristics of this communication revolution have profound implications for health communication, education, and promotion in transforming how people learn about and act on health information and interact with health professionals. One is the multiplication of platforms through which information is distributed by different groups and accessed by different audiences, raising fundamental questions about the definitions of *mass communication* and *mass media* (Viswanath et al., 2012). Broad audiences no longer need to tune into the national nightly news to learn the results of a new medical study. Instead, audiences can find health-relevant information on hundreds of cable channels; on countless internet sites, wikis, and blogs; and through social media outlets such as Facebook and Twitter, where friends and acquaintances curate information for their social networks.

Another important change is the shift in the traditional command-and-control approach to the generation and distribution of health information content (Viswanath et al., 2012). In the past, *big media* performed a gatekeeping function, influencing much of what the public learned about subjects or events and defining worldviews for audiences. When information production is decentralized and even individuals can generate health information (whether accurate or not) worldwide, our traditional notions of "expertise" are challenged, as are the traditional boundaries of disciplines and geographies. As a result, information about developments in health and medicine, and their implications for health education and behavior, increasingly are not disseminated and interpreted in a controlled and calibrated manner by expert gatekeepers but, instead, by anyone who has an opinion and the means to express it. Communication systems of the analog world could be characterized as the expert-dominated and organizationally controlled mass production and delivery of information to end users: audiences who had little interaction with the information producers. In the digital world, communication systems enable end-user creation, control, and high interactivity, where information delivery can be tailored and customized to users' perspectives and expectations. With limited mass population–level information sharing and more self-selection of information, the polarized information environment may draw the public further apart in their attitudes, opinions, and behaviors, rather than building a focus on commonalities or broader consensus (Baum, 2011).

These changes (proliferation of platforms, less gatekeeping, and greater grassroots participation in health information generation and distribution) have led to the production and dissemination of larger amounts of health information than in the past. Judging what is true and untrue, or even harder, where the untruths lie within something that may be mostly true, in this ocean of information is a major challenge for health, social, and political systems as well as for individuals. This places a greater onus on individuals to be informed consumers—coping with the tide of information, processing it for relevance and accuracy, and acting on it. Being an informed consumer is particularly difficult when the public information environment surrounding health often provides conflicting information (Nagler, 2014) or highly technical information, thus lending greater importance to the resources—cognitive, social, and material—one brings to coping with the information deluge. In addition, what is accepted as truth in the health sciences is itself a moving target, as research reveals new insights almost daily.

Further, demands on consumer health access and action arising from these developments in information and communication technologies have brought to the fore classic divides that pervade our society. The social determinants of health that contribute to communication inequalities—differences among social groups in accessing, processing, acting on, and benefiting from health information and health services—become especially important in light of new modes of information dissemination (Niederdeppe, Bigman, Gonzales, & Gollust, 2013; Viswanath, 2011; Viswanath & Ackerson, 2011). These divides continue despite the penetration of technologies such as cell phones as people, especially those from lower SES groups, can experience interruption in communication and information services for nonpayment or other reasons.

The information and communication technologies revolutions also offer important opportunities for health promotion and communication, with the potential to overcome traditional divides and barriers and to provide more customized and tailored information to different audiences. Moreover, these technologies facilitate the creation of content by consumers. As we study health communication and its effects on health, these developments challenge our understanding and application of theories and models of communication, including our understanding of media institutions, definitions and characteristics of audiences, and media effects. These developments form the background for the rest of this chapter.

Overview of Mass Communication Theories

The impact of mass communication is everywhere and is central to understanding human behavior. Theory is an important guide in applied communication, because it provides a framework that organizes important variables into relationships, some of which can be manipulated or modified, permitting us to predict health outcomes. However, no single theory explains and predicts all communication outcomes, given the complexity and changing nature of communication technologies (Bryant & Miron, 2004). Communication processes and effects can operate simultaneously, with synergy on different levels, converging to shape behaviors. While communication studies may be organized in many ways, the ecological framework of levels of analysis (see Chapter Three) provides a way to organize our thinking about communication factors, processes, and outcomes from the micro to the macro levels (Table 17.1). Rather than identifying and discussing discrete theories in depth, much of the discussion in this chapter will focus on hypotheses and models of media influence that emerge from multiple disciplines. In the context of the interdisciplinarity of health communication, over multiple decades several communication-centric hypotheses have been developed and empirically tested, as we discuss next.

Individual-Level Models

At the individual level of analysis, media studies emphasize the effects of media exposure on a person's motivations, cognitions, opinions, attitudes, and behaviors. In understanding media exposure effects at the individual level, research often draws from health behavior theories, as identified here. Research also draws from information processing theories, such as the Elaboration Likelihood Model, and message effect theories such as *framing* (Bryant, Zillman, & Oliver, 2002).

Table 17.1   Selected Communication Theories and Levels of Analysis

Level of Analysis	Microlevel Analysis (e.g., media effects on individuals)	Macrolevel Analysis (e.g., media effects on and through communities and social systems)
Theory or concept	1. Expectancy-value theories/Integrated Behavioral Model 2. Social Cognitive Theory 3. Information processing theories 4. Message effect theories and persuasion	1. Knowledge gap 2. Agenda setting 3. Definition, framing of social issues 4. Cultivation studies 5. Risk communication
Major studies, reviews	1. Fishbein & Cappella, 2006 2. Bryant & Zillman, 1994 3. Cappella & Rimer, 2006 4. Palmgreen & Donohew, 2002; Zillman, 2006	1. Tichenor, Donohue, & Olien, 1970; Viswanath & Finnegan, 1996 2. Kosicki, 1993 3. Bryant & Miron, 2004; Scheufele & Tewksbury, 2007 4. Gerbner, Gross, Morgan, Signorelli, & Bryant 1994 5. Rimer, Glanz, & Rasband, 2001; McComas, 2006
Disciplinary origin	1–4: Psychology 1–4: Social psychology	1. Sociology—structural/Functionalism social conflict 2. Sociology, psychology, political science 3. Sociology/social construction of knowledge 4. Sociology of mass society 5. Sociology, psychology

Theories of Communication Effects on Behaviors

Several theories that are often used in health behavior and health education offer explanations for media effects at the individual level. For example, variants of expectancy-value theories, including the Health Belief Model (Chapter Five), Theory of Reasoned Action, and Theory of Planned Behavior (Chapter Six), propose pathways of behavior change through changes in attitudes and beliefs. All these theories emphasize that people's behaviors are driven by some interactive combination of beliefs, feelings toward performing a behavior, and subjective norms about the behavior. Media communications may be targeted either to change these beliefs or to reinforce them.

Fishbein and colleagues (Fishbein & Cappella, 2006) attempted to bring these different theories together in the Integrative Behavioral Model (IBM) (see Chapter Six) and applied that model in the context of explaining media effects on marijuana use and sexual behavior. The key proposition of this model is that media effects vary depending on the behavior and population under study and on the relative importance of the determinants. Also, media messages can be targeted, depending on which set of beliefs could most likely influence behavioral intentions.

Information Processing Theories

Information processing theories focus on how media messages may lead to changes in attitudes or to reinforcement of existing attitudes. There are several relevant theories. The most commonly used are the dual process models such as the Elaboration Likelihood Model (ELM) and the Heuristic-Systematic Processing Model (HSM) (Bryant & Zillman, 1994). Both assume that persuasive messages—such as antismoking messages—are processed in either of two ways. On the one hand, a central or a systematic processing route involves the deliberate, thoughtful weighing of message arguments, and the changes accompanying such processing are likely to be more enduring. On the other hand, peripheral or heuristic processing occurs in low motivation conditions, and the recipient relies on peripheral cues, such as the celebrity status of a spokesperson pitching a product. A related classification distinguishes those who alter their beliefs based on additional information (known as online processors) versus those who store information in their memory (memory-based processors) (Brinol & Petty, 2005). These individual differences in processing style show promise as predictors of which individuals will be more or less influenced by media information delivered at different points in time (Druckman & Leeper, 2012).

Message Effects Theories

Research on message effects examines how the formats and construction of messages interact with audience characteristics to influence information processing and impact (Cappella & Rimer, 2006). The most commonly investigated elements comprise framing, exemplification, and narratives. *Framing* has multiple definitions from multiple disciplinary origins, but communication scholars generally refer to one or the other of the following two. First, framing can refer to presenting logically equivalent information in different ways, as Tversky and Kahneman did in framing disease risk information in terms of "lives lost" or "lives gained" (Tversky & Kahneman, 1981). This work launched a productive research agenda examining the effects of health messages framed positively or negatively that continues to this day. Second, framing can refer to problem definition, the outcome of a competitive process in which frame sponsors define the terms of a debate, often invoking the cause of, solutions to, and moral valence of a particular issue in society (Chong & Druckman, 2007; Entman, 1993). This type of framing is sometimes called *issue framing*. For instance, obesity could be framed as a problem of individuals behaving poorly (e.g., failing to diet or failing to exercise) or as a problem of social structures and of the food and beverage industry producing an obesogenic social environment that unfairly constrains individual opportunities to make healthy choices (Barry, Brescoll, & Gollust, 2013). Messages can also arouse emotions (e.g., fear, guilt, and anger), either intentionally or unintentionally, with variable influences on message effectiveness and message processing (see, e.g., Dillard & Nabi, 2006).

Exemplars in messages provide specific details to illustrate a general class of events. For example, a news story on childhood immunization may describe the case of a particular parent who chose to vaccinate her child against hepatitis B. Some research shows that exemplars are more effective when they are simple, emotional, and concrete (Zillman, 2006). However, evidence is mixed on the use of exemplars to influence health-related outcomes. Although some research suggests that exemplars of specific individuals can produce heightened emotional engagement and empathetic response (Slovic, 2007), other research suggests that the focusing of news stories on individuals leads to an individualization of social problems, heightening individual blame and reducing support for policy (Barry et al., 2013; Iyengar, 1991).

Extensions of exemplars, *narratives* are among the most powerful and visible message structures. Recognizing the limited effectiveness of standard health promotion tools, public health practitioners have increasingly turned to narrative forms of communication—embedding persuasive health messages in stories—to improve public health (Hinyard & Kreuter, 2007). When health information is conveyed in a story (including characters, plot, conflict, and resolution), research suggests that audience members may be more likely to engage in a target behavior or change their attitudes, compared to what they do when receiving information communicated through more traditional didactic messages and formats (i.e., statistics or evidence and exhortations or arguments) (Green & Brock, 2000; Kreuter et al., 2007; Niederdeppe et al., 2013). The persuasive potential of narrative interventions is supported by social cognitive theory (see Chapter Nine): after observing a model behavior (even if conveyed as fictional), individuals are more likely to attempt it. They may believe social norms are more supportive of the behavior when they see others, particularly people similar to them, engaging in it (Ajzen & Fishbein, 1980). Narrative interventions may be particularly effective for health behaviors that individuals are likely to resist, such as getting vaccines or cancer screenings (Kreuter et al., 2007). The theory of *transportation* (Green & Brock, 2000) posits that when individuals become immersed in a narrative's plot and/or characters, they are less likely to resist a message because they may not necessarily identify its persuasive intent, and their cognitive capacity becomes so absorbed in the emotional aspects of the story that they have reduced motivation and ability to counterargue (Green & Brock, 2000; Kreuter et al., 2007). While the mechanisms that explain the impact of narratives are well thought out and empirically tenable, we know very little about how to construct narratives that will change audience cognitions, attitudes, and behaviors.

Audience Characteristics

Certain individual characteristics, such as personality traits, values, and information processing style, limit or enhance the effectiveness of media communication at shaping attitude or behavior change. Understanding such audience characteristics allows message designers to target messages more effectively. For example, sensation seeking is a personality trait that is characterized by the search for novelty, thrill seeking, and impulsive decision making (making risky behaviors more likely) and that influences attention, processing, and comprehension of messages (Palmgreen & Donohew, 2002). Messages with high sensation value have been used effectively in discouraging drug use and promoting safe sex (Stephenson & Southwell, 2006). Other researchers have examined the match between message content and the values orientation of the audience, generally finding that messages that resonate with particular social or political values are more persuasive (Shen & Edwards, 2005). The theory of reactance

(Brehm, 1966) posits that any persuasive message (particularly one that threatens individuals' perceptions of freedom) may arouse a motivation, called *reactance*, to reject the advocacy (Dillard & Shen, 2005). Such a response can produce backlash effects, such as when adolescents report increasing interest in a risky health behavior after exposure to a health risk message (Fishbein, Hall-Jamieson, Zimmer, Von Haeften, & Nabi, 2002). The theory of biased processing (also known as *motivated reasoning*) offers a complementary explanation for reactance, explaining that people are motivated to evaluate the strength and credibility of messages differently depending on their predisposing attitudes and beliefs (Taber & Lodge, 2006). Nyhan, Reifler, Richey, and Freed (2014) used biased processing theory to explain why health messages countering claims of vaccine side effects are ineffective among those who are against vaccines to start with.

In summary, a variety of communication theories focus on explaining how attitudes and behaviors could be changed at the individual level and the types of message formats and interactions with audience characteristics that could lead to such changes. These theories draw extensively from and contribute to other disciplines, including social and cognitive psychology and political science.

Interpersonal and Social Network Models

Interpersonal diffusion of information and influence (persuasion) has attracted considerable attention, starting with the famous "two-step flow" study by Katz and Lazarsfeld (1955), who posited that media effects are less likely to be direct and, instead, are more likely to flow through interpersonal interactions. Subsequently, work in the Diffusion of Innovations (Rogers, 2003; also see Chapter Sixteen) and social network (Chapter Eleven) traditions documented the role played by interpersonal networks in the flow of innovations and information relating to health, among other areas. The role of interpersonal and small-group communication has evolved into two distinct though occasionally overlapping streams of work in health communication. One stream of this research focuses on patient-provider communication (see Chapter Thirteen).

Given the extensive discussion on social networks (in Chapter Eleven) and patient-provider communication (in Chapter Thirteen), here we will focus on how media effects are mediated by interpersonal conversations that moderate and modify media influences on health (Southwell & Yzer, 2009). This latter tradition has become more important with the emergence of social media and the Internet, which offer new possibilities for disseminating and interpreting health information and offering social support (Chapter Ten). Communication studies have demonstrated that interpersonal channels and organizational participation increase knowledge about a variety of health topics, such as cardiovascular disease (Viswanath, Randolph Steele, & Finnegan, 2006), in addition to providing social support. For instance, a health communication intervention showed that peers can nominate others for mammography screening successfully (Southwell, Slater, Nelson, & Rothman, 2012). Interpersonal communications within broad social networks may enhance the chances of exposure to health-promoting information (Ackerson & Viswanath, 2009).

Organizational-Level Models

The academic study of communication in organizations originated first as part of management studies in industrial and organizational psychology and sociology. The focus was on the role of communication in the functioning of rational organizations and goal achievement. Today, the field analyzes "a process through which people, acting together, create, sustain, and manage meanings through the use of verbal and nonverbal signs and symbols within a particular context" (Conrad & Poole, 2012). Others have described the principal focus as "a concern with collective action, agency, messages, symbols and discourse" (Mumby & Stohl, 1996). While it is tempting to think of organizations as large and corporate, scholars in this arena are careful to note that smaller groups with members collaborating for the achievement of common goals are also included, such as community-based nonprofits, start-up companies, and so on. But whatever the context, understanding the role of communication externally and internally in organizations is important because as units in communities, nations, and societies, organizations are powerful sources of influence in shaping values, attitudes, and beliefs and also sources of cultural socialization into norms and behaviors (Lammers & Barbour, 2006). For example, in the health arena, scholars have examined communication within health care organizations, looking at such factors as the prevalence of provider communication competencies and their relationship to patient behavior, satisfaction, and adherence to recommended regimens. Scholars have also examined how health organizations themselves frame, shape, and change patient-provider relationships. While these are analyses of internal communication processes and effects, organizations' external power and use of persuasion to shape public policy and set public agendas can also be studied (Zhan & Tang, 2013).

Macrolevel Models

A strong body of work in communication studies examines the role of social context and community structures—such as racial or socioeconomic composition and access to community resources—in how health communication messages are generated, received, interpreted, and acted upon. This is a natural fit for *mass communication* with its societal reach across populations. We next discuss some exemplar macrolevel theories and hypotheses.

Agenda Setting and Framing

For some time, communication researchers have focused on the influence of mass media on public opinion, especially in politics and policymaking. Early writers such as Walter Lippman (1922) saw the media's behavior as a "restless searchlight" panning from one issue to the next while seldom lingering long on any single issue. Later researchers such as Bernard Berelson (1948) noted that while the media influence public opinion, the reverse is also true: public opinion influences what the media report. Paul Lazarsfeld and colleagues (Lazarsfeld, Berelson, & Gaudet, 1948) noted that media attention confers status upon issues and raises their importance. These insights coalesced in the 1970s as a focus on the mass media's powerful role in setting the public agenda of important issues and problems, presenting a number of

Table 17.2   Agenda-Setting Concepts, Definitions, and Applications

Concept	Definition	Application
Media agenda setting	Institutional roles, factors, and process that influence "the definition, selection, and emphasis of issues in the media."	Working with media professionals to understand their work needs and routines in gathering and reporting news.
Public agenda setting	The link between issues portrayed in the media and the public's issue priorities.	Working with media professionals in advocacy or partnership contexts to build the public agenda for important health issues.
Policy agenda setting	The link between issues developed in policymaking institutions and issues portrayed by the media.	Working with community leaders and policymakers to build the importance of health issues on the media's and public's agendas.
Problem identification or definition	Factors and processes leading to identification of an issue by social institutions.	Community leaders, advocacy groups, and/or organizations mobilize to define an issue and modes of solution or basis for action.
Framing	Organized public discourse about an issue leading to the selection and emphasis of some characteristics and dimensions and the exclusion of others.	Public health advocacy groups "package" an important health issue for the media and the public (e.g., secondhand smoke framed as the public's involuntary exposure to toxic pollutants contrasted with the "smokers' rights" emphasis of tobacco advocates).

opportunities for public health applications (Bryant & Miron, 2004) (see Table 17.2). Kosicki (1993) identified three types of agenda-setting research: (1) public agenda setting that examines the link between media portrayal of issues and their impact on issue priorities assigned by the public, (2) policy agenda setting that examines the connection between media coverage and the legislative agendas of policymaking bodies, and (3) media agenda setting that focuses on factors that influence the media to cover certain issues.

Later research suggested refinements to agenda-setting theory (Shah, McLeod, Gotlieb, & Lee, 2009; Takeshita, 2006), as initial correlational studies have given way to more empirically sophisticated designs with clearer causal links (Iyengar & Kinder, 1987; McCombs, 2004) and concepts have been clarified. Researchers now agree that the media not only tell us what is important in a general way, they also provide ways of thinking about specific issues through the signs, symbols, terms, and sources they use to define the issue in the first place. In this view, public problems are social constructions (Borah, 2011). That is, groups, institutions, and advocates compete to identify problems, to move them onto the public agenda, *and* to define the issues symbolically (Entman, 1993). This refinement suggests that the media's agenda-setting function is not completely independent but is built by various community groups, institutions, and advocates. This has applications for those in public health who seek to use the media to raise public salience and awareness of specific problems. Current research in this arena is bringing agenda-setting theory together with the concepts of framing and priming (Scheufele & Tewksbury, 2007). Framing concerns how an issue is characterized, especially in the news, whereas priming encourages audiences to alter the standards they apply to evaluating outcomes related to an issue.

Communication Inequalities and Health

Secular trends in health, left to themselves, result in profound inequalities among social classes, races, and ethnicities across the entire continuum of health, from prevention to diagnosis, treatment, and survival (Phelan, Link, & Tehranifar, 2010). These observed inequalities are attributed to social determinants, such as socioeconomic position, political power, race or ethnicity, geography, social cohesion, racism, working conditions, and/or social and health policies (Berkman & Kawachi, 2000) or to people's being at the intersection of multiple social status categories (Williams et al., 2012).

In parallel, communication inequalities, defined as differences among social classes in the generation, processing, and distribution of information among social groups and in the access to and capacity to use the information among individuals (Viswanath, 2006), have attracted attention. Inequalities manifest at multiple levels, ultimately leading to an impact on organizations, social networks, and individuals (see Chapter Three).

For example, communication inequalities among social groups and institutions have been specifically observed among organizations. Illustrative are the figures for the marketing and promotional budget of the tobacco industry ($5 billion a year) or for the food and beverage industry that has spent approximately $2 billion per year marketing to children (Kovacic, 2008). These huge marketing and promotional budgets, particularly through their sophisticated use of media such as video games (Chester, 2009) and social media such as Facebook or Twitter (Richardson & Harris, 2011), result in an information environment that may contradict public health messaging, and exposure to such information may lead to confusion among the public. More important, these marketing communications and promotions contribute to health inequalities, owing to sophisticated strategies targeting vulnerable groups such as children (Powell, Schermbeck, Szczypka, Chaloupka, & Braunschweig, 2011) and minorities (Grier & Kumanyika, 2010).

Communication inequalities also have been documented extensively across several communication dimensions at the individual level including access to and use of a variety of media (Viswanath & Ackerson, 2011); attention to health information (Viswanath, 2005; Viswanath & Ackerson, 2011); information seeking (Galarce et al., 2011); information avoidance (McCloud, Jung, & Viswanath, 2013); health outcomes, including knowledge (Hwang & Jeong, 2009; Tichenor et al., 1970; Viswanath & Finnegan, 1996); and end-of-life communications among patients, providers, and families (Mack, Paul, Viswanath, & Prigerson, 2010). In almost all cases, it was observed that people in higher socioeconomic position, whites, and those in white-collar employment are more likely to access and use information and communication technologies, including the Internet and broadband, to their advantage—a trend often labeled the *digital divide* or *digital inequality* (DiMaggio, Hargittai, Celeste, & Shafer, 2004; Viswanath et al., 2012).

Emerging research shows that communication inequalities are contributing to health inequalities, as observed in attitudes and behaviors with regard to AIDS in India (Ackerson, Ramanadhan, Arya, & Viswanath, 2012), rural Ethiopia (Bekalu & Eggermont, 2013), and fourteen sub-Saharan African countries (Jung, Arya, & Viswanath, 2013). One dimension of inequalities that has been extensively studied over the last thirty-five years, under the rubric of the knowledge gap hypothesis, will be discussed next.

The Knowledge Gap Hypothesis

Conventional wisdom long held that persistent social problems could be resolved through public education alone. However, knowledge and information, it turned out, are distributed unequally across populations. These findings were presented as the knowledge gap hypothesis by Minnesota researchers Tichenor, Donohue, and Olien (1970), who proposed that an increasing flow of information into a social system (from a media campaign, for example) would be more likely to benefit groups of higher socioeconomic status (SES) than those of lower SES. Moreover, increasing the information available in the system would only exacerbate already existing differences between these groups. They supported this proposition with studies of several topics, including health. The disturbing implications were, of course, that public campaigns would only perpetuate inequities. Because this called into question the entire basis of guided social change efforts, it attracted the attention of scholars and policymakers.

The knowledge gap hypothesis advanced the thinking about media effects in at least two important ways. It contradicted the conventional wisdom that communication campaigns could be a simple panacea for social problems, and it suggested that media have differential impacts on audiences that can be traced to differences in social class and social structure conditions in communities. It was thus one of the first media studies hypotheses to draw attention to the role of the social environment in shaping the media impact on individuals (Viswanath & Finnegan, 1996).

Fortunately, subsequent studies found that knowledge gaps were not intractable. Researchers discovered a variety of contingent and contributory conditions that could affect knowledge gaps and also present opportunities for applications in public health campaigns (Table 17.3): content domains, channel influence, social conflict and community mobilization, the structure of communities, and individual motivational factors (Viswanath & Finnegan, 1996).

Cross-Level Models: Risk Communication

Communication about risk is of special concern in public health, because it is about dangers that need to be described, assessed, and managed for reduction or prevention of some negative outcome (McComas, 2006). Research on risk communication concerns how individuals and groups perceive, process, and act upon their understanding of risk. It also addresses how the media and other powerful institutions shape these processes.

Scholars focus on understanding cognitive mechanisms and developing expert and mental models of communication, issues of confusion and misinformation (Weinstein, 2000), the efficacy of individualized counseling and tailoring (Rimer et al., 2001), and the advantages to intensive, calibrated, and directed communication (Rimer & Glassman, 1999). Researchers also emphasize the cognitive mechanisms by which individuals are exposed to and attend to information about risk, how they interpret risk information in relation to themselves, and

Table 17.3   Knowledge Gap Definitions and Opportunities for Application in Public Health Campaigns

Concept	Definition	Application
Knowledge gap	Difference in measured knowledge between groups of differing socioeconomic status (SES) over time.	Potential unintended consequence of public health interventions that could increase SES-based differences over time.
Knowledge	Factual and interpretive information leading to understanding or usefulness for taking informed action.	Communication of factual and interpretive information about causes and prevention of disease and skills for health improvement.
Information flow	Degree of availability of information on an issue or topic in a social system such as a community.	Increasing community opportunities (through multiple media and other channels) to encounter health information and knowledge.
Socioeconomic status	Population units or subunits characterized on the basis of differing education, income, wealth, or occupation.	Emphasis on information of interest and use to differing SES groups; emphasis on channel strategies designed especially to reach low-SES groups.
Social structure, pluralism	Differentiation and interdependence among community subsystems including social institutions, organizations, interest groups, and other centers of power and influence that maintain the social system; often influenced by size of the community (the larger the community, the greater the differentiation).	Highly differentiated communities increase competition for public attention to health information. While level of communication activity required is often more intensive than in a smaller, less differentiated community, public health resources seldom permit dominating the information flow; emphasis is on targeting of media and other strategies to reach groups of interest.
Social conflict	Opposition or disagreement over an issue or problem, often representing a struggle for power and influence between social groups or leaders.	Controversy attracts media attention, especially in highly differentiated communities; it tends to increase public interest and may lead to equalizing information on a topic across SES groups.
Mobilization	Organized activity seeking to focus community power and influence to address a problem or issue.	Media publicity about a public health issue is frequently driven by the actions of social groups and leaders; increases public attention, and may lead to equalizing information across SES groups.
Motivation	Factors influencing individuals to attend to and act upon information and knowledge (e.g., personal interest, involvement, self-efficacy).	Emphasis on strategies to increase motivational factors to acquire and act upon information and knowledge.

finally, whether and how they act upon risk information to alter their behavior (Glanz & Yang, 1996; Weinstein, 2000).

Significant developments in the study of risk have also occurred at the community level of analysis. Studies of risk communication have focused on the interaction of populations and social institutions, such as government agencies, advocacy groups, and the mass media, in the formation and management of public opinion and policymaking about risk. Here, risk communication studies owe much of their theoretical basis to the agenda-setting and agenda-building perspectives as well as to research on the definition and framing of public issues (Glanz & Yang, 1996; Sandman, 1987).

Public definitions of risk usually include some form of scientifically assessed risk information (*objective risk*), mediated by the political and social context of the risk. Social conflict is a critical variable in drawing attention to social problems and leading to arousal and increased salience of the issue. This can have both negative and positive consequences, depending on whether the actual risk is low or high and whether public outrage is low or high. Outrage can have the effect of quickly propelling important information through the population at all socioeconomic levels. Where outrage is low, one might expect to find socioeconomic group differences in knowledge about risk. Either situation may have an impact on policymaking about risk where the public is well or ill informed. Further, a community's definition of risk can be crucial to social action by powerful actors, as can be seen in the case of AIDS in Africa. In the best case, strategic communication about risk accomplishes positive goals of adding social value (Palenchar & Heath, 2007). In the worst case, it is capable of destructive and dangerous unintended outcomes.

Applications

In this section we discuss two specific applications that draw on developments and hypotheses discussed in the chapter. The first application illustrates how developments in information and communication technologies (ICTs), specifically mobile phones, could be used to promote health. The second application discusses how a significant public health issue, HPV and cervical cancer, could be addressed by drawing on communication science.

Application 1: mHealth—Use of Mobile Phones in Health

The communication revolution (Viswanath, 2005) has led to swift changes in how people generate and receive information, resulting in an increase in the development of innovative strategies to reach individuals with health information. The use of mobile technology in health interventions, often termed *mHealth*, has great potential to influence the way interventions are delivered, including collecting real-time data and providing personalized feedback (Nilsen et al., 2012). Due to their portability and nearly continuous availability, mobile phones address constraints of space and time that may hinder more traditional forms of mass media communication (Viswanath et al., 2012). As of 2013, 91 percent of the U.S. adult population owned some sort of cell phone, with 56 percent of adults owning smartphones (Smith, 2013). The nearly ubiquitous availability of cell phones in the United States increases the promise of this medium for reaching diverse segments of the population (Fjeldsoe, Marshall, & Miller, 2009). The portability and relatively low cost of many of these devices has opened the door for low-income individuals to access the web and other information in ways not possible when relying on broadband internet connection alone, thus addressing the digital divide. Accordingly, the worldwide penetration of cell phones has gone up manyfold in the developed and developing worlds, though the penetration in the developing countries continues to lag the rates in the developed world (Viswanath et al., 2012). Furthermore, the use of this technology allows for the personalization, or *tailoring*, of relevant information, so that it will resonate with the receiver.

A popular feature of mobile phones for health research is their ability to send short, succinct text messages that are instantly available to the intended audience. This short message service, or SMS, is a growing feature in many interventions owing to its ability to convey health messages in simple language (Fjeldsoe, Miller, & Marshall, 2012). One example is the Australian intervention MobileMums, in which lower SES, postpartum women received a twelve-week, theoretically driven program to increase physical activity (Fjeldsoe, Miller, & Marshall, 2010). The intervention was created in part to address the need to develop delivery methods for physical activity interventions that could be accessed more equally across sociodemographic groups.

The researchers used Social Cognitive Theory (SCT) to structure their intervention (see Chapter Nine), drawing heavily on the principle of *reciprocal determinism* and emphasizing the way cognitions, environmental perceptions, and behaviors interact (Fjeldsoe et al., 2012). Participants were randomized to an intervention or control group, and all participants received an initial face-to-face consultation with a trained behavioral counselor to set physical activity goals. Intervention group participants then received a twelve-week intervention that contained an additional telephone consultation at six weeks, a goal-setting refrigerator magnet for self-monitoring, and forty-two personally tailored short text messages providing behavioral and cognitive strategies to increase physical activity. These texts targeted constructs of SCT throughout the intervention, emphasizing outcome expectancies, environmental opportunities for physical activity, self-efficacy, social support, and goal-setting skills. Messages also provided weekly goal checks, in which a text asked participants to indicate whether they had reached their goal. Based on participants' responses, they either received positive reinforcement or advice on how to reach their goal for the following week. Participants also nominated a social support person to help them reach their goals. (See Table 17.4.)

Intervention participants increased their moderate to vigorous physical activity frequency by 1.82 days per week, and their walking for exercise by 1.08 days per week by the end of the intervention. Posttrial interviews with the women indicated that program satisfaction was high and that participants appreciated the way MobileMums focused on their needs, provided messages that prompted them to exercise, and gave them information about local exercise opportunities. MobileMums is currently being evaluated in a larger, community-based randomized controlled trial (Fjeldsoe et al., 2012). Given their potential to reach

Table 17.4   Example of MobileMums Content

Theoretical Construct	Example of SMS Content
Self-efficacy	Lee talk 2 Kevin about watching the kids while u exercise. U could set a regular time each week so plans r in place.
Outcome expectancy	Did u know exercise helps u sleep better & stress less? Get out there & feel the difference.
Goal-setting skills	Hi Lee. Ur treat 4 reaching this week's exercise goal is a bubble bath. It's a treat u deserve so work 4 it.
Social support	Lee. Make a deal with Susie 2 watch the kids while u do exercise then return the favor.
Perceived environmental opportunity for physical activity	Lee. Free walking group 4 mums starts Mon 25th June at 9:30 am in Apex Park near the lake. Prams welcome. Join the Group.

Note: All names are pseudonyms: Lee = participant; Kevin = support person; Susie = potential exercise partner.
Source: Fjeldsoe, Miller, & Marshall, 2010, p. 104.

diverse audiences, SMS components have also been included in trials for diabetes management (Franklin, Waller, Pagliari, & Greene, 2006), physical activity (Kim & Glanz, 2013), and smoking cessation (Naughton, Prevost, Gilbert, & Sutton, 2012), among other health behaviors. A recent meta-analysis showed that the SMS interventions had statistically significant outcomes on health behaviors for smoking cessation and physical activity but not for other behaviors (Head, Noar, Iannarino, & Grant Harrington, 2013). Use of theory to construct messages did produce a significantly stronger effect compared to interventions that did not use theory. Also, as this intervention modality is relatively new, it is important to look to emerging research for new findings.

Application 2: Communication and HPV Vaccine

Communication about the human papillomavirus (HPV) vaccination in the United States illuminates many of the themes described earlier. A sexually transmitted infection, HPV is extremely prevalent, infecting nearly 79 million Americans (Centers for Disease Control and Prevention, 2013), and two vaccines are available (Gardasil, manufactured by Merck, and Cervarix, manufactured by GSK) that target strains of HPV associated with cervical cancer. Vaccination uptake has not met targets, with only 37.6 percent of adolescent females and 13.9 percent of adolescent males having received all three doses of the vaccine as of 2013 (Elam-Evans et al., 2014; National Cancer Institute, 2014). Because of this inadequacy in uptake of the vaccine relative to its potential for cancer prevention, researchers have examined the many potential influences on vaccine uptake. Communication (including patient-provider communication, parental communication, and mass media communication and marketing) has been identified as a major factor of interest, both in the public health literature and by national public health experts. Mass communication played a major role in the introduction and dissemination of the vaccines; a high-profile, direct-to-consumer marketing campaign by Merck reached large numbers of the target audience of teenage girls (Leader et al., 2011) and the news media devoted significant attention to the issue as well. One study identified over two thousand news articles appearing about the HPV vaccine in local newspapers between 2006 and 2007 (Fowler, Gollust, Dempsey, Lantz, & Ubel, 2012). Given the young age of the CDC recommended target groups, new information technologies have also featured in this communication landscape, with discussions about the HPV vaccine appearing on blogs and social media (Briones, Nan, Madden, & Waks, 2012).

Empirical researchers have leveraged several health communication theories in their approaches to understanding the role of mass communication in HPV vaccine utilization and in assessing why, despite high awareness of the vaccine, uptake has not met the expectations of public health officials. In the following section, we describe how framing and biased processing have featured in the literature surrounding HPV vaccine communication.

Framing

Several researchers have examined the role of *framing* in shaping HPV vaccine attitudes and behaviors. For instance, Leader, Weiner, Kelly, Hornik, and Cappella (2009) found that framing the purpose of the vaccine as cancer prevention, versus sexually transmitted infection prevention, led to women's higher intentions to receive the vaccine. In a subsequent study, Krieger and Sarge (2013) examined potential mediators of the link between vaccine framing and people's behaviors, suggesting that framing the vaccine as genital wart prevention increased young women's intentions to talk with their physicians by increasing their self-efficacy. Another opportunity for framing involves presenting different attributes of the vaccine. Bigman, Cappella, and Hornik (2010) applied a version of loss-gain frames to examine how equivalent ways of presenting the vaccine's effectiveness (as 70% effective or as 30% ineffective) affects attitudes. They found that those exposed to the positive frames believed the vaccine to be more effective and were more supportive of vaccine requirements for school attendance than those exposed to the logically equivalent but negatively framed message.

Information Processing

Other research suggests that *biased processing* based on political characteristics may shape public attitudes, behaviors, and information response related to HPV vaccines. Two studies showed that individuals identifying as politically liberal were more accepting than political conservatives of vaccines (Constantine & Jerman, 2007; Stupiansky, Rosenthal, Wiehe, & Zimet, 2010). Media and political debate over legislation to mandate the vaccine tended to discuss outcry over the vaccine among certain groups, based on their concerns about the sexual transmission of HPV, potential for vaccine side effects, involvement of the vaccine manufacturer in policymaking, and government overreach in vaccine mandates (Colgrove, Abiola, & Mello, 2010). As a potential consequence of this politically charged information environment, another study showed that political ideology influenced how different groups were exposed to mass media information (Gollust, Attanasio, Dempsey, Benson, & Fowler, 2013), suggesting that biased processing of HPV vaccine information may be in play.

Summary

The digital age is changing communication capacities that interact with the ecologies shaping human health activity and behavior at all levels—dyadic, family, organizational, community, societal, and cultural. Communication at each level (dyadic, group, and mass population) occurs in a context. Understanding context is key to applying behavioral and communication theories in health settings, particularly in a changing media environment; to understanding the dynamics of processes, effects, and outcomes; and to proactively shaping them through campaigns and interventions. As discussed here and elsewhere in this book, each level is part of a systemic ecology of forces and conditions shaping our behavior that forms the essence of context. Theory is an important guide in applied communication because it provides a framework that organizes important variables into relationships, some of which can be manipulated or modified, permitting us to predict health outcomes. Planning communication to change health behavior successfully on a population or community level requires using theory and empirical research to, for instance, segment audiences, tailor effective messages, and examine multiple interacting levels of effects. The effective application of communication theory in health will thus depend on the goals of change at each level. For example, the health communication strategies you would use when seeking to build support for a change in public policy among legislators are likely to be different from those you would use to persuade reluctant mothers to have their infants regularly vaccinated.

There are methodological challenges in health communication as well, especially in the measurement of effect and impact. In the analog world of relatively isolated community media systems, one could craft quasi-experimental studies comparing outcomes in intervention and comparison communities in order to look at the effect of health communication campaigns. This approach derived from classic empirical models focusing on treatment and control conditions, where the latter were kept carefully isolated from the former. In the world of digital communication and increasingly interlinked communities and national and global systems, this controlled design is less possible. Designs with a focus on time series and longitudinal analyses are one direction in research methods. Big data methods are also emerging as digital technologies, such as Google Analytics, facilitate the collection and analysis of vast amounts of data to examine trends and directions in content, search methods, and even public opinion. The challenges here are how to make sense and meaning out of complexity.

These and other factors will guide the future research agenda in health communication in the context of the ecological model of health that informs much of this book. Other promising influences in the future of health communication research may include emerging advances in neurology and brain science, especially if they can provide new understandings of stages of brain development, information processing, and communication dynamics and behavior affecting health. How increasingly interactive audiences themselves shape health information will continue to be an important part of work in this arena. Together, these research advances could lead to more useful and effective communication strategies across the life course, with the ultimate goal of improved population health.

References

Ackerson, L. K., Ramanadhan, S., Arya, M., & Viswanath, K. (2012). Social disparities, communication inequalities, and HIV/AIDS-related knowledge and attitudes in India. *AIDS Behavior, 16*(7), 2072–2081.

Ackerson, L. K., & Viswanath, K. (2009). Communication inequalities, social determinants, and intermittent smoking in the 2003 Health Information National Trends Survey. *Preventing Chronic Disease, 6*(2), A40.

Ajzen, I., & Fishbein, M. (1980). *Understanding attitudes and predicting social behavior.* Englewood Cliffs, NJ: Prentice Hall.

Barry, C. L., Brescoll, V. L., & Gollust, S. E. (2013). Framing support for childhood obesity policies: The effects of individualizing the problem. *Political Psychology, 34*(3), 327–349.

Baum, M. A. (2011). Red state, blue state, flu state: Media self-selection and partisan gaps in swine flu vaccinations. *Journal of Health Politics, Policy and Law, 36*(6), 1021–1059.

Bekalu, M., & Eggermont, S. (2013). Determinants of HIV/AIDS-related information needs and media use: Beyond individual-level factors. *Health Communication, 28*(6), 624–636.

Berelson, B. (1948). Communications and public opinion. In W. Schramm (Ed.), *Communications in modern society*. Urbana: University of Illinois Press.

Berkman, L., & Kawachi, I. (2000). *Social epidemiology*. New York: Oxford University Press.

Bigman, C. A., Cappella, J. N., & Hornik, R. C. (2010). Effective or ineffective: Attribute framing and the human papillomavirus (HPV) vaccine. *Patient Education and Counseling, 81*(Suppl.), S70–S76.

Borah, P. (2011). Conceptual issues in framing theory: A systematic examination of a decade's literature. *Journal of Communication, 61*(2), 246–263.

Brehm, J. W. (1966). *A theory of psychological reactance*. New York: Wiley.

Brinol, P., & Petty, R. E. (2005). Individual differences in persuasion. In D. Albarracín, B. Johnson, & M. Zanna (Eds.), *The handbook of attitudes and attitude change* (pp. 575–616). Hillsdale, NJ: Erlbaum.

Briones, R., Nan, X., Madden, K., & Waks, L. (2012). When vaccines go viral: An analysis of HPV vaccine coverage on YouTube. *Health Communication, 27*(5), 478–485.

Bryant, J., & Miron, D. (2004). Theory and research in mass communication. *Journal of Communication, 54*(4), 662–704.

Bryant, J., & Zillman, D. (1994). *Media effects: Advances in theory and research*. Hillsdale, NJ: Erlbaum.

Bryant, J. Z., Zillman, D., & Oliver, M. B. (2002). *Media effects: Advances in theory and research*. Hillsdale, NJ: Erlbaum.

Cappella, J. N., & Rimer, B. K. (Eds.). (2006). The role of theory in developing effective health communications (Special issue). *Journal of Communication, 56*, S1–S279.

Centers for Disease Control and Prevention. (2013). *Genetic HPV infection—fact sheet*. Retrieved from http://www.cdc.gov/std/hpv/stdfact-hpv.htm

Chester, J.M.K. (2009). *Digital marketing: Opportunities for addressing interactive food and beverage marketing to youth*. Berkeley, CA: Berkeley Media Studies Group.

Chong, D., & Druckman, J. N. (2007). Framing theory. *Annual Review of Political Science, 10*, 103–126.

Colgrove, J., Abiola, S., & Mello, M. (2010). HPV vaccination mandates: Lawmaking amid political and scientific controversy. *New England Journal of Medicine, 363*(8), 785–791.

Conrad, C., & Poole, M. S. (2012). *Strategic organizational communication: Into the 21st century*. Fort Worth, TX: Harcourt Brace.

Constantine, N. A., & Jerman, P. (2007). Acceptance of human papillomavirus vaccination among Californian parents of daughters: A representative statewide analysis. *Journal of Adolescent Health, 40*(2), 108–115.

Dillard, J. P., & Nabi, R. L. (2006). The persuasive influence of emotion in cancer prevention and detection messages. *Journal of Communication, 56*(Suppl. 1), S123–S139.

Dillard, J. P., & Shen, L. J. (2005). On the nature of reactance and its role in persuasive health communication. *Communication Monographs, 72*(2), 144–168.

DiMaggio, P., Hargittai, E., Celeste, C., & Shafer, S. (2004). Digital inequality: From unequal access to differentiated use. *Social Inequality*, 355–400.

Druckman, J. N., & Leeper, T. J. (2012). Learning more from political communication experiments: Pretreatment and its effects. *American Journal of Political Science, 56*(4), 875–896.

Elam-Evans, L. D., Yankey, D., Jeyarajah, J., Singleton, J. A., Curtis, C. R., MacNeil, J., & Hariri, S. (2014). National, regional, state, and selected local area vaccination coverage among adolescents aged 13–17 years—United States, 2013. *Morbidity and Mortality Weekly Report, 63*(29), 625–633.

Entman, R. (1993). Framing: Toward clarification of a fractured paradigm. *Journal of Communication, 34*(4), 51–85.

Fishbein, M., & Cappella, J. (2006). The role of theory in developing effective health communication. *Journal of Communication, 56*(Suppl. 1), S1–S17.

Fishbein, M., Hall-Jamieson, K., Zimmer, E., Von Haeften, I., & Nabi, R. (2002). Avoiding the boomerang: Testing the relative effectiveness of antidrug public service announcements before a national campaign. *American Journal of Public Health, 92*(2), 238–245.

Fjeldsoe, B. S., Marshall, A. L., & Miller, Y. D. (2009). Behavior change interventions delivered by mobile telephone short-message service. *American Journal of Preventive Medicine, 36*(2), 165–173.

Fjeldsoe, B. S., Miller, Y. D., & Marshall, A. L. (2010). MobileMums: A randomized controlled trial of an SMS-based physical activity intervention. *Annals of Behavioral Medicine, 39*(2), 101–111.

Fjeldsoe, B. S., Miller, Y. D., & Marshall, A. L. (2012). Social cognitive mediators of the effect of the MobileMums intervention on physical activity. *Health Psychology, 32*(7), 729–738.

Fowler, E. F., Gollust, S. E., Dempsey, A. F., Lantz, P. M., & Ubel, P. A. (2012). Issue emergence, evolution of controversy, and implications for competitive framing: The case of the HPV vaccine. *International Journal of Press/Politics, 17*(2), 169–189.

Franklin, V. L., Waller, A., Pagliari, C., & Greene, A. (2006). A randomized controlled trial of sweet talk, a text-messaging system to support young people with diabetes. *Diabetic Medicine, 23*(12), 1332–1338.

Galarce, E. M., Ramanadhan, S., Weeks, J. C., Schneider, E., Gray, S., & Viswanath, K. (2011). Class, race, ethnicity and information needs in post-treatment cancer patients. *Patient Education and Counseling, 85*(3), 432–439.

Gerbner, G., Gross, L., Morgan, M., Signorelli, N., & Bryant, J. (1994). *Growing up with television: The cultivation perspective.* Hillsdale, NJ: Erlbaum.

Glanz, K., & Yang, H. (1996). Communicating about risk of infectious diseases. *JAMA, 275*(3), 253–256.

Gollust, S. E., Attanasio, L., Dempsey, A., Benson, A. M., & Fowler, E. F. (2013). Political and news media factors shaping public awareness of the HPV vaccine. *Women's Health Issues, 23*(3), e143–e151.

Green, M. C., & Brock, T. C. (2000). The role of transportation in the persuasiveness of public narratives. *Journal of Personality and Social Psychology, 79*(5), 701–721.

Grier, S. A., & Kumanyika, S. (2010). Targeted marketing and public health. *Annual Review of Public Health, 31*, 349–369.

Head, K. J., Noar, S. M., Iannarino, N. T., & Grant Harrington, N. (2013). Efficacy of text message-based interventions for health promotion: A meta-analysis. *Social Science & Medicine, 97*, 41–48.

Hinyard, L. J., & Kreuter, M. W. (2007). Using narrative communication as a tool for health behavior change: A conceptual, theoretical, and empirical overview. *Health Education & Behavior, 34*(5), 777–792.

Hwang, Y., & Jeong, S. (2009). Revisiting the knowledge gap hypothesis: A meta-analysis of thirty-five years of research. *Journalism & Mass Communication Quarterly, 86*(3), 513–532.

Iyengar, S. (1991). *Is anyone responsible?* Chicago: University of Chicago Press.

Iyengar, S., & Kinder, D. R. (1987). *News that matters.* Chicago: University of Chicago Press.

Jung, M., Arya, M., & Viswanath, K. (2013). Effect of media use on HIV/AIDS-related knowledge and condom use in sub-Saharan Africa: A cross-sectional study. *PLoS ONE, 8*(7), e68359.

Katz, E., & Lazarsfeld, P. (1955). *Personal influence.* New York: Free Press.

Kim, B., & Glanz, K. (2013). A motivational text messaging walking program for older African Americans: A pilot study. *American Journal of Preventive Medicine, 44*, 71–75.

Kosicki, G. M. (1993). Problems and opportunities in agenda-setting research. *Journal of Communication, 43*(2), 100–127.

Kovacic, W. E. (2008). *Marketing food to children and adolescents: A review of industry expenditures, activities, and self-regulation: A Federal Trade Commission report to Congress.* Washington, DC: Federal Trade Commission.

Kreuter, M. W., Green, M. C., Cappella, J. N., Slater, M. D., Wise, M. E., Storey, D., . . . Woolley, S. (2007). Narrative communication in cancer prevention and control: A framework to guide research and application. *Annals of Behavioral Medicine, 33*(3), 221–235.

Krieger, J. L., & Sarge, M. A. (2013). A serial mediation model of message framing on intentions to receive the human papillomavirus (HPV) vaccine: Revisiting the role of threat and efficacy perceptions. *Health Communication, 28*(1), 5–19.

Lammers, J. C., & Barbour, J. B. (2006). An institutional theory of organizational communication. *Communication Theory, 16*(3), 356–377.

Lazarsfeld, P., Berelson, B., & Gaudet, H. (1948). *The people's choice.* New York: Columbia University Press.

Leader, A. E., Cashman, R., Voytek, C. D., Baker, J. L., Brawner, B. M., & Frank, I. (2011). An exploratory study of adolescent female reactions to direct-to-consumer advertising: The case of the human papillomavirus (HPV) vaccine. *Health Marketing Quarterly, 28*(4), 372–385.

Leader, A. E., Weiner, J. L., Kelly, B. J., Hornik, R. C., & Cappella, J. N. (2009). Effects of information framing on human papillomavirus vaccination. *Journal of Women's Health, 18*(2), 225–233.

Lippman, W. (1922). *Public opinion.* New York: MacMillan.

Mack, J. W., Paul, M. E., Viswanath, K., & Prigerson, H. G. (2010). Racial disparities in the outcomes of communication on medical care received near death. *Archives of Internal Medicine, 170*(17), 1533–1540.

McCloud, R., Jung, M., & Viswanath, K. (2013). Class, race and ethnicity and information avoidance among cancer survivors. *British Journal of Cancer, 108*(10), 1949–1956.

McComas, K. A. (2006). Defining moments in risk communication research: 1996–2005. *Journal of Health Communication, 11*(1), 75–91.

McCombs, M. (2004). *Setting the agenda: The mass media and public opinion.* Cambridge, UK: Polity Press.

Mumby, D. K., & Stohl, C. (1996). Disciplining organizational communication studies. *Management Communication Quarterly, 10*(1), 50–72.

Nagler, R. H. (2014). Adverse outcomes associated with media exposure to contradictory nutrition messages. *Journal of Health Communication, 19*(1), 24–40.

National Cancer Institute. (2014). *Accelerating HPV vaccine uptake: Urgency for action to prevent cancer. A report to the President of the United States from the president's cancer panel.* Retrieved from http://deainfo.nci.nih.gov/advisory/pcp/annualreports

Naughton, F., Prevost, T., Gilbert, H., & Sutton, S. (2012). Randomized controlled trial evaluation of a tailored leaflet and SMS text message self-help intervention for pregnant smokers (MiQuit). *Nicotine & Tobacco Research, 14*(5), 569–577.

Neuman, R. (1999). Broadcasting and bandwidth. *Economics of Science, Technology, and Innovation, 15*, 215–236.

Niederdeppe, J., Bigman, C. A., Gonzales, A. L., & Gollust, S. E. (2013). Communication about health disparities in the mass media. *Journal of Communication, 63*(1), 8–30.

Nilsen, W., Santosh, K., Shar, A., Varoquiers, C., Wiley, T., Riley, W., . . . Atienza, A. (2012). Advancing the science of mHealth. *Journal of Health Communication, 17*(Suppl. 1), 5–10.

Nyhan, B., Reifler, J., Richey, S., & Freed, G. L. (2014). Effective messages in vaccine promotion: A randomized trial. *Pediatrics, 133*(4), e835–e842.

Palenchar, M. J., & Heath, R. L. (2007). Strategic risk communication: Adding value to society. *Public Relations Review, 33*, 120–129.

Palmgreen, P., & Donohew, L. (2002). Effective mass media strategies for drug abuse prevention campaigns. In Z. Sloboda & W. Bukoski (Eds.), *Effective strategies for drug abuse prevention.* New York: Plenum Press.

Phelan, J. C., Link, B. G., & Tehranifar, P. (2010). Social conditions as fundamental causes of health inequalities: Theory, evidence, and policy implications. *Journal of Health and Social Behavior, 51*(Suppl.), S528–S540.

Powell, L. M., Schermbeck, R. M., Szczypka, G., Chaloupka, F. J., & Braunschweig, C. L. (2011). Trends in the nutritional content of television food advertisements seen by children in the United States: Analyses by age, food categories, and companies. *Archives of Pediatrics & Adolescent Medicine, 165*(12), 1078–1086.

Richardson, J., & Harris, J. L. (2011, November). *Food marketing and social media: Findings from fast food FACTS and sugary drink FACTS.* Paper presented at the American University Digital Food Marketing Conference, Washington, DC.

Rimer, B. K., Glanz, K., & Rasband, G. (2001). Searching for evidence about health education and health behavior interventions. *Health Education & Behavior, 28*(2), 231–248.

Rimer, B. K., & Glassman, B. (1999). Is there a use for tailored print communications in cancer risk communication? *Journal of National Cancer Institute Monographs, 25*, 140–148.

Rogers, E. M. (2003). *Diffusion of innovations* (5th ed.). New York: Free Press.

Sandman, P. M. (1987). Risk communication: Facing public outrage. *US Environmental Protection Agency Journal, 13*, 21–22.

Scheufele, D. A., & Tewksbury, D. (2007). Framing, agenda-setting and priming: The evolution of three effects models. *Journal of Communication, 57*(1), 9–20.

Shah, D., McLeod, D., Gotlieb, M., & Lee, N. (2009). Framing and agenda setting. In R. Nabi & M. Oliver (Eds.), *The Sage handbook of media processes and effects* (pp. 83–98). Thousand Oaks, CA: Sage.

Shen, F. Y., & Edwards, H. H. (2005). Economic individualism, humanitarianism, and welfare reform: A value-based account of framing effects. *Journal of Communication, 55*(4), 795–809.

Slovic, P. (2007). If I look at the mass I will never act: Psychic numbing and genocide. *Judgment and Decision Making, 2*(2), 79–95.

Smith, A. (2013). *Smartphone ownership 2013* (Pew Research Center report). Retrieved from http://www .pewinternet.org/Reports/2013/Smartphone-Ownership-2013.aspx

Southwell, B. G., Slater, J. S., Nelson, C. L., & Rothman, A. J. (2012). Does it pay to pay people to share information? Using financial incentives to promote peer referral for mammography among the underinsured. *American Journal of Health Promotion, 26*(6), 348–351.

Southwell, B. G., & Yzer, M. C. (2009). When (and why) interpersonal talk matters for campaigns. *Communication Theory, 19*(1), 1–8.

Stephenson, M. T., & Southwell, B. (2006). Sensation-seeking, the activation model, and mass media health campaigns. *Journal of Communication, 56*(Suppl. 1), S38–S56.

Stupiansky, N. W., Rosenthal, S. L., Wiehe, S. E., & Zimet, G. D. (2010). Human papillomavirus vaccine acceptability among a national sample of adult women in the USA. *Sexual Health, 7*(3), 304–309.

Taber, C. S., & Lodge, M. (2006). Motivated skepticism in the evaluation of political beliefs. *American Journal of Political Science, 50*(3), 755–769.

Takeshita, T. (2006). Current critical problems in agenda-setting research. *International Journal of Public Opinion Research, 18*(3), 275–296.

Tichenor, P. J., Donohue, G. A., & Olien, C. N. (1970). Mass media flow and differential growth in knowledge. *Public Opinion Quarterly, 34*(2), 159–170.

Tversky, A., & Kahneman, D. (1981). The framing of decisions and the psychology of choice. *Science, 211*(4481), 453–458.

Viswanath, K. (2005). The communications revolution and cancer control. *Nature Reviews: Cancer, 5*(10), 828–835.

Viswanath, K. (2006). Public communications and its role in reducing and eliminating health disparities. In G. E. Thomson, F. Mitchell, & M. Williams (Eds.), *Examining the health disparities research plan of the National Institutes of Health: Unfinished business* (pp. 215–253). Washington, DC: Institute of Medicine.

Viswanath, K. (2011). Cyberinfrastructure: An extraordinary opportunity to bridge health and communication inequalities? *American Journal of Preventive Medicine, 40*(5, Suppl. 2), S245–S248.

Viswanath, K., & Ackerson, L. (2011). Race, ethnicity, language, social class, and health communication inequalities: A nationally-representative cross-sectional study. *PLoS ONE, 6*(1), e14550.

Viswanath, K., & Finnegan, J. R. (1996). The knowledge gap hypothesis: Twenty-five years later. In B. Burleson (Ed.), *Communication yearbook* (Vol. 19, pp. 187–227). Thousand Oaks, CA: Sage.

Viswanath, K., Nagler, R. H., Bigman-Galimore, C. A., Jung, M., McCauley, M., & Ramanadhan, S. (2012). The communications revolution and health inequalities in the 21st century: Implications for cancer control. *Cancer Epidemiology, Biomarkers & Prevention, 21*(10), 1701–1708.

Viswanath, K., Randolph Steele, W., & Finnegan, J. R. (2006). Social capital and health: Civic engagement, community size, and recall of health messages. *American Journal of Public Health, 96*(8), 1456–1461.

Weinstein, N. D. (2000). Perceived probability, perceived severity, and health-protective behavior. *Health Psychology, 19*(1), 65–74.

Williams, D. R., Kontos, E. Z., Viswanath, K., Haas, J. S., Lathan, C., MacConaill, L., . . . Ayanian, J. Z. (2012). Integrating multiple social statuses in health disparities research: The case of lung cancer. *Health Services Research, 47*(3, Pt. 2), 1255–1277.

Zhan, X., & Tang, S. Y. (2013). Political opportunities, resource constraints and policy advocacy of environmental NGOs in China. *Public Administration, 91*(2), 381–399.

Zillman, D. (2006). Exemplification effects in the promotion of safety and health. *Journal of Communication, 56*(Suppl. 1), S221–S237.

PART FIVE

USING THEORY IN RESEARCH AND PRACTICE

CHAPTER 18

INTRODUCTION TO USING THEORY IN RESEARCH AND PRACTICE

The Editors

One of the greatest challenges for public health professionals is to learn to analyze the *fit* of a theory or model for issues and populations of interest. A working knowledge of a handful of theories, preferably from different levels of intervention (e.g., individuals and communities), and the ways in which they have been applied is a first step. Mastering the challenges of using theories appropriately and effectively is the logical next step. Effective practice depends on marshaling the most appropriate theory (or theories) and practice strategies for a given situation. Theory-based research and evaluation further require designs, measures, and procedures appropriate to the health problem, context, and unique population at hand, as well as the development and implementation of promising or proven interventions.

No one theory or model will be right in all cases. Depending on the unit of practice and type of health behavior or issue, different theoretical frameworks will be appropriate, practical, and useful. Often more than one theory is needed to adequately address an issue. For comprehensive health behavior change programs, this is almost always true. It is also evident in the use and description of applied theories found in the professional literature.

The preceding sections of this book make clear that theories often overlap, and that some fit easily within broader models. Generally, theories can be used most effectively when they are integrated into a comprehensive planning framework. Such a system assigns a central role to research as input; it determines the situation and needs of the population to be served, the resources available, and the progress and effectiveness of the program at various stages. Planning is a continuous process in which new information is constantly gathered to build or improve the program.

The chapters in Part Five give specific examples of how theories can be combined for greater impact. Chapter Nineteen, by L. Kay Bartholomew and colleagues, describes two well-developed planning models, PRECEDE-PROCEED and Intervention Mapping, that can be used to integrate and apply diverse theoretical frameworks. Both models take comprehensive approaches that begin with assessing the problem and population and continue to evaluation, based on a theoretically informed logic model.

In Chapter Twenty, Kevin Volpp and his coauthors present the rationale for and the key constructs of applying behavioral economics to health improvement programs. Behavioral economics has roots in classical economics and expected utility theory, blended with a grounding in theories and evidence from psychology and sociology. The authors illustrate the broad applicability of behavioral economics constructs and provide examples of specific applications to interventions to facilitate weight loss and improve medication adherence.

In Chapter Twenty-One, J. Douglas Storey and colleagues describe the purpose, key components, and methods of social marketing. They illustrate the application of social marketing in a family health program in Egypt and an ambitious social marketing program in Uganda that addresses the multiple problems of HIV/AIDS, malaria, family planning, and maternal and child health.

This chapter provides highlights from each of the remaining chapters in this section, discusses emerging developments and challenges, and comments on the state of the art in the use of theory in health behavior research and practice. Using theory thoughtfully and appropriately is not simple but it can be rewarding. This discussion aims to provoke thought and debate and stimulate further reading, rather than to provide definitive answers or prescriptions for the field.

Theory-Based Planning Models

In Chapter Nineteen, Bartholomew, Markham, Mullen, and Fernández, describe two models for systematic development of theory- and evidence-based health promotion programs: the PRECEDE-PROCEED Model and Intervention Mapping. They explicitly illustrate the ways that behavior change theories can be applied and incorporated into a systematic planning process and note the challenges of applying the models. As with some of the theories discussed in earlier chapters, using these planning models can be a demanding and laborious process for practitioners and community groups. But when mastered, it can lead to the development of effective, appropriate health behavior change programs.

A key premise of this chapter is that while health behavior theories are critical tools, they do not substitute for adequate planning and research. However, theories do help us to interpret problem situations and plan feasible, promising interventions and appropriate program evaluations. Because we can use theories to articulate the assumptions behind intervention strategies, theories can be helpful in pinpointing intermediate steps that should be assessed in evaluations.

The PRECEDE-PROCEED Model has as its raison d'être the systematic application of theory and previous research to assessment of local needs, priorities, circumstances, and resources (Green et al., 1994). Phase 3 of this model focuses on examining factors that shape behavioral actions and environmental factors. Theories help to guide examination of predisposing, enabling, and reinforcing factors for particular behaviors. For example, constructs from the Health Belief Model might help researchers to understand why some women do not get mammograms (see Chapter Five). PRECEDE-PROCEED also can be used in conjunction with the Transtheoretical Model of change to design stage-appropriate health messages (see Chapter Seven). The concepts of priority, changeability, and community preferences should be considered along with analytical and empirical findings about health behavior determinants. For example, health experts concerned with effecting distribution of safe drinking water must understand how people in the recipient communities think about water sources and what beliefs might be amenable to change. These ideas are also consistent with concepts presented in earlier chapters on community engagement and implementation and dissemination.

Bartholomew and colleagues also describe Intervention Mapping (IM), a framework for developing theory- and evidence-based health behavior or education programs, and illustrate how IM has been applied. Intervention Mapping (Bartholomew, Parcel, Kok, Gottlieb, & Fernandez, 2011) is composed of five steps that are complementary to the planning phases of the PRECEDE-PROCEED Model. Intervention Mapping can be helpful in guiding program planners toward explicit specifications for using both theory and empirical findings to develop effective health behavior interventions.

Behavioral Economics

Behavioral economics has its foundations in classical economics and expected utility theory, blended with a grounding in theories and evidence from psychology and sociology. Behavioral economics has received growing attention in recent years, with applications in several fields in which anticipated costs and benefits play a central role: labor markets, wage policies, savings and retirement plans and policies, and organizational behavior (Camerer, Loewenstein, & Rabin, 2004; Diamond & Vartianen, 2007). Its application to health behavior and health care utilization is emerging rapidly, as described in Chapter Twenty.

Behavioral economics aims to increase the explanatory power of economics by grounding that approach in psychological and social foundations. It is not a single theory per se, but uses insights from cognitive psychology, sociology, and decision analysis (Camerer et al., 2004). Behavioral economics recognizes that people make decision errors in weighing the costs and benefits of their actions, and that message framing can influence how people react to persuasive communications. Key implications from behavioral economics for health behavior change suggest that incentives can improve health behaviors, but also, importantly, that the way incentives are delivered can matter more than the amount of incentives. This idea, which is also consistent with applied behavioral analysis and Social Cognitive Theory (Chapter Nine), has been used in health behavior intervention research by the chapter authors and others with substantial success.

In Chapter Twenty, Volpp, Loewenstein, and Asch report on successful interventions that used incentives and feedback to improve weight loss success and medication adherence. These authors also noted an important limitation: that once incentives were no longer provided, behavior changes were not maintained. This has been a constant in most studies of incentives, which have been used in many programs over the years. Unless behavior change is internally motivated by individuals and not merely a response to a reinforcement, once the incentive has been applied, the desired behavior stops. Behavioral economics does not delve specifically into the arena of habitual behaviors and maintenance, though this is a future direction for researchers in this field. An interesting prospect would be to blend behavioral economics with central tenets of Self-Determination Theory, which posits that maintenance of behaviors over time requires that patients internalize values and skills for change (Ryan & Deci, 2000).

Social Marketing

Social marketing is a process that promotes desired voluntary behaviors among members of a target market by offering attractive benefits and/or reducing barriers associated with healthful choices. It involves the adaptation of commercial marketing technologies to promote socially desirable goals. In Chapter Twenty-One, Storey, Hess, and Saffitz take a fresh look at social marketing. They emphasize how social marketing can be applied within a strategic health communication framework and link key theories of health communication and health behavior to the effective practice of social marketing.

When using social marketing, success is most likely when marketers accurately determine the perceptions, needs, and wants of target markets and satisfy them through the design, communication, pricing, and delivery of appropriate, competitive, and visible offerings. The process is consumer-driven, not only expert-driven. This orientation is consistent with principles of community organization, and its product development approach parallels the innovation development process of diffusion theory. At the same time, it shares an economic perspective with behavioral economics, a field of inquiry that relates individual behaviors to economic variables (Bickel & Vuchinich, 2000). Another parallel between social marketing and behavioral economics is that each is adapted from a more mature and extensive field: social marketing uses some principles from commercial marketing and behavioral economics builds on classic economic theory.

Like the PRECEDE-PROCEED Model and Intervention Mapping, social marketing provides a framework to identify what drives and maintains behavior, and what factors might drive and maintain behavior change. It also requires identification of potential intermediaries, channels of distribution and communication, and actual and potential competitors. As the chapter authors indicate, theories of health behavior can help to guide the analytical process in social marketing and aid in the formulation of intervention strategies and materials. The authors explicitly illustrate four theories that contribute to social marketing approaches: the Theory of Planned Behavior, the extended parallel processing model, Social Cognitive Theory and its observational learning construct, and Diffusion of Innovations. Because of their focus on understanding consumers (or target audiences) from the consumers' point of view, social marketing models are robust for use in diverse and unique populations, including disadvantaged groups and ethnic minorities, and in many countries. In fact, it is often thought that social marketing programs tend to be inherently culturally sensitive because they follow a consumer-oriented process. In social marketing it is always important to identify and fulfill demand—that is, to "start where the people are."

Cross-Cutting Propositions About Using Theory

Here we offer some key cross-cutting propositions to readers to put the use of health behavior theory in perspective. These ideas are germane to the review and discussion of the chapters in this section and throughout this book.

1. Researchers and practitioners should not confuse *using* or *applying* theory with testing theory or developing theory. They are fundamentally different activities even though complementary.

2. Testing the efficacy or effectiveness of theory-based interventions does not constitute testing a theory or theories per se.

3. It is likely that the strongest interventions will be built from multiple theories. The most replicable and transparent interventions will be built in a way that the contributions of each theory can be understood.

4. When combining theories, it is important to clearly think through the unique contribution of each different theory to the combined model. If this is not done carefully or well, the "new" combined approach may be redundant, overlapping, and hard to interpret in the context of established theories.

5. Rigorous tests of theory-based interventions, including measurements and analyses of mediators and moderators, are the building blocks of the evidence base in health behavior change.

6. Theory use, testing, and development will be enhanced by the use of shared instruments and reporting. The more researchers and practitioners can build on past efforts, the more they are likely to advance the public's health. We recommend employing adaptations of the protocol concept used in clinical research so that the measures used with particular theories and the ways in which theory is turned into interventions are transparent and accessible. The opportunity to offer online materials to supplement journal publications makes this increasingly feasible.

7. Theory, research, and practice are parts of a continuum for understanding the determinants of behaviors, testing strategies for change, and disseminating effective interventions (see Chapters Sixteen and Nineteen).

8. There is as much to learn from failure as there is to learn from success. Researchers and practitioners who develop and test theory-based interventions should publish their findings when they are negative and when they are positive.

9. There is no substitute for knowing the audience. This applies to the conduct of fundamental research to understand determinants of health behavior as much as it applies to developing health promotion programs for specific individuals, groups, and communities. Participatory research and program design improve the odds of success.

The authors of the remaining three chapters in Part Five describe tools, strategies, models, and issues that are critical to consider when applying theories. This section of *Health Behavior: Theory, Research, and Practice* tackles the complexity of health behavior and health promotion at its multiple levels. A basic theme is that if intervention strategies are based on a carefully researched understanding of the determinants of behavior and environments, and if systematic approaches to tailoring, targeting, implementation, and evaluation are used, the chances are good that programs will be effective. And when they are not effective, then there should be good information about why they did not work. Understanding past failure is critical to future success.

Moving Forward

After one becomes familiar with some contemporary theories of health behavior, the challenge is to use them within a comprehensive planning process. Researchers and practitioners can increase the odds of success by examining health and behavior at multiple levels, as articulated in ecological models (Chapter Three).

At its simplest, an ecological perspective emphasizes two main options: change people and/or change the environment. The most powerful approaches will use both of these options together (Smedley & Syme, 2000). The activities most directly tied to changing *people* are derived from individual-level theories like the Health Belief Model, Transtheoretical Model of change, and Integrated Behavioral Model. In contrast, activities aimed at changing the *environment* draw on community-level theories. In between are Social Cognitive Theory, theories of social support and social networks, and interpersonal communication models. Each of these focuses on reciprocal relations among persons or between individuals and their environments.

Theoretical frameworks are guides in the pursuit of successful change efforts, maximizing researchers' and practitioners' flexibility and helping them to apply abstract concepts of theory in ways that are most useful in diverse work settings and situations. Knowledge of theory and comprehensive planning systems offers a great deal of help in this pursuit. Other key elements of effective programs are a good program-to-audience match; accessible and practical information; active learning and participant involvement; and skill building, practice, and reinforcement. Strong interventions will often, although not always, be built on theory, yet theory alone cannot lead to effective interventions. Theory helps you to ask the right questions, and effective planning enables you to zero in on the right elements in relation to a specific problem. Still, theory must be turned into effective interventions, and these must be applied with fidelity and evaluated well. A lot happens between theory and behavior change. Effective use of theory for practice and research requires practice, but it can yield important dividends in efforts to enhance the health of individuals and populations. In the end, we should ask ourselves whether our work has made a difference. Developing better theories is a means to that end.

In the first edition of *Health Behavior and Health Education*, Irwin M. Rosenstock said, "it would be the height of folly to predict the future needs of health education [and health behavior] research and practice, at least without the assistance of an outstanding California astrologer or the Great Kreskin" (Rosenstock, 1990, p. 405). Times have changed, and indeed, scientific advances and new technology have dramatically altered our lives. Every day, we find ourselves adapting to life with new technologies, which are appearing at an astonishing pace. They have changed our understanding about the health risks we confront, the information we can obtain, day-to-day priorities and worries, relationships, and the ways we communicate.

The modern field of health behavior dates back only about eighty years, and progress has accelerated most rapidly in the past thirty years. As the authors of the chapters in this book have shown, many of the early ideas of social and behavioral theorists serve as solid foundations for our work today. To continue to accelerate our progress, we should stand on the shoulders of the pioneers in the field, equip ourselves to be explorers, address today's problems with new tools, and anticipate the challenges of the future.

References

Bartholomew, L. K., Parcel, G. S., Kok, G., Gottlieb, N. H., & Fernández, M. E. (2011). *Planning health promotion programs: An intervention mapping approach* (3rd ed.). San Francisco: Jossey-Bass.

Bickel, W. K., & Vuchinich, R. E. (Eds.). (2000). *Reframing health behavior change with behavioral economics*. Mahwah, NJ: Erlbaum.

Camerer, C. F., Loewenstein, G., & Rabin, M. (Eds.). (2004). *Advances in behavioral economics*. Princeton, NJ: Princeton University Press.

Diamond, P., & Vartianen, H. (Eds.). (2007). *Behavioral economics and its applications*. Princeton, NJ: Princeton University Press.

Green, L. W., Glanz, K., Hochbaum, G. M., Kok, G., Kreuter, M. W., Lewis, F. M., . . . , Rosenstock, I. M. (1994). Can we build on, or must we replace, the theories and models in health education? *Health Education Research, 9*, 397–404.

Rosenstock, I. M. (1990). The past, present, and future of health education. In K. Glanz, F. M. Lewis, & B. K. Rimer (Eds.), *Health behavior and health education: Theory, research, and practice*. San Francisco: Jossey-Bass.

Ryan, R. M., & Deci, E. L. (2000). Self-determination theory and the facilitation of intrinsic motivation, social development, and well-being. *American Psychologist, 55*, 68–78.

Smedley, B. D., & Syme, S. L. (Eds.). (2000). *Promoting health: Intervention strategies from social and behavioral research*. Washington, DC: National Academies Press.

CHAPTER 19

PLANNING MODELS FOR THEORY-BASED HEALTH PROMOTION INTERVENTIONS

L. Kay Bartholomew
Christine Markham
Pat Mullen
María E. Fernández

In the development of interventions to change behaviors and/or environments, a framework or model enables program planners to apply theories of health behavior and their constructs to address health and health behavior problems. Once factors contributing to desirable change are understood, the framework can also guide the choice of leverage points to produce that change. The purpose of a framework or model is to guide planners to identify the full range of constructs that may be relevant to one or more target behavior(s) and outcomes. Program developers may use constructs from multiple theories in describing a problem or devising solutions, and they may also use constructs that are not explicitly theory based (Fishbein et al., 2001; Noar & Zimmerman, 2005). We use the terms *framework* and *model* interchangeably throughout this chapter to mean a structure that elicits a hypothesized set of relationships among constructs and one or more behavior(s) or environmental factor(s) leading to health outcomes.

Health professionals and researchers who develop, implement, and evaluate interventions often approach theory in a way that is fundamentally different from that of researchers interested in theory generation or single-theory testing. A researcher or practitioner who wants to find a solution to a public health problem in a real-world situation will apply a problem-driven, applied behavioral

KEY POINTS

This chapter will:

- Describe two models for systematic development of theory- and evidence-based health promotion programs: the PRECEDE-PROCEED Model and Intervention Mapping.

- Present steps for using planning models to facilitate systematic use of theory and evidence when designing health promotion interventions.

- Give examples of using the two models to integrate theory and evidence into program planning.

- Provide two case studies that show the full sequence of using PRECEDE-PROCEED and Intervention Mapping for intervention development.

or social science approach using one or multiple theories, empirical evidence, and new research both to assess the problem and to solve or prevent the problem (Buunk & Vugt, 2008). In this problem-focused approach to using theory, the main criteria for success are health outcomes rather than theory testing or development. Intervention planners make many choices (e.g., where in a system to intervene and/or how to intervene) in the development of an intervention, and theories are one tool to enable better choices. Both the PRECEDE-PROCEED Model and Intervention Mapping are tools that help guide the selection of constructs and theories to optimize change in the behavioral and environmental factors that influence health.

To develop theory- and evidence-based interventions, researchers and practitioners using PRECEDE-PROCEED and Intervention Mapping can build diagrams depicting *logic models*. Logic models depict proposed causal relationships among variables related to health problems and their solutions. A *logic model of the problem* or *theory of the problem* depicts plausible causal explanations of a problem. A *logic model of change, theory of change*, or *intervention theory* refers to a plausible causal pathway of the mechanisms of change proposed for an intervention (Buunk & Vugt, 2008; Glanz, Rimer, & Viswanath, 2008; Rossi, Lipsey, & Freeman, 2004). For example, a logic model (theory) of the *problem* might depict, with boxes and arrows, the motivational and environmental factors that influence a certain health behavior. In contrast, a logic model (theory) of *change* would include change methods aimed at factors related to health-promoting behavior change and improved health outcomes.

The next two sections describe the PRECEDE-PROCEED Model and Intervention Mapping. Before we describe the steps of these two planning frameworks, it is important to point out several processes that should always be used in health promotion planning and that are explicitly included or implied in both frameworks. From the days of the earliest work on PRECEDE (prior to the addition of PROCEED), many sources of wisdom in health promotion planning have recommended meaningful attention to the participation of stakeholders, in-depth consideration of theories and theoretical constructs, and attention to cultural appropriateness (Green, Kreuter, Deeds, & Partridge, 1980). Ideally, planners will follow principles of collaboration that include striving to understand personal and institutional histories; to promote multiple stakeholder involvement; to recognize diverse members' expertise; and to promote equity in decision making and shared learning (Israel, Eng, Schulz, & Parker, 2005; Minkler & Wallerstein, 2010; also see Chapter Fifteen). Both PRECEDE-PROCEED and Intervention Mapping can be used with a wide range of theories for describing health problems and devising solutions.

The PRECEDE-PROCEED Model

The PRECEDE-PROCEED Model, which has been a cornerstone of health promotion practice for more than three decades, can help to guide the process of designing, implementing, and evaluating health behavior change programs (Green et al., 1980; Green & Kreuter, 2005). PRECEDE-PROCEED can be thought of as a *road map*, and behavior change theories as the specific *directions* to a destination. The road map presents all the possible avenues, while the theory suggests certain avenues to follow. The map's main purpose is to provide a structure for *applying* theories and concepts systematically in the planning and evaluating of health behavior change programs (Gielen et al., 2008).

A population-based planning framework that is ecological in its perspective, the PRECEDE-PROCEED Model (Green & Kreuter, 1991, 1999, 2005) has been used for planning hundreds of programs (Aboumatar et al., 2012; Buta et al., 2011; Cole & Horacek, 2009; Hazavei, Sabzmakan, Hasanzadeh, Rabiei, & Roohafza, 2012; Li et al., 2009). When developed in the 1970s, PRECEDE began to influence the health education field toward an outcome-focused approach to planning. By this we mean that rather than having people jumping into applying solutions to health problems, PRECEDE-PROCEED promotes in-depth understanding of the community or other population or target audience and its needs, as well as both the proximal determinants of health and quality-of-life problems and the more distant contextual causes. Its use leads to planning interventions that are specifically targeted to these desired outcomes and causes and provides a structure for systematically applying theories and concepts.

The first three phases of PRECEDE help planners to develop a logic model (theory) of the problem (Figure 19.1). They guide an analysis of the causes of health problems at multiple ecological levels and help planners focus on determinants of health-related behavior and environment (Gómez, Seoane, Varela-Centelles, Diz, & Takkouche, 2009; Peacock, Pogrel, & Schmidt, 2008). The socioecological model, which focuses on the interrelationships among individuals with their biological, psychological, and behavioral characteristics and their

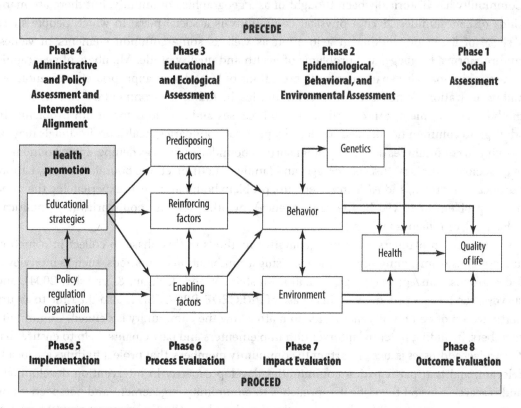

Figure 19.1   PRECEDE-PROCEED Planning Model

environments, drives the perspective underlying the importance of including the environment in a logic model of the problem (Bronfenbrenner, 1979; Kok, Gottlieb, Commers, & Smerecnik, 2008; also see Chapter Three).

These ecological levels can influence both individual behavior and environments. In an example of children's consumption of sugar-sweetened beverages, parents' provision of sodas to their child would be in the interpersonal level of the ecological model; lack of policy concerning sodas in school vending machines would be at the organizational level; social norms for soda consumption, at the community level; and laws restricting sales of oversized sodas at food stores and restaurants, at the societal level. In another example, in a hospital-based study to reduce health care–associated infections, inadequate hand hygiene by health care providers (individual level) and lack of enforcement of hand hygiene guidelines and contaminated environmental surfaces and equipment (organizational level) were all found to contribute to the transmission of multidrug-resistant organisms (Aboumatar et al., 2012). Similarly, in a study of work-related musculoskeletal disorders among supermarket cashiers, prolonged standing at a workstation, lack of managerial compliance to federal ergonomic guidelines, and poor architectural design of the workstation all contributed to work-related health problems (Wasilewski, Mateo, & Sidorovsky, 2007).

In the PRECEDE-PROCEED Model Phase 1—social assessment, participatory planning, and situation analysis—planners try to understand the community in which they are working. Community has historically been thought of as a geographic community, but there are many kinds of communities. Even a physical community is a social place in which people share a sense of living or working in a location as well as some common elements of values, culture, norms, language, and problems of health and quality of life. Members of geographic communities may also share common perceptions of boundaries, appropriate representation, and prioritizations of needs. Further, communities, including environmental elements such as the built environment, can contribute to both causes and solutions for health problems. In addition to communities defined partially by physical boundaries, health professionals may be working in communities defined by other sorts of boundaries, such as demographic boundaries (e.g., socioeconomic status, gender, age, and family structure), ethnic boundaries (e.g., Latino, European American, and African American), problem boundaries (e.g., experiencing the same health problem or served by the same agency), or other identity boundaries (e.g., political, behavioral, or religious identity).

Intervention planners often use qualitative methods in this phase to collect information and opinions from community members. Using a combination of methods, such as interviews, focus groups, concept mapping (Trochim, Milstein, Wood, Jackson, & Pressler, 2004), and surveys, can be very productive. This phase of PRECEDE-PROCEED is also the time to assure participation of community members, no matter how the community is defined. Community members, including potential intervention implementers and participants, help to ensure that the project addresses issues important to community members, that project findings are locally relevant, and that participating communities develop capacity in intervention development and research. Several theoretical approaches to community engagement and perspectives on community structure and needs can be helpful at this phase (Bartholomew et al., 2011). A few examples of theories that can help with perspectives on communities and needs are systems theories (Goodson, 2009; National Cancer Institute, 2007), theories regarding social networks (Heaney & Israel, 2008), and constructs of social capital and community capacity (Green & Kreuter, 2005; Wendel et al., 2009). Other theories, for example, stakeholder theories (Foster-Fishman, Nowell, & Yang, 2007) and coalition theories (Butterfoss, Kegler, & Francisco, 2008) can give guidance for community engagement. Table 19.1 shows examples of theories often used in the various phases of PRECEDE-PROCEED.

In Phase 2, epidemiological assessment, the planner begins building a logic model of the health problem from right to left, usually starting with descriptions of health problems and

Table 19.1   PRECEDE-PROCEED Model as a Structure for Using Theories and Constructs

Examples of Theories and Principles, by Ecological Level	Phase 1: Social Assessment	Phase 2: Epidemiological, Behavioral, and Environmental Assessment	Phase 3: Educational and Ecological Assessment	Phase 4: Administrative and Policy Assessment and Intervention Alignment
Community level				
Participation and relevance: e.g., stakeholder theory, theories of power, coalition theories	X	X	X	X
Community assessment: e.g., systems theories, social capital, and community capacity	X	X	X	X
Intervention: e.g., community organization, community mobilization, organizational change, Diffusion of Innovations		X		X
Interpersonal level				
Social Cognitive Theory		X	X	X
Adult learning		X	X	
Interpersonal communication			X	
Social networks and social support			X	
Individual level				
Social Cognitive Theory		X	X	
Theories of self-regulation		X	X	
Goal setting and planning			X	
Health Belief Model			X	
Transtheoretical Model of behavior change (Stages of Change)			X	
Theory of Reasoned Action				
Theory of Planned Behavior				
Information processing				

related quality of life in the community. When completed, the model is read from left to right as a causal model of the health and quality-of-life problems. The epidemiological analysis includes health problems and their related quality-of-life impact, behavioral causes of the health problems, and environmental causes of the health problem or risk behavior. Reducing or eliminating health problems should be the intention of a health education or promotion intervention. For example, if premature mortality and morbidity from health care–associated infections are the health problem, loss of productive years and increased health care costs begin to define the quality-of-life issues for the individual and for society. The behavioral analysis typically includes what the at-risk group does that increases risk of experiencing the health problem. In the case of secondary and tertiary prevention, the analysis investigates what individuals do that increases the risk of disability or death from a health problem they already have. For example, lack of adherence to prescribed dietary, physical activity, and medication guidelines is a major barrier to the proper treatment of diabetes and can lead not only to the disease but also to increased disease burden (morbidity or mortality).

The environmental analysis includes conditions in the social, physical, and biological environments that influence the health problem directly or through its behavioral causes. In most analyses of health problems, the environment plays a significant and modifiable role in causing the problem, either directly, such as through exposure to lead-based paint or lead-contaminated dust in lead poisoning, or indirectly through behavior, such as lack of smoking bans in the workplace.

Several theories are useful when describing behavior and environment. For example, Social Cognitive Theory (see Chapter Nine) focuses on the reciprocal interaction of behavior and environment. Also, some theories are important for specifying the details of the behavior targeted for change. For example, Self-Regulation Theory (Vohs & Baumeister, 2011), theories of goal setting and planning (Gollwitzer & Sheeran, 2006), and the Transtheoretical Model of behavior change (Stages of Change) (Prochaska, 2013; see Chapter Seven) are theories that can help with understanding the steps people engage in to change behavior (see Table 19.1).

At this phase, planners can usually begin to describe the problems in the community and their causes with existing data sources (e.g., local, state, and national health surveys; disease registries; and medical claims). Data from these sources are generally available electronically, and many sources provide extensive resources for both access and interpretation (e.g., the National Health Information Center, at www.health.gov/nhic; the National Library of Medicine databases and electronic resources, at www.nlm.nih.gov/databases; and the National Center for Health Statistics, at www.cdc.gov/nchs).

In Phase 3, ecological and educational assessment, health professionals explore the factors that produce the behavioral and environmental conditions described in Phase 2. Here, the question is, what antecedent and reinforcing factors encourage the risk behaviors or environmental conditions that cause or contribute to the health problem? Green and Kreuter (2005) describe these factors as *predisposing factors*, "a person or population's knowledge, attitudes, beliefs, values, and perceptions that facilitate or hinder motivation for change" (p. 14); *reinforcing factors*, "the rewards received and the feedback the learner receives from others following adoption of a behavior" (p. 15); and *enabling factors*, "those skills, resources, or barriers that can help or hinder the desired behavioral changes as well as environmental changes" (p. 15). For example, in their hospital-based study to reduce health care–associated infections, Aboumatar et al. (2012) found that antecedent factors such as lack of knowledge and skeptical attitudes about the risk of multidrug-resistant organisms contributed to poor compliance, and Wasilewski et al. (2007) found that employees did not feel susceptible to or believe in the seriousness of musculoskeletal disorders (determinants from the Health Belief Model) (see Chapter Five), and that this was coupled with lack of managerial support and ergonomic problems in the workplace.

Describing the determinants of behavior is a process that can benefit significantly from "thinking with theory." Constructs from the Health Belief Model (perceived severity and susceptibility, barriers and benefits, cues to action, and self-efficacy) (Chapter Five), the Theory of Planned Behavior (attitudes, subjective norms, intention, and perceived behavioral control) (Chapter Six), and Social Cognitive Theory (self-efficacy, behavioral capability, outcome expectations, reinforcement, observational learning, and reciprocal determinism) (Chapter Nine) all address determinants of behavior. These determinants of behavior apply both to the at-risk group and to those agents responsible for environmental conditions (see Table 19.1).

The original PRECEDE model had a separate category of nonbehavioral factors, such as the natural history of disease (Green et al., 1980). These were nonmodifiable factors that nevertheless should be considered in a needs assessment because they may influence factors that can be changed. They also may provide the social or biological context for behaviors of an at-risk group or of those who influence environmental conditions. In the current PRECEDE-PROCEED model, genetics is in the model as a factor that is not yet (often) modifiable but may be quite important in understanding the health problem and various affected groups (Green & Kreuter, 2005).

In Phase 4, administrative and policy assessment and intervention alignment, the question is, what program components and interventions are needed to effect the changes specified in the previous phases? Does this program have the organizational, policy, and administrative capability and resources to develop and implement the program? Green and Kreuter (2005) offer recommendations from the extensive program development literature for "intervention matching, mapping, pooling and patching" (p. 197) at this stage of planning. Specifically, building a comprehensive program requires (1) *matching* the ecological levels to broad program components; (2) *mapping* specific interventions based on theory and prior research and practice to specific predisposing, enabling, and reinforcing factors; (3) *pooling* prior interventions and community-preferred interventions that might have less evidence to support them; and if necessary, (4) *patching* those interventions to fill gaps in the evidence-based best practices. In the previous phase, theories were mostly helpful to understand why people engage in risky behaviors, why environmental risk factors exist, and why change might occur. In this phase, intervention planners will use theory to apply change methods. A key challenge of creating an intervention that produces change is using theory to target the correct determinants of behavior and environment in the previous phase. At Phase 4, the challenge is to continue to use theory to choose the powerful methods to promote the desired change within an organizational and/or political context. Theories of organizational change (Butterfoss, Kegler, & Francisco, 2008) may be especially useful at this stage of the planning process.

Moving into final PROCEED phases, the planner prepares for implementation (Phase 5) by developing the necessary training, materials, and resources to support program delivery. Data collected in the first four phases of PRECEDE-PROCEED are used to guide specific inservice content or skills development so that program facilitators have the capacity and resources to implement the proposed program. In Phases 6 to 8, the planner develops data collection plans to conduct process, impact, and outcome evaluations, respectively (Green & Kreuter, 2005). *Process evaluation* determines the extent to which the program was implemented according to protocol. *Impact evaluation* assesses change in predisposing, reinforcing, and enabling factors, as well as in the behavioral and environmental factors. Finally, *outcome evaluation* determines the effect of the program on health and quality-of-life indicators. Typically, the measurable objectives that are written in each phase of PRECEDE-PROCEED serve as milestones against which accomplishments are evaluated.

Intervention Mapping

PRECEDE-PROCEED is the foundation for the Intervention Mapping approach to health promotion planning. Intervention Mapping builds on the logic model of the problem developed in PRECEDE and expands on PROCEED to add detail to the process of intervention development. Intervention Mapping focuses on defining determinants of behavioral and environmental change and matching theory-based change methods to the determinants (Bartholomew, Parcel, & Kok, 1998). Intervention Mapping has guided the development of health promotion programs for many different health problems. Recent examples include antiretroviral treatment adherence (de Bruin, Hospers, de Borne, Kok, & Prins, 2005), physical activity (Brug, Oenema, & Ferreira, 2005), smoking (Dalum, Schaalma, & Kok, 2012), obesity (Lloyd, Logan, Greaves, & Wyatt, 2011), cancer screening (Byrd et al., 2012), chronic disease self-management (Detaille, van der Gulden, Engels, Heerkens, & van Dijk, 2010), HIV prevention (Munir, Kalawsky, Wallis, & Donaldson-Feilder, 2013), vaccination (Kok et al., 2011), and sexual and relationship health (Mkumbo et al., 2009; Newby, Bayley, & Wallace, 2011). Others have explicitly used Intervention Mapping to guide community-based participatory research (Belansky, Cutforth, Chavez, Waters, & Bartlett-Horch, 2011); to better understand what specific parts of interventions produce change, that is, the "active ingredients" (Brendryen, Kraft, & Schaalma, 2010; Kok & Mesters, 2011); and to adapt and implement evidence-based interventions (Tortolero et al., 2010).

Each step of Intervention Mapping comprises several tasks (Figure 19.2). The completion of the tasks in each step leads to products that inform the subsequent step, and the completion of all steps creates a blueprint, or *map*, for designing, implementing, and evaluating an intervention. Even though the depiction of Intervention Mapping is one of sequential, cumulative steps, the process is iterative rather than strictly linear.

In Step 1 (logic model [theory] of the problem), the developers of Intervention Mapping recommend that the first step of program planning be to use PRECEDE to conduct a

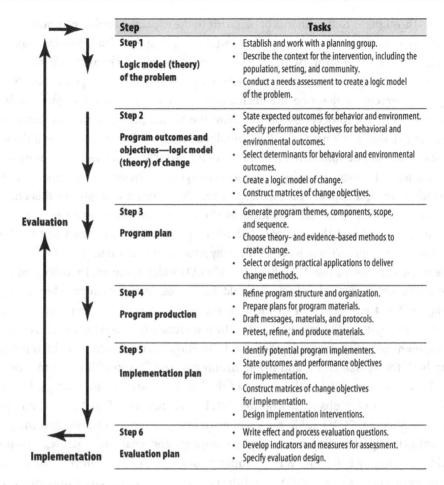

Step	Tasks
Step 1 **Logic model (theory) of the problem**	• Establish and work with a planning group. • Describe the context for the intervention, including the population, setting, and community. • Conduct a needs assessment to create a logic model of the problem.
Step 2 **Program outcomes and objectives—logic model (theory) of change**	• State expected outcomes for behavior and environment. • Specify performance objectives for behavioral and environmental outcomes. • Select determinants for behavioral and environmental outcomes. • Create a logic model of change. • Construct matrices of change objectives.
Step 3 **Program plan**	• Generate program themes, components, scope, and sequence. • Choose theory- and evidence-based methods to create change. • Select or design practical applications to deliver change methods.
Step 4 **Program production**	• Refine program structure and organization. • Prepare plans for program materials. • Draft messages, materials, and protocols. • Pretest, refine, and produce materials.
Step 5 **Implementation plan**	• Identify potential program implementers. • State outcomes and performance objectives for implementation. • Construct matrices of change objectives for implementation. • Design implementation interventions.
Step 6 **Evaluation plan**	• Write effect and process evaluation questions. • Develop indicators and measures for assessment. • Specify evaluation design.

Evaluation

Implementation

Figure 19.2   Intervention Mapping Overview
Source: Adapted from Bartholomew et al., 2011.

needs assessment, which will result in the development of a logic model of the problem, as shown in Figure 19.1 and described in Figure 19.2 (Bartholomew et al., 2011). The developers of Intervention Mapping use a modified version of PRECEDE in this step: they combine predisposing and reinforcing factors (Figure 19.1) into one category of personal determinants—those cognitive and emotional factors that lead to either the behavior of the risk group or the behaviors of persons in the environment. Enabling factors (those environmental conditions that make the behavior of the at-risk group either easier or more difficult) are included in the environment box of the logic model. The same theories mentioned earlier in discussing the development of the PRECEDE model are relevant in Step 1 of Intervention Mapping.

In Step 2 of Intervention Mapping (program outcomes and objectives—the logic model [theory] of change), health professionals use theory and evidence to describe the targets of change for the intervention. These are hypothesized causal pathways from the planned intervention through the determinants of behavior to the expected health-promoting behaviors of both the at-risk group and the environmental change agents (those individuals who are able to create change in environmental factors) and ultimately to changes in health outcomes. This step builds directly on the previous step. Once the health care professionals who are planning the intervention describe the health problem and its causes, the question becomes, "What needs to change to decrease or eliminate the health problem and the behavioral and environmental risks?" Looking at the logic model of the problem, planners will decide, first, which behavioral and environmental factors are most strongly associated with improvement in health outcomes (relevance) and which are most changeable. For example, in the middle school sexual health education application called *It's Your Game*, described later in this chapter, the planners targeted delayed sexual initiation as the main behavioral outcome for the at-risk group. They then analyzed this complex behavior to detail the components of the behavior, termed *performance objectives* (e.g., to avoid risky situations that might lead to sex).

As described earlier for the PRECEDE-PROCEED model, there are theories that are useful for considering what specific behavior should be the target for change whether a planner is thinking of the at-risk group or of those in the environment who can create change. For example, Social Cognitive Theory emphasizes the interaction between person and environment and is congruent with the emphasis of this Intervention Mapping step on the importance of change in both the at-risk group and the environment (see Chapter Nine). Some theories are particularly helpful in specifying the details of the behavior targeted for change. For example, Self-Regulation Theory (Vohs & Baumeister, 2011) and theories of goal setting and planning (Gollwitzer & Sheeran, 2006) guide the planner to break behavior change into the processes of self-monitoring, goal setting, planning, performing, and evaluating strategies—processes that could apply to any behavior. When thinking about the behavior of persons or groups in the environment, such as organizations, political entities, or communities, theories at a higher ecological level can be helpful. These include theories that address social support and social networks (Uchino, 2009; also see Chapter Ten), stage of organizational change (Butterfoss et al., 2008), and community organization (Minkler & Wallerstein, 2004; also see Chapter Fifteen) (see Figure 19.3).

The next task in this step is to use theory, empirical evidence, and new data to understand the hypothesized determinants of the behavior changes for the at-risk group and for the environmental agents. These determinants answer the question of *why* the person at risk or the environmental agent would make a behavior change. We label these as hypothesized because, even though interventions are based on causal assumptions ("if we do *x*, *y* will happen"), the factors designated as possible determinants of behavior are often derived from a mix of research types and theories. Planners may have evidence from cross-sectional and longitudinal surveys and experiments as well as from perceptions of their communities and the planning team. They should be skeptical about the causal direction based on cross-sectional studies where behavior and assumed determinants are measured at the same time. It could be possible that the causal direction is reversed or even multidirectional. For example, does depression lead to obesity, or obesity to depression? This question is impossible to answer without longitudinal research.

At-Risk Group

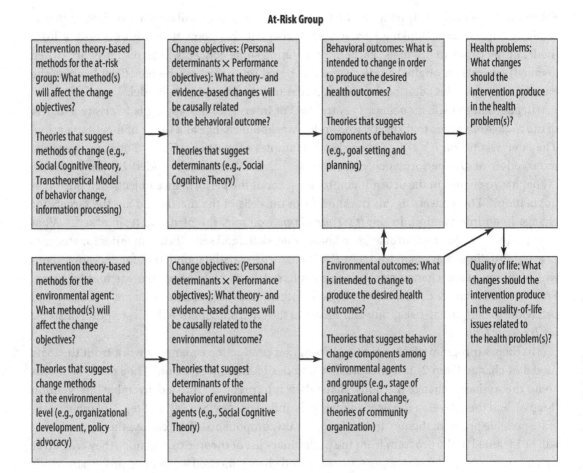

Figure 19.3   Logic Model (Theory) of Change

Planners will also use theory to posit factors that may influence the behaviors of interest. In the applied work of thinking about the determinants of behavior, there is no mandate to specify a *single* theory, and a decision about which theories and/or constructs to include begins with a review of the previous research on factors that have been shown to be related to the behavior of interest. Some of the studies found will be theory-based, and others will be atheoretical. As described earlier regarding the PRECEDE model, several theories are routinely used in health promotion to examine proposed determinants of behavior (e.g., Social Cognitive Theory, the Theory of Planned Behavior/Theory of Reasoned Action, and the Health Belief Model). For example, when Bartholomew and Mullen (2011) conducted a brief review of why dentists did or did not conduct oral cancer screening, they found evidence for the influence of Social Cognitive Theory constructs of skills, knowledge of what to do and how to do it, and self-efficacy. Furthermore, they found that some patient and provider beliefs can be defined by the Social Cognitive Theory construct of outcome expectations—"if I do *x*, *y* will happen."

For example, "If I talk to my patients about an oral cancer exam, I will increase their awareness." So, in reality, we are "thinking harder with theory" at this point than we were in the logic model of the problem discussed earlier. Interpreting some concepts in terms of theory (when justified) even when original studies were not based on theory can be beneficial because the entire theory provides additional constructs that may be added to the model.

In addition to logic modeling, a central tool of Intervention Mapping is to create a matrix of the *change objectives* that specify *who* and *what* should change as a result of the intervention. The later section on *It's Your Game* shows examples of matrices. Change objectives are the intersection of the performance objectives and the determinants guided by the question, "What has to change in the determinant to bring about the performance objective in the target population?" The answers to this question form the cells of the matrix and are the targets for change in an intervention. In the *It's Your Game* example, the planning team asked, "What does the intervention have to change in knowledge, skills, and self-efficacy in order for students to avoid situations that might lead to sex?" The matrices are the foundation for decisions about which theory-based change methods (also referred to as *techniques*; see Michie, Johnston, Francis, Hardeman, & Eccles, 2008) will likely influence change in determinants of the targeted behaviors in both the at-risk group and agents in the environment (see the description of Step 2 for *It's Your Game*).

In Step 3 (program plan) and Step 4 (program production), planners work from the logic model of change (Step 2) to conceptualize and design the intervention. They make decisions about theory-based change methods, shape their interpretation into a deliverable intervention (Step 3), and then develop the needed materials and messages (Step 4). In Step 3, planners generate possible program themes and major program components. They choose the methods that will be included in the program from the preliminary list of theoretical methods they created as a part of the logic model of change. A theory-based change method is a defined process by which theories postulate, and empiric research provides evidence for, the ways in which interventions can influence change in the determinants of behavior of individuals, groups, or social structures. Determinants of behavior almost always include many factors other than knowledge and awareness; therefore methods must include processes to influence factors other than simple knowledge. Theory-based methods are likely to form a major foundation for an intervention's *active ingredients*, because they have been matched directly to the change objectives. Table 19.2 lists a sampling of theory-based change methods and gives definitions for them.

For example, the planners guiding the *It's Your Game* project (Tortolero et al., 2010) considered many different methods that could influence a change objective, but they ultimately chose a limited number of methods that could be feasibly implemented in the program environment. As planners figure out how to deliver a program and write its content, they must consider parameters for the use of each method. Parameters are theory or research-derived "instructions" for effective use of a method. For example, a role model must be credible to the observer, must demonstrate clearly the skill to be learned, and must be positively reinforced (Bandura, 1986).

A planning group must also be very meticulous at this stage, because links between change methods and the determinants of behavior and environment can easily be lost in this crucial

Table 19.2   Samples of Theory-Based Change Methods

Theoretical Method (Theory)	Definition
Determinant: skills and self-efficacy	
Modeling (Social Cognitive Theory)	Enabling someone to observe an appropriate model performing the behavior and being reinforced
Reward and reinforcement (Social Cognitive Theory)	Offering contingent valued consequences (only if the behavior is performed)
Guided practice, skills training, and feedback (Social Cognitive Theory; learning theory, goal setting)	Prompting individuals to rehearse and repeat the behavior various times, discuss the experience, and provide feedback
Determinant: knowledge	
Imagery (theories of information processing)	Providing familiar physical or verbal images as analogies to a less familiar process
Advance organizers (theories of information processing)	Presenting an overview of the material that enables a learner to activate relevant schemas so that new material can be associated
Elaboration (theories of information processing, Elaboration Likelihood Model)	Stimulating the learner to add meaning to the information that is processed
Determinant: attitudes	
Repeated exposure (theories of learning)	Making a stimulus or message repeatedly accessible to an individual
Self-reevaluation (Transtheoretical Model)	Encouraging combining both cognitive and affective assessments of one's self-image with and without an unhealthy behavior
Environmental reevaluation (Transtheoretical Model)	Encouraging realizing the negative impact of the unhealthy behavior and the positive impact of the healthful behavior
Shifting perspective (theories of stigma and discrimination)	Encouraging taking the perspective of the other
Determinant: social influence and perceived social norms	
Provide opportunities for social comparison (Social Comparison Theory)	Facilitating observation of nonexpert others in order to evaluate one's own opinions and performance abilities
Information about others' approval (Theory of Planned Behavior/Theory of Reasoned Action)	Providing information about what others think about the person's behavior and whether others will approve or disapprove of any proposed behavior change

step. One reason for this planning hazard is that the theories used to understand or predict a behavior may offer little or no guidance on how to change determinants related to the behavior. Other theories may be needed for this purpose. For example, the Health Belief Model suggests the importance of perceived susceptibility in predicting action, but offers little guidance about how to change this belief (see Chapter Five). Social Cognitive Theory, in contrast, offers specific methods for affecting change in determinants (see Chapter Nine).

These chosen theory-derived change methods are then matched with practical delivery strategies and woven into a coherent program with a defined scope and sequence. The final delivered intervention will often be a multicomponent and possibly multilevel program targeting change in both at-risk groups and environmental agents. Each part of the program may require materials and messages. One challenge of Intervention Mapping Step 4 is translation: optimizing the odds of getting the materials and messages "right" in order to deliver the methods and practical applications as effectively as possible so that the change objectives can be accomplished.

In Step 5 (implementation plan), planners have another opportunity to use theory and evidence systematically in program development and implementation. Potentially effective health promotion programs will have no impact if they are not implemented and will not reach as far as desired in the populations for which they are intended if they are not sustained or widely disseminated (Glasgow, Klesges, Dzewaltowski, Estabrooks, & Vogt, 2006). The developers of Intervention Mapping suggest that without a planned dissemination intervention to ensure appropriate adoption, implementation, maintenance, and sustainability, a health promotion program is likely to be less widely used than it could have been, or used with less fidelity (also see Chapter Sixteen). For new programs, demonstration projects, and research projects, the focus of Step 5 is on planning for program use in initial testing of the program's efficacy or effectiveness. If the program is shown to be effective, then its ultimate degree of impact on public health will depend on populations' degree of exposure to the program, and developers can use Step 5 to plan for larger program dissemination.

In this step, planners repeat the processes of considering needs, performance objectives, and determinants—but this time for the program adopters, implementers, and maintainers. Working with potential adopters and implementers as core members of the planning group from the beginning of a project, in addition to compiling matrices of change objectives in order to fully understand the reasons that they may implement a program, can form the foundation for developing program components that directly affect implementation.

In Step 6 (evaluation plan), planners propose process and outcome evaluation methods. The evaluation plan is based on the products from the previous Intervention Mapping steps. A wealth of literature is available from which to learn the basics of program evaluation (Patton, 2008; Rossi et al., 2004; Wholey, Hatry, & Newcomer, 2010). Thinking about the evaluation is a parallel process with program planning, and should begin along with the work on the needs assessment and logic model of the problem. Most evaluation texts (see Rossi et al., 2004; Wholey et al., 2010) include program planning or understanding the program as the first part of the evaluation process. They ask questions about the program's logic and design to determine evaluability. For example: Is there a need for the program? Have the right target groups been identified? Do stakeholders agree on the program objectives? Is the program theory, that is, the logic model of change, flawed? Have appropriate delivery channels been selected? Such questions are suggested to avoid wasting resources on programs with insufficient planning. Programs that have been developed using a systematic framework such as Intervention Mapping are likely to perform well in this initial step of evaluation. The logic of the intended program effects will be transparent.

Once the logic of the program is understood, evaluations determine whether the intervention was successful in meeting program goals and objectives (effects or outcomes evaluation), and why the intervention was or was not successful (process evaluation). Using the output from each Intervention Mapping step, planners determine evaluation questions, indicators and measures, and an appropriate research design to ensure that findings can be appropriately attributed to the program under consideration.

The general focus of evaluation questions for each Intervention Mapping step is shown in the following list:

Step 1: Did the program have an effect on health or quality-of-life factors?

Step 2: Did the program have an effect on behavioral and environmental change as specified in the program plan? (Measurement of this change should follow the performance objectives.) Did the program affect the determinants of behavior or environmental conditions? (Measurement of this change should follow the change objectives [on the matrices], organized by determinant.)

Step 3: Were the theory-based change methods included in the program appropriate to influence change? Were the theory-based change methods and practical applications implemented as intended in the program design and according to the theoretical guidance for their use?

Step 4: Were the program components acceptable to the target population?

Step 5: Was the program delivered as intended (with fidelity)? What was the extent of the program's reach to the intended populations?

Applying the PRECEDE-PROCEED Model and Intervention Mapping

The following applications illustrate how researchers have used the PRECEDE-PROCEED Model and Intervention Mapping, respectively, as theory- and evidence-based planning models to develop, implement, and evaluate two distinct health promotion interventions.

Application 1: A Youth Mental Health Community Awareness Campaign

The Compass Strategy program is an example of an application of the PRECEDE-PROCEED model to develop, implement, and evaluate a successful youth mental health community awareness campaign in Melbourne, Australia. Details of the development process and results from a quasi-experimental trial have been reported elsewhere (Wright, McGorry, Harris, Jorm, & Pennell, 2006).

Findings from a population assessment with youth, focus groups with youth affected by mental health disorders and their parents, and consultations with service providers informed the needs assessment and intervention development (Wright et al., 2006). A project development group comprising representatives from key stakeholder groups, including mental health service providers, general practitioners, and local, state, and Commonwealth government departments, reviewed these data and provided ongoing consultation during the implementation and evaluation phases.

Social and Epidemiological Assessment

Most mental disorders typically first present during adolescence and young adulthood, and they are often characterized by comorbidity (Kessler, Berglund, Demler, Jin, & Walters, 2005). These specific disorders and this age group were considered an important target for improving mental health, as early detection and treatment at the time of first onset have been found to improve long-term outcomes (Kupfer, Frank, & Perel, 1989) and reduce the risk of future illness episodes (Kroll, Harrington, Jayson, Fraser, & Gowers, 1996). The project team found that over a quarter (26%) of Australian youth aged sixteen to twenty-four report having a mental health disorder (Australian Bureau of Statistics, 2008). Related quality-of-life issues include school failure, poor social and family functioning, and high rates of enduring disability (McGorry, 2010). In 2009, the financial cost of mental illness among Australian youth aged twelve to twenty-five was AU$10.6 billion; the value of lost well-being (disability and premature death) was a further AU$20.5 billion (Access Economics, 2009). The team set objectives for increasing rates of early detection and treatment for mental health disorders to lead to better health and quality-of-life outcomes.

Previous studies had indicated that recognition of depression, and especially psychosis, was limited, although such recognition is an essential step for effective help seeking (Wright et al., 2005). Help seeking at the earliest possible stage is essential for the early receipt of treatment. However, rates of help seeking were also low, particularly in relation to mood disorders. Thus, based on the literature and focus group findings, the most important and changeable behavioral factors for early detection and treatment were identified as (1) recognition of the problem, (2) seeking help for the problem, (3) delivery of appropriate treatment, and (4) treatment compliance. Given that other agencies were already targeting treatment delivery and compliance, the project development group decided to focus on recognition and help seeking behavior as key behavioral targets for youth.

In the environmental assessment, the project development group considered social and physical factors that might influence the health outcome directly or indirectly via behavior. Physical factors, such as the accessibility and availability of mental health services, were already being addressed. Thus social support and social norms associated with youth's recognition of the problem and with help seeking for mental health services were identified as the key environmental target.

Educational and Ecological

Based on the literature and findings from the focus groups and youth population survey, the key predisposing factors that impeded recognition and help seeking were limited knowledge of signs, symptoms, and treatment availability; low perceived susceptibility and severity; perceived barriers to help seeking; and stigma related to mental health disorders. Reinforcing factors identified by youth and the literature indicated a role for social support from family, friends, teachers, counselors, and lay leaders. However, focus group data and input from service providers indicated that these social support individuals often faced the same barriers to action as the youth did; they had limited knowledge of signs and symptoms and a perception that youth had low susceptibility. Enabling factors included the need to increase the availability of mental health information and to enhance behavioral skills related to recognition and help seeking (Figure 19.4).

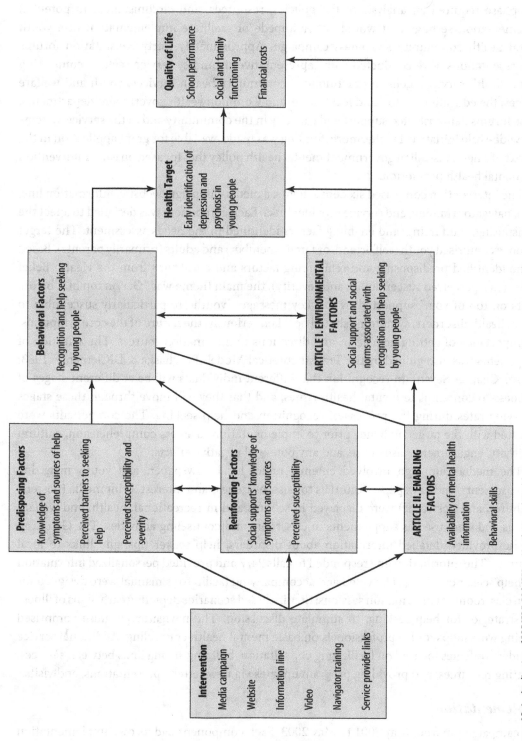

Figure 19.4 Application of PRECEDE-PROCEED to Youth Mental Health Awareness

Source: Adapted from Wright et al., 2006.

The following text boxes appear within the figure:

Quality of Life
School performance
Social and family functioning
Financial costs

Health Target
Early identification of depression and psychosis in young people

Behavioral Factors
Recognition and help seeking by young people

ARTICLE I. ENVIRONMENTAL FACTORS
Social support and social norms associated with recognition and help seeking by young people

Predisposing Factors
Knowledge of symptoms and sources of help
Perceived barriers to seeking help
Perceived susceptibility and severity

Reinforcing Factors
Social supports' knowledge of symptoms and sources
Perceived susceptibility

ARTICLE II. ENABLING FACTORS
Availability of mental health information
Behavioral skills

Intervention
Media campaign
Website
Information line
Video
Navigator training
Service provider links

Administrative and Policy Assessment and Intervention Alignment

This phase required an analysis of the policies, resources, and circumstances in potential implementation settings that would either impede or facilitate implementation of a youth mental health community awareness campaign. Approximately thirty consultation forums and presentations were conducted with representatives from key service sectors, comprising mental health services, general practitioners, community health services, youth and welfare services, the education sector, and local, state, and Commonwealth government departments. These forums demonstrated support and capacity in the community and in the service systems for a wide-scale initiative. Furthermore, funding was made available for grant application in the context of a new Australian government mental health policy that focused on early intervention and mental health promotion.

The intervention comprised six components: a media campaign, website, information line, video, navigator training, and service provider links. Each component was designed to affect the predisposing, reinforcing, and enabling factors identified in the needs assessment. The target audience comprised youth (self, friend, or family member) and adults (primarily parents). Based on the identified predisposing and reinforcing factors and constructs from the Health Belief Model (e.g., perceived susceptibility and severity), the main theme was "Get on top of it before it gets on top of you," supported by five key messages: youth are particularly susceptible to mental health disorders, symptoms should be taken seriously, the nature of the core symptoms, the importance of getting help early, and directions to information sources. The selection of components was also guided by the Transtheoretical Model (Prochaska & DiClemente, 1983; also see Chapter Seven), in recognition that different individuals will be at different stages of readiness to contemplate mental health issues, and that they will move through these stages at varying rates during the process of recognition and help seeking. The components were pretested with the target audience prior to implementation to assess comprehension, cultural sensitivity, engagement, ease of use, and any potential negative effects.

The media campaign involved cinema, radio, local newspaper, and youth magazine advertisements, and newspaper editorials to raise awareness and interest. Print media (posters, brochures, and postcards) were displayed in schools and in recreational, health, and welfare settings and were used as supplements in classroom and counseling activities. The Getontop website provided detailed information about disorders, help seeker tips, and links to local resources. The information line responded to calls 24/7 and provided personalized information and help seeker coaching. The video and accompanying facilitator's manual were designed for use in classrooms or information sessions; they included scenarios depicting early signs of illness and strategies for help seeking, to stimulate discussion. The navigator program comprised training workshops for lay professionals on basic mental health counseling. Additional service provider strategies focused on facilitating consultation, building strong links between services, updating resources, and providing program updates via newsletters, presentations, and visits.

Implementation

The campaign ran from May 2001 to May 2003. Each component had its own implementation plan to ensure effective and coordinated delivery. The media campaign targeted high-impact periods, such as school holidays, to maximize exposure for youth and parents. Print media, the navigator program, and service provider strategies were delivered primarily during the school semester. Thus the campaign proceeded in waves of intensity with a varying number of components being implemented at any given time. This helped to ensure wide-scale coverage and reduced the risk of message burnout.

Process, Impact, and Outcome Evaluation

Process evaluation data were collected to document whether the campaign was being implemented as designed and to allow for real-time adjustments. Program reach and effectiveness were assessed by monitoring hits to the website and calls to the information line. Distribution rates were used to assess the number of media activities, print materials, and service provider materials distributed.

During the first fourteen months of the campaign, the website and information line averaged 465 visits and 28 calls per month, respectively; over 7,000 cinema and 195 radio advertisements were aired; twenty-one weeks of youth magazine advertisements and 15 newspaper advertisements (average circulation 20,000 per advertisement) were circulated; and 15,000 postcards, 600 posters, and 20,000 stickers were distributed to schools and/or health care services. The Strategy Compass newsletter was distributed to 532 services, and 157 service providers requested Compass materials.

Impact evaluation was conducted using a quasi-experimental design. A cross-sectional telephone survey was conducted before and fourteen months after the start of the campaign. Randomly selected samples of 600 youth aged twelve to twenty-five from the experimental region and 600 youth in the same age range from a comparison region were surveyed at each time point. Outcomes measured included the targeted behaviors (e.g., correct recognition of mental health disorder, and active help seeking) and the predisposing, reinforcing, and enabling factors (e.g., perceived barriers to help seeking, perceived likelihood of discrimination, and helpfulness ratings of professionals and medications), and exposure to mental health campaigns.

Among youth in the experimental regions, the campaign had a statistically significant, positive impact on self-identified depression, help seeking for depression in the previous year, correct estimate of the prevalence of mental health disorders, increased awareness of suicide risk, a reduction in perceived barriers to help seeking, and an increased awareness of mental health campaigns, compared to youth in the comparison region. For example, after the campaign, a greater percentage of youth in the experimental regions correctly estimated the prevalence of mental health issues compared to youth in the comparison region (24.7%, vs. 22.8%), and were more likely to perceive themselves to be at risk for suicide than the other youth were (20.4% vs. 17.8%).

Application 2: It's Your Game. . . Keep It Real

It's Your Game. . . Keep It Real is a sexual health education program for middle school students (Markham et al., 2012; Tortolero et al., 2010) that was developed using Intervention Mapping. School-based programs offer an efficient strategy to reach youth with the aim of reducing adolescent risky sexual behaviors that may lead to sexually transmitted infections (STIs), including the human immunodeficiency virus (HIV) and human papillomavirus (HPV), and to teen pregnancy. However, development and delivery of sexual health education programs at the middle school level present several challenges, including the heterogeneity of students' physical and social development, and community needs and sensitivities regarding sexual health education at this age. This example describes how program planners used the Intervention Mapping process to develop an innovative, theory-based sexual education program that addresses the diverse needs of middle school students.

The planning team engaged multiple community partners throughout program development, including members from local medical, religious, and community service organizations, school district personnel, parents, and teenagers. They used several community engagement methods to gain input: (1) formation of a community advisory board and a teen advisory board, (2) use of focus groups with parents and teenagers from the priority population, and (3) use of school district presentations and meetings. These methods helped to ensure program sensitivity to the needs of the priority population (see Chapter Fifteen).

Step 1: Logic Model (Theory) of the Problem

The population for the initial *It's Your Game* project comprised predominantly African American and Hispanic middle school students attending a large, urban school district in the south-central United States. All students attended middle schools with high participation in the free or reduced-price school lunch program, which is an indicator of low socioeconomic status.

Using the PRECEDE model to guide the needs assessment, the team used secondary data sources, empirical literature reviews, and community input to describe health problems and quality-of-life issues related to sexual risk behaviors that may begin in middle school. Minority youth are disproportionately affected both by teen births and STIs (Centers for Disease Control and Prevention [CDC], 2013; Hamilton & Ventura, 2012). Teen pregnancy is a major factor in dropping out of high school and welfare dependency and also in negative outcomes for children of teens (Hoffman, 2006; Shuger, 2012).

Examining behavioral factors, the team identified early sexual initiation as a risk factor for STIs and teen pregnancy. Nationally in 2011, 47 percent of high school students reported ever having sex; of these, 40 percent said they did not use a condom at last intercourse, 15 percent had had four or more partners, and 9 percent had experienced dating violence (CDC, Division of Adolescent and School Health, 2013). Other behaviors, such as dating older partners and low health care use, increase the risk of adverse health outcomes (Marin, Kirby, Hudes, Gomez, & Coyle, 2003). Environmental factors, such as low parental communication about sexual health and low parental monitoring and also state policies on minors' access to health care services (The Guttmacher Institute, 2013) also affect adolescent sexual behaviors. Finally, many psychosocial determinants, such as knowledge, self-efficacy, and outcome expectations, also influence adolescent behavior (Kirby, Lepore, & Ryan, 2005). These findings are evidence of the need for effective sexual education for those in the early years of adolescence.

Step 2: Program Outcomes and Objectives—Logic Model (Theory) of Change

Working from their logic model of the problem, the team developed a logic model of change and matrices of change objectives to guide the program's content and evaluation. Behavioral and environmental outcomes, descriptions of what middle school youth will do, and what environmental changes will occur as a result of the program are displayed in Table 19.3, along with the details of the specific behaviors students and parents would have to perform to achieve these outcomes (performance objectives).

The next task in developing the logic model of change is to use health and empirical research to identify why program participants would accomplish the performance objectives. The planning group for *It's Your Game* used Social Cognitive Theory (see Chapter Nine), a literature review, and data from the needs assessment to answer the question, "Why would a participant perform a particular behavior?" The team then developed a matrix of change objectives by asking, "What needs to change related to this determinant to influence this performance objective?" For example: "What needs to change about outcome expectations regarding sexual behavior to decide not to have sex?" Table 19.4 depicts a partial matrix for students and for parents. It displays all the relevant determinants but only three of the performance objectives and related change objectives.

Steps 3 and 4: Program Plan and Program Production

The *It's Your Game* team selected potential theory-based methods that had been shown to be effective for sex education and matched them to specific change objectives in the matrices (Coyle et al., 1996; Coyle, Kirby, Marin, Gómez, & Gregorich, 2004). These methods comprised information transfer, active learning, modeling, group discussion, persuasive communication, scenario-based risk information, skills training with guided practice, anticipated regret, and goal setting.

The team then translated these theory-based change methods into practical program components to be implemented via multiple communication channels and vehicles, including group-based classroom lessons, individual journaling and computer-based lessons tailored by gender and sexual experience, parent-child take-home activities, and parent newsletters. The planners wrote content (messages) appropriate for twenty-four fifty-minute lessons, with twelve lessons in seventh grade and twelve lessons in eighth grade. The computer activities included interactive skills-training exercises, peer role model videos, and real-world-style teen serials with online student feedback to reinforce and supplement activities in the group-based classroom lessons. Each grade level included three take-home activities to facilitate parent-child communication and a parent newsletter.

The seventh-grade curriculum was structured to begin with lessons on general decision making or life skills, founded on a self-regulatory, decision-making paradigm or theme: *select* (students select their personal rules or limits), *detect* (students recognize challenges to these rules), and *protect* (students avoid situations that challenge these rules and use refusal skills to protect these rules). These three steps would enable students to keep their game (their life) real (healthy), initially by setting rules for general risk behaviors (e.g., not using drugs

Table 19.3   Step 2: Behavioral Outcomes, Environmental Outcomes, and Performance Objectives for *It's Your Game. . . Keep It Real*

Outcomes	Associated Performance Objectives
Behavioral outcomes: students will. . .	
1. Choose not to have sex.	Decide to not have sex. Communicate personal limits regarding sex. Avoid situations that could lead to sex. Refuse to have sex.
2. Use condoms correctly and consistently if having sex.	Make the decision to use condoms. Buy or obtain a free condom. Carry condoms. Negotiate the use of a condom with every partner. Use a condom correctly. Maintain condom use with every partner every time you have sex.
3. Use effective method of contraception along with condoms if having sex.	Make decision to use birth control. Choose appropriate birth control method. Negotiate use of birth control method each time you engage in sex. Use chosen birth control method effectively and consistently.
4. [For students who have sex.] Get tested and counseled for HIV, STI, and pregnancy.	Make the decision to get tested. Make appointment to get tested by health care provider. Keep appointment to get tested. Obtain test results. Obtain and follow through with health care if necessary. Notify partner(s) of test results. Maintain testing behavior over time.
5. Have healthy relationships with their friends, girlfriends, or boyfriends.	Evaluate past, current, and potential relationships. Communicate expectations about healthy relationships. Avoid relationships with friends, boyfriends/girlfriends that are not healthy. Get out of relationships with friends, boyfriends/girlfriends that are not healthy.
Environmental outcomes: parents will. . .	
1. Communicate with child about sexual health topics.	Plan to discuss dating, healthy relationships, and sexual behaviors with child. Identify and create appropriate time and location to talk to child. Discuss advantages of abstinence. Discuss refusal skills. Discuss avoidance of risky situations. Discuss alternatives to having sex. Discuss use of condoms and other contraceptive methods. Listen to child's feelings and opinions calmly and nonjudgmentally. Answer child's questions or concerns. Maintain open channel of communication with child over time.
2. Monitor child's time, friendships, and dating activities.	Limit child's unsupervised time. Establish rules on how child spends time, friendships, and dating. Discuss rules with child. Ask child where he [or she] is going, with whom, and what they will be doing. Discuss with child and other parents about the potential exposure to risk at the location where the child will be. Obtain and update list of names and phone numbers of child's friends, boyfriends, and girlfriends. Review child's Internet and other media use. Evaluate if activity is appropriate. If activity is inappropriate, negotiate an alternative activity with child. Maintain monitoring behaviors over time.

Table 19.4   Partial Matrix for Behavioral Outcome 1: Student Chooses Not to Have Sex

Performance Objectives	Determinants				
	Knowledge	Skills	Self-Efficacy	Perceived Norms	Outcome Expectations
The middle school student will. . .					
1. Decide to not have sex	Define the different types of sex (anal, oral, and vaginal sex).	Demonstrate ability to make the decision to not have sex.	Express confidence in ability to make the decision to not have sex.	State that most middle school students do not have sex.	State that abstaining from sex will help in achieving life goals, self-respect, and respect for others.
2. Communicate personal limits regarding sex.	Describe what is a personal limit. List your personal limits regarding sex. List ways to communicate personal limits to friends/ boyfriend/ girlfriend.	Demonstrate ability to communicate to friends or boyfriend/girlfriend your personal limit to wait to have sex.	Express confidence in ability to communicate to friends or boyfriend/girlfriend your personal limit to wait to have sex.	State that other teens communicate their personal limits regarding sex to friends/ boyfriend/girlfriend.	State that communicating your personal limits will decrease risk of HIV/STI and pregnancy. State that telling personal limits will lead to better relationship with boyfriend/girlfriend.
3. Avoid situations that might lead to sex.	Identify signs (feeling pressure to do something, lack of adult supervision, alcohol and drugs) and situations (places, peers, times) that make it hard to say no.	Demonstrate ability to identify signs and situations that may make it hard to say no to sex. Demonstrate ability to avoid these situations.	Express confidence in ability to identify signs and situations that may make it hard to say no to sex. Express confidence in ability to avoid these situations.		State that avoiding a high-risk situation will help you to not have sex.

and not stealing); then the steps would be applied more specifically to sexual situations. The eighth-grade lessons continued to apply the paradigm to sexual situations, along with activities on healthy dating relationships and contraception and testing messages for all students.

Step 5: Implementation Plan

Program planners faced three main challenges regarding program adoption, implementation, and sustainability: (1) obtaining support at the school district and local school levels for program adoption, (2) identifying and training teachers for program delivery, and (3) facilitating the sustainability of *It's Your Game* within a school district. As in Step 2, they wrote behavioral outcomes and performance objectives for each challenge. They also identified relevant determinants, methods and practical applications, and delivery vehicles to facilitate program adoption, implementation, and sustainability. These steps, initially taken to understand how to promote robust implementation of the program for the evaluation trials, also provided the foundation for ongoing program dissemination once effectiveness was established. *It's Your Game. . . Keep*

It Real is now nationally recognized as an effective sexual health education program (U.S. Department of Health and Human Services, Office of Adolescent Health, 2013) and has been adopted by school districts across the United States, reaching over 33,000 middle school students. Much of the program's success may be attributed to the use of Intervention Mapping to systematically guide program development and dissemination.

Step 6: Evaluation Plan

It's Your Game was evaluated in two randomized controlled trials with urban middle school students (Markham et al., 2012; Tortolero et al., 2010). Each trial involved a cohort of predominantly African American and Hispanic students followed from seventh grade into ninth grade. In the first trial ($n = 907$), control group students experienced more statistically significant negative outcomes compared to students in the intervention group. They were 1.29 times more likely to initiate sex by the ninth grade, and students who were sexually active had had a higher frequency of vaginal sex in the past three months (adjusted relative risk $= 1.30$) compared to students who received *It's Your Game*. No other statistically significant outcomes were reported among the much smaller number of sexually active youth. Students who received *It's Your Game* had more positive changes in determinants of change. These included having more positive beliefs about abstinence, perceiving fewer of their friends as engaging in sex, having greater condom and HIV/STI knowledge and more positive condom norms, and reporting less exposure to risky situations (Tortolero et al., 2010). The second trial ($n = 627$) reported similar effects on behavior and its determinants as well as positive reductions in unprotected sex. Students who received *It's Your Game* were significantly less likely to engage in unprotected sex at last vaginal intercourse compared to students in the control group (Markham et al., 2012).

Summary

This chapter presented two models for developing theory-based health promotion interventions: the PRECEDE-PROCEED Model and Intervention Mapping. These frameworks are used extensively in health promotion planning, with PRECEDE coming into use in the late 1970s and Intervention Mapping in the late 1990s. Both frameworks take an ecological approach to planning, and provide guidance for the use of theory both to understand health problems and to plan interventions that influence the determinants of these problems. Both also start with the important assumption that a diagnostic process should be undertaken before program components are selected.

These models have been used to guide community-based work and are flexible enough to be useful tools for community-based participatory research (Belansky et al., 2011). Because they do not specify or restrict which theories and constructs should be used to understand problems and create solutions, they are appropriate for a wide range of health problems and have been used extensively to address health disparities and problems in underresourced communities worldwide (Mkumbo et al., 2009). These frameworks have also been applied to influence the detailed reporting of health promotion interventions (Bartholomew & Mullen, 2011), to understand theory-based change methods at the community level (Kok, Gottlieb, Panne, & Smerecnik, 2012), and to guide adaptation of evidence-based interventions in new settings (Bartholomew et al., 2011).

References

Aboumatar, H., Ristaino, P., Davis, R., Thompson, C. B., Maragakis, L., Cosgrove, S. M., & Perl, T. (2012). Infection prevention promotion program based on the PRECEDE model: Improving hand hygiene behaviors among healthcare personnel. *Infection Control and Hospital Epidemiology*, 33(2), 144–151.

Access Economics. (2009). *The economic impact of youth mental illness and the cost-effectiveness of early intervention*. Canberra: Access Economics.

Australian Bureau of Statistics. (2008). *National survey of mental health and wellbeing: Summary of results*. Canberra: Author.

Bandura, A. (1986). *Social foundations of thought and action: A social cognitive theory*. Englewood Cliffs, NJ: Prentice Hall.

Bartholomew, L. K., & Mullen, P. D. (2011). Five roles for using theory and evidence in the design and testing of behavior change interventions. *Journal of Public Health Dentistry*, 71(Suppl. 1), S20–S33.

Bartholomew, L. K., Parcel, G. S., & Kok, G. (1998). Intervention mapping: A process for developing theory- and evidence-based health education programs. *Health Education & Behavior*, 25(5), 545–563.

Bartholomew, L. K., Parcel, G. S., Kok, G., Gottlieb, N. H., & Fernández, M. E. (2011). *Planning health promotion programs: An intervention mapping approach* (3rd ed.). San Francisco: Jossey-Bass.

Belansky, E. S., Cutforth, N., Chavez, R. A., Waters, E., & Bartlett-Horch, K. (2011). An adapted version of intervention mapping (AIM) is a tool for conducting community-based participatory research. *Health Promotion Practice*, 12(3), 440–455.

Brendryen, H., Kraft, P., & Schaalma, H. (2010). Looking inside the black box: Using intervention mapping to describe the development of the automated smoking cessation intervention "Happy Ending." *Journal of Smoking Cessation*, 5(01), 29–56.

Bronfenbrenner, U. (1979). *The ecology of human development: Experiments by nature and design*. Cambridge, MA: Harvard University Press.

Brug, J., Oenema, A., & Ferreira, I. (2005). Theory, evidence and intervention mapping to improve behavior nutrition and physical activity interventions. *International Journal of Behavioral Nutrition and Physical Activity*, 2(1), 2.

Buta, B., Brewer, L., Hamlin, D. L., Palmer, M. W., Bowie, J., & Gielen, A. (2011). An innovative faith-based healthy eating program: From class assignment to real-world application of PRECEDE/PROCEED. *Health Promotion Practice*, 12(6), 867–875.

Butterfoss, F. D., Kegler, M. C., & Francisco, V. T. (2008). Mobilizing organizations for health promotion: Theories of organizational change. In K. Glanz, B. K. Rimer, & K. Viswanath (Eds.), *Health behavior and health education: Theory, research, and practice* (4th ed., pp. 335–362). San Francisco: Jossey-Bass.

Buunk, A. P., & Vugt, M. V. (2008). *Applying social psychology: From problems to solutions*. Thousand Oaks, CA: Sage.

Byrd, T. L., Wilson, K. M., Smith, J. L., Heckert, A., Orians, C. E., Vernon, S. W., & Fernández, M. E. (2012). Using intervention mapping as a participatory strategy: Development of a cervical cancer screening intervention for Hispanic women. *Health Education & Behavior, 39*(5), 603–611.

Centers for Disease Control and Prevention. (2013). *Diagnoses of HIV infection and population among young adults aged 20–24 years, by race/ethnicity, 2010—46 states.* Atlanta: Author. Retrieved from http://www.cdc.gov/hiv/pdf/statistics_surveillance_Adolescents.pdf

Centers for Disease Control and Prevention, Division of Adolescent and School Health. (2013). *High school Youth Risk Behavior Survey (YRBS), 2013.* Atlanta: Author. Retrieved from http://www.cdc.gov/healthyyouth/yrbs/overall.htm

Cole, R. E., & Horacek, T. (2009). Applying PRECEDE-PROCEED to develop an intuitive eating nondieting approach to weight management pilot program. *Journal of Nutrition Education and Behavior, 41*(2), 120–126.

Coyle, K., Kirby, D., Parcel, G., Basen-Engquist, K., Banspach, S., Rugg, D., & Weil, M. (1996). Safer choices: A multicomponent school-based HIV/STD and pregnancy prevention program for adolescents. *Journal of School Health, 66*(3), 89–94.

Coyle, K. K., Kirby, D. B., Marin, B. V., Gómez, C. A., & Gregorich, S. E. (2004). Draw the line/respect the line: A randomized trial of a middle school intervention to reduce sexual risk behaviors. *American Journal of Public Health, 94*(5), 843–851.

Dalum, P., Schaalma, H., & Kok, G. (2012). The development of an adolescent smoking cessation intervention—an intervention mapping approach to planning. *Health Education Research, 27*(1), 172–181.

de Bruin, M., Hospers, H., de Borne, H. W., Kok, G., & Prins, J. (2005). Theory- and evidence-based intervention to improve adherence to antiretroviral therapy among HIV-infected patients in the Netherlands: A pilot study. *AIDS Patient Care & STDs, 19*(6), 384–394.

Detaille, S. I., van der Gulden, J.W.J., Engels, J. A., Heerkens, Y. F., & van Dijk, F. J. (2010). Using intervention mapping (IM) to develop a self-management programme for employees with a chronic disease in the Netherlands. *BMC Public Health, 10*(1), 353.

Fishbein, M., Triandis, H. C., Kanfer, F. H., Becker, M., Middlestadt, S. E., & Eichler, A. (2001). *Factors influencing behavior and behavior change.* In A. Baum, T. A. Revenson, & J. E. Singer (Eds.), *Handbook of health psychology* (pp. 3–17). Mahwah, NJ: Erlbaum.

Foster-Fishman, P. G., Nowell, B., & Yang, H. (2007). Putting the system back into systems change: A framework for understanding and changing organizational and community systems. *American Journal of Community Psychology, 39*(3–4), 197–215.

Gielen, A. C., McDonald, E. M., Gary, T. L., & Bone, L. R. (2008). Using the PRECEDE-PROCEED model to apply health behavior theories. In K. Glanz, B. K. Rimer, & K. Viswanath (Eds.), *Health behavior and health education: Theory, research, and practice* (4th ed., pp. 402–433). San Francisco: Jossey-Bass.

Glanz, K., Rimer, B. K., & Viswanath, K. (Eds.). (2008). *Health behavior and health education: Theory, research, and practice* (4th ed.). San Francisco: Jossey-Bass.

Glasgow, R. E., Klesges, L. M., Dzewaltowski, D. A., Estabrooks, P. A., & Vogt, T. M. (2006). Evaluating the impact of health promotion programs: Using the RE-AIM framework to form summary measures for decision making involving complex issues. *Health Education Research, 21*(5), 688–694.

Gollwitzer, P. M., & Sheeran, P. (2006). Implementation intentions and goal achievement: A meta-analysis of effects and processes. In M. P. Zanna (Ed.), *Advances in experimental social psychology* (Vol. 38, pp. 69–119). San Diego: Academic Press.

Gómez, I., Seoane, J., Varela-Centelles, P., Diz, P., & Takkouche, B. (2009). Is diagnostic delay related to advanced-stage oral cancer? A meta-analysis. *European Journal of Oral Sciences, 117*(5), 541–546.

Goodson, P. (2009). *Theory in health promotion research and practice: Thinking outside the box.* Sudbury, MA: Jones & Bartlett.

Green, L. W., & Kreuter, M. W. (1991). *Health promotion planning: An educational and environmental approach.* Mountain View, CA: Mayfield.

Green, L. W., & Kreuter, M. W. (1999). *Health promotion planning: An educational and ecological approach* (3rd ed.). Mountain View, CA: Mayfield.

Green, L. W., & Kreuter, M. W. (2005). *Health program planning: An educational and ecological approach* (4th ed.). New York: McGraw-Hill.

Green, L. W., Kreuter, M. W., Deeds, S. G., & Partridge, K. B. (1980). *Health education planning: A diagnostic approach.* Palo Alto, CA: Mayfield.

The Guttmacher Institute. (2013). *State policies in brief: An overview of minors' consent law.* Retrieved from http://www.guttmacher.org/statecenter/spibs/spib_OMCL.pdf

Hamilton, B. E., & Ventura, S. J. (2012). *Birth rates for US teenagers reach historic lows for all age and ethnic groups* (Data Brief Number 89). Atlanta: US Department of Health and Human Services, Centers for Disease Control and Prevention, National Center for Health Statistics.

Hazavei, S.M.M., Sabzmakan, L., Hasanzadeh, A., Rabiei, K., & Roohafza, H. (2012). The effects of an educational program based on PRECEDE model on depression levels in patients with coronary artery bypass grafting. *ARYA Atherosclerosis, 8*(1), 36.

Heaney, C. A., & Israel, B. A., (2008). Social networks and social support. In K. Glanz, B. K. Rimer, & K. Viswanath (Eds.), *Health behavior and health education: Theory, research, and practice* (4th ed., pp. 189–210). San Francisco: Jossey-Bass.

Hoffman, S. D. (2006). *By the numbers: The public costs of teen childbearing.* Washington, DC: National Campaign to Prevent Teen Pregnancy.

Israel, B. A., Eng, E., Schulz, A. J., & Parker, E. A. (2005). Introduction to methods in community-based participatory research for health. In B. A. Israel, E. Eng, A. J. Schulz, & E. A. Parker (Eds.), *Methods in community-based participatory research for health* (pp. 3–26). San Francisco: Jossey-Bass.

Kessler, R. C., Berglund, P., Demler, O., Jin, R., & Walters, E. E. (2005). Lifetime prevalence and age-of-onset distributions of DSM-IV disorders in the National Comorbidity Survey replication. *Archives of General Psychiatry, 62*(6), 593–602.

Kirby, D., Lepore, G., & Ryan, J. (2005). *Sexual risk and protective factors—factors affecting teen sexual behavior, pregnancy, childbearing and sexually transmitted disease: Which are important? Which can you change?* Washington, DC: National Campaign to Prevent Teen Pregnancy.

Kok, G., Gottlieb, N. H., Commers, M., & Smerecnik, C. (2008). The ecological approach in health promotion programs: A decade later. *American Journal of Health Promotion, 22*(6), 437–442.

Kok, G., Gottlieb, N. H., Panne, R., & Smerecnik, C. (2012). Methods for environmental change: An exploratory study. *BMC Public Health, 12*, 1037.

Kok, G., & Mesters, I. (2011). Getting inside the black box of health promotion programmes using intervention mapping. *Chronic Illness, 7*(3), 176–180.

Kok, G., van Essen, G. A., Wicker, S., Llupia, A., Mena, G., Correia, R., & Ruiter, R. A. (2011). Planning for influenza vaccination in health care workers: An intervention mapping approach. *Vaccine, 29*(47), 8512–8519.

Kroll, L., Harrington, R., Jayson, D., Fraser, J., & Gowers, S. (1996). Pilot study of continuation of cognitive-behavioral therapy for major depression in adolescent psychiatric patients. *Journal of the American Academy of Child & Adolescent Psychiatry, 35*(9), 1156–1161.

Kupfer, D. J., Frank, E., & Perel, J. M. (1989). The advantages of early treatment intervention in recurrent depression. *Archives of General Psychiatry, 46*(9), 771–775.

Li, Y., Cao, J., Lin, H., Li, D., Wang, Y., & He, J. (2009). Community health needs assessment with precede-proceed model: A mixed methods study. *BMC Health Services Research, 9*, 181.

Lloyd, J. J., Logan, S., Greaves, C. J., & Wyatt, K. M. (2011). Evidence, theory and context—using intervention mapping to develop a school-based intervention to prevent obesity in children. *International Journal of Behavioral Nutrition and Physical Activity, 8*, 73.

Marin, B., Kirby, D., Hudes, E., Gomez, C., & Coyle, K. (2003). Youth with older boyfriends and girlfriends: Associations with sexual risk. In B. Albert, S. Brown, & C. Flanigan (Eds.), *14 and younger: The sexual behavior of young adolescents* (pp. 83–90). Washington, DC: National Campaign to Prevent Teen Pregnancy.

Markham, C. M., Tortolero, S. R., Peskin, M. F., Shegog, R., Thiel, M., Baumler, E. R., & Robin, L. (2012). Sexual risk avoidance and sexual risk reduction interventions for middle school youth: A randomized controlled trial. *Journal of Adolescent Health, 50*(3), 279–288.

McGorry, P. (2010). A promising future for youth mental health. *Australian Medical Student Journal, 1*(1), 5.

Michie, S., Johnston, M., Francis, J., Hardeman, W., & Eccles, M. (2008). From theory to intervention: Mapping theoretically derived behavioural determinants to behaviour change techniques. *Applied Psychology, 57*(4), 660–680.

Minkler, M., & Wallerstein, N. (2004). Improving health through community organization and building: A health education perspective. In M. Minkler (Ed.), *Community organizing and community building for health* (2nd ed., pp. 26–50). New Brunswick, NJ: Rutgers University Press.

Minkler, M., & Wallerstein, N. (2010). *Community-based participatory research for health: From process to outcomes.* San Francisco: Jossey-Bass.

Mkumbo, K., Schaalma, H., Kaaya, S., Leerlooijer, J., Mbwambo, J., & Kilonzo, G. (2009). The application of intervention mapping in developing and implementing school-based sexuality and HIV/AIDS education in a developing country context: The case of Tanzania. *Scandinavian Journal of Public Health, 37*(Suppl. 2), 28–36.

Munir, F., Kalawsky, K., Wallis, D. J., & Donaldson-Feilder, E. (2013). Using intervention mapping to develop a work-related guidance tool for those affected by cancer. *BMC Public Health, 13*, 6.

National Cancer Institute (2007). Greater than the sum: Systems thinking in tobacco control. Bethesda, MD: Department of Health and Human Services, National Institutes of Health, National Cancer Institute.

Newby, K., Bayley, J., & Wallace, L. (2011). "What should we tell the children about relationships and sex?"© : Development of a program for parents using intervention mapping. *Health Promotion Practice, 12*(2), 209–228.

Noar, S. M., & Zimmerman, R. S. (2005). Health behavior theory and cumulative knowledge regarding health behaviors: Are we moving in the right direction? *Health Education Research, 20*(3), 275–290.

Patton, M. Q. (2008). *Utilization-focused evaluation* (4th ed.). Los Angeles: Sage.

Peacock, Z. S., Pogrel, M. A., & Schmidt, B. L. (2008). Exploring the reasons for delay in treatment of oral cancer. *Journal of the American Dental Association, 139*(10), 1346–1352.

Prochaska, J. O. (2013). Transtheoretical model of behavior change. In M. D. Gellman & J. R. Turner (Eds.), *Encyclopedia of behavioral medicine* (pp. 1997–2000). New York: Springer.

Prochaska, J. O., & DiClemente, C. C. (1983). Stages and processes of self-change in smoking: Towards an integrative model of change. *Journal of Consulting and Clinical Psychology, 51*(3), 390–395.

Rossi, P. H., Lipsey, M. W., & Freeman, H. E. (2004). *Evaluation: A systematic approach* (7th ed.). Thousand Oaks, CA: Sage.

Shuger, L. (2012). *Teen pregnancy and high school dropout: What communities can do to address these issues.* Washington, DC: National Campaign to Prevent Teen and Unplanned Pregnancy and America's Promise.

Tortolero, S. R., Markham, C. M., Peskin, M. F., Shegog, R., Addy, R. C., Escobar-Chaves, S. L., & Baumler, E. R. (2010). It's Your Game: Keep It Real: Delaying sexual behavior with an effective middle school program. *Journal of Adolescent Health, 46*(2), 169–179.

Trochim, W. M., Milstein, B., Wood, B. J., Jackson, S., & Pressler, V. (2004). Setting objectives for community and systems change: An application of concept mapping for planning a statewide health improvement initiative. *Health Promotion Practice, 5*(1), 8–19.

Uchino, B. (2009). Understanding the links between social support and physical health: A life-span perspective with emphasis on the separability of perceived and received support. *Perspectives on Psychological Science, 4*(3), 236–255.

U.S. Department of Health and Human Services, Office of Adolescent Health. (2013). Who are the current OAH grantees? Retrieved from http://www.hhs.gov/ash/oah/grants/grantees/tier1-tx-the.html

Vohs, K. D., & Baumeister, R. F. (Eds.). (2011). *Handbook of self-regulation: Research, theory, and applications* (2nd ed.). New York: Guilford Press.

Wasilewski, R. M., Mateo, P., & Sidorovsky, P. (2007). Preventing work-related musculoskeletal disorders within supermarket cashiers: An ergonomic training program based on the theoretical framework of the PRECEDE-PROCEED model. *Work, 28*(1), 23–31.

Wendel, M. L., Burdine, J. N., McLeroy, K. R., Alaniz, A., Norton, B., & Felix, M.R.J. (2009). Community capacity: Theory and application. In R. J. DiClemente, R. A. Crosby, & M. C. Kegler (Eds.), *Emerging theories in health promotion practice and research* (2nd ed., pp. 277–302). San Francisco: Jossey-Bass.

Wholey, J. S., Hatry, H. P., & Newcomer, K. E. (Eds.). (2010). *Handbook of practical program evaluation* (3rd ed.). San Francisco: Jossey-Bass.

Wright, A., Harris, M. G., Wiggers, J. H., Jorm, A. F., Cotton, S. M., Harrigan, S.,. . . McGorry, P. D. (2005). Recognition of depression and psychosis by young Australians and their beliefs about treatment. *Medical Journal of Australia, 183*(1), 18–23.

Wright, A., McGorry, P. D., Harris, M. G., Jorm, A. F., & Pennell, K. (2006). Development and evaluation of a youth mental health community awareness campaign—The Compass Strategy. *BMC Public Health, 6*, 215.

CHAPTER 20

BEHAVIORAL ECONOMICS AND HEALTH

Kevin Volpp
George Loewenstein
David Asch

Experts estimate that noncommunicable diseases (NCDs), including hypertension, tobacco use, physical inactivity, unhealthy diet, obesity, and alcohol overuse, account for as many as two-thirds of all deaths worldwide and are substantially or primarily driven by behavioral choices (Flegal, Graubard, Williamson, & Gail, 2005; Mokdad, Marks, Stroup, & Gerberding, 2004; World Health Organization, 2011). Similarly, the potential benefits of many advances in health care, such as cancer screening, childhood immunization, and pharmacological management of chronic conditions, are limited by poor adherence (Kripalani, Yao, & Haynes, 2007). One year following myocardial infarction, about half of patients prescribed medications to lower their cholesterol have stopped taking them—even when those drugs are provided free (Jackevicius, Mamdani, & Tu, 2002). There is a large gap between what is theoretically achievable and what is actually achieved.

Recognizing that there are many reasons why people do not take action to improve their health, behavior change experts have focused efforts on changing both individual behaviors and environments in ways that will support health (Glanz & Bishop, 2010). Policymakers have similarly instituted strategies targeted at individual behavior such as incentives, and environmental strategies such as mandated food labeling. For example, Section 2705 of the Affordable Care Act allows employers to provide incentives of up to 50 percent of total premiums based on outcomes such as reduced body mass index (BMI), lowered blood pressure

KEY POINTS

This chapter will discuss the following:

- Behavioral economics provides a better descriptive and predictive model of human behavior than standard economics.

- A key implication of behavioral economics is that program designers should be aware of and take account of common decision errors to optimize program effectiveness.

- The goal of health-improvement programs is to improve health, not to save money. All programs—whether therapeutic or preventive—should be judged by whether they improve health at a reasonable cost.

or cholesterol, and smoking cessation, an approach that could put as much as $300 billion worth of employee health incentives in play annually (Madison, Schmidt, & Volpp, 2013).

Many of the approaches being used have built-in limitations, having been designed around the pervasive view that health care decisions are rationally based economic transactions and that rational people will dispassionately assess the net present value of the costs and benefits of alternative paths and pursue the best path forward. When incentives are used, there is often an assumption that all that matters is the magnitude of the incentives and that the design, feedback frequency, saliency, and framing do not matter. These approaches seem generally well suited to supporting the health of people who behave as economists assume they do, but may be less effective in supporting the health of broader populations. Public health programs, including those involving financial incentives, would likely be more effective if designed based not on how perfectly rational people *ought* to make health decisions but rather on how real people *actually* make them.

A Brief Description of Behavioral Economics and How It Differs from Classical Economics

Behavioral economics has been getting increasing attention because of its conceptual appeal for describing and influencing human behavior. In addition, it has considerable potential to offer relatively low-cost and unobtrusive solutions to some of the most serious problems facing our society, such as undersaving, overeating, and other unhealthy behaviors. Behavioral economics builds on neoclassical economics that has at its core expected utility theory (also see the chapters in Part Two for more discussion of this theory). Expected utility theory presumes to describe both how people make decisions and how such decisions should be made. In essence, the framework of neoclassical economics posits that individuals are rational expected utility maximizers, meaning that they are able to dispassionately address decision alternatives, calculate the probabilities of utility or disutility for different outcomes, and then, through a process of backward induction, decide which decision has the highest net present value. It is a process of weighing different outcomes where the weights are based on the probabilities of the different outcomes (Neumann & Morgenstern, 1953).

Expected utility maximization is a powerful construct, but it has some important limitations. It presumes that people are fully rational, driven primarily by self-interest, and have stable preferences (Kahneman, 2011). When it comes to health behaviors, this assumption is problematic. The inference that problems like obesity are simply a reflection of individuals' preferences represents an underappreciation of the complexity of such health problems. As a result, standard economics lacks methods to suggest creative ways to address them. It further ignores that preferences often change over time, predicated on an individual's starting point (reference point), and are heavily influenced by other factors such as what those in the individual's social network are doing. Under conventional economics, regulatory interventions, including targeted taxes and subsidies, are permissible only in situations characterized by externalities or other market failures: that is, costs, such as secondhand cigarette smoke, that an individual's actions impose on others.

Table 20.1 Traditional Versus Behavioral Economics

Traditional Economics	Behavioral Economics
Core theory: expected utility maximization.	Core theory: prospect theory.
Assumes people have perfect rationality.	Recognizes that people make decision errors.
Starting point and assessment are independent.	Assessment depends on starting point.
Framing doesn't matter.	Framing affects assessment even when utilities are the same.
People have stable preferences.	People's preferences are inconsistent over time.
People discount the future at constant rates.	People discount the near future to a greater degree and engage in time inconsistent discounting.
Interventions should occur only when people's actions adversely affect others (negative externalities).	Interventions should be considered when people will harm their future selves (internalities).
Regulations and policies should be generally geared to protecting people from the actions of others.	Regulations and policies should often be geared to protecting people from themselves.

Over the past several decades, leaders in behavioral economics have described ways in which people's decisions differ from standard economic models (see Table 20.1). Although economists such as Herb Simon mapped out concepts of *bounded rationality* in the 1950s (Simon, 1955), and Maurice Allais in 1953 laid out the Allais paradox (to a group of leading economists) as a contradiction of standard expected utility maximization (Allais, 1953), the publication of Prospect Theory by Kahneman and Tversky (1979) is widely credited with being seminal in the development of behavioral economics. Prospect Theory provided an overarching conceptual framework for describing what Kahneman and Tversky and others had observed in a number of studies about human behaviors that could not be explained by expected utility theory. In essence, Prospect Theory has several important components: (1) the way people feel about a set of possible outcomes depends on their starting point (this is also known as *reference dependence*, meaning that decision makers evaluate outcomes as gains or losses depending on their starting, or reference, point); (2) people's sensitivity to both gains and losses may diminish depending on their starting point; and (3) people exhibit loss aversion: that is, the disutility of a loss is much stronger than the utility of an equivalent gain (Kahneman, 2011; Kahneman & Tversky, 1979). Another important implication of this theory is that people *over*weight small probabilities (referred to as *nonlinear probability weighting*).

The importance of reference points is nicely illustrated by an example Kahneman gives in his book *Thinking, Fast and Slow* (Kahneman, 2011). Consider two people who today each have $4 million. Standard models would consider them to have roughly equivalent utility of wealth. However, imagine that as of yesterday one of the two had $1 million and the other had $7 million. Clearly, the person who had $1 million yesterday should be ecstatic today and the one who had $7 million yesterday should be despondent. Diminishing sensitivity to changes in wealth (or utility more broadly) is illustrated by this example: consider the utility of getting an extra $500 when your wealth is $1 million as opposed to if you have no money. The utility of this extra $500 is much greater if you have no (or very little) money than if you already have a lot.

The fact that people's utility for money varies by how much they already have is consistent with expected utility theory. However, expected utility theory does not account for the observation that how people think about utility varies between gains and losses of the same amount. Utility theory would simply compare the two states of wealth, but empirically it has been shown that the disutility of losing money is much greater than the utility of gaining the same amount of money. A number of studies have shown that people have what Kahneman calls a *loss aversion ratio*, in a range of 1.5 to 2.5 (Novemsky & Kahneman, 2005). For example, when offered a 50-50 chance of winning $150 or losing $100, most people would not voluntarily enter into this gamble, because the potential pain of losing $100 is greater than the joy of winning $150. Yet under standard expected utility maximization, it would be a no-brainer to take this gamble because the expected utility is 0.5 (–$100) + 0.5 ($150), or $25.

Furthermore, people tend to be risk averse when it comes to gains, but risk seeking in the domain of losses. Whether choices are framed as losses or gains has a big influence on what people choose. This is illustrated by the famous "Asian disease example" (Tversky & Kahneman, 1981). Let's presume you are in charge of a public health department and you are confronted with the following situation:

> Imagine that the United States is preparing for the outbreak of an unusual Asian disease, which is expected to kill 600 people. Two alternative programs to combat the disease have been proposed. Assume that the exact scientific estimates of the consequences of the program are as follows:

> If program A is adopted, 200 people will be saved.

> If program B is adopted, there is a one-third probability that 600 people will be saved and a two-thirds probability that no one will be saved.

Given these choices, a substantial majority (about 70%) choose A. Removing uncertainty favors the sure bet of saving 200 lives.

Now consider the following options.

> If program A' is adopted, 400 people will die.

> If program B' is adopted, there is a one-third probability that no one will die and a two-thirds probability that 600 people will die.

About 70 percent of people choose option B'. However, these two choices—between A and B and between A' and B'—are, from an expected utility standpoint, exactly the same choice. When outcomes are viewed as gains, decision makers tend to avoid gambles and are risk averse. When choosing between two bad outcomes, however, decision makers tend to take a gamble (be risk seeking). This highlights the importance of framing. Often, a decision will inadvertently be presented without considering that how it is framed will likely have a significant impact in terms of what people choose.

Further work in behavioral economics reveals other limitations to expected utility theory. Another central observation from behavioral economics is the concept of *hyperbolic discounting*. While it is standard in conventional economics to assume that people discount the future, behavioral economists have mapped out ways in which people tend to discount outcomes nearer in time more than those further off in time. Thus, discounting also tends to be inconsistent over time, in contrast to standard economic models (Laibson, 1997; O'Donoghue & Rabin, 1999).

By recognizing the prevalence of less than perfectly rational behavior, behavioral economics points to a large category of situations in which policy intervention might be justified. This category is characterized by *internalities*—that is, costs, such as the long-run health consequences of smoking on smokers, that people impose on themselves (Tversky & Kahneman, 1981; Novemsky & Kahneman, 2005). Internalities abound because people make decision errors, and behavioral economists have described many common ones, such as those that we describe next.

A Framework for Thinking About Behavioral Economics

Behavioral economists have proposed an *asymmetric paternalism* approach to public policy (Camerer, Issacharoff, Loewenstein, O'Donoghue, & Rabin, 2003; Thaler & Sunstein, 2003). This approach is paternalistic in the sense of attempting to help individuals achieve their own goals, in effect protecting them from themselves, in contrast to conventional forms of regulation designed to prevent individuals from harming others. Asymmetric paternalism differs from more heavy-handed forms of paternalism in attempting to protect people without limiting freedom of choice. It is asymmetric in the sense of helping individuals who are prone to making irrational decisions, while not restricting the freedom of choice of those making informed, deliberate decisions. For example, arranging the presentation of food in a cafeteria line so that the healthy foods appear first is likely to increase the amount of healthy food chosen, without depriving those who want the unhealthy foods of the opportunity to purchase them (Thaler & Sunstein, 2003). People who believe that individuals behave optimally should not object to asymmetric paternalism, because it does not limit freedom, while those who accept the limits of human rationality should endorse such measures.

Whereas traditional economics justifies seemingly poor decisions as reflections of some implied but hidden rational choice, behavioral economics sees our seemingly poor decisions as errors. Many of us have trouble dieting, exercising, and saving money and are prone to procrastination even when the cumulative consequences are severe. Many commercial enterprises exploit these decision errors (Issacharoff & Delaney, 2006; Loewenstein & Haisley, 2008; Loewenstein & O'Donoghue, 2006). Credit card companies and automobile manufacturers lure new customers with "$0 down" and fleeting but tempting teaser rates of "0% interest," playing on the common propensity to focus on the present rather than on the future. Banks earn revenue by charging high fees (generally not prominent in program descriptions) for minor mistakes such as account overdrafts or breaches of minimum balance rules. States market lottery tickets that return $0.45 on the dollar and promote these games in ways that ignore probabilities with messages such as "you can't win if you don't play."

Table 20.2   Key Decision Errors and Suggestions for Addressing Them

Present-biased preferences	Feedback needs to be relatively immediate.
Nonlinear probability weighting	Probabilistic rewards (lotteries) can be efficient ways to motivate.
Overoptimism and loss aversion	Getting people to precommit and put money at risk is an effective motivational tool.
Peanuts effect	Delivering rewards in bundles avoids having many small rewards.
Narrow bracketing	Framing rewards in terms of effort per day is preferable to offering them per month or year.
Regret aversion	Anticipated regret can be used to augment motivation.
Defaults/status quo bias	A choice architect can set defaults to create environments that shift the path of least resistance to favor healthy choices.
Rational-world bias	Recognize that simply providing information and assuming people will act rationally likely will not result in the desired behaviors.

The promise of behavioral economics for population health is that many of the same messages, incentives, and choice structures used so effectively to lure people into situations where they may be exploited can be redirected to attract them to healthier choices that improve their long-term well-being. Decision errors affect policymakers as well, with broader ramifications for the types of policies that are developed and adopted. Following are discussions of some key decision errors and how knowledge of them can be used to enhance the effectiveness of programs aimed at improving health behaviors, particularly in regard to incentive design (Table 20.2 summarizes these ideas).

A central lesson from the field of behavioral economics is that *how incentives are delivered can matter more than their objective magnitude* (Loewenstein, Asch, & Volpp, 2013; Volpp, Pauly, Loewenstein, & Bangsberg, 2009). There are ways of delivering large incentives that make them ineffective in changing behavior, and also ways to deliver small incentives that greatly magnify their effectiveness. This observation is a source of optimism, implying that with careful design we can leverage relatively small investments to improve public health. Of course, in public health, perhaps more than in banking, people are concerned about the potential of actual or perceived coercion on behavioral decisions. This is an important consideration, and care should be taken in designing incentive strategies and messages to avoid any sense of coercion.

Present-Biased Preferences

The decision error that most impedes healthy behaviors is *present bias* (Ainslie, 1975; Frederick, Loewenstein, & O'Donoghue, 2002; Loewenstein, 1992; Loewenstein & Angner, 2003; Loewenstein, O'Donoghue, & Rabin, 2003; O'Donoghue & Rabin, 1999). Present bias derives from two important behavioral tendencies: to overweight immediate costs and benefits relative to those occurring in the future, and to take a more evenhanded approach to delayed costs and benefits. We are much more willing to begin dieting *tomorrow* than today because the overweighting of immediate costs deters us from undertaking the deprivation of dieting immediately, and our more balanced perspective on delayed deprivation makes us willing to impose these costs on ourselves in the future.

Although present-biased preferences typically promote unhealthy behaviors, policymakers can use them for beneficial effects. The motivational impact of benefits and costs, such as rewards for good behavior and punishments for bad behavior, can be increased substantially if they are made immediate. These consequences should coincide as closely as possible with the timing of the behaviors they are meant to encourage or deter. Funds for this could be provided by employers or insurers for whom this might be a cost-effective way to improve worker health and productivity (Warner, Smith, Smith, & Fries, 1996).

Such programs have been shown to have dramatic effects in the area of drug addiction (Bigelow & Silverman, 1999; Higgins, 1999). This is particularly striking, because many individuals with drug addiction already face major adverse consequences, such as loss of livelihood and disenfranchisement from their families; yet these costs are often insufficient to motivate abstinence. Similarly, small incentives offered on proof of abstinence have succeeded in tripling smoking cessation rates where the far larger but delayed incentive of improved health has failed (Volpp, Troxel, et al., 2009). Small, daily, lottery-based incentives have greatly increased medication adherence and weight loss (Haisley, Volpp, Pellathy, & Loewenstein, 2012; Kimmel et al., 2012; Volpp, John, et al., 2008; Volpp, Loewenstein, et al., 2008), in part because they bring immediate rewards (money, excitement) to a situation in which the benefits of avoiding ill health are typically distant and uncertain (Loewenstein, Asch, et al., 2013).

Thus, rather than requiring individuals to make decisions based on consideration of their long-term best interests, it might be useful to change the short-term incentives so that beneficial actions are also easier to choose. Some school districts have begun to use this approach, banning or making less accessible various products, such as soda and candy from vending machines, so that the cost of obtaining them now includes a walk off campus. In addition, people's willingness to commit to future changes can be leveraged by giving them choices between health-benefiting and health-harming behaviors before they actually have to act on them. An example of this is scheduling gym visits and laboratory tests to monitor cholesterol ahead of time and having patients voluntarily agree, also in advance, to pay financial penalties for last-minute cancellations.

Nonlinear Probability Weighting

People tend to put disproportionate weight on outcomes that have a small probability of occurring, but are insensitive to variations in probability at the low end of the probability scale—for example, between a 0.001 and a 0.00001 chance of winning a prize—even though the probabilities differ by several orders of magnitude (Sunstein, 2002). Such overweighting of small probabilities is partly responsible for the enormous attraction of lottery tickets. Like present-biased preferences, this overweighting can be used to advantage in public health interventions.

We have designed lottery-based reward systems in a variety of programs aimed at motivating diverse health behaviors (described more fully later) (Kimmel et al., 2012; Volpp, John, et al., 2008). These interventions exploit overweighting of small probabilities and also play on other psychological insights. Because people tend to be motivated by both the experience of past rewards and the prospect of future rewards (Camerer & Ho, 1999), these lottery-based systems provide frequent small payoffs and infrequent large payoffs. This approach has been demonstrated to be effective in a variety of areas, including helping people to lose weight (in one study, 52.6% of people receiving frequent small rewards achieved their sixteen-week weight loss goals compared with about 10.5% in the control group) and to reduce medication nonadherence (from about 23% to about 3%) (Volpp, John, et al., 2008; Volpp, Loewenstein, et al., 2008).

Overoptimism and Loss Aversion

We discuss the errors of overoptimism and loss aversion together, because they work very well in concert with each other. For most people (depressed people being an exception), overoptimism refers, naturally, to being overoptimistic about life outcomes (Sharot, 2011). It is especially pronounced in the context of people's predictions about their own likelihood of exerting self-control, sometimes referred to as the *false hope syndrome* (Sharot, 2011). Although in some contexts overoptimism seems to be beneficial, it can also result in suboptimal patterns of behavior. For example, people prefer paying a flat rate for gym memberships, even though they would spend less if they were to pay on a per-visit basis, in part because they overestimate their future gym attendance (Della Vigna & Malmendier, 2002).

Loss aversion reflects the tendency to put greater weight on losses than on similarly sized gains (Kahneman, Knetsch, & Thaler, 1991; Tversky & Kahneman, 1991). It can produce a variety of undesired behaviors, from excessive risk aversion to the tendency for people to hold on too long to losing investments, such as houses or stocks (O'Dean, 1998; Shefrin & Statman, 1985; Weber & Chapman, 2005).

Loss aversion can be utilized in the design of programs with sticks (which are losses) rather than carrots (which are gains). However, programs with sticks can seem more punitive than organizations are willing to appear, and public health settings may offer few opportunities to deploy them. Nevertheless, it is possible to take advantage of loss aversion by designing programs in which people voluntarily put their own money at risk in the service of achieving health behavior goals that they themselves desire.

In our research, we have exploited a combination of overoptimism and loss aversion to help people lose weight. We gave them the opportunity to participate in deposit contracts, in which they could deposit $0.01 to $3.00 per day of their own money, which we matched 1:1. Participants reported their weight daily and received the sum of their deposit and the matching funds each day they were on track to meeting their monthly weight loss target, but they forfeited both amounts if they were not on track (Volpp, John, et al., 2008). The deposit contract leveraged participants' overoptimistic self-predictions of how much weight they would lose as well as their loss aversion once the deposits were made. In this sixteen-week study, average weight loss was 14.0 pounds in the deposit group compared with 3.9 pounds in the control group ($p = 0.006$). We extended this work in a thirty-two-week study and found that weight loss was sustained for the duration of the intervention (8.7 vs. 2.2 pounds in the control group; $p = 0.04$). Although these results were promising, to be effective as a population health strategy this approach needs to achieve high ongoing participation rates, which poses a challenge for the organizations that have been using it.

Peanuts Effects

Small gains or losses are not motivating (Markowitz, 1952; Prelec & Loewenstein, 1991; Weber & Chapman, 2005). This observation challenges health behavior change programs that emphasize efforts to repeatedly achieve small changes, as weight loss programs do. It is easy for a patient to rationalize that no single cigarette causes lung cancer. No single trip to the gym prevents heart disease. If we see each event on its own, it is easier to understand such self-destructive patterns of behavior as cigarette smoking, weight gain, and cell phone use or texting while driving. The pleasure of smoking a cigarette or eating a dessert and the convenience and engagement of conducting business or socializing in otherwise "dead" time are immediate and tangible, whereas the costs—increased risks of developing lung cancer, being overweight, or having a car accident—seem inappreciably small. Across a lifetime or a population, however, these effects are not small at all.

The tendency to underweight small events can also make it easier for people to put away small sums for retirement savings in short cycle lengths or to make small periodic investments in their health via medication adherence. In each of these efforts, we need to think asymmetrically. In our incentive programs we should provide frequent (often daily) feedback on rewards because of present-biased preferences, but when we are *delivering* financial rewards, we want to bundle them. To use the peanuts effect to advantage, one might alert people to their rewards daily but then deliver them monthly to create larger aggregate payments.

Narrow Bracketing

Narrow, or *choice*, *bracketing* refers to the process of grouping individual choices together into sets. When making choices, we bracket them either *broadly*, by considering all of the consequences together (as standard economic theory assumes), or *narrowly*, by making each decision in isolation (Read, Loewenstein, & Rabin, 1999). People tend to bracket narrowly and to focus on the local consequences of the most immediately available choices while ignoring the aggregate costs and benefits over a long time horizon (Herrnstein & Prelec, 1992; Sabini & Silver, 1982). Bracketing effects interact with other errors and biases and can be used to induce these other biases. For example, the peanuts effect is more likely to occur when costs or benefits are framed narrowly, so an exercise goal may seem less onerous if it is expressed as miles per day rather than hundreds of miles per month or year.

Regret Aversion

People really dislike regretting decisions they have made (Connolly & Butler, 2006), often voicing laments such as "if only I had. . . " Many people, moreover, anticipate possible future regret and seek to make decisions today that reduce that risk. The avoidance of anticipated regret is a useful exception to present-biased preferences (also see Chapter Four for discussion of this issue). This understanding underlies the success of the Dutch postal code lottery, in which winning postal codes are selected and those living within the selected areas who have purchased tickets receive prizes. Those who did not purchase tickets learn that they would have received a prize had they done so (Zeelenberg & Pieters, 2004). Individuals see their neighbors winning large prizes that they do not share, and their desire to avoid future regret drives lottery participation.

Anticipated regret has been shown to affect a variety of preventive behaviors, such as the significant increase in vaccination use among people who have experienced illness after failing to get vaccinated (Chapman & Coups, 2006). In our lottery-based incentive programs that aim to increase health-promoting behaviors, we notify both winners and losers. We tell people they would have won had they only taken their medication, checked their blood pressure, or lost weight in the previous period (Kimmel et al., 2012; Volpp, John, et al., 2008).

Defaults Status Quo Bias

The *default*, or *status quo*, bias reflects our tendency to take the path of least resistance—to continue doing what we have been doing, or to do what comes automatically, even when superior alternatives exist (Johnson & Goldstein, 2003; Kahneman et al., 1991; Samuelson & Zeckhauser, 1988). Defaults have been blamed for a wide range of suboptimal outcomes, from the failure of employees to put aside retirement funds in companies whose default contribution rate is zero (Gneezy & Potters, 1997; Madrian & Shea, 2001; Thaler & Benartzi, 2004) to suboptimal allocation between investment alternatives (Thaler, Tversky, Kahneman, & Schwartz, 1997) to excessive consumption of French fries and large sodas as part of "supersized" meals at fast food franchises (Halpern, Ubel, & Asch, 2007; Loewenstein, Brennan, & Volpp, 2007; Thaler & Sunstein, 2003). In Western European countries that have opt-in policies for organ donation—that is, the default is nonparticipation (as in the United States)—donation rates tend to be in the range of 10 percent. In contrast, in countries with opt-out policies, in which citizens are automatically enrolled as organ donors unless they actively choose not to be, organ donation rates are often close to 99 percent (Johnson & Goldstein, 2003). Defaults have been shown to increase the rate at which patients with terminal lung diseases choose comfort-oriented plans of care (Halpern et al., 2013), and they could be used more widely to encourage the choice of beneficial health options.

A *choice architect* (a person who makes decisions on how choices are presented to the end user) can use defaults tactically, such as changing scheduled automatic prescription refills from thirty to ninety days (or longer) for patients requiring lifelong chronic disease therapy or changing the default option for fast food restaurants' combination meals from large sodas to small sodas or water to help propel people toward self-beneficial behaviors (Halpern et al., 2007; Loewenstein et al., 2007). Such approaches would cost nothing, would preserve freedom of choice, and could change behavior substantially.

Rational-World Bias

Perhaps the most prominent decision error affecting health-related behaviors is the tendency of some well-meaning public health officials and private sector benefit designers to make policy decisions based on an assumption that people's choices are considered and rational. When this in turn leads to assumptions that the provision of information is all that is needed for optimal decision making, it follows that when financial incentives are offered, the amount is assumed to be all that really matters. Human behavior is far more complex.

One significant manifestation of the rational-world bias is the complexity of health insurance plans. Health insurance is complicated for many reasons, including insurance companies' desire to shield themselves from costs and, possibly, to shroud information that might be perceived as unfavorable (Gabaix & Laibson, 2006). A major rationale for this complexity is the inclusion of benefit design elements that incentivize patients to engage in desired cost-minimizing and health-maximizing behaviors. For these built-in incentives to exert their desired influence, however, patients must understand the incentives they are facing, and there is considerable evidence that they do not (Frank & Lamiraud, 2009; Handel & Kolstad, 2013). In recent research (Loewenstein, Friedman, et al., 2013), we found that most consumers in our studies lacked an understanding of the most basic insurance concepts, such as deductibles, copays, and coinsurance, and, when given a simplified version of a traditional insurance plan, were unable to compute the costs they would incur for basic services.

Applications of Behavioral Economics

This section provides two examples of applying the concepts of behavioral economics to health behavior change, looking at weight loss interventions over time and at efforts to improve medication adherence.

Application 1: Weight Loss Interventions

Early Studies of the Impact of Incentives on Weight Loss

In a series of studies, starting in the 1970s, Jeffery and others examined the impact of incentives on weight loss (Jeffery, Gerber, Rosenthal, & Lindquist, 1983; Jeffery, Thompson, & Wing, 1978). While some of the studies had methodological deficits, the underlying hypothesis came from the observation that participants who deposited money and other valuables with a therapist, and signed contracts in which the return of their valuables was contingent on progress toward prespecified weight loss goals, lost large amounts of weight (Mann, 1972). Deposits were large ($200 in 1974 dollars, about $1,000 in current dollars).

A downside of the approach used in these studies is selection bias. It is likely that contracts with high penalties deter a substantial portion of high-risk potential participants—due to either insufficient funds or lack of motivation—from entering. In later research, Jeffery et al. (1983) tested the effects of different contract amounts on either individual or group weight loss. Mean weight loss was large in all three groups but did not differ significantly based on contract size. However, the proportion of participants who reached the goal of losing thirty pounds was significantly higher in the larger dollar groups. In another study that tested the use of increasing payments ($5, $10, $20, $40, or $75) for each five-pound increment of weight loss (Jeffery, Bjornson-Benson, Rosenthal, Kurth, & Dunn, 1984), the researchers found that the increasing payments resulted in larger weight losses during the weight loss phase but that a maintenance program without payments did not prevent weight gain.

Jeffrey and colleagues found that paying participants for weight loss using direct payments was less effective than deposit contracts. In a randomized trial, these authors found that cash payments up to $25 per week for making 100 percent of proportional progress toward a goal, $12.50 for 50 percent of the goal, and $2.50 for not gaining weight did not result in greater weight loss in the payment group than among control subjects (Jeffery et al., 1993).

Studies that have shown no effects on either initial weight loss or maintenance typically have used incentives of a small magnitude or were targeted at behaviors, like attendance at weight loss programs, that in and of themselves do not ensure weight loss (Jeffery, Wing, Thorson, & Burton, 1998; Wing & Anglin, 1996). In recent years, weight loss incentives have become a common feature in programs used by employers and health plans, and a variety of start-ups, like stickk.com and dietbet.com, use deposit contracts as a way of trying to help people lose weight.

Recent Studies of Financial Incentives for Weight Loss

More recently, building on the first generation of studies described above, our team has conducted several financial incentives studies for weight loss. We generally have found significant increases in weight loss using different types of incentives. The remaining challenge is how to achieve maintenance of these effects postintervention.

Our first study provided proof of the concept that daily lottery-type incentives and precommitment contract incentives are highly effective in achieving initial weight loss over sixteen weeks (lottery = 13.1 lbs. lost, p-value for lottery vs. control = .014; deposit contract = 14.0 lbs. lost, p-value for contract vs. control = .003) (see Figure 20.1). However, over the following three months, participants regained

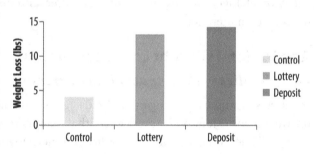

Figure 20.1 Weight Loss in Groups Receiving Incentives Versus Control Group

most of the weight they had lost. We were not sure whether this was because we had framed the period after the intervention as a period of maintenance as opposed to ongoing weight loss, or whether this was simply because the incentives had ended. In a subsequent eight-month trial, we tested two different types of deposit contracts: one that featured an eight-month weight loss program, the other had a weight loss program for six months followed by two months of maintenance. This study showed no difference in mean weight loss during the intervention between the two groups based on framing, and both were successful in achieving a mean weight loss of about ten pounds (John et al., 2011). Subsequent tests included a study that showed greater effectiveness for team competitive versus individual incentives, though there was a confound in that participants in the teams had the potential to win more money than those in the individual arms of the study (Kullgren et al., 2013).

In ongoing work, we are currently conducting the first study that, to our knowledge, rigorously tests in an employer setting two alternatives to a standard incentive design. The standard design is a premium adjustment in the following year based on achievement of a biometric goal: for example, a BMI of 25. The alternative designs are (1) a premium adjustment immediately upon achievement of goals, or (2) a behavioral economic approach that uses the same amount of incentive dollars but offers daily lotteries for which people are eligible when their weigh-ins are at or below a trajectory consistent with their six-month goals. We are also conducting two studies in partnership with Weight Watchers using Weight Watchers members. One study is a four-arm randomized controlled trial (RCT) testing the impact of differing degrees of employer subsidies toward the cost of Weight Watchers membership on program participation and weight loss. In the second study, we are looking at incentives for maintenance of weight loss. Weight Watchers members who have initial success in losing weight (5 kg over four to six months) are randomly assigned to either standard Weight Watchers, daily lottery-type incentives or daily fixed payments. The findings of these studies will refine our understanding of the effects of different types of incentive designs on weight loss and maintenance.

Application 2: Efforts to Improve Medication Adherence

Numerous studies have shown that at least one-third of patients fail to adhere to medication regimens. One approach to improving medication adherence is to change some of the underlying defaults by, for example, using ninety-day prescriptions for chronic illness medications as opposed to thirty-day prescriptions. It seems logical that adherence rates would be higher over a year if people had to get refills three times as opposed to eleven times—the latter requirement provides more opportunities to forget or experience delays in filling prescriptions. Ninety-day prescriptions could be set up as the default and patients or their providers could opt out if desired. Of course, opt-out defaults are not always possible. If a large pharmacy benefits manager wanted to encourage automatic refills for patients on long-term medication, she or he might not be able to have members opt out of such a system because of the potential that those who missed the implications of the opt-out would then be surprised or angry about charges for automatic refills. In one study, switching from an opt-in system to a system that embedded a choice (yes or no) within the refill process and highlighted the advantages in terms of convenience ("we can send your refills to you automatically or you can get your refills manually if you prefer") resulted in more than twice as many patients choosing to be in the automatic refill program (Keller, Harlam, Loewenstein, & Volpp, 2011).

We conducted a series of studies (Sen et al., 2014) using daily, lottery-based financial incentives to improve medication adherence (Kimmel et al., 2012; Volpp, Lowenstein, 2008). The first two studies were pilots that tested the impact of a lottery with a daily expected value (EV) of $5 and $3, respectively, on medication adherence among patients on warfarin, a blood thinner used to prevent strokes in people at high risk. Participants were eligible for the lottery daily if they took their warfarin correctly, and they were informed of their winnings the next day. In the first pilot (EV of $5 per day) over 979 patient-days of warfarin use, the proportion of incorrect pill taking was 2.3 percent (97.7% adherence), compared with a historic mean of 22 percent incorrect pill taking in this population. In the second pilot (EV of $3 per day) over

813 patient-days of warfarin use, the overall mean adherence was 98.4 percent (i.e., 1.6% days nonadherent), similar to the $5 a day pilot.

We then conducted a two-arm RCT of lotteries for warfarin adherence that, in the subgroup with well-controlled anticoagulation at baseline (i.e., an international normalized ratio [INR] within therapeutic range), demonstrated no impact of the lottery incentive. However, among the a priori subgroup with baseline INRs below the therapeutic range, there was a significant reduction in out-of-range INRs in the lottery arm versus the control arm (adjusted OR 0.39 [95% CI, 0.25–0.62]) (Kimmel et al., 2012). This study highlighted the importance of targeting interventions to nonadherent patients and provided evidence from an RCT that lottery incentives can be effective in achieving improved clinical outcomes. However, this outcome left open the question of to what degree these effects were due to the incentives, given the fact that the incentive also constituted a daily reminder. Subsequently, we have been conducting a four-arm, National Heart, Lung, and Blood Institute–funded RCT testing the impact of daily lotteries and daily reminders in a 2 × 2 factorial design on warfarin adherence. Another important area of active investigation is in testing ways to improve habit formation and leverage social influences.

A major challenge is determining the optimal method to reach patients and reinforce their behavior each day if we want to significantly improve medication adherence. Even patients with chronic illnesses may spend only a few hours a year with a doctor or nurse, but they spend about 5,000 waking hours a year doing just about everything else (Loewenstein & O'Donoghue, 2006). Those 5,000 hours when they live their lives and make choices about what to eat and whether to exercise, smoke, take their medications, or visit the doctor are typically ignored by the U.S. health care system. This occurs, in part, because current approaches to U.S. health care financing support health care during visits to the doctor but not between those visits, and also because "hovering over" people during the hours between visits is personnel intensive, often requiring nurses to telephone or to visit patients or to staff telemedicine programs. Hovering also requires a fair amount of the very kind of engagement in their own health and health care that is so often missing in the patients these interventions aim to reach.

A key lesson from behavioral economics is that if you want to affect a behavior that occurs frequently (such as taking a medication), you need to engage the person at nearly the same frequency. That degree of engagement would have been impossible or prohibitively expensive before people became accustomed to using their cell phones and other devices regularly. Today an increasing number of pill bottles, glucometers, scales, and other devices that transmit information are available, and they can be used to provide feedback to patients and providers. However, the technology alone is unlikely to lead to sustained changes in behavior. A patient who is nonadherent to medication is likely also to be nonadherent to using a new electronic device, unless the provision of the device is accompanied by engagement strategies that apply behavioral economics concepts (Sen et al., 2014). In testing daily use rates of wireless glucometers and blood pressure cuffs in a population of patients with poorly controlled blood sugar, we found that patients who were randomized to be asked to use their wireless glucometer or blood pressure cuff daily had used these devices only 50 percent of the time by the end of a three-month period, whereas patients randomized to receive daily lotteries conditional on device use utilized their devices more than 80 percent of the time and achieved better glycemic control (Sen et al., 2014).

Value-Based Insurance Design: An Emerging Issue for Behavioral Economics

A surprising and unfortunate feature of many health insurance plans is that they require patients to pay some or all costs out of pocket for a number of high-value elements of care and hence discourage the use of this care; two examples are the treatment of hypertension and the use of statins by patients with diabetes—care that is widely seen as worth its cost. By requiring consumers to pay "first dollar" for initial health expenditures, high-deductible (also known as consumer-driven) insurance plans intend to make consumers more cost conscious and thus better shoppers for health care services. However, as a RAND health insurance study famously showed (Kripalani et al., 2007) and other research also concluded (Jackevicius et al., 2002), high-deductible health plans are as likely to discourage the use of high-value services as the use of low-value services. Because patients lack knowledge about which tests or services are high value and which are low value, and do not have information about the relationship between price and quality, such plans discourage spending on *all* tests and services, including those of high value. In effect, the baby is thrown out with the bathwater.

Value-based insurance design—which involves discounting, or making free, services deemed to be high in value—is an attempt to fine-tune the blunt incentives inherent in deductibles and copayments. Value-based insurance design was inspired by research that showed the use of higher copayments significantly reduced the use of services such as prescriptions but ultimately raised costs because the lower rates of medication adherence led to higher rates of emergency department visits and adverse outcomes (Jackevicius et al., 2002). Extrapolating from these results, it was natural to conclude that lowering cost sharing for high-value activities, such as taking medications for chronic conditions, would increase adherence and reduce long-term costs. The Affordable Care Act incorporates a kind of value-based insurance design in its requirement that preventive services be offered to patients at no charge.

Up to the present time, value-based insurance design has not lived up to its promise. The economic impact of value-based insurance design depends on whether it can make enough people adherent who were previously nonadherent—and on the health and cost consequences of that improved adherence—to offset the loss of the copayments from those who were already adherent. Although some experimental tests of value-based insurance design have found that copayment reductions increase adherence, those effects have typically been small, in the range of 3 to 6 percentage points (Chernew et al., 2008; Choudhry, 2011; Gibson et al., 2011; Maciejewski, Farley, Parker, & Wansink, 2010). Even among patients who had experienced recent heart attacks and were given their cardiovascular medications for free, average adherence was only about 45 percent (Choudhry et al., 2011). One reason for these disappointing results may be what is known as the "dog that didn't bark" problem (Tversky & Kahneman, 1981). People who are nonadherent don't notice that their copays have been reduced because they have not been using (and thus not paying for) the service.

Indeed, one of the valuable lessons learned from efforts to introduce value-based insurance design has been a reminder of the asymmetry of the forces that surround patient engagement. Based on conventional economic reasoning, it might seem reasonable to assume that decreasing copayments would create effects equal and opposite to those of increasing copayments. If we build on understandings developed from behavioral economic research, however, we realize that framing matters and that losses (in this case, of the higher copayments intended to reduce use) loom larger in patients' minds than gains (lowered copayments). We also need to recognize that the people who would be deterred by higher copayments are different from the people who might become adherent with lower copayments, because the first group consists of those who take their medications whereas the second group consists of those who do not. Behavioral economic thinking, therefore, helps to explain what in fact has been observed: increasing copayments on the one hand and decreasing them on the other do not have opposite effects that are similar in magnitude.

Value-based insurance design is an appealing idea. But the benefits of value-based insurance design could be increased through the application of ideas from behavioral economics, such as making simple changes in reward delivery to increase salience (e.g., retaining the copay but sending a rebate) and sending communications from insurers to patients so that even those who are nonadherent are aware of the benefit.

Summary

Individual and population health outcomes would be greatly advanced if people were able to weigh the present and future costs of their actions carefully and dispassionately and had the necessary information and self-control to implement behavioral plans and overcome decision errors that contribute to unhealthy behaviors. Few people can do that, however, so behavior change interventions and public health policies should not be structured around such a rational model of behavior.

The potential for using understandings of human motivation rooted in behavioral economics to improve health behavior is substantial. Behavioral economics has much to offer in terms of prevention as its concepts can aid in developing and testing innovations that can keep people healthy. A shift of research expenditures, which are disproportionately allocated to treatment (97%) rather than to prevention (3%), also could tip the balance toward strategies more likely to improve population health.

A key challenge is that, in part because of present bias, preventive services often are covered only if they show a positive return on investment. Treatments are not held to the same standard, however; in fact, the cost of treatments is not even allowed to be considered in Medicare coverage decisions. This leads to overinvestment in treatments of low value and underinvestment in prevention. The same standard for assessing the impact of health programs, with the goal of achieving the most health possible with the available resources (Volpp, Asch, & Loewenstein, 2012) could be used for both preventive and therapeutic services, with the potential to improve preventive health behavior.

The efforts of the Behavioural Insights Team in the United Kingdom have attracted attention. Making government "smarter" by performing randomized tests of the impact of different kinds of messaging and then choosing defaults that are likely to improve health is worthwhile and should continue to be part of government processes, but it is important that efforts to improve health not stop there, because there are additional pathways and opportunities for achieving important health goals. For example, raising taxes on cigarettes and other unhealthy goods where it is in the public interest to consume less is a powerful economic policy tool. Behavioral economics can help make such policies more effective but is not a substitute for them (Loewenstein & Ubel, 2010).

The implications of choosing defaults wisely are also recognized by many private sector organizations that aim to shift the path of least resistance toward healthier choices. Setting up defaults in benefit design to favor health plans that provide better coverage of preventive services, changing the environment in workplaces to make it easier to take the stairs, and serving more healthful food in cafeterias represent approaches to leading people gently toward individual and population goals.

In short, there is a great deal of opportunity for behavioral economics to improve health behavior and health care utilization. Whether in health care delivery settings or in private or public sector organizations, there will be benefits from carefully considering the choice environment and whether defaults can be chosen that increase the likelihood of improved health. It can be recognized that many decision makers have short-term time horizons and that the key question regarding any health program is whether it leads to improved health at a reasonable price, not whether it saves money in the short term. Adopting this perspective will increase uptake of health improvement programs more generally. Concepts and tools from behavioral economics will be an important part of efforts to improve population health in the future.

References

Ainslie, G. (1975). Specious reward: A behavioral theory of impulsiveness and impulse control. *Psychological Bulletin, 82,* 463–496.

Allais, P. M. (1953). Le comportement de l'homme rationnel devant le risque: critique des postulats et axiomes de l'école Américain. [Rational man's behaviour in the presence of risk: Critique of the postulates and axioms of the American school]. *Econometrica, 21*(4), 503–546.

Bigelow, G. E., & Silverman, K. (1999). Theoretical and empirical foundations of contingency management treatments for drug abuse. In S. T. Higgins & K. Silverman (Eds.), *Motivating behavior change among illicit drug users* (pp. 15–30). Washington, DC: American Psychological Association.

Camerer, C., & Ho, T.-H. (1999). Experience-weighted attraction learning in normal form games. *Econometrica, 67,* 837–874.

Camerer, C., Issacharoff, S., Loewenstein, G., O'Donoghue, T., & Rabin, M. (2003). Regulation for conservatives: Behavioral economics and the case for "asymmetric paternalism." *University of Pennsylvania Law Review, 151*(3), 1211–1254.

Chapman, G. B., & Coups, E. J. (2006). Emotions and preventive health behavior: Worry, regret, and influenza vaccination. *Health Psychology, 25*(1), 82–90.

Chernew, M. E., Shah, M. R., Wegh, A., Rosenberg, S. N., Juster, I. A., Rosen, A. B.,. . . Fendrick, A. M. (2008). Impact of decreasing copayments on medication adherence within a disease management environment. *Health Affairs, 27*(1), 103–112.

Choudhry, N. K., Avorn, J., Glynn, R. J., Antman, E. M., Schneeweiss, S., Toscano, M.,. . . Shrank, W. H. (2011). Full coverage for preventive medications after myocardial infarction. *New England Journal of Medicine, 365*(22), 2088–2097.

Connolly, T., & Butler, D. U. (2006). Regret in economic and psychological theories of choice. *Journal of Behavioral Decision Making, 19*(2), 148–158.

Della Vigna, P., & Malmendier, L. (2002). Paying not to go to the gym. *American Economic Review, 96,* 694–719.

Flegal, K. M., Graubard, B. I., Williamson, D. F., & Gail, M. H. (2005). Excess deaths associated with underweight, overweight, and obesity. *JAMA, 293*(15), 1861–1867.

Frank, R., & Lamiraud, K. (2009). Choice, price competition and complexity in markets for health insurance. *Journal of Economic Behavior & Organization, 71,* 550–562.

Frederick, S., Loewenstein, G., & O'Donoghue, T. (2002). Time discounting and time preference: A critical review. *Journal of Economic Literature, 40*(2), 351–401.

Gabaix, X., & Laibson, D. (2006). Shrouded attributes, consumer myopia, and information suppression in competitive markets. *Quarterly Journal of Economics, 121,* 505–540.

Gibson, T. B., Wang, S., Kelly, E., Brown, C., Turner, C., Frech-Tamas, F.,. . . Mauceri, E. (2011). A value-based insurance design program at a large company boosted medication adherence for employees with chronic illnesses. *Health Affairs, 30,* 109–117.

Glanz, K., & Bishop, D. B. (2010). The role of behavioral science theory in development and implementation of public health interventions. *Annual Review of Public Health, 31,* 399–418.

Gneezy, U., & Potters, J. (1997). An experiment on risk taking and evaluation periods. *Quarterly Journal of Economics, 112*(2), 631–645.

Haisley, E., Volpp, K. G., Pellathy, T., & Loewenstein, G. (2012). The impact of alternative incentive schemes on completion of health risk assessments. *American Journal of Health Promotion, 26*(3), 184–188.

Halpern, S., Loewenstein, G., Volpp, K., Cooney, E., Vranas, K., Quill, C.,. . . Bryce, C. (2013). Default options in advance directives influence how patients set goals for end-of-life care. *Health Affairs, 32*(2), 408–417.

Halpern, S. D., Ubel, P. A., & Asch, D. A. (2007). Harnessing the power of default options to improve health care. *New England Journal of Medicine, 357*(13), 1340–1344.

Handel, B., & Kolstad, J. (2013). *Health insurance for humans: Information frictions, plan choice and consumer welfare* (National Bureau of Economic Research Working Paper No. 19373). Cambridge, MA: National Bureau of Economic Research.

Herrnstein, R. J., & Prelec, D. (1992). Melioration. In G. Loewenstein & J. Elster (Eds.), *Choice over time* (pp. 235–263). New York: Russell Sage.

Higgins, S. T. (1999). Applying behavioral economics to the challenge of reducing cocaine abuse. In F. J. Chaloupka, M. Grossman, W. K. Bickel, & H. Saffer (Eds.), *The economic analysis of substance use and abuse* (pp. 157–174). Cambridge, MA: National Bureau of Economic Research.

Issacharoff, S., & Delaney, E. F. (2006). Credit card accountability. *University of Chicago Law Review, 73,* 157–182.

Jackevicius, C. A., Mamdani, M., & Tu, J. V. (2002). Adherence with statin therapy in elderly patients with and without acute coronary syndromes. *JAMA, 288*(4), 462–467.

Jeffery, R. W., Bjornson-Benson, W. M., Rosenthal, B. S., Kurth, C. L., & Dunn, M. M. (1984). Effectiveness of monetary contracts with two repayment schedules of weight reduction in men and women from self-referred and population samples. *Behavior Therapy, 15*, 273–279.

Jeffery, R. W., Gerber, W. M., Rosenthal, B. S., & Lindquist, R. A. (1983). Monetary contracts in weight control: Effectiveness of group and individual contracts of varying size. *Journal of Consulting and Clinical Psychology, 51*(2), 242–248.

Jeffery, R. W., Thompson, P. D., & Wing, R. R. (1978). Effects on weight reduction of strong monetary contracts for calorie restriction or weight loss. *Behavior Research and Therapy, 16*(5), 363–369.

Jeffery, R. W., Wing, R. R., Thorson, C., & Burton, L. R. (1998). Use of personal trainers and financial incentives to increase exercise in a behavioral weight-loss program. *Journal of Consulting and Clinical Psychology, 66*(5), 777–783.

Jeffery, R. W., Wing, R. R., Thorson, C., Burton, L. R., Raether, C., Harvey, J., & Mullen, M. (1993). Strengthening behavioral interventions for weight loss: A randomized trial of food provision and monetary incentives. *Journal of Consulting and Clinical Psychology, 61*(6), 1038–1045.

John, L., Loewenstein, G., Troxel, A., Norton, L., Fassbender, J., & Volpp, K. G. (2011). Financial incentives for extended weight loss: A randomized, controlled trial. *Journal of General Internal Medicine, 26*(6), 621–626.

Johnson, E. J., & Goldstein, D. (2003). Do defaults save lives? *Science and Justice, 302*(5649), 1338–1339.

Kahneman, D. (2011). *Thinking, fast and slow*. New York: Farrar, Straus & Giroux.

Kahneman, D., Knetsch, J. L., & Thaler, R. H. (1991). The endowment effect, loss aversion, and status quo bias: Anomalies. *Journal of Economic Perspectives, 5*(1), 193–206.

Kahneman, D., & Tversky, A. (1979). Prospect theory: An analysis of decision under risk. *Econometrica, 47*, 263–291.

Keller, P. A., Harlam, B., Loewenstein, G., & Volpp, K. G. (2011). Enhanced active choice: A new method to motivate behavior change. *Journal of Consumer Psychology, 21*, 376–383.

Kimmel, S. E., Troxel, A. B., Loewenstein, G., Brensinger, C. M., Jaskowiak, J., Doshi, J. A.,. . . Volpp, K. (2012). Randomized trial of lottery-based incentives to improve warfarin adherence. *American Heart Journal, 164*(2), 268–274.

Kripalani, S., Yao, X., & Haynes, R. B. (2007). Interventions to enhance medication adherence in chronic medical conditions: A systematic review. *Archives of Internal Medicine, 167*(6), 540–549.

Kullgren, J. T., Troxel, A. B., Loewenstein, G., Asch, D. A., Norton, L. A., Wesby, L.,. . . Volpp, K. G. (2013). Individual- versus group-based financial incentives for weight loss: A randomized, controlled trial. *Annals of Internal Medicine, 158*(7), 505–514.

Laibson, D. I. (1997). Golden eggs and hyperbolic discounting. *Quarterly Journal of Economics, 62*, 443–477.

Loewenstein, G. (1992). The fall and rise of psychological explanation in the economics of intertemporal choice. In G. Loewenstein & J. Elster (Eds.), *Choice over time* (pp. 3–34). New York: Russell Sage.

Loewenstein, G., & Angner, E. (2003). Predicting and indulging changing preferences. In G. Loewenstein, D. Read, & R. Baumeister (Eds.), *Time and decision: Economic and psychological perspectives on intertemporal choice* (pp. 351–391). New York: Russell Sage.

Loewenstein, G., Asch, D. A., & Volpp, K. G. (2013). Behavioral economics holds potential to deliver better results for patients, insurers, and employers. *Health Affairs, 32*(7), 1244–1250.

Loewenstein, G., Brennan, T., & Volpp, K. G. (2007). Asymmetric paternalism to improve health behaviors. *JAMA*, *298*(20), 2415–2417.

Loewenstein, G., Friedman, J. Y., McGill, B., Ahmad, S., Linck, S., Sinkula, S.,. . . Volpp, K. (2013). Consumers' misunderstanding of health insurance. *Journal of Health Economics*, *32*(5), 850–862.

Loewenstein, G., & Haisley, E. (2008). The economist as therapist: Methodological issues raised by "light" paternalism. In A. Caplin & A. Schotter (Eds.), *Perspectives on the future of economics: Positive and normative foundations* (Vol. 1, pp. 210–248). Oxford, UK: Oxford University Press.

Loewenstein, G., & O'Donoghue, T. (2006). We can do this the easy way or the hard way: Negative emotions, self-regulation, and the law. *University of Chicago Law Review*, *73*, 183–206.

Loewenstein, G., O'Donoghue, T., & Rabin, M. (2003). Projection bias in predicting future utility. *Quarterly Journal of Economics*, *118*, 1209–1248.

Loewenstein, G., & Ubel, P. (2010, July 15). Economics behaving badly. *The New York Times*, p. A31.

Maciejewski, M. L., Farley, J. F., Parker, J., & Wansink, D. (2010). Copayment reductions generate greater medication adherence in targeted patients. *Health Affairs*, *29*(11), 2002–2008.

Madison, K., Schmidt, H., & Volpp, K. G. (2013). Smoking, obesity, health insurance, and health incentives in the Affordable Care Act. *JAMA*, *310*(2), 143–144.

Madrian, B. C., & Shea, D. F. (2001). The power of suggestion: Inertia in 401(k) participation and savings behavior. *Quarterly Journal of Economics*, *116*(4), 1149–1525.

Mann, R. A. (1972). The behavior-therapeutic use of contingency contracting to control an adult behavior problem: Weight control. *Journal of Applied Behavior Analysis*, *5*(2), 99–109.

Markowitz, H. (1952). The utility of wealth. *Journal of Political Economy*, *60*, 151–158.

Mokdad, A. H., Marks, J. S., Stroup, D. F., & Gerberding, J. L. (2004). Actual causes of death in the United States, 2000. *JAMA*, *291*(10), 1238–1245.

Neumann, J. V., & Morgenstern, O. (1953). *Theory of games and economic behavior*. Princeton, NJ: Princeton University Press.

Novemsky, N., & Kahneman, D. (2005). The boundaries of loss aversion. *Journal of Marketing Research*, *42*, 119–128.

O'Dean, T. (1998). Are investors reluctant to realize their losses? *Journal of Finance*, *53*(5), 1775–1798.

O'Donoghue, T., & Rabin, M. (1999). Doing it now or later. *American Economic Review*, *89*(1), 103–124.

Prelec, D., & Loewenstein, G. (1991). Decision making over time and under uncertainty: A common approach. *Management Science*, *37*, 770–786.

Read, D., Loewenstein, G., & Rabin, M. (1999). Choice bracketing. *Journal of Risk and Uncertainty*, *19*, 171–197.

Sabini, J., & Silver, M. (1982). *Moralities of everyday life*. Oxford, UK: Oxford University Press.

Samuelson, W., & Zeckhauser, R. (1988). Status quo bias in decision making. *Journal of Risk and Uncertainty*, *1*, 7–59.

Sen, A., Sewell, T., Riley, E., Stearman, B., Bellamy, S., Hu, M.,. . . Volpp, K. (2014). Financial incentives for home-based health monitoring: A randomized controlled trial. *Journal of General Internal Medicine*, *29*(5), 770–777.

Sharot, T. (2011). *The optimism bias*. New York: First Vintage Books.

Shefrin, H., & Statman, M. (1985). The disposition to sell winners too early and ride losers too long. *Journal of Finance*, *40* (777–790).

Simon, H. A. (1955). A behavioral model of rational choice. *Quarterly Journal of Economics, 69*, 99–118.

Sunstein, C. R. (2002). Probability neglect: Emotions, worst cases, and law. *Yale Law Journal, 112*, 61–107.

Thaler, R. H., & Benartzi, S. (2004). Save more tomorrow: Using behavioral economics to increase employee saving. *Journal of Political Economy, 112*(1), S164–S187.

Thaler, R. H., & Sunstein, C. R. (2003). Libertarian paternalism. *American Economic Review, 93*(2), 175–179.

Thaler, R. H., Tversky, A., Kahneman, D. R., & Schwartz, A. (1997). The effect of myopia and loss aversion on risk taking: An experimental test. *Quarterly Journal of Economics, 112*, 647–661.

Tversky, A., & Kahneman, D. (1981). The framing of decisions and the psychology of choice. *Science, 211*(4481), 453–458.

Tversky, A., & Kahneman, D. R. (1991). Loss aversion in riskless choice: A reference-dependent model. *Quarterly Journal of Economics, 106*(4), 1039–1061.

Volpp, K., Asch, D., & Loewenstein, G. (2012). Evaluating health care programs: Asking the wrong question. *JAMA, 307*(20), 2153–2154.

Volpp, K. G., John, L. K., Troxel, A. B., Norton, L., Fassbender, J., & Loewenstein, G. (2008). Financial incentive-based approaches for weight loss: A randomized trial. *JAMA, 300*(22), 2631–2637.

Volpp, K. G., Loewenstein, G., Troxel, A., Doshi, J., Price, M., Laskin, M., & Kimmel, S. K. (2008). A test of financial incentives to improve warfarin adherence. *BMC Health Services Research, 8*, 272.

Volpp, K. G., Pauly, M. V., Loewenstein, G., & Bangsberg, D. (2009). P4P4P: An agenda for research on pay for performance for patients. *Health Affairs, 28*(1), 206–214.

Volpp, K. G., Troxel, A. B., Pauly, M. V., Glick, H. A., Puig, A., Asch, D. A.,. . . Audrain-McGovern, J. (2009). A randomized, controlled trial of financial incentives for smoking cessation. *New England Journal of Medicine, 360*(7), 699–709.

Warner, K. E., Smith, R. J., Smith, D. G., & Fries, B. E. (1996). Health and economic implications of a work-site smoking-cessation program: A simulation analysis. *Journal of Occupational and Environmental Medicine, 38*(10), 981–992.

Weber, B. J., & Chapman, G. B. (2005). Playing for peanuts: Why is risk seeking more common for low-stakes gambles? *Organizational Behavior and Human Decision Processes, 97*, 31–46.

Wing, R. R., & Anglin, K. (1996). Effectiveness of a behavioral weight control program for blacks and whites with NIDDM. *Diabetes Care, 19*(5), 409–413.

World Health Organization. (2011). *Global status report on noncommunicable diseases 2010.* Geneva: Author.

Zeelenberg, M., & Pieters, R. (2004). Consequences of regret aversion in real life: The case of the Dutch postcode lottery. *Organizational Behavior & Human Decision Processes, 93*(2), 155–168.

CHAPTER 21

SOCIAL MARKETING

J. Douglas Storey
Ronald Hess
Gary Saffitz

In the more than half a century since G. D. Wiebe (1951–1952) posed his famous question "Why can't you sell brotherhood like soap?" the concept of social marketing has gained enormous appeal for health promotion and social change programs, in part because it evokes the perceived power of ubiquitous and successful commercial advertising. But this analogy is complicated. Not only is commercial marketing, of which advertising is an important component, a highly sophisticated and complex undertaking, it is also hugely expensive and not always successful. Marketers of soap typically have much larger budgets than marketers of brotherhood, as well as much larger infrastructures dedicated primarily to the marketing function. They also are more often focused on selling specific brands (e.g., Trojans™) than on generating demand for a product category (e.g., condoms) or a class of behavior (e.g., contraception) that could be practiced in more than one way. Furthermore, the ultimate goal of commercial marketing, even campaigns that try to broadly shape markets, almost always involves—directly or indirectly—purchasing behaviors. Social marketing, in contrast, usually aims to influence a broad range of outcomes, including attitudes and social priorities, as well as behaviors in the public interest. Philip Kotler (Kotler & Armstrong, 2010) supported the application of social marketing to diverse noncommercial domains such as health and the performing arts and argued that the social marketing perspective fosters innovation in both commercial

KEY POINTS

This chapter will:

- Define social marketing, its basic principles, and how those principles can be applied within a strategic health communication framework.

- Link commonly used theories of health communication and health behavior to the effective practice of social marketing.

- Describe the uses of research in the formative, implementation, and evaluation stages of social marketing programs.

- Provide examples of international social marketing programs that illustrate how principles and processes can come together to achieve social change and behavior change.

and noncommercial marketing. This broadening has continued in recent years. Lefebvre makes the case for *transformative* social marketing (Domegan, Collins, Stead, McHugh, & Hughes, 2013; Lefebvre, 2012; Peattie, Peattie, & Thomas, 2012), in which whole markets are reshaped "through social action, regulation, or leveraging and realigning market forces of supply and demand" (Lefebvre, 2012, p. 123), using the fundamental principles of commercial marketing. As social marketing has evolved, key perspectives, principles, and tactics from commercial marketing have been adapted to improve the strategic value of health communication; the goal is to increase the likelihood that people can and will make healthy choices—sometimes in spite of themselves—and in the long run, improve social conditions.

The influence of social marketing has been such that in the early twenty-first century most health promotion programs that attempt to achieve population-level impact use multiple, mutually reinforcing tactics, including aspects of social marketing. What distinguishes social marketing from other health promotion and health communication approaches? (See Chapter Seventeen on this topic also.) Why should one consider social marketing as a strategy for influencing health behavior? How can the efficiency and effectiveness of social marketing be optimized? The rest of this chapter will address these questions, starting with a definition of social marketing, and drawing substantially on examples of integrated social marketing programs in non-U.S. settings, including Indonesia, Egypt, and Uganda.

Definition of Social Marketing

Social marketing as a field began to take shape in the late 1960s (Kotler & Levy, 1969). The term itself is usually attributed to Kotler and Zaltman (1971), who originally defined it as "a social influence technology involving the design, implementation and control of programs aimed at increasing the acceptability of a social idea or practice in one or more groups of target adopters" (Kotler & Roberto, 1989, p. 24). Some of the earliest applications of social marketing may have occurred in the field of public health, specifically in family planning campaigns in India in the 1960s (Harvey, 1999). Since then, it has evolved through extensive application and scholarship. Journals, websites, textbooks, institutes, university courses, and funding from the nonprofit sector and from foreign assistance donors continue to drive this evolution.

Andreasen's definition continues to be one of the most concise yet comprehensive: "Social marketing is the *application of commercial marketing technologies* to the analysis, planning, execution and evaluation of programs *designed to influence the voluntary behavior* of target audiences in order *to improve their personal welfare and that of their society*" (Andreasen, 1994, p. 11; emphasis added). These three highlighted aspects—the use of a marketing perspective to influence voluntary behavior for individual and social good—lie at the heart of all social marketing efforts. The *focus* on outcomes that improve personal and social *welfare* is the primary feature that distinguishes social from commercial marketing.

To the features noted by Andreasen, Maibach, Rothschild, and Novelli (2002) add another one derived from Bagozzi (1974, 1978) and Rothschild (2000): the mutual fulfillment of self-interest through voluntary exchange. Voluntary exchange, from a consumer's view, means that the interaction fulfills a felt need or desire, the perceived cost (social, economic, or physical) of

Table 21.1   Comparisons Between Social Marketing and Commercial Marketing

	Social Marketing	Commercial Marketing
Primary locus of benefit	Individuals. Social and political leaders. Professionals. Society at large.	Marketing organization. Stockholders. Producer of marketed goods.
Types of outcomes	Behaviors that increase personal and social welfare. Knowledge, attitudes, norms, values, and consumer self-image addressed to inform behavioral decisions. Gratifications more likely to be delayed. Benefits tend to be longer term.	Purchasing behaviors. Attitudes toward and image of product. Consumer self-image. Norms and values addressed to the extent that they affect purchases. Gratifications may be more immediate. Benefits tend to be shorter term.
Characteristics of audiences	Tend to be less affluent, more diverse, more in need of social services, and harder to reach. Segmented by psychographic attributes and relationship to or involvement with product.	Tend to be more affluent, more connected to media, and easier to reach. Typically segmented by psychographic and demographic attributes and relationship to or involvement with product.
Voluntary exchange	Includes weighing of economic and social costs and benefits. More emphasis on nonmonetary exchange. Costs of marketing organizations usually subsidized. Expectation that information about the product is complete and that choices are fully informed.	More emphasis on monetary exchange. May include weighing of social costs and benefits, mostly for consumer. Expectation that information about the commercial product is true, but biased in favor of the product.
Market perspective	Products tend to be less tangible and more complex. Competition tends to be more varied and less tangible. Economic factors (e.g., purchasing power) tend to be less important.	Products tend to be more tangible. Competition tends to be more tangible and categorical. Economic factors (e.g., purchasing power) tend to be more important.

which does not outweigh the perceived gain. Voluntary exchange from a marketer's point of view means providing a good or service that is in *the marketer's* best interest, that is, it is not provided at a loss. In commercial settings, this means that the cost of providing and promoting a product or service is more than offset by what consumers pay in exchange for it. In the case of social marketing, however, consumers and marketers presumably share the same goal, namely, increasing benefits to society as a whole. Unlike commercial marketing organizations, social marketers often are obliged to serve all audience members in need, not just those in a position to pay for a product. A summary of some key distinctions between social and commercial marketing is provided in Table 21.1.

While debates over the definition of social marketing will no doubt continue, social marketing is now a well-developed area of scholarship and practice. For example, the Centers for Disease Control and Prevention (CDC) maintains a website dedicated to social marketing, the Gateway to Health Communication and Social Marketing Practice, complete with tools, templates, and guidelines for research, systematic planning, audience segmentation, and theoretical work, as well as access to information about current campaigns, publications, and other professional resources (CDC, 2007). And social marketing continues to be the subject of extensive research. A Google Scholar search in September 2014 produced 7,530 links to articles, books, and book chapters dated since 2013 that referred to both "social marketing" and "health," illustrating that social marketing in health is clearly an active focus of scholarship and practice.

Basic Principles of Social Marketing

In this section, we describe five principles that have made social marketing popular and effective as a health promotion strategy: (1) focusing on behavioral outcomes, (2) prioritizing consumers' rather than marketers' benefits, (3) maintaining an ecological perspective, (4) developing a strategic *marketing mix* of communication elements according to the four P's of marketing, and (5) using audience segmentation to identify meaningful differences among consumers that affect their response to the product or service being offered.

Focusing on Behavior

In the past, social *products* were defined broadly to include ideas (e.g., family planning, environmental conservation), attitudes (e.g., preference for small family size, approval of recycling), services (e.g., family planning clinics, recycling centers), and behaviors (e.g., using hormonal contraceptives, recycling glass bottles). But Andreasen (1994, 2006) and others argue that the proper objective of social marketing is to influence behavior. It is not enough to promote products or services; people must obtain and use them. In the commercial world, soft drink manufacturers would fail if their business goal was merely to promote awareness of or positive attitudes toward their products; consumers must purchase them. Yet the commercial marketing organization is largely indifferent to how its products are used or whether they are used at all, as long as the products are bought. In social marketing, *use* of the product is of much greater importance, because usually it is use, rather than possession per se, that confers benefit. A condom marketing campaign would have to be judged unsuccessful, even if millions of condoms were distributed, if they were not used as they were meant to be—to prevent disease and pregnancy. In other words, the focus on behavior is inextricably linked to the second principle, consumer benefit.

Prioritizing Consumer Benefits

A general dimension of communication campaigns, *locus of benefit* (Rogers & Storey, 1987), refers to whether successful achievement of program objectives benefits primarily the program designers or the program audience. Although consumers *may* benefit from commercial advertising campaigns, the driving force behind them is to create profit for the producers of consumer goods and their stockholders. In contrast, social marketing campaigns benefit primarily members of the campaign audience or society at large in the form of better health or a cleaner and more stable environment. There may be little, if any, immediate benefit to the government agency running a health campaign if consumers change their health behavior, except in the sense that a healthier populace means a lower burden of disease and fewer demands on public health resources. The transformative marketing perspective (Lefebvre, 2012), which emphasizes co-creation of value by marketers and consumers with common goals, blurs this distinction somewhat because benefits (and costs) are mutually shared. Nevertheless, consumer or societal benefit is paramount.

Maintaining a Market Perspective

Another principle of social marketing that sets it apart from other forms of persuasive communication is the concept of the market itself. First, a market perspective requires adoption of a *consumer orientation*; that is, markets revolve around consumer needs and desires and the ways in which decisions are made to satisfy those needs. Second, the functioning of markets is dependent on the *flow of information* about products that are available, what they cost, how they can be used, what benefits they provide, and where to obtain them. Third, promoted products always face *competition* for the consumer's attention and resources in a dynamic marketplace of ideas, priorities, and choices. Therefore marketing communication explicitly acknowledges the environment where decisions are made and develops strategies to increase desirability or relative value so that the product can compete favorably with other options that consumers have.

Some social marketing approaches refer to strategies addressing an *upstream* focus on infrastructural change (such as policy or regulatory change) or a *downstream* focus on individual change (such as changes in knowledge, attitudes, or practices) (Andreasen, 2006). Often, upstream and downstream strategies need to be coordinated in order to change upstream structural conditions that pose downstream barriers to individual change. This is consistent with ecological models (see Chapter Three). Paisley and Atkin (2013), for example, describe the interrelated three E's of public communication campaign strategy: engineering, enforcement, and education. The upstream engineering of automotive safety, for example, includes features such as automatic seatbelt reminders and technologies for hands-free cell phone use to prevent traffic accidents. But engineering approaches must be supported by the upstream enforcement of seatbelt laws and laws against cell phone use while driving, as well as the downstream education of the public about those laws, about penalties that can result from noncompliance, and about the effectiveness of laws in reducing death and bodily harm.

Determining Marketing Mix with the Four P's

Another distinguishing characteristic of social marketing approaches is consideration of the proper combination of strategic elements, often described in terms of the four P's: product, price, place, and promotion (Kotler & Armstrong, 2010). These are closely interwoven in an effective strategy, but each draws attention to different aspects of the marketing ecosystem.

Product

Rather than thinking of *products* as physical objects (e.g., antiretroviral AIDS drugs, recycling centers), marketers think of them as a constellation of benefits—advantages or gains that result from practicing the recommended behavior—that can be offered to consumers to make the use of those products enticing (Tapp & Spotswood, 2013). To identify the most important bundle of benefits to offer, social marketers conduct research to understand the current behaviors of consumer groups and how a new or alternative behavior can be made more attractive or valuable. Consider a campaign to make it easier for restaurant patrons to identify and choose healthier foods on the menu. Adding certain menu items labeled as "heart healthy" or "light" to distinguish them from other choices defines those products in terms of the benefits they offer ("the Greek salad not only looks tasty, it has lower fat content"). The attributes or benefits that define a product in the mind of the consumer may be physical, economic, social, psychological, or some combination thereof.

Price

Price refers to the perceived costs or barriers associated with the product being offered and is an essential aspect of the voluntary exchange dynamic. Costs can be monetary, social, or psychological. Will maintaining a low-fat diet require buying more expensive foods? Will an exercise program cut into time spent with family? Consumers weigh the perceived costs of a behavior against its perceived benefits, sometimes casually and sometimes with great care and attention, before making a decision to purchase a product or adopt a behavior (see Chapter Five). Social marketers try to set an attractive price or influence the perceived cost-benefit ratio in order to tip the balance in favor of the promoted behavior.

Consider a campaign to increase the practice of caging chickens to prevent the birds and the backyard poultry farmers in Indonesia who work with them from becoming infected with the H5N1 virus that causes avian influenza. Free ranging of chickens is generally cheaper than keeping birds caged because it costs less to feed them and because building cages requires some investment of time and materials. By encouraging the use of local materials such as split bamboo rather than more expensive wire fencing, the anticipated price of caging is lowered, thereby making the behavior appear more affordable. Furthermore, by pairing the idea of lower cost with the desirable benefits of protecting one's investment and the health of one's family, the cost-benefit ratio of the behavior becomes more favorable.

Place

Place refers to where the consumer is reached with the product and information about it and where the voluntary exchange takes place. Distribution channels for the product (if there is a physical object to be used, such as oral contraceptives or diet aids), or for information about how to use it, must be chosen to maximize the convenience of the "buying" experience for the consumer. Convenience may include such things as the product's location in physical or virtual space, the times at which it is available, and the time and effort it takes to find and access the product. In the case of commercial products, place might include a retail outlet, door-to-door delivery through outreach workers (or a salesforce) and social networks. Products, services, and/or the opportunities to take action must be placed where targeted consumer groups gather, and must be displayed conveniently within those locations to maximize attention. For example, placing condom vending machines and messages about preventing sexually transmitted diseases in the restrooms of nightclubs and twenty-four-hour convenience stores increases the likelihood that the idea of—as well as the means to practice—safer sex will be available at a convenient place and at a time of elevated risk for some consumers.

Many placement options are available to social marketers, including point-of-purchase advertising, advertising in broadcast media, interpersonal channels in the community, message placement at public sporting or holiday events, direct mail, telemarketing, and many more. The best placement option is determined from up-to-date information about which channels are being used and when by the greatest numbers of the intended audience. The growth of interactive, web-based technologies has dramatically expanded the virtual space within which consumers can access and choose from a nearly unlimited range of products and personalize their purchasing experience. This in turn extends the lifetime of product placement and the *long tail* (Anderson, 2006) of profit or social benefit.

Maibach, Abroms, and Marosits (2007) underscore the importance of place when they describe the social marketing perspective in terms of a socioecological "people and places" framework that situates audiences and choices within geographic, economic, and cultural spaces that determine access to and the relevance and value of the product. This requires a thorough understanding, obtained through systematic research, of individual-level factors (such as outcome expectancy, self-efficacy, motivations, demographic characteristics, social relationships, media habits, and emotions), as well as the characteristics of the location within which decisions are made, such as availability of products and services, physical features of the environment, laws and regulations, and the overall content of the symbolic environment.

Promotion

Promotion refers to the communication and messaging elements of a social marketing program, to the forms and content of information provided, and the ways that communication and messages are formatted, sequenced, reinforced, and complemented by other elements of the marketing mix. Promotional strategies may provide information about the other P's, such as the features of the product and benefits the consumer can expect, how barriers to product use can be overcome, and where the product can be obtained or practiced.

Different consumer groups may respond better to one promotional strategy than to another. For example, teenagers who value their independence may respond better to smoking cessation messages that depict tobacco addiction as a "bully" than to messages that emphasize health statistics (U.S. Food and Drug Administration, 2014). Whatever the issue may be, promotional approaches must be selected to correspond with audience preferences and information processing styles. An enormous catalog of message strategies is available to choose from, many of which are described in a 2006 special issue of the *Journal of Communication* (Cappella & Rimer, 2006).

Using Audience Segmentation

The principle of audience segmentation refers to the identification of relatively homogeneous subgroups and the development of marketing strategies customized to the characteristics of each subgroup. Different subgroups require different strategies because they value different benefits associated with a product, prioritize price considerations differently, seek and obtain product information or social support for behavior change through different channels, and respond more readily to some message formats than others. Segmentation strategies typically consider the socioeconomic, cultural, geographic, psychographic, and age characteristics of an audience as well as patterns of use (e.g., high or low, frequent or infrequent, experienced or inexperienced) to identify clusters that respond or relate in similar ways to a product (see Grunig, 1989, and Slater & Flora, 1991, for examples of segmentation approaches).

Consider an adolescent reproductive health campaign focused on reducing teenage pregnancy. Within the age range of fourteen to eighteen years, for example, some individuals are sexually active and some are not. An audience segmentation strategy for teenage pregnancy prevention based on sexual activity status might focus on condom use for teens who are sexually active and abstinence or delay of sexual debut for teens who are not sexually active. Each product would have its own bundle of benefits, product and message placement, description of costs and benefits, and promotional strategy (perhaps using different types of role models) appropriate for the target audience.

The Role of Social Marketing in a Strategic Communication Framework

As long ago as the late 1950s, the World Health Organization (WHO) promoted efforts to define health and well-being in a way that went beyond the narrow disease prevention perspective, stating that health is "a state of complete mental, physical, and social well-being and not merely the absence of disease" (WHO, 1958). Consistent with this view, social marketing communication must be grounded in underlying social, political, and economic conditions, which together define the market. In all societies, health communication occurs within three principal domains: the sociopolitical environment, health service delivery systems, and among individuals in communities and households (Pollock & Storey, 2012; Storey, Figueroa, & Kincaid, 2005; United States Agency for International Development [USAID], 2001). Communication within each of these domains combines to change audiences and institutions over time, making the environment more supportive of healthy practices, improving the performance of health services, and increasing the likelihood of preventive health practices. To the extent that these changes are durable, improved health outcomes can be sustained. (For more discussion of multilevel thinking about health education and health behavior, see Chapter Three.)

Obviously, not all social marketing programs engage with all levels of the market ecology, but within this larger framework, approaches can be selected depending on needs and resources. Program planners can think of these as *product-driven* approaches, *consumer- or demand-driven* approaches, and *market-driven* approaches.

Product-Driven Approaches

Product-driven approaches aim to increase the appeal of a product and differentiate it positively from alternatives. *Branding* can help to achieve this. In commercial marketing, branding identifies a product category and associates it with desirable attributes: consider Nike athletic gear, Apple iPhones, and the like. Noncommercial "products" have brand identities too: the World Wildlife Federation, Amnesty International, and the International Red Cross Society are examples of noncommercial popular, internationally recognized brands. Commercial marketers offer products with a consistent bundle of promised benefits (e.g., quality or creativity). Consumers come to expect those benefits and return to the products again and again in anticipation of predictable outcomes. Social marketers use similar branding tactics.

In 1988, Indonesia's highly successful national family planning program introduced the Blue Circle (*Lingkaran Biru*) (see the supplementary materials website for this book) as the brand image for products and services provided by urban, private sector doctors and midwives, then expanded this branding to cover a range of products and services available everywhere in the nation (Mize & Robey, 2006; Piotrow, Kincaid, Rimon, & Rinehart, 1997). Eventually, the Blue Circle logo appeared in an enormous variety of ways: with the letters KB (*Keluarga Berencana*, or "family planning"); on signs indicating hospitals, clinics, pharmacies, and other facilities where contraceptives and services were available; on contraceptive packaging; on posters, billboards, and televised public service announcements promoting providers who offered value-added Blue Circle services; on car wheel covers; and as decoration on village gates to indicate the community's support for families choosing to practice family planning. Even old automobile tires were painted blue and mounted on fence posts lining country roads.

Consumer-Driven Approaches

Consumer-driven approaches go beyond promoting the product itself to building demand for the product so that maintaining behavioral momentum shifts from the marketing organization to consumers. One strategy for achieving and sustaining consumer demand is to target social norms (Burchell, Rettie, & Patel, 2013; Haines, 1998; Linkenbach, 1999). This approach is based on the theory that much behavior is influenced by perceptions about what is typical or socially acceptable and the perceived sanctions or rewards that result respectively from deviating from or complying with those norms (Cialdini, 2012; Perkins & Berkowitz, 1986; Yanovitzky & Rimal, 2006). Evoking thoughts of important reference groups or significant others (Ajzen, 1991), sometimes in a more general sense ("other teens your age") and sometimes in a very personal way through group activities within peer networks can bring norms into focus and encourage compliance with them (see Chapter Eleven for further discussion of social networks).

Unfortunately, misperception of norms is common. The perceived frequency of behavior (descriptive norm) is likely to be underestimated when behaviors are less publicly visible, as in the case of taboo or illegal behaviors like sex or drug use. Frequency is likely to be overestimated in the case of highly publicized behaviors like alcohol abuse on college campuses. But social norms marketing can be used to inform people about the actual frequency of positive behaviors within groups they care about in order to create salient social pressure (injunctive norms) or shift perceptions of relatively rare but dramatically visible negative behaviors. A program might even introduce and promote a new norm and reinforce its practice by spreading images of it in the mass media, thereby increasing perceived support in the social environment (Kincaid, 2004).

Consider again the Blue Circle in Indonesia. Almost nonstop national and local campaigns over more than twenty years contributed to a rapid increase in contraceptive use from 23 percent of married women in 1977 to 58 percent in 2012 and a drop in the total fertility rate from 5.6 to 2.6 average number of births in a woman's lifetime during the same period (Statistics Indonesia et al., 2013). By the late 1990s, family planning and small family size had become so ingrained that even the economic crisis and political instability that Indonesia suffered from 1998 to 2002 had little effect on contraceptive use rates, even though commodities became more expensive and harder to obtain (Frankenberg, Sikoki, & Suriastini, 2003; Storey & Schoemaker, 2006).

Market-Driven Approaches

Market-driven approaches are an extension of consumer- (or demand-) driven ones. Consumer demand is important when many choices exist. For example, responsible consumption of alcoholic beverages, especially around holiday periods, competes against the allure of drinking portrayed in a flood of seasonal advertising that emphasizes the camaraderie of alcohol consumption. A market-driven approach to responsible drinking must position its product (alcohol-free social interaction) as normative or as an attractive alternative to the competition.

The Role of Theory and Research in Social Marketing

Social marketing is a strategic approach to social and behavior change. It is not a theory of change, but it uses theories to understand audiences and develop strategies to facilitate change.

The Use of Theory

Many health behavior theories are available to guide the planning and evaluation of social marketing programs (as discussed in detail in the other chapters in this book). Some theories operate exclusively at an individual level, while others focus somewhat more on interpersonal, group, or even structural levels. Key ideas and applications of four key theories often used in social marketing research and design are summarized in Table 21.2.

Theories offer insights into determinants of behavior that can be confirmed through formative research. For example, according to Diffusion of Innovations theory (see Chapter Sixteen), the adoption of a new behavior is more rapid when it (1) is perceived to have a relative advantage over current behavior; (2) is compatible with one's daily routine, priorities, and values; (3) seems relatively easy to adopt or practice; (4) can be tried without great risk before committing to it; and (5) can be observed in action to see what outcomes others experience

Table 21.2   Applications of Major Theories and Research in Social Marketing

Theoretical Framework	Applications of Framework		
	Identify Motives for Action	**Identify Message Strategies**	**Identify Target Audiences**
Extended Parallel Processing Model (EPPM) (Witte, 1994)	• To what extent is the health issue thought to pose a serious and personal threat (costs of inaction)? • To what extent are proposed actions perceived to be effective (response efficacy or benefit of action)? • How do people perceive their ability to enact the behavior (personal efficacy)?	• Create messages that increase understanding of the threat and explain or demonstrate how responses can effectively reduce the threat. • Create messages that explain how to carry out the recommended response. • Explain how to overcome barriers to the recommended response.	• Segment audiences into categories representing levels of perceived threat and efficacy.
Theory of Reasoned Action/Theory of Planned Behavior (Azjen, 1991; Fishbein & Yzer, 2003; also see Chapter Six)	• What are the advantages (benefits) and disadvantages (costs), both personal and social, of a health behavior?	• Change beliefs about and evaluations of consequences (costs and benefits) of action. • Change perceptions of subjective norms. • Change motivations to comply with subjective norms.	• Define primary audiences (those who would benefit from attitude change). • Define secondary audiences (significant others of those to be influenced).
Social Cognitive Theory (Bandura, 1986; also see Chapter Nine)	• What perceived personal and social incentives or reinforcements (benefits) affect learning and action? • What perceived personal and social barriers (costs) affect learning and action?	• Provide models of effective action that are appealing and compelling. • Encourage rehearsal and trial of the behavior. • Provide feedback and reinforcement for behavioral attempts. • Provide incentives for performance of the proposed behavior.	• Define primary audiences (those who would benefit from attitude change). • Define secondary audiences (potential role models and advocates).
Diffusion of Innovations (Rogers, 2003; also see Chapter Sixteen)	• How do members of the audience perceive the behavioral innovation? • What relative advantages (benefits) does it offer? • How complex or risky is it (costs)? • Can consequences (costs and benefits) of the behavior be observed? • Is the behavior compatible with current practices (costs)? • What social influences or networks exist in the environment that encourage or discourage the action (social costs and benefits)?	• Show and explain the benefits of the proposed action. • Explain how to do it in simple terms. • Show how the new behavior fits with or grows out of current practices. • Encourage those who already practice the behavior to advocate it to others.	• Segment audience according to perceptions of the behavior. • Target people who are key network members (opinion leaders).

before trying it oneself (Rogers, 1995). By examining the perceived characteristics of a product among potential consumers, marketers can design a message strategy to reinforce positive perceptions and change negative perceptions in order to increase the likelihood of acceptance and adoption.

Social marketers also use theories to segment audiences in meaningful ways. For example, the Extended Parallel Processing Model (EPPM) and its close cousin the Risk Perception Attitude Framework describe the interaction between perceived threat and perceived efficacy, which influence information seeking or avoidance (Rimal & Real, 2003) and behavioral decision making (Witte, 1994). Splitting the threat and efficacy dimensions into low and high categories creates a two-by-two typology of audience segments. Consider the backyard poultry farmer in Indonesia again. If the farmer knows that over 80 percent of those birds infected with avian flu in Indonesia will die, but feels confident that protective equipment and hygienic poultry handling practices are effective and feasible ways to avoid infection, then she or he is more likely to take protective action, compared to another farmer who is neither concerned about the disease nor confident in the proposed solutions or in his or her ability to implement them. A communication strategy for the lower fear/lower efficacy segment might focus on increasing realistic risk perceptions and educating about protective actions. For the higher fear/higher efficacy segment, a communication strategy might focus simply on cues to action during the rainy season, when avian flu outbreaks are more likely to occur.

Various stage theories of behavior change, such as the Transtheoretical Model (Prochaska & DiClemente, 1992; also see Chapter Seven), also can be used to identify segments of the overall audience who may be at different stages of change and to tailor messages accordingly: some may be barely aware of a health issue, while others may be knowledgeable and capable of responding but lack motivation to act or to sustain healthy behavior over time.

Multiple audience segments may be addressed within an integrated marketing strategy through the use of multiple models representing distinct segments, tailored persuasive strategies, or personalized channels of communication (Kalyanaraman & Sundar, 2006). Technologies increasingly make it possible to target more and more tightly defined segments, even individuals, making the information delivered more personally relevant and engaging. For example, a recent meta-analysis of forty studies, by Lustria et al. (2013), found consistent evidence that web-based tailoring of health information (mostly around nutrition, physical activity, and smoking) resulted in better health outcomes than generic messages.

The Uses of Research

Research plays a role across all stages of health programs, from design through implementation to impact evaluation (see Chapter Nineteen for more on theory-based planning models). Because consumer decision making and behavior are complex and situational, systematic research into the conditions and dynamics of targeted behaviors—rather than inspired guesswork—helps validate program planning decisions, increases the likelihood that programs will succeed, and makes it possible to attribute change to specific aspects of the strategy.

Design Phase

During the design phase of a program, sociobehavioral research helps planners determine the prevalence of the problem overall and among specific subaudiences; select audiences to target in order to achieve maximum individual and societal benefit; identify the unique communication needs, media habits, and preferences of the different audience segments; catalog the social, cultural, and structural or environmental factors that positively or negatively influence behavior; and identify sources of personal influence over the behavior of audience members. At a structural level, organizational research and environmental scans help identify organizations or social institutions that influence the intended audiences and might be engaged as partners to support the program, as well as the communication and media channels that are available. Qualitative and quantitative concept testing and message pretesting are essential research steps in the design process that help planners explore the four P's, determine an optimum marketing mix, and craft compelling messages.

Implementation

During implementation, data can be collected to monitor the timing and completeness of activities as well as progress toward goals. Monitoring or process evaluation provides answers to such questions as these: Is the program being implemented as designed? Are activities and materials reaching the intended audience? Is the timing of activities and message distribution going as planned? Is the program beginning to have impact? Does the program need adjustment and fine-tuning at midcourse? Sometimes programs can take advantage of existing data collection systems or activities, such as

- Media reach data: often available for purchase from commercial research firms like AC Nielson in many markets or from the broadcast logs of radio and television stations.

- Health service statistics: routinely collected by health service providers, these data are often publicly available in the government sector and can be used to trace longitudinal trends in services utilized or commodities distributed.

- Web analytics: websites and social media often can be designed to automatically generate data about user traffic, types of information users seek, search patterns, and so on that can reveal who is being reached with what kinds of information.

Finally, *during the evaluation phase* of the program, population-based sociobehavioral and cost-effectiveness research helps determine how well a program is meeting its objectives. It can explain why a program is effective (or not)—including the effects of different activities or messages on different audience segments—determine the magnitude of change, and demonstrate what aspects of the program contributed to those changes. It can measure the cost of achieving specific outcomes or impacts and indicate which parts of the program should be continued or strengthened.

For an example of how compelling good research can be in the practice of social marketing, consider the concept of return on investment (ROI): what a program can expect to gain for the resources expended to promote a product or behavior. Naturally, marketers wish to gain more than they spend, or at least to break even. In commercial settings, on the one hand, the monetary cost of producing, promoting, and distributing a product or service must be more than offset by what consumers pay in exchange for it. Social marketers, on the other hand, often are obliged to serve all audience members in need, not just those in a position to pay for a product, so they may offer products for free or at subsidized prices in order to increase benefits to society. The marketing of subsidized contraceptives for low-income consumers and free distribution of condoms for HIV/AIDS prevention are examples of this. The more subsidized contraceptives or condoms that are distributed, the more costly it is for the organization because consumers pay little or nothing in return for them. But the presumed public benefit of increased contraceptive or condom use is considered to offset the mounting cost of commodities as uptake increases. The social marketing organization and its donors may tolerate a financial loss (cost of commodities and distribution) if the social benefits to society (e.g., lower birth rates or fewer HIV infections) are judged to offset those costs. However, those social benefits are rarely quantified in monetary terms. Increasingly, members of the donor community (USAID and the Bill and Melinda Gates Foundation, in particular) are trying to get a better handle on how to calculate ROI.

Several studies have illustrated how to do this through cost-effectiveness analysis of HIV prevention communication campaigns in South Africa. Kincaid and Parker (2008) used data from a population-based survey that measured program exposure, preventive behaviors, and seroprevalence/HIV status to estimate that 701,495 HIV infections were *prevented* between 2000 and 2005 as a result of protective behavior attributable to the campaign. Extrapolating from the average $8,000 lifetime cost of providing government subsidized antiretroviral therapy to one HIV-positive patient, they calculated that the $2.3 million national campaign would save the South African government $5.6 billion in health care costs over twenty years. A similar analysis estimated a $1.1 billion savings resulting from 132,066 infections averted due to condom use at first sex among youth (Kincaid, Babalola, & Figueroa, 2014). These are powerful arguments for investment in preventive health campaigns.

International Social Marketing Applications

In this section, we profile two health communication programs from a social marketing perspective: the integrated Communication for Healthy Living (CHL) family health program in Upper Egypt (2002–2010) and the work of the Uganda Health Marketing Group (UHMG), an indigenous social marketing company founded in 2006 to address a wide range of infectious diseases. We describe how each program reflects the five principles of social marketing (focusing on behavior, not products; focusing on consumer benefits; maintaining an ecological market perspective; optimizing market mix through use of the four P's; and using audience segmentation), as well as how each used theory and research to guide decision making. We also describe some impact data from each program to illustrate how social marketing programs can be evaluated.

Case Study 1: Communication for Healthy Living 2002–2010 (Egypt)

Communication for Healthy Living (CHL) was an integrated health communication program in Egypt funded by the United States Agency for International Development (USAID). Begun in 2002, CHL built on more than twenty-five years of USAID support to Egypt's Ministry of Health and Population (MOHP) and Ministry of Information–State Information Services (MOI-SIS).

Focus on Behavior

The project prioritized contraceptive use as a primary behavioral goal, but positioned it within a cycle of family health behaviors, using marriage as the entry point for the communication strategy. Newlywed couples immediately face health issues related to reproduction, including whether or not to delay the first pregnancy. When the first pregnancy occurs, new behaviors become relevant: protecting the prenatal health of the mother and the fetus, preparing for safe delivery, and delivery with the assistance of a doctor or trained midwife. After delivery, postpartum care for the mother and postnatal care for the infant, initiation of breastfeeding and postpartum initiation of contraception to delay a subsequent pregnancy become relevant, followed by infant feeding practices and immunization. As the family matures, other lifestyle behaviors become important, such as routine hand washing, preventing infectious diseases (hepatitis, HIV/AIDS, and avian influenza), exercising, smoking cessation, and avoidance of secondhand smoke.

CHL publicized the availability of health services and promoted the purchase and use of over-the-counter products such as oral contraceptives, hand soap, and feminine hygiene products, but positioned these as ways to achieve behavioral goals, not as consumer products per se.

Focus on Consumer Benefit

The signature theme that branded all CHL messages and activities was *Sahetak Sarwetak* ("Your Health Is Your Wealth"). Messaging focused on the benefits of life stage behaviors: longer birth spacing results in better maternal and child health, immunization and breastfeeding improve the mental and physical development of infants, avoidance of secondhand smoke reduces cardiovascular disease and cancer risk, and so on. CHL positioned each behavior as an informed choice that people make in order to protect their greatest asset—good health—a deeply held value that emerged strongly in precampaign formative research.

Maintaining a Market Perspective

CHL reflected a market perspective in several ways, most notably through its private sector pharmacy initiative, known as *Isaal Istashir* (*Ask-Consult*). This campaign invited consumers to "ask and consult" their local pharmacists about family health information and appropriate products wherever they saw the *Ask-Consult* logo. By 2009, *Ask-Consult* had built a national network of over 30,000 private sector neighborhood pharmacists who associated with the project in order to improve their level of services and products and to increase their sales.

Ask-Consult competed for consumer attention through national television advertising, public relations activities, point-of-sale promotions, direct mail, and contests. Messages promoted positive behaviors and appropriate health products for family planning, hygiene, and maternal and child health. CHL also attracted more than two dozen national and international corporate partners, such as Fine (household paper products), Procter & Gamble (household cleaning and hygiene products), Schering and Organon (pharmaceuticals), Vodafone (telecommunications), and Durex (condoms), who participated in and donated a total of $6.3 million in support of training, public events, and product giveaways.

Focus on the Four P's

Product   As noted here, CHL products were a set of life stage–appropriate behaviors (family planning, maternal and child health, and healthy lifestyle practices) bundled together under the *Sahetak Sarwetak* umbrella. For example, less than half of Egyptian women use contraceptives after the birth of their first child, even though delaying the second pregnancy has health benefits for both the mother and the newborn child. CHL messages described the health benefits of longer spacing between pregnancies as a way of countering the pressures newlyweds face from in-laws to have more children, and also described the economic pressures that more children create.

Price   CHL reduced the real and perceived cost of everyday health behaviors in part by making access to quality health information and products easier through conveniently located local pharmacies. Messaging explained the negative costs associated with inaction (e.g., failing to protect pregnant women and infants from secondhand smoke can result in lower birth weight and lower growth rates) in order to influence the perceived cost-benefit ratio associated with asking friends not to smoke in your home.

Place   Outreach activities included community events, home visits, contests, and birth preparedness and infant feeding classes at public health clinics. Print materials for both health service providers and clients were distributed nationwide to more than 5,000 public sector clinics, to private sector pharmacies, through a network of NGOs, and in birthing hospitals.

Promotion   Messages were customized to different audience segments and health topics. On issues where baseline knowledge was limited, messages were more informational. For example, few people knew about the link between hepatitis C infection and the reuse of syringes, so some messages encouraged parents to ask their doctor to use only disposable syringes to prevent the transmission of blood-borne diseases. Entertainment-education events and media programming embedded health messages within game shows, children's shows like *Alam Simsim* (the Egyptian *Sesame Street*), and local news coverage of wedding celebrations to maximize attention and emotional appeal. Some examples of CHL messages are displayed in Figure 21.1.

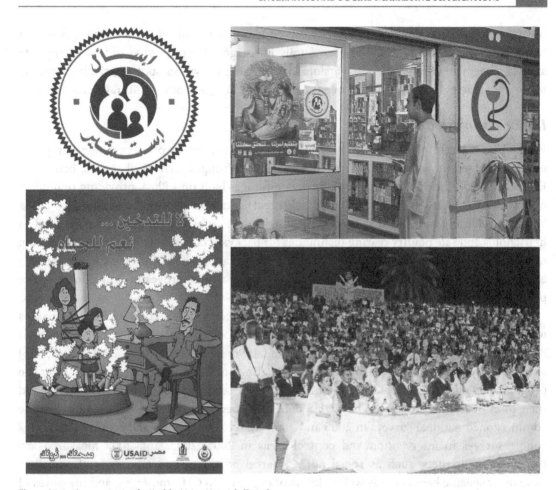

Figure 21.1 Communication for Healthy Living Materials (Egypt)

Messages were spread through multiple channels, including national and regional TV, radio, the press, telephone hotlines, the Internet, community-based performing arts, publicity events, community meetings, home visits, and clinic-based counseling. CHL cultivated relationships with print, TV, and radio journalists to encourage accurate and timely reporting about the national health agenda. Large-scale publicity events, such as regional "newlywed celebrations" for hundreds of local couples and guests, received extensive free national media coverage. Popular television game shows featuring newlywed couples added quiz questions about family health, reaching a national audience of fifteen million viewers. Finally, various interactive media were made available, such as national telephone hotlines on HIV/AIDS and a searchable online database of health information with materials in Arabic and English.

Audience Segmentation

CHL segmented its audience by life stage, as well as by urban-rural differences and gender. Newlywed couples were a primary target audience, as were pregnant, postpartum, and breastfeeding women, couples with one or two children, and children between the ages of four to six years. Behaviors relevant to each family life stage were promoted to the appropriate audience segment, while different versions of the same television spot about birth spacing featured characters reflecting urban or rural dress, language, and other cultural characteristics.

Use of Theory and Research

Formative research for CHL drew on constructs from several theories, and messaging was developed based on what research indicated were the strongest drivers of specific behaviors. For example, on the one hand, avian influenza messages built on EPPM, providing reminders of how dangerous H5N1 infections could be (threat), but emphasizing the actions that could be taken (efficacy) to avoid that threat, such as hygienic preparation of poultry for food in households and safe poultry rearing techniques for backyard chicken farmers. Family planning messages, on the other hand, drew on the Theory of Planned Behavior (see Chapter Six) by emphasizing beliefs about the benefits of birth spacing and of progestin-only contraceptive pills for breastfeeding mothers.

During the design phases of CHL, in-depth audience segmentation and trend analysis was conducted, using publicly available Egyptian Demographic and Health Survey (EDHS) data (El-Zanaty, Hussein, Shawky, Way, & Kishor, 1996; El-Zanaty & Way, 2001, 2004, 2006) and commercially available pharmaceutical marketing and media monitoring data. After the program launched in 2002, CHL systematically used several data sources to monitor and then to evaluate the program. The EDHS data described trends at the national level, while commissioned national surveys in 2005 and 2007 (CHL, 2005, 2006a) and repeated measures cohort surveys in intervention and control areas in 2004, 2005, and 2007 measured key theoretical constructs, such as social norms, perceived threat and efficacy, and perceived benefits of specific behaviors, as well as levels of exposure to CHL messages, and measures of knowledge, attitudes, and self-reported behaviors related to CHL objectives. This theory-based evaluation allowed the project to determine not just whether or not the program worked but also to understand what was working and why.

National survey data showed that use of contraception after the birth of the first child increased from 55 percent of married women under the age of thirty in 2000 to 74 percent in 2008 (El-Zanaty & Way, 2001, 2006, 2009). Similar gains were seen in use of prenatal care services, medically assisted delivery, and birth spacing longer than 2.5 years. Sixty-seven percent of adults over age fifteen could recall *Sahetak Sarwetak*; 70 percent could recall *Ask-Consult* (CHL, 2006a). The same survey found that 71 percent of adults had initiated at least one new behavior to protect themselves from avian influenza and that the mean number of protective behaviors increased with the number of CHL messages recalled (CHL, 2006a).

Commercially purchased media ratings data helped the project track the reach of CHL's media offerings and the impact of the *Ask-Consult* promotions: according to PARC media monitoring reports, CHL TV spots reached an estimated thirty-two million adults between the ages of fifteen and forty-nine in 2004 (CHL, 2006b).

Pharmaceutical sales data from 2002 through 2009 were used to show that sales of contraceptives promoted by CHL increased dramatically: sales of one-month injectable contraceptives increased sevenfold, while sales of progestin-only contraceptive pills for breastfeeding mothers doubled.

Finally, nongovernmental organizations working as outreach partners at the community level collected extensive monitoring data on maternal and child health, including infant birth weights, immunization coverage, and malnutrition. These data showed that the percentage of malnourished infants in focal villages where intensive community outreach occurred had declined from 26 percent to 5 percent over the life of the project.

CHL project funding ended in December 2010. Barely a month later, unrest related to the Arab Spring movement began in Egypt, causing disruption of civil services. Nevertheless, some aspects of CHL that had been well institutionalized, such as the *Ask-Consult* network, survived the political upheaval. In 2013, at the time of this writing, *Ask-Consult*—now called *AskConsult for Health* (AC4H)—continued to operate without donor funding by competing successfully for its own social marketing contracts. It still maintained support for the pharmacy network but had also expanded its work into support for a broader range of health communication activities, including producing materials for a school-based hygiene program in Cairo and Alexandria, designing a workplace wellness program for Shell Oil Egypt, designing a university-based viral hepatitis prevention campaign, and supplying technical assistance to tobacco control efforts, thus demonstrating the possible sustainability of a well-designed, well-managed social marketing organization.

Case Study 2: Uganda Health Marketing Group (2006–2013)

The case of the Uganda Health Marketing Group (UHMG) illustrates the broad transformative approach to social marketing described in this chapter, even as it fits a classic programmatic definition of a project or organization that uses "marketing principles and techniques to influence a target audience to voluntarily accept, reject, modify, or abandon a behavior for the benefit of individuals, groups, or society as a whole" (Kotler, Roberto, & Lee, 2002). UHMG is an indigenous, self-sustaining, not-for-profit organization founded in 2006. Like *Ask-Consult* in Egypt, it was established through a USAID-funded project (AFFORD) with the goals of growing the market for health in Uganda and helping the country achieve its Millennium Development Goals (MDGs) for maternal health. Uganda is making progress toward these goals, but still falls short of targets for maternal and child mortality and the spread of HIV/AIDS and malaria (United Nations, 2013). To close these gaps, UHMG is using an integrated supply-and-demand approach: creating demand and value for health products and services as well as access to them within a wider framework of healthy living. UHMG's vision is to enable all Ugandans to "live the Good Life," by meeting their health needs in four key areas: HIV/AIDS, malaria prevention and treatment, family planning, and maternal and child health.

Focus on Behavior

UHMG focuses on changing household behaviors in order to drive uptake of health products and services. The Good Life brand promises good health achieved through behavioral solutions, that is, the use of services and products. For example, the malaria component goes beyond promoting the use of bed nets for malaria prevention; it also encourages testing and treatment practices for malaria among people with symptoms. Project messaging is designed to increase household knowledge about the symptoms of malaria, accurate assessment of malaria risks, routine vigilance related to those risks, and timely response to symptoms. Reinforcing its *Don't Guess, First Test* campaign, the project also supports UHMG-affiliated service centers by training personnel in malaria counseling and stocking the centers with affordable rapid diagnostic test (RDT) kits and artemisinin-based combination therapy (ACT) treatments.

Focus on Consumer Benefit

The Good Life motto embodies the ultimate benefit that can be achieved by healthy practices and the proper use of health products and services: achieving and maintaining one's own health and that of one's family. Each promoted behavior is associated with particular benefits. For example, HIV testing for married couples helps them have an HIV-free baby, while proper prenatal care and delivery at a health facility reduces risks of maternal and neonatal morbidity and mortality and use of short-term contraceptive methods enables couples to space births farther apart to protect the health of the children and their mother.

Maintain a Market Perspective

UHMG considers the whole market by analyzing market need and opportunity; by segmenting its audiences and messaging according to age, gender, and health needs; by offering product and service solutions at scale; and by maintaining a self-sustaining business model. For example, a core business activity of UHMG is to procure, warehouse, distribute, and sell affordable health products, covering the cost of goods sold with revenues to maintain sustainability. Including this logistics dimension is relatively rare in international social marketing projects.

Focus on the Four P's

Product   Consistent with Tapp and Spotswood's (2013) suggestion to broaden the concept of *product* to include benefits and outcomes resulting from behavior, UHMG sells an array of tangible health products, but describes them as ways to achieve the Good Life: the opportunity to delay a pregnancy, the diagnosis and treatment of a child ill from malaria, purer household drinking water, and an HIV-free baby. Every product that UHMG offers is linked explicitly and clearly to a consumer benefit and value, defined by and tailored to what a particular household needs.

UHMG promotes and supports health services that facilitate behaviors, including a network of 200 private sector Good Life Clinics throughout the country, where clients can find trained providers, affordable commodities, and integrated services covering family planning, maternal and child health, malaria prevention and treatment, and HIV prevention, testing, and treatment services. Finally, UHMG markets a range of affordable health and pharmaceutical supplies through the private sector. This generates gross revenues of over $3 million per year, exceeding expenditures and leaving UHMG financially sustainable. Products distributed by UHMG include its own brands as well as third-party commercial brands and other USAID-subsidized social marketing brands.

Price Spotswood and Tapp (2013) stress the cultural embeddedness of behaviors and the attendant *costs* of behavior change in terms of social, economic, and cultural capital (Bourdieu, 1993). So while UHMG uses survey data to set prices for commodities (AFFORD, 2013), it also considers perceived social costs and benefits of adopting certain behaviors. For example, UHMG focuses messages about prevention of mother-to-child transmission (PMTCT) of HIV on the importance of couples' counseling sessions and of men getting tested with their pregnant partners. This helps lower the potentially high social cost of a pregnant woman being tested alone and then having to face—without a supportive partner—the additional burden of disclosing the results, negotiating with her partner to also be tested, and encountering the risk of social stigma. UHMG trains its Good Life service providers as well as volunteers from the local community to encourage couples' testing as a norm.

Place Place entails considerations of timing and social opportunity. Certain family-oriented UHMG products (such as ZinKid, RestORS, and NewFem contraceptives) are made available nationwide through drug shops, clinics, and pharmacies, while other products such as the youth-oriented Condom "O" are distributed through nightclubs and bars in urban Kampala. For certain high-risk populations at the most isolated ends of the supply chain, such as fishermen with high HIV prevalence, UHMG uses community outreach. For example, in a two-day event for fishing communities on Lake Victoria, UHMG promoted products and services for HIV/AIDS, family planning, malaria, and maternal and child health through small-group discussions, demonstrations, video shows, participatory games, educational skits, and condom demonstrations. STAR-EC, a local service delivery partner, provided counseling and testing for HIV, male circumcision for men who tested HIV-negative, prenatal care and counseling for PMTCT of HIV, antiretroviral treatment for clients who tested HIV-positive, treatment for sexually transmitted infections, and screening and referral for TB treatment. Malaria tests were provided, contraceptive implants were inserted, children were immunized, and eye care was provided.

Promotion While it delivers products and services nationwide, UHMG is probably best known for its media campaigns like *Get Off the Sexual Network* (HIV), *Smart Choices* (family planning methods campaign), *GeNext* (family planning youth campaign), and *Have an HIV-Free Baby* (PMTCT of HIV). These are well known and widely discussed (AFFORD, 2013) and delivered through an integrated, transmedia approach that ties them together under the unifying Good Life platform. Communication channels include broadcast media and outdoor advertising for maximum reach and local cues to action, distribution of messages, and the creation of networks through social media and mobile health/SMS platforms, as well as community mobilization at group, peer-to-peer, and individual levels, including one-on-one clinical counseling.

Audience Segmentation

UHMG's choice of products and services was dictated initially by its funded mandate to address specific health issues, but these issues naturally target different age, gender, and stage of life audience segments. For example, the *GeNext* family planning campaign was geared toward sexually active youth, encouraging the use of contraceptives to avoid unintended pregnancy and to establish a new generation of Ugandans who took control of their lives and wisely planned for their futures. The *Smart Choices* family planning campaign, in contrast, was geared to slightly older, established or married couples, encouraging them to find the contraceptive method that matched their fertility intentions (e.g., desired family size and optimum timing of pregnancies). Within the *Smart Choices* campaign, audiences were further segmented by parity (the number of children they already have) because this determines the appropriateness of shorter term versus longer term contraception methods: young couples having a first child are encouraged to consider a short-term method like hormonal pills to delay pregnancy in the short term, while couples having achieved their desired family size are encouraged to consider long-term methods such as implants or IUDs in order to prevent additional childbearing.

In the realm of HIV, the *Get Off the Sexual Network* campaign targeted younger adults with multiple sexual partners in an effort to reduce multiple serial or concurrent partnerships, while the *Have an HIV-Free Baby* campaign targeted pregnant women and their partners with messages about getting tested for HIV together and initiating treatment if necessary to prevent transmission of the virus to the unborn child. Pregnant couples were also targeted by the *Saving Mothers, Giving Life* campaign, which encouraged birth preparedness and medically assisted delivery. New parents were the audience for such products as ZinKids and RestORS, which help children under five years old survive bouts of diarrhea, while families with older children were targeted by *The Power of Day One*, a campaign encouraging rapid care seeking and treatment within twenty-four hours for suspected cases of malaria. Some examples of UHMG materials are shown in Figure 21.2.

Use of Theory and Research

UHMG used several theoretical frameworks to guide formative research for program design and message development. For example, EPPM, with its focus on threat and efficacy perceptions, informed messages for the *Saving Mothers, Giving Life* campaign about the unrecognized dangers of delivering a baby at home and the safer option of delivering at a clinic or hospital with the help of medically trained service providers. The concept of role modeling from Social Learning Theory was used to craft messages for the *Get Off the Sexual Network* campaign: characters were featured in messages illustrating safer and riskier sexual behaviors. Diffusion of Innovations and the Theory of Planned Behavior were used to frame the relative advantages and positive consequences (the *value exchange*) of having fewer sexual partners, including social stability and emotional peace of mind.

Research also played a key role in monitoring and evaluation. UHMG purchases local media reach data from IPSOS-SYNOVATE, an international market research firm. These data indicated a 78 percent reach (IPSOS-SYNOVATE, 2013), meaning that roughly 12.5 million

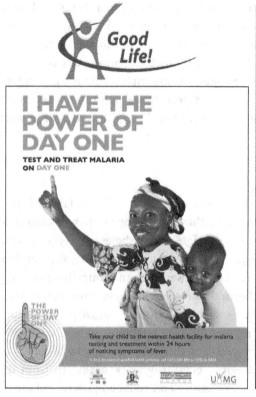
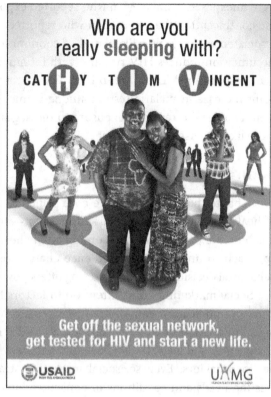

Figure 21.2 UHMG Social Marketing Campaigns

adult Ugandans heard a UHMG health message. In addition, a national monthly retail audit conducted in 2013 indicated availability of key products at a high percentage of outlets: Protector condoms (at 79% of outlets), PilplanPlus oral contraceptives (85%), and Injectaplan Depo-Provera (78%).

To evaluate the impact of UHMG campaigns, a population-based survey was conducted in October 2012 ($n = 7{,}542$ men and women, aged fifteen to fifty-four) (AFFORD, 2013). It covered a wide range of topics, including self-reported exposure to the campaigns and the channels used to deliver them, and measured theory-informed factors, including knowledge, attitudes, risk and efficacy perceptions, perceived norms, and behaviors related to family planning, sexual behavior, HIV/AIDS, malaria, and maternal and child health.

Because a randomized controlled study design cannot be used for a full-coverage national campaign, a propensity score matching (PSM) technique (Babalola & Kincaid, 2009) was used to strengthen causal attribution. PSM identifies predictors of exposure from survey data, uses them to calculate the likelihood of or propensity for exposure for each respondent, then averages the percentage difference in behavior across groups of exposed and unexposed respondents at comparable levels of propensity. This produces an unbiased estimate of the net effect of campaign exposure.

The results from using this approach indicated that women exposed to UHMG family planning messages were 11 percentage points more likely to report contraceptive use than were unexposed women. Men who reported exposure were 7 percentage points more likely to use contraception than were men who reported no exposure. Exposure to HIV messages was associated with a higher likelihood of condom use at last sex and with knowledge that male circumcision reduces HIV risk and with intention to get circumcised (among uncircumcised male respondents). Exposure to UHMG malaria messages was associated with a 4 percentage point increase in malaria testing among women and an 8 percentage point increase among men. People who reported exposure to messages about Aquasafe, RestORS, and ZinKid were more likely to use these products.

Summary

This chapter has introduced the core principles and some examples of the social marketing of health behaviors. Social marketing is not—anymore than other approaches described in this book—a panacea for overcoming public health challenges. Nevertheless, in its systematic approach to understanding audience characteristics and the market structure surrounding behavioral decisions, social marketing offers powerful guidelines for communication planning.

Social marketing draws attention to factors beyond the individual level and toward ways that communication can affect—even transform—social conditions through policy change (e.g., fluoridation of water or iodization of salt), legislation (e.g., seatbelt use), and normative change (e.g., reduced HIV/AIDS stigma), thereby facilitating the voluntary uptake of beneficial health behaviors. Even so, social marketing strategies necessarily work backward from the existing needs and conditions of consumers' lives to identify and reduce barriers and create structures that facilitate beneficial behavior. In both commercial and social marketing, it is sometimes necessary to build or create value, but in social marketing it is always important to identify and fulfill demand. The social marketing perspective also encourages planners to optimize the four P's. Creating appealing messages about the product is important, but this must be done together with considerations of the cost-benefit ratio, where the exchange is likely to take place, what forces compete against the product for attention and resources, and how the entire social ecology of decision making affects health choices and sustained health outcomes.

One of the enduring appeals of social marketing approaches is its family resemblance to commercial advertising, which is both widely loathed and widely admired. This resemblance should not be discounted or rejected owing to the best of high-minded intentions. Commercial advertising can be highly imaginative and often has its finger on the pulse of popular culture. So even though creativity and cultural resonance may not be enough, by themselves, to sell brotherhood or achieve other highly desirable social improvements, when they are combined with the systematic application of the social marketing principles described in this chapter, they may be.

References

AFFORD. (2013). *Uganda Joint Behavior Change communication survey report 2012*. Kampala: Johns Hopkins Center for Communication Programs.

Ajzen, I. (1991). The theory of planned behavior. *Organizational Behavior and Human Decision Processes, 50*(2), 179–211.

Anderson, C. (2006). *The long tail: Why the future of business is selling less of more*. New York: Hyperion.

Andreasen, A. (1994). Social marketing: Definition and domain. *Journal of Public Policy & Marketing*, *13*(1), 108–114.

Andreasen, A. (2006). *Social marketing in the 21st century*. Thousand Oaks, CA: Sage.

Babalola, S., & Kincaid, D. (2009). New methods for estimating the impact of health communication programs. *Communication Methods and Measures*, *3*(1), 61–83.

Bagozzi, R. P. (1974). Marketing as an organized behavioral system of exchange. *Journal of Marketing*, *38*(4), 77–81.

Bagozzi, R. P. (1978). Marketing as exchange: A theory of transactions in the marketplace. *American Behavioral Scientist*, *21*, 535–556.

Bandura, A. (1986). *Social foundation of thought and action: A social cognitive theory*. Upper Saddle River, NJ: Prentice Hall.

Bourdieu, P. (1993). *The field of cultural production: Essays on art and literature*. New York: Columbia University Press.

Burchell, K., Rettie, R., & Patel, K. (2013). Marketing social norms: Social marketing and the "social norm approach." *Journal of Consumer Behaviour*, *12*, 1–9.

Cappella, J. N., & Rimer, B. K. (Eds.). (2006). Integrating behavior change and message effects theories in cancer prevention, treatment, and care (Special issue). *Journal of Communication*, *56*(Suppl. 1), S1–S279.

Centers for Disease Control and Prevention. (2007). *Gateway to health communication and social marketing practice*. Atlanta: Author. Retrieved from http://www.cdc.gov/healthcommunication

Cialdini, R. B. (2012). The focus theory of normative conduct. In P. Van Lange, A. Kruglanski, & E. Higgins (Eds.), *Handbook of theories of social psychology* (pp. 295–313). London: Sage.

Communication for Healthy Living. (2005). *Egypt health communication survey*. Cairo: Zanaty & Associates and Health Communication Partnership.

Communication for Healthy Living. (2006a). *Egypt health communication survey*. Cairo: Zanaty & Associates and Health Communication Partnership.

Communication for Healthy Living. (2006b). *Year three progress report*. Baltimore: Johns Hopkins Center for Communication Programs.

Domegan, C., Collins, K., Stead, M., McHugh, P., & Hughes, T. (2013). Value co-creation in social marketing: Functional or fanciful? *Journal of Social Marketing*, *3*(3), 239–256.

El-Zanaty, F., Hussein, E. M., Shawky, G. A., Way, A. A., & Kishor, S. (1996). *Egypt demographic and health survey 1995*. Calverton, MD: National Population Council [Egypt] and Macro International Inc.

El-Zanaty, F., & Way, A. A. (2001). *Egypt demographic and health survey 2000*. Calverton, MD: Ministry of Health and Population [Egypt], National Population Council, and ORC Macro.

El-Zanaty, F., & Way, A. A. (2004). *2003 Egypt interim demographic and health survey*. Cairo: Ministry of Health and Population [Egypt], National Population Council, E1-Zanaty and Associates, and ORC Macro.

El-Zanaty, F., & Way, A. A. (2006). *Egypt demographic and health survey 2005*. Cairo: Ministry of Health and Population, National Population Council, El-Zanaty and Associates, and ORC Macro.

El-Zanaty, F., & Way, A. A. (2009). *Egypt demographic and health survey 2008*. Cairo: Ministry of Health and Population, National Population Council, El-Zanaty and Associates, and ORC Macro.

Fishbein, M., & Yzer, M. (2003). Using theory to design effective health behavior interventions. *Communication Theory, 13*(2), 164–183.

Frankenberg, E., Sikoki, B., & Suriastini, W. (2003). Contraceptive use in a changing service environment: Evidence from Indonesia during the economic crisis. *Studies in Family Planning, 34*(2), 103–116.

Grunig, J. E. (1989). Publics, audiences, and market segments: Segmentation principles for campaigns. In C. T. Salmon (Ed.), *Information campaigns: Balancing social values and social change* (pp. 199–228). Thousand Oaks, CA: Sage.

Haines, M. P. (1998). Social norms: A wellness model for health promotion in higher education. *Wellness Management, 14*(4), 1–10.

Harvey, P. D. (1999). *Let every child be wanted: How social marketing is revolutionizing contraceptive use around the world.* Westport, CT: Auburn House.

IPSOS-SYNOVATE. *Media monitoring and unduplicated reach.* UHMG Program Reports, April–June 2013.

Kalyanaraman, S., & Sundar, S. (2006). The psychological appeal of personalized content in web portals: Does customization affect attitudes and behavior? *Journal of Communication, 56*(1), 110–132.

Kincaid, D. L. (2004). From innovation to social norm: Bounded normative influence. *Journal of Health Communication, 9*(1), 37–57.

Kincaid, D. L., Babalola, S., & Figueroa, M. E. (2014). HIV communication programs, condom use at sexual debut, and HIV infections averted in South Africa, 2005. *Journal of Acquired Immune Deficiency Syndrome, 66*(Suppl. 3), S278–S284.

Kincaid, D. L., & Parker, W. (2008). *National AIDS communication programs, HIV prevention behavior and HIV infections averted in South Africa, 2005.* Pretoria: Johns Hopkins Health and Education in South Africa.

Kotler, P., & Armstrong, G. (2010). *Principles of marketing* (13th ed.). Upper Saddle River, NJ: Prentice Hall.

Kotler, P., & Levy, S. J. (1969). Broadening the concept of marketing. *Journal of Marketing, 33*, 10–15.

Kotler, P., & Roberto, N. L. (1989). *Social marketing: Strategies for changing public behavior.* New York: Free Press.

Kotler, P., Roberto, N. L., & Lee, N. R. (2002). *Social marketing: Improving the quality of life.* Thousand Oaks, CA: Sage.

Kotler, P., & Zaltman, G. (1971). Social marketing: An approach to planned social change. *Journal of Marketing, 35*, 3–12.

Lefebvre, R. C. (2012). Transformative social marketing: Co-creating the social marketing discipline and brand. *Journal of Social Marketing, 2*(2), 118–129.

Linkenbach, J. W. (1999). Application of social norms marketing to a variety of health issues. *Wellness Management, 15*(3), 7–8.

Lustria, M. L., Noar, S. M., Cortese, J., van Stee, S. K., Gluekauf, R. L., & Lee, J. (2013). A meta-analysis of web-delivered tailored health behavior change interventions. *Journal of Health Communication, 18*(9), 1039–1069.

Maibach, E., Abroms, L., & Marosits, M. (2007). Communication and marketing as tools to cultivate the public's health: A proposed "people and places" framework. *BMC Public Health, 7*, 88.

Maibach, E., Rothschild, M., & Novelli, W. (2002). Social marketing. In K. Glanz, B. K. Rimer, & L. F. Marcus (Eds.), *Health behavior and health education: Theory, research, and practice* (3rd ed., pp. 437–461). San Francisco: Jossey-Bass.

Mize, L., & Robey, B. (2006). *A 35 year commitment to family planning in Indonesia: BKKBN and USAID's historic partnership.* Baltimore: Johns Hopkins Bloomberg School of Public Health, Center for Communication Programs.

Paisley, W., & Atkin, C. (2013). Public communication campaigns: The American experience. In R. Rice & C. Atkin (Eds.), *Public communication campaigns* (4th ed., pp. 21–33). Thousand Oaks, CA: Sage.

Peattie, S., Peattie, K., & Thomas, R. (2012). Social marketing as transformational marketing in public services. *Public Management Review, 14*(7), 987–1010.

Perkins, H. W., & Berkowitz, A. D. (1986). Perceiving the community norms of alcohol use among students: Some research implications for campus alcohol education programming. *International Journal of the Addictions, 21*(9–10), 961–976.

Piotrow, P. T., Kincaid, D. L., Rimon, J. G., & Rinehart, W. (1997). *Health communication: Lessons from family planning and reproductive health.* Westport, CT: Praeger.

Pollock, J. C., & Storey, J. D. (2012). Comparing health communication. In F. Esser & T. Hanitzsch (Eds.), *Handbook of comparative communication research* (pp. 161–182). New York: Taylor & Francis.

Prochaska, J., & DiClemente, C. (1992). The transtheoretical approach. In J. C. Norcross & M. R. Goldfield (Eds.), *Handbook of psychotherapy integration.* New York: Basic Books.

Rimal, R., & Real, K. (2003). Perceived risk and efficacy beliefs as motivators of change: Use of the risk perception attitude (RPA) framework to understand health behaviors. *Human Communication Research, 29*(3), 370–399.

Rogers, E. M. (1995). *Diffusion of innovations* (4th ed.). New York: Free Press.

Rogers, E. M. (2003). *Diffusion of innovations* (5th ed.). New York: Free Press.

Rogers, E. M., & Storey, J. D. (1987). Communication campaigns. In C. Berger & S. Chaffee (Eds.), *Handbook of communication science* (pp. 814–846). Thousand Oaks, CA: Sage.

Rothschild, M. L. (2000). Carrots, sticks, and promises: A conceptual framework for the management of public health and social issue behaviors. *Social Marketing Quarterly, 6*(4), 86–114.

Slater, M., & Flora, J. A. (1991). Health lifestyles: Audience segmentation analysis for public health interventions. *Health Education Quarterly, 18*(2), 221–233.

Statistics Indonesia (Badan Pusat Statistik–BPS), National Population and Family Planning Board (BKKBN), Kementerian Kesehatan (Kemenkes–MOH), & ICF International. (2013). *Indonesia demographic and health survey 2012.* Jakarta: Author.

Storey, J. D., Figueroa, M. E., & Kincaid, D. L. (2005). *Health competence communication: A systems approach to sustainable preventive health* (Technical report). Baltimore: Johns Hopkins Bloomberg School of Public Health, Center for Communication Programs.

Storey, J. D., & Schoemaker, J. (2006, May). *Communication, normative influence and the sustainability of health behavior over time: A multilevel analysis of contraceptive use in Indonesia, 1997–2003.* Paper presented at the Annual Conference of the International Communication Association, Dresden, Germany.

Tapp, A., & Spotswood, F. (2013). From the 4Ps to COM-SM: Reconfiguring the social marketing mix. *Journal of Social Marketing, 3*(3), 206–222.

United Nations. (2013). *The millennium development goals report: 2013.* New York: Author.

United States Agency for International Development. (2001). *Draft concept paper: Communication activity approval document.* Washington, DC: United States Agency for International Development, Office of Population and Reproductive Health.

U.S. Food and Drug Administration. (2014). FDA launches its first national public education campaign to prevent, reduce youth tobacco use (News release). Retrieved from http://www.fda.gov/newsevents/newsroom/pressannouncements/ucm384049.htm

Witte, K. (1994). Fear control and danger control: A test of the Extended Parallel Processing Model (EPPM). *Communication Monographs, 61*, 113–134.

World Health Organization. (1958). WHO definition of health. Retrieved from http://who.int/about/definition/en/print.html

Yanovitzky, I., & Rimal, R. N. (2006). Communication and normative influence: An introduction to the special issue. *Communication Theory, 16*(1), 1–6.